SYMPTOM-BASED DIAGNOSIS
IN PEDIATRICS

SECOND EDITION

SYMPTOM-BASED DIAGNOSIS IN PEDIATRICS

Samir S. Shah, MD, MSCE

Director, Division of Hospital Medicine
Cincinnati Children's Research Foundation
  Endowed Chair
Attending Physician in Hospital Medicine &
  Infectious Diseases
Cincinnati Children's Hospital Medical Center
Professor, Department of Pediatrics
University of Cincinnati College of Medicine
CINCINNATI, OHIO

Stephen Ludwig, MD

Professor of Pediatrics
Associate Chief Medical Officer for Education
Perelman School of Medicine
University of Pennsylvania
Division of General Pediatrics & Pediatric
  Emergency Medicine
The Children's Hospital of Philadelphia
PHILADELPHIA, PENNSYLVANIA

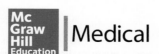

New York Chicago San Francisco Athens London Madrid Mexico City
Milan New Delhi Singapore Sydney Toronto

Symptom-Based Diagnosis in Pediatrics, Second Edition

Previous edition, titled *Pediatric Complaints and Diagnostic Dilemmas: A Case-Based Approach,* copyright © 2004 by Lippincott Williams & Wilkins.

1 2 3 4 5 6 7 8 9 0 CTP/CTP 18 17 16 15 14 13

ISBN 978-0-07-160174-0
MHID 0-07-160174-0

This book was set in Utopia by Cenveo® Publisher Services.
The editors were Alyssa K. Fried and Peter J. Boyle.
The production supervisor was Catherine H. Saggese.
Production management was provided by Sandhya Gola, Cenveo Publisher Services.
China Translation & Printing Services, Ltd., was printer and binder.
This book is printed on acid-free paper.

Library of Congress Cataloging-in-Publication Data

Symptom-based diagnosis in pediatrics / [edited by] Samir S. Shah, Stephen Ludwig.—Second edition.
        p. ; cm.
    Preceded by: Pediatric complaints and diagnostic dilemmas. c2004.
    Includes bibliographical references and index.
    ISBN 978-0-07-160174-0 (book : alk. paper)—ISBN 978-0-07-160175-7 (ebook)
    I. Ludwig, Stephen, 1945- editor of compilation.   II. Shah, Samir S., editor of compilation.
III. Title.
    [DNLM: 1. Pediatrics—Case Reports.   2. Adolescent Medicine—Case Reports.   3. Adolescent.
4. Child.   5. Diagnostic Techniques and Procedures—Case Reports.   6. Infant.   7. Signs and
Symptoms—Case Reports. WS 200]
  RJ50
  618.92'0075—dc23
                                                                                    2013022618

To my wife, Kara, and my children, Siddharth, Avani, and Anika
—SSS

To my wife, Zella, and her three adoring grandsons, Jack, Seneca, and Rainer
—SL

CONTENTS

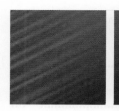

CONTENTS BY DIAGNOSIS

CONTRIBUTORS

Paul L. Aronson, MD
Attending Physician
Section of Emergency Medicine
Yale-New Haven Children's Hospital
Assistant Professor of Pediatrics
Yale School of Medicine
NEW HAVEN, CONNECTICUT
Chapters 3, 7, and 13

Megan Aylor, MD
Assistant Professor of Pediatrics
Oregon Health & Science University
PORTLAND, OREGON
Chapters 2 and 5

Gil Binenbaum, MD, MSCE
Assistant Professor of Ophthalmology
Children's Hospital of Philadelphia
Perlman School of Medicine
University of Pennsylvania
PHILADELPHIA, PENNSYLVANIA
Chapter 18

Debra Boyer, MD
Assistant Professor of Pediatrics
Boston Children's Hospital
Division of Respiratory Diseases
BOSTON, MASSACHUSETTS
Chapters 4 and 14

Alicia Casey, MD
Instructor of Medicine
Harvard Medical School
Boston Children's Hospital
BOSTON, MASSACHUSETTS
Chapters 4 and 14

Marina Catallozzi, MD, MSCE
Assistant Professor of Pediatrics
Section of Adolescent Medicine
Division of General Pediatrics
Department of Pediatrics
Columbia University College of Physicians &
    Surgeons
Assistant Professor of Population and Family Health
Heilbrunn Department of Population & Family
    Health
Mailman School of Public Health
Columbia University
NEW YORK, NEW YORK
Chapter 7

Amy Feldman, MD
Fellow, Pediatric Gastroenterology, Hepatology,
    and Nutrition
Children's Hospital Colorado
AURORA, COLORADO
Chapters 3 and 17

Evan S. Fieldston, MD, MBA, MSHP
Assistant Professor of Pediatrics
Perelman School of Medicine
University of Pennsylvania
Children's Hospital of Philadelphia
PHILADELPHIA, PENNSYLVANIA
Chapters 1 and 5

Todd A. Florin, MD, MSCE
Assistant Professor of Pediatrics
University of Cincinnati College of Medicine
Attending Physician
Division of Emergency Medicine
Cincinnati Children's Hospital Medical Center
CINCINNATI, OHIO
Chapters 1, 3, and 4

Pratichi K. Goenka, MD
Attending Physician
Children's Hospital of Philadelphia
PHILADELPHIA, PENNSYLVANIA
Inpatient Care Network
University Medical Center of Princeton at Plainsboro
PLAINSBORO, NEW JERSEY
Chapters 12, 13, 14, and 19

Dustin R. Haferbecker, MD
Clinical Assistant Professor
University of Washington School of Medicine
Pediatric Hospitalist
Mary Bridge Children's Hospital
TACOMA, WASHINGTON
Chapter 1

Maya A. Jones, MD, MPH
Fellow, Emergency Medicine
Children's Hospital of Philadelphia
PHILADELPHIA, PENNSYLVANIA
Chapters 5, 6, and 10

Lianne Kopel, MD
Division of Respiratory Diseases
Boston Children's Hospital
BOSTON, MASSACHUSETTS
Chapters 4 and 14

Brandon C. Ku, MD
Instructor of Pediatrics
Perelman School of Medicine
University of Pennsylvania
Attending Physician
Children's Hospital of Philadelphia
Division of Emergency Medicine
PHILADELPHIA, PENNSYLVANIA
Chapters 6 and 13

Christine T. Lauren, MD
Assistant Professor of Clinical
Dermatology and Clinical Pediatrics
Columbia University Medical Center
Department of Dermatology
NEW YORK, NEW YORK
Chapter 9

Stephen Ludwig, MD
Professor of Pediatrics
Associate Chief Medical Officer for Education
Perelman School of Medicine
University of Pennsylvania
Division of General Pediatrics & Pediatric
Emergency Medicine
Children's Hospital of Philadelphia
PHILADELPHIA, PENNSYLVANIA
Chapters 6, 10, and 13

Christina L. Master, MD
Associate Director
Primary Care Sports Medicine Fellowship
Attending Physician
Divisions of General Pediatrics and Orthopedics
and Sports Medicine
Children's Hospital of Philadelphia
PHILADELPHIA, PENNSYLVANIA
Chapter 17

Pamela A. Mazzeo, MD
Clinical Associate in Pediatrics
Perelman School of Medicine
University of Pennsylvania
Attending Physician
Division of General Pediatrics
Children's Hospital of Philadelphia
PHILADELPHIA, PENNSYLVANIA
Chapter 5

Jennifer L. McGuire, MD
Instructor, Neurology
Children's Hospital of Philadelphia
Perelman School of Medicine
University of Pennsylvania
PHILADELPHIA, PENNSYLVANIA
Chapter 8

Jeanine Ronan, MD
Assistant Professor of Clinical Pediatrics
Perelman School of Medicine
University of Pennsylvania
Co-Director, Pediatrics Clerkship
Children's Hospital of Philadelphia
PHILADELPHIA, PENNSYLVANIA
Chapter 16

Stacey R. Rose, MD
Attending Physician
Division of General Pediatrics
Children's Hospital of Philadelphia
PHILADELPHIA, PENNSYLVANIA
Clinical Assistant, Professor of Pediatrics
Perelman School of Medicine
University of Pennsylvania
PHILADELPHIA, PENNSYLVANIA
Chapter 15

Kara N. Shah, MD, PhD
Director, Division of Pediatric Dermatology
Cincinnati Children's Hospital Medical Center
Associate Professor of Pediatrics and
    Dermatology
University of Cincinnati College of Medicine
CINCINNATI, OHIO
Chapter 9

Samir S. Shah, MD, MSCE
Director, Division of Hospital Medicine
Cincinnati Children's Research Foundation
    Endowed Chair
Attending Physician in Hospital Medicine &
    Infectious Diseases
Cincinnati Children's Hospital Medical
    Center
Professor, Department of Pediatrics
University of Cincinnati College of Medicine
CINCINNATI, OHIO
Chapters 11, 12, 18, and 19

Tregony Simoneau, MD
Division of Respiratory Diseases
Boston Children's Hospital
BOSTON, MASSACHUSETTS
Chapters 4 and 14

Phillip Spandorfer, MD
Assistant Professor
Division of Emergency Medicine
Children's Hospital of Philadelphia
Department of Pediatrics
University of Pennsylvania School of Medicine
PHILADELPHIA, PENNSYLVANIA
Chapter 2

Sanjeev K. Swami, MD
Attending Physician
Division of Infectious Diseases
Nemours/Alfred I. duPont Hospital for Children
WILMINGTON, DE
Clinical Assistant Professor
Jefferson Medical College
PHILADELPHIA, PENNSYLVANIA
Chapters 5, 6, and 7

Rebecca Tenney-Soeiro, MD
Assistant Professor of Clinical Pediatrics
Children's Hospital of Philadelphia
Perelman School of Medicine
PHILADELPHIA, PENNSYLVANIA
Chapters 11, 12, and 19

Matthew Test, MD
Division of Hospital Medicine
University of Cincinnati College of Medicine
CINCINNATI, OHIO
Chapters 2 and 19

Nathan Timm, MD
Emergency Medicine
Cincinnati Children's Hospital Medical Center
    and Department of Pediatrics
University of Cincinnati College of Medicine
CINCINNATI, OHIO
Chapters 2 and 8

Phuong Vo, MD
Assistant Professor of Pediatrics
Division of Respiratory Diseases
Boston Children's Hospital
BOSTON, MASSACHUSETTS
Chapters 4 and 14

Amy T. Waldman, MD, MSCE
Assistant Professor of Neurology
Children's Hospital of Philadelphia
Perelman School of Medicine
University of Pennsylvania
PHILADELPHIA, PENNSYLVANIA
Chapters 16 and 19

Heidi C. Werner, MD
Fellow
Division of Emergency Medicine
Boston Children's Hospital
Instructor of Pediatrics
Harvard Medical School
BOSTON, MASSACHUSETTS
Chapters 12 and 13

Joanne N. Wood, MD, MSHP
Attending Physician
Children's Hospital of Philadelphia
Assistant Professor of Pediatrics
Perelman School of Medicine
University of Pennsylvania
PHILADELPHIA, PENNSYLVANIA
Chapters 3 and 9

Kamillah N. Wood, MD, MPH
Assistant Professor, Pediatrics
George Washington University School of Medicine
   and Health Sciences
WASHINGTON, DC
Chapters 3, 6, and 9

Stephanie Zandieh, MD, MS
Assistant Professor
Division of Pediatric Pulmonology
NYU Langone Medical Center
NEW YORK, NEW YORK
Chapter 4

PREFACE

The conceptual framework for this book is based on a traditional model of medical education: case-based learning. The case-based model is still very relevant, perhaps even more relevant, in the changing environment of physician training and education and advancing medical technology which combine to make it less likely that an individual physician will witness the evolution of a complex case from start to finish.

By understanding what happens in individual cases, one is able to generalize to similar situations and incorporate basic principles into practice. We are taught the classic signs and symptoms of innumerable diseases and disorders in the course of our medical training to develop skills in pattern recognition. From repetitive review of these patterns, we learn the elements of these common conditions. As the stages of medical education advance, one becomes more oriented to the expectations and, ultimately, exceptions in these routine patterns. It is appreciating the occurrence of deviations from this pattern, however minor, that leads to more advanced diagnostic skills. The astute physician detects variance from the typical pattern to make the more unusual or exceptional diagnosis.

In the education of pediatric house officers at the Children's Hospital of Philadelphia, there is a tradition of special rounds for the senior residents. The senior rounds are organized and conducted by the chief residents and supported by the faculty. It is within the context of these educational seminars that our residents are able to move and mature from pattern recognition to pattern deviation. We hope that in this effort they will move from good pediatricians to exceptional pediatricians.

This book represents a collection of many of those cases presented at the Children's Hospital of Philadelphia senior rounds. Most cases start with common complaints on the part of the child or parent. The cases presented in this text have common complaints, but, despite the protean presenting signs and symptoms, evolve into challenging diagnostic dilemmas. Each chapter in this book begins with a definition of a complaint, exploration of associated signs and symptoms that bring the patient to the physician, and discussion of questions associated with the complaint. The chapters then include a series of cases, each with twists and turns, that illustrate how to identify which children with common presenting complaints may have unusual or uncommon conditions. The cases are accompanied by clinical or radiologic images to enhance learning and retention. Following each case presentation, there is discussion of a broad differential diagnosis, commentary about which particular elements of that case led to the final diagnosis, and detailed discussion about the diagnosis in question, including epidemiology, signs and symptoms, diagnostic evaluation, and treatment.

For the book to be enjoyed most, we suggest the reader review each case and try to arrive at his or her own differential diagnosis and plan of evaluation, then read on and find out how the "mystery" was solved. An alternate way to use this book is to conduct your own group discussion or senior rounds by having one member of the group present a case and lead a discussion while using the text to facilitate dialogue.

Samir S. Shah
Stephen Ludwig

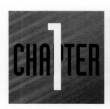

CHAPTER 1

WHEEZING

DUSTIN R. HAFERBECKER

DEFINITION OF THE COMPLAINT

Noisy breathing in infants is a common presenting complaint. The first step toward formulating a differential diagnosis is to characterize the type of sound heard. Stertor, a low-pitched rattling inspiratory noise, is caused by obstruction of airway above the level of the larynx. It is frequently heard in infants with nasal congestion and is often of little consequence. Stridor, a harsh, high-pitched respiratory sound typically heard on inspiration, often indicates laryngeal obstruction. Wheezing, a musical sound heard on expiration, is caused by partial obstruction of the lower airway. In young children, sometimes expiratory noises cannot be easily distinguished from inspiratory ones, and at times both may be present. Among these causes of noisy breathing, wheezing is the most common of clinical significance.

COMPLAINT BY CAUSE AND FREQUENCY

The causes of wheezing in childhood vary by age (Table 1-1) and may also be grouped in categories based on the following criteria: (1) Anatomic (extrinsic or intrinsic to the airway), (2) Inflammatory/Infectious, (3) Genetic/Metabolic, or (4) Miscellaneous causes (Table 1-2).

CLARIFYING QUESTIONS

A thorough study of the child's history is essential to arrive at an accurate diagnosis in a child who presents with wheezing. Consideration of age at onset, course and pattern of illness, and associated clinical features provides a useful framework for creating a differential diagnosis. The following questions may help provide clues to the diagnosis:

- What was the age at onset of wheezing?
  —Onset at birth or during early infancy suggests congenital structural abnormalities. Congenital diaphragmatic hernias are usually detected on prenatal ultrasound. Vascular rings and aberrant vessels can cause wheezing or other respiratory symptoms early in life. Infants <2 years of age are more susceptible to lower respiratory infection, such as bronchiolitis, whereas adolescents are more likely to have asthma or infection caused by atypical bacteria, such as *Mycoplasma pneumoniae*.

- Is the wheezing a new onset or recurrent?
  —The initial episode of wheezing in a previously healthy infant in conjunction with symptoms of upper respiratory tract infection usually indicates bronchiolitis. A sudden onset of wheezing is also characteristic of anaphylaxis; particularly in the presence of urticaria, stridor, or pertinent environmental exposures. Recurrent episodes of wheezing may suggest gastroesophageal reflux. However, if precipitated by upper respiratory infections, recurrent wheezing may suggest reactive airways disease. Recurrent wheezing or "difficult to control asthma" should lead to a consideration of cystic fibrosis, immotile cilia syndrome, recurrent aspiration, immune deficiency, or anatomic abnormalities.

- Is the wheezing episodic or persistent?
  —Persistent wheezing suggests mechanical obstruction from a variety of causes, such as

1

TABLE 1-1.	Causes of wheezing in childhood by age.	
Disease Prevalence	**Neonate/Infant**	**School Age/Adolescent**
Common	Bronchiolitis Asthma	Asthma
Less Common	Pulmonary aspiration –Gastroesophageal reflux –Swallowing dysfunction Foreign body aspiration Bronchopulmonary dysplasia Cystic fibrosis	Foreign body aspiration Anaphylaxis Cystic fibrosis
Uncommon	Congenital heart disease Defective host defenses –Immune deficiency –Immotile cilia syndrome Congenital structural anomalies –Tracheobronchomalacia –Vascular ring –Lobar emphysema –Cystic abnormalities –Tracheoesophageal fistula	Defective host defenses Mediastinal tumors Enlarged mediastinal lymph nodes Parasitic infection Pulmonary hemosiderosis α1-antitrypsin deficiency

airway foreign body, congenital airway narrowing, or external compression by a mediastinal mass or vascular anomaly.

- Was the episode of wheezing preceded by choking or gagging?

—Aspiration of a foreign body is sometimes associated with the sudden onset of symptoms after gagging or choking. Foreign body aspiration is most common in children between the ages of 1 and 4 years. Symptoms depend on the size and location of the foreign body. The wheezing may

TABLE 1-2.	Causes of wheezing in childhood by mechanism.		
Anatomic	Extrinsic to airway –Lymphadenopathy –Tumor –Diaphragmatic hernia –Vascular ring/aberrant vessel Intrinsic to airway –Tracheobronchomalacia –Foreign body aspiration –Endobronchial tuberculosis –Vocal cord dysfunction –Bronchopulmonary dysplasia –Congestive heart failure/ pulmonary edema –Pulmonary cysts –Congenital lobar emphysema –Pulmonary sequestration	**Inflammatory/ Infectious (Cont.)**	Bronchitis Pneumonia –*Mycoplasma pneumoniae* –*Chlamydophila pneumoniae* –Aspiration pneumonia Bronchiectasis Bronchial papillomas Hypersensitivity pneumonitis α1-antitrypsin deficiency Pulmonary hemosiderosis
		Genetic/Metabolic	Cystic fibrosis Immotile cilia syndrome –Kartagener syndrome Metabolic disturbances –Hypocalcemia –Hypokalemia
Inflammatory/ Infectious	Asthma/reactive airways disease Bronchiolitis –Respiratory syncytial virus –Influenza viruses A and B –Parainfluenza viruses –Adenovirus –Human metapneumovirus –Rhinovirus –Coronaviruses	**Miscellaneous**	Psychosomatic illness –Emotional laryngeal wheezing

be unilateral and secondary bacterial infection may occur.

- Was the wheezing preceded by upper respiratory tract infection?
—Antecedent upper respiratory tract infection is suggestive of an underlying inflammatory or infectious etiology.

- What is the child's weight and height?
—Features suggestive of cystic fibrosis include failure to thrive, steatorrhea, or recurrent infections.

- Is there a history of recurrent bacterial infection?
—Children with cystic fibrosis often have recurrent respiratory tract infections. Ciliary dyskinesis is associated with frequent cough, sinusitis, and otitis media.

- Is there a history of preterm birth or did the child require mechanical ventilation or prolonged supplemental oxygen after birth?
—Bronchopulmonary dysplasia chronic lung disease of prematurity should be considered.

- Are there allergic shiners, Dennie lines, nasal crease, or atopic dermatitis?
—The presence of atopy increases the likelihood of asthma.

- Are symptoms exacerbated by feeding?
—Gastroesophageal reflux and tracheoesophageal fistula should be considered. H-type tracheo-esophageal fistulas may not be accompanied by esophageal atresia.

- Was the mother tested for sexually transmitted diseases during pregnancy?
—*Chlamydia trachomatis* pneumonia may present during the second month of life with nonpurulent conjunctivitis, wheezing, and pneumonia without fever.

- Is there a family history of wheezing or asthma?
—A family history of asthma in either or both parents increases the risk of the patient having asthma to 2-3 times above the baseline prevalence.

SUGGESTED READING

1. Bjerg A, Hedman L, Perzanowski MS, et al. Family history of asthma and atopy: in-depth analyses of the impact on asthma and wheeze in 7- to 8-year-old children. *Pediatrics* 2007;120:741-748.

The following cases represent less common causes of wheezing in childhood.

CASE 1-1

Eight-Month-Old Girl

DUSTIN R. HAFERBECKER

HISTORY OF PRESENT ILLNESS

The patient was an 8-month-old girl who presented to the emergency department for the third consecutive day with parental complaints of wheezing and cough. Two days prior to admission she was examined in the emergency department, diagnosed with bronchiolitis and otitis media and discharged on amoxicillin, nebulized albuterol, and prednisolone. One day prior to admission, she was again evaluated in the emergency department for continued wheezing and cough which improved with nebulized albuterol.

A chest radiograph demonstrated hyperinflation and peribronchiolar thickening. There was no cardiomegaly or pleural effusion. On the day of admission, her cough was accompanied by two episodes of perioral cyanosis. She had decreased oral intake and urine output and was febrile to 39.7°C at home.

MEDICAL HISTORY

The girl's history was remarkable for frequent episodes of wheezing since 5 months of age. She had received nebulized albuterol intermittently, including every 4 hours for the past month, without significant improvement in her wheezing. Her cough was worse at night but did not seem to be worse with feeding or supine positioning. Her birth history was unremarkable and the prenatal ultrasound was reportedly normal.

PHYSICAL EXAMINATION

T 38.3°C; RR 60/min; HR 110 bpm; BP 110/55 mmHg; SpO$_2$ 100% in room air

Height 25th percentile; Weight 25th percentile; Head circumference 25th percentile

Initial examination revealed a well-nourished, acyanotic infant in moderate respiratory distress. Physical examination was remarkable for purulent rhinorrhea and buccal mucosal thrush. Moderate intercostal and subcostal retractions were present. There was fair lung aeration with diffuse expiratory wheezing. No murmurs or gallops were heard on cardiac examination and femoral pulses were palpable. No hepatomegaly or splenomegaly was present.

DIAGNOSTIC STUDIES

Laboratory analysis revealed 14 600 white blood cells/mm^3 with 38% segmented neutrophils, 53% lymphocytes, and no band forms. The hemoglobin was 11.0 g/dL and there were 580 000 platelets/mm^3. Electrolytes, blood urea nitrogen, and creatinine were normal. Polymerase chain reaction performed on nasopharyngeal aspirate was negative for *Bordetella pertussis*. Antigens of adenovirus, influenza A and B viruses, parainfluenza virus types 1, 2, and 3, and respiratory syncytial virus were not detected by immunofluorescence of nasopharyngeal washings. However, respiratory syncytial virus subsequently grew in viral culture of the nasopharyngeal aspirate. Blood and urine cultures were subsequently negative.

COURSE OF ILLNESS

The patient was diagnosed with bronchiolitis, and her tachypnea and wheezing improved over time. She was treated with nebulized albuterol and oral prednisolone, with unclear benefit. She was discharged after 3 days of hospitalization, receiving albuterol every 4 hours as needed. A radionuclide milk scan was scheduled on an outpatient basis to assess the presence of gastroesophageal reflux and pulmonary aspiration.

Ten days later the patient returned to the emergency room with increased wheezing and recurrence of fever. She had poor oral intake which had not improved significantly since the last admission and was now accompanied by frequent emesis. She was admitted for treatment and further evaluation. Her radionuclide milk scan which had been performed between admissions revealed gastroesophageal reflux without pulmonary aspiration. During her current admission, careful examination of the chest radiograph suggested the diagnosis (Figures 1-1A and B). Magnetic resonance imaging (MRI) of the chest confirmed this diagnosis (Figure 1-1C).

DISCUSSION CASE 1-1

DIFFERENTIAL DIAGNOSIS

The causes of recurrent or persistent wheezing in infant are diverse. Common causes of recurrent wheezing in infancy include bronchiolitis, reactive airways disease, and gastroesophageal reflux with microaspiration. Less commonly, recurrent wheezing is caused by congenital abnormalities of the lung or respiratory tract (congenital cystic adenomatous malformations, tracheoesophageal fistula), diaphragmatic abnormalities (paralysis of the diaphragm, congenital diaphragmatic hernia), cystic fibrosis, or immunologic defects (congenital absence of thymus, DiGeorge syndrome or other 22q11 deletion syndromes, chronic granulomatous disease, gamma globulin deficiencies). Rarely, anomalies of the major arterial branches of the aorta or pulmonary blood vessels may compress the trachea and bronchi of the infant causing acute or progressive respiratory distress. The features of this case which prompted additional evaluation included recurrent episodes of wheezing, incomplete resolution of wheezing despite prolonged beta-agonist therapy, and episodes of cyanosis.

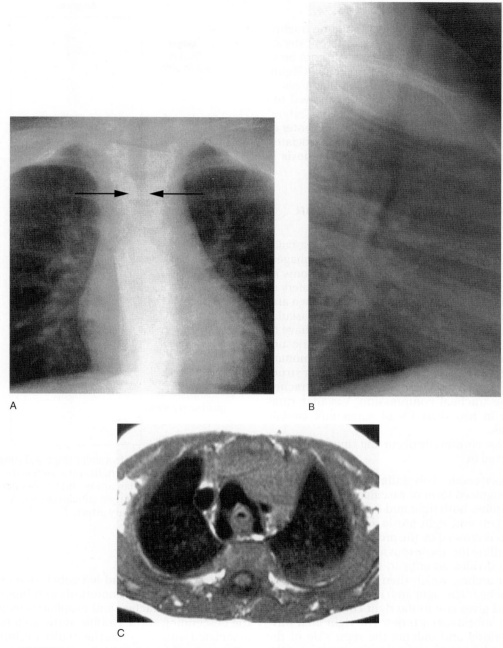

FIGURE 1-1. **A.** Antero-posterior chest radiograph. **B.** Lateral chest radiograph. **C.** Chest MRI.

DIAGNOSIS

The chest radiographs revealed a midline trachea with bilateral indentations in the anteroposterior projection (Figure 1-1A, arrows) and anterior bowing of the trachea on the lateral projection (Figure 1-1B). These findings suggested the diagnosis of double aortic arch. MRI of the chest showed the bifurcation of this double arch as the "horseshoe" structure surrounding the trachea in the center of the image (Figure 1-1C). There were no associated structural defects of the heart. **The diagnosis is double aortic arch.**

INCIDENCE AND ANATOMY OF VASCULAR RINGS AND SLINGS

Vascular anomalies, commonly referred to "vascular rings and slings," can cause tracheal or esophageal compression leading to respiratory symptoms or feeding difficulty. The term *vascular ring* refers to any aortic arch anomaly in which the trachea and esophagus are completely surrounded by vascular structures. The vascular structures do not have to be patent. For example, a ligamentum arteriosum may complete a ring. A vascular or pulmonary sling refers to an anomaly in which vascular structures only partially surround the lower trachea but cause tracheal compression. Vascular rings are seen in less than 1% of congenital cardiac anomalies.

The most commonly occurring rings and slings are depicted in Figure 1-2.

Double aortic arch. This is the most common clinically recognized form of vascular ring and, as the name implies, both right and left aortic arches are present. Left and right aortic arch refer to which bronchus is crossed by the arch, not to which side of the midline the aortic root ascends. The ascending aorta divides anterior to the trachea into left and right arches, which then pass on either side of the trachea. The right arch is usually higher and larger and gives rise to the right common carotid and right subclavian arteries. The right arch travels posteriorly and indents the right side of the trachea and the right and posterior portions of the esophagus, as it passes behind the esophagus to join the left arch at the junction of the left-sided descending aorta. The left arch gives rise to the

Anatomy

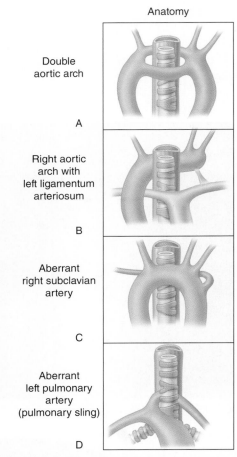

Double aortic arch

A

Right aortic arch with left ligamentum arteriosum

B

Aberrant right subclavian artery

C

Aberrant left pulmonary artery (pulmonary sling)

D

FIGURE 1-2. Anatomy of vascular rings and slings: **(A)** double aortic arch; **(B)** right aortic arch with anomalous left subclavian artery and left ligamentum arteriosum; **(C)** aberrant right subclavian artery; and **(D)** aberrant left pulmonary artery.

left common carotid and left subclavian arteries. The left arch is located anteriorly and indents the left side of the trachea and esophagus as it joins the descending aorta. Double aortic arch is rarely associated with congenital heart disease, but when present tetralogy of Fallot is the most common, and transposition of the great arteries is occasionally seen. Surgical division of one of the arches, usually the smaller one, is curative. Respiratory symptoms may persist for months postoperatively because of prolonged deformity of the tracheobronchial tree.

Aberrant right subclavian artery. This is also known as left aortic arch with retroesophageal right subclavian artery. It is the most common aortic arch malformation noted on postmortem examination. The incidence of this abnormality in the general population is approximately 0.5%. Aberrant right subclavian artery was found in 0.9% of 3427 consecutive patients undergoing cardiac catheterization at The Children's Hospital of Philadelphia. It represented 20% of aortic arch anomalies found at catheterization. It is also seen in approximately one-third of Down syndrome patients with congenital heart disease. The left aortic arch has a normal course to the left and anterior to the trachea. However, the right subclavian artery arises as the last branch of the arch and runs posteriorly from the descending thoracic aorta to reach the right arm, passing obliquely up to and right behind the esophagus and indenting it posteriorly. Although most patients with this anomaly are asymptomatic, an older patient may complain of dysphagia. Symptomatic anterior tracheal compression results if there is a common origin of both carotid arteries in conjunction with a retroesophageal aberrant right subclavian artery. Rarely, an anomalous right subclavian artery in association with a left aortic arch, retroesophageal descending aorta, and right ligamentum arteriosum produces a symptomatic vascular ring.

Right aortic arch with anomalous left subclavian artery and left ductus arteriosus or ligamentum arteriosum. The aortic arch passes to the right of the trachea, becomes retroesophageal, and descends on left. The first branch is the left carotid artery, the second is the right carotid artery, the third the right subclavian artery, and the fourth the left subclavian artery, which arises from the descending aorta. The ductus arteriosus originates from a retroesophageal diverticulum of the descending aorta, courses to the left and connects to the pulmonary artery. Patients are usually asymptomatic. However, some patients present with wheezing or stridor because of tracheal compression and require surgical division of the ligamentum arteriosum. Older children with dysphagia

may require relief of esophageal compression by actual division of the aortic arch. The retroesophageal portion is mobilized and reanastomosis of ascending and descending portions of the aorta is completed using a graft.

Aberrant left pulmonary artery (pulmonary sling). A normal pulmonary artery is absent, and the left lung is supplied by an anomalous left pulmonary artery arising from the distal right pulmonary artery. The vessel courses to the right of the trachea and then passes between the trachea and esophagus, causing compression of the right main stem bronchus, trachea, and esophagus. The resulting compression of the right main stem bronchus and trachea leads to airway obstruction, primarily affecting the right lung. Two-thirds of affected infants present in the first month of life with wheezing, stridor, or apnea. Dysphagia is rare. There may be associated collapse or hyperinflation of the right lung. Aberrant left pulmonary artery is frequently associated with complete cartilaginous rings in the distal trachea, resulting in tracheal stenosis. It usually appears as an isolated abnormality but can be associated with other congenital cardiac defects, particularly tetralogy of Fallot. Surgical repair involves division of the left pulmonary artery from the right and reanastomosis in front of the trachea. Bronchoscopy is performed at the time of surgical repair because of the frequent association of complete cartilaginous rings causing tracheal stenosis.

CLINICAL PRESENTATION OF VASCULAR RINGS AND SLINGS

Most infants present with symptoms in early infancy. Superimposed viral infection with edema of the trachea or bronchi may account for or contribute to the respiratory symptoms. Asymptomatic infants, particularly those with aberrant right subclavian artery, are sometimes diagnosed incidentally on chest radiograph during a viral respiratory illness.

The symptoms of a vascular ring or sling are due to tracheal compression and, to a lesser degree, to esophageal compression. Symptoms of tracheal compression include wheezing, stridor, and apnea. Some infants hyperextend their necks to reduce tracheal compression.

Symptoms related to esophageal compression include emesis, choking, and nonspecific feeding difficulties in infants, and dysphagia in older children. Less severe obstructions may present with recurrent respiratory infections as a result of aspiration or inadequate clearing of respiratory secretions.

DIAGNOSTIC APPROACH

Clinicians should have a high index of suspicion for a vascular anomaly in the evaluation of an infant with recurrent wheezing. Chest radiograph and barium esophagogram should be considered in the initial evaluation.

Chest radiograph. The diagnosis of a vascular ring may be suspected prior to barium esophagogram. Chest radiograph should be examined to assess laterality of the aortic arch and for evidence of tracheal or bronchial compression. The following features on chest radiograph are suggestive of a vascular anomaly and require additional evaluation: (1) A midline trachea in which there is no rotation of the patient or a sharp indentation on the right side of the trachea above the carina suggests a right aortic arch. The normal infant's trachea is slightly displaced to the right by the normal left arch. (2) Lateral displacement of the right mediastinal pleural line indicates a right descending aorta. (3) Anterior bowing of the trachea rather than a normal posterior convexity on the lateral view indicates compression (Figure 1-1B). Generalized or focal areas of hyperinflation because of tracheal or bronchial compression can be mistakenly diagnosed as a foreign body aspiration.

Barium esophagogram. Patients with swallowing difficulties should undergo a barium swallow as part of the initial evaluation. Abnormal compression of the middle part of the esophagus posteriorly (vascular ring) or anteriorly (pulmonary sling) is typically evident.

Magnetic resonance angiography (MRA) and computed tomography angiography (CTA). Both MRA and CTA have been shown to provide excellent anatomic details and are helpful in planning reconstructive procedures.

Angiogram and transthoracic echocardiogram. In the absence of any other cardiac defect, catheter-based angiography has essentially become obsolete because of advances in three-dimensional renderings of MRA and CTA data. Transthoracic echocardiography is important to detect associated congenital cardiac defects but is less reliable at delineating vascular and tracheal anatomy.

Bronchoscopy. This enables direct visualization of compression on the trachea and is indicated when tracheal stenosis is present or suspected.

TREATMENT

Surgical management is necessary to relieve symptomatic obstruction of trachea and esophagus. Surgery should also be considered when the infant has frequent respiratory infections or poor weight gain. The infant with severe preoperative respiratory symptoms is likely to have postoperative tracheomalacia from prolonged compression by the vascular ring. However, feeding difficulties resolve rapidly.

SUGGESTED READINGS

1. Dillman JR, Attili AK, Agarwal PP, et al. Common and uncommon vascular rings and slings: a multi-modality review. *Pediatr Radiol.* 2011;41:1440-1454.
2. Berdon WE, Baker DH. Vascular anomalies and the infant lung: rings, slings, and other things. *Semin Roentgen.* 1972;7:39-63.
3. Edwards JE. Malformations of the aortic arch system manifested as "vascular rings." *Lab Invest.* 1953;2:56-75.
4. Goldstein WB. Aberrant right subclavian artery in mongolism. *Am J Roentgenol Radium Ther Nucl Med* 1965;95:131-134.
5. Hawker RE, Celermajer JM, Cartmill TB, Bowdler JD. Double aortic arch and complex cardiac malformations. *Br Heart J.* 1972;34:1311-1313.
6. Moes CAF, Freedom RM. Rare types of aortic arch anomalies. *Pediatr Cardiol.* 1993;14:93-101.
7. Weinberg PM. Aortic arch anomalies. In: Emmanouilides GC, Riemenschneider TA, Allen HD, Gutgesell HP, eds. *Moss and Adams Heart Disease in Infants, Children, and Adolescents, Including the Fetus and Young Adult.* 5th ed. Baltimore: Williams & Wilkins; 1995:810-837.

CASE 1-2

Three-Year-Old Boy

DUSTIN R. HAFERBECKER

HISTORY OF PRESENT ILLNESS

A 3-year-old boy was referred to the emergency department for evaluation of wheezing, cough, and increased work of breathing. He had been well until 3 days prior to admission, when he developed rhinorrhea and cough without fever. Nebulized albuterol was prescribed for wheezing and retractions, with little improvement. On the day of admission, the child's respiratory distress had continued and his cough had worsened and was accompanied by mild sternal discomfort exacerbated by coughing. He had received nebulized albuterol every 4 hours during the day of admission without significant relief. There was no vomiting or diarrhea. The onset of wheezing was not accompanied by an episode of choking or gagging. There was no history of trauma.

MEDICAL HISTORY

The boy's medical history was unremarkable. There were no previous episodes of wheezing. He was born at 39 weeks gestational age without perinatal complications. There was no family history of atopic dermatitis or asthma.

PHYSICAL EXAMINATION

T 37.7°C; RR 52/min; HR 130 bpm; BP 108/70 mmHg; SpO$_2$ 95% in room air

Weight 50th percentile

Physical examination revealed a fair-haired Caucasian boy in mild respiratory distress. On examination, there was no conjunctival injection or chemosis. Clear rhinorrhea was present. He had mild intercostal and subcostal retractions. His lung examination revealed dullness to percussion, diminished breath sounds, and prominent wheezing at the left base. There was good aeration without wheezing, rales, or rhonchi in the remainder of the left lung and throughout the right side. An I/VI vibratory systolic ejection murmur was present at the left sternal border. His abdomen was thin and soft with active bowel sounds and no organomegaly or palpable mass. The remainder of the physical examination was normal.

DIAGNOSTIC STUDIES

Laboratory analysis revealed 15 100 white blood cells/mm^3 with 0% band forms, 52% segmented neutrophils, 33% lymphocytes, and 5% eosinophils. Hemoglobin, platelet count, electrolytes, blood urea nitrogen, and creatinine were normal.

COURSE OF ILLNESS

The patient's lung examination did not change with the administration of nebulized albuterol. A chest radiograph revealed the diagnosis as indicated in Figure 1-3.

DISCUSSION CASE 1-2

DIFFERENTIAL DIAGNOSIS

The most likely cause of a first episode of wheezing in a 3-year-old boy, particularly in the context of an upper respiratory infection, is asthma. Foreign body aspiration should also be strongly suspected in this age group, especially if there are asymmetries on lung examination. Less common causes in this age group include anaphylaxis, which is typically associated with urticaria or other features of a systemic allergic response, and airway compression due to mediastinal tumors, lymph nodes, or other structures. In the immunocompromised host, *Pneumocystis jiroveci* (formerly *P. carinii*) pneumonia often presents with tachypnea, wheezing, and respiratory distress in the absence of fever. Children with cystic fibrosis usually have poor weight gain, pancreatic insufficiency, and recurrent respiratory symptoms. The characteristics of this case that prompted additional evaluation included hypoxemia, progressive respiratory

FIGURE 1-3. Chest radiograph. **A.** Antero-posterior view. **B.** Lateral view.

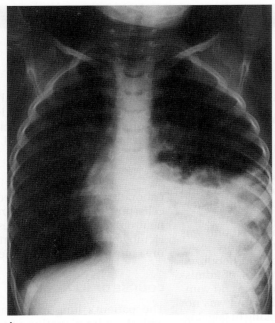
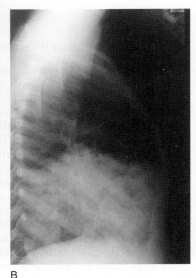

A

B

distress that was unresponsive to beta-agonist therapy, and the presence of focal wheezing evident on lung examination.

DIAGNOSIS

The chest radiograph (Figure 1-3) revealed a heterogeneous opacity overlying the lower half of the left lung consistent with the appearance of both small and large bowel in the thorax. The mediastinal structures are displaced rightward. **The diagnosis is postero-lateral congenital diaphragmatic (Bochdalek) hernia with delayed presentation.**

INCIDENCE AND EPIDEMIOLOGY

Congenital diaphragmatic hernia (CDH) is a simple anatomic defect in which a hole in the diaphragm allows abdominal viscera to herniate into the thorax. CDH defects are usually left-sided (80%). The incidence of CDH is estimated to be 1 per 2000 to 5000 births. While most cases of CDH are diagnosed prenatally or during the neonatal

period, approximately 10%-20% have delayed presentation (age >1 month). They are thought to occur most often as a sporadic developmental anomaly, although familial cases have been reported. The recurrence risk in a first-degree relative is approximately 2%. Approximately 40% of liveborn patients who have CDH have one or more associated anomalies including cardiac (60%), genitourinary (23%), gastrointestinal (17%), central nervous system (14%), and chromosomal (10%) (Table 1-3). Infants with isolated CDH are more likely to be premature, macrosomic, and male.

TABLE 1-3.	The prevalence of associated anomalies detected in 40% of patients with congenital diaphragmatic hernia.
Abnormality	*Prevalence*
Cardiac	60%
Genitourinary	23%
Gastrointestinal	17%
Central nervous system	14%
Chromosomal	10%

Population-based studies of CDH among live-born, stillborn, and spontaneously aborted fetuses suggest that approximately 30% of fetuses who have CDH will die before birth, usually from chromosomal or lethal nonpulmonary malformations. Among fetuses with prenatally diagnosed CDH and without major associated anomalies, early term delivery (i.e., 37 weeks compared with 39-41 weeks gestational age) may confer a survival advantage. In CDH, the location of the defect may also affect postnatal survival and the development of chronic lung disease. In one study, more neonates with left-sided CDH died of severe pulmonary hypertension despite extracorporeal membrane oxygenation. Fewer neonates with right-sided CDH died, yet higher degrees of pulmonary hypoplasia and oxygen requirement were observed despite extracorporeal membrane oxygenation.

Congenital diaphragmatic hernias may vary in size and occur in various portions of the diaphragm. Types of CDH include postero-lateral (Bochdalek) (59.5%), antero-medial (Morgagni) (2.6%), hiatal (23.3%), and eventration (14.6%). Postero-lateral diaphragmatic hernias result from an absence or defective fusion of the septum transversum dorsally and pleuroperitoneal membrane postero-laterally. There appear to be two groups of patients with delayed presentations of postero-lateral CDH. In the first group, the defect is long-standing, but the viscera are confined by a hernia sac or obturated by a solid organ. Presentation occurs when the sac ruptures or the intraabdominal pressure is raised, causing the viscera to herniate. A previously normal chest radiograph is supportive. The second group also has a congenital defect but only present when a complication of the herniated contents such as volvulus, strangulation, or acute or recurrent respiratory distress develops.

CLINICAL PRESENTATION

Many patients with CDH are diagnosed antenatally by ultrasound. In such instances, other congenital anomalies, particularly those affecting the cardiovascular and central nervous systems, should be sought. The presentation of CDH in the neonatal period is determined primarily by the severity of the pulmonary hypoplasia and pulmonary hypertension. The most severely affected infants show obvious respiratory signs within the first 24 hours of life. Classically, these infants are born with a scaphoid abdomen and develop progressive respiratory distress as swallowed air causes intestinal distension followed by worsening lung compression and mediastinal shift. These infants may have cyanosis, increased work of breathing, and respiratory failure.

In contrast, the presentation of diaphragmatic hernia outside the neonatal period is extremely varied, and may be associated with misleading clinical and radiologic assessments. Children who have CDH with delayed presentation may have recurrent respiratory distress, chronic pulmonary infection, or acute gastrointestinal symptoms caused by gastric volvulus or intestinal obstruction.

DIAGNOSTIC APPROACH

Prenatal ultrasound. CDH may be diagnosed by ultrasound during routine obstetric screening or during investigation of polyhydramnios, which may complicate up to 80% of pregnancies in which CDH occurs. The accuracy of prenatal diagnosis varies, depending on the site of the lesion and the presence of corroborating criteria, such as mediastinal shift and abnormal fetal abdominal anatomy. The diagnosis is suggested strongly by the presence of a fluid-filled stomach or intestine at the level of the four-chamber view of the heart.

Fetal MRI. In cases where CDH is expected based on ultrasound but remains unclear, fetal MRI has the potential to assist in the diagnosis. The additional information provided by MRI may also be helpful in counseling the family regarding potential value of prenatal and postnatal interventions.

Associated studies. Once the diagnosis of CDH in a neonate has been confirmed, a careful search for associated anomalies should be performed. Additional studies to consider include renal and cranial ultrasonography, echocardiography, and karyotyping.

Chest radiograph. The diagnosis is confirmed by a chest radiograph that demonstrates loops of intestine within the chest. The location of the gastric bubble should also be noted, and its position can be confirmed by placement of a nasogastric tube. Occasionally, a large multicystic lung lesion such as congenital cystic adenomatoid malformation will have the appearance of a CDH on plain radiography. In these instances, ultrasonographic visualization of an intact diaphragm or computed tomographic scan of the chest may be necessary. In an older child, the radiographic appearance of CDH may be misinterpreted pneumothorax, pneumatocele, or lobar consolidation.

Upper gastrointestinal barium series. Confirmative barium studies represent an unnecessary delay in appropriate therapy for the neonate. However, in the older child they serve to confirm the diagnosis. Additionally, up to 30% of children with delayed presentation of CDH have associated abnormalities of bowel fixation or rotation requiring repair.

TREATMENT

Prenatal care. Antenatal diagnosis of CDH has allowed optimal immediate care of affected infants. Birth at a tertiary care center that has pediatric surgery and neonatology services as well as advanced strategies for managing respiratory failure, including extracorporeal membrane oxygenation (ECMO), usually is most appropriate. A spontaneous vaginal delivery should be anticipated unless obstetric issues dictate otherwise.

Fetal therapy. The role of in utero surgery for CDH remains controversial. Fetal intervention is currently focused on temporary occlusion of the fetal trachea for those fetuses who have CDH and liver herniation above the diaphragm in an attempt to correct the severe pulmonary hypoplasia often associated with CDH. Normally, fetal lungs produce a continuous flow of fluid that exits the trachea into the amniotic space. In the presence of tracheal obstruction, the lungs grow, and there is gradual reduction of herniated viscera back into the abdomen. Following a period of intrauterine tracheal occlusion sufficient to cause a reversal of pulmonary hypoplasia, the fetus is delivered and maintained on placental support until the tracheal obstruction is relieved and an adequate neonatal airway is established. Other forms of antenatal therapy include the development of pharmacologic strategies that target pulmonary growth and development.

Delivery room and intensive care. Immediate resuscitation includes prompt endotracheal intubation, avoidance of bag-mask ventilation, placement of a nasogastric tube to provide intestinal decompression, and ongoing care in an intensive care nursery by individuals experienced in the management of the newborn who has CDH.

Surgical repair in the neonate. Historically, neonates who had CDH were rushed to the operating room under the mistaken belief that decompression of the lungs by reduction of the abdominal viscera offered the greatest chance of survival. This disorder is no longer thought to require immediate surgery because the primary problem after birth is not herniation of abdominal viscera into the chest but severe pulmonary hypoplasia and associated pulmonary hypertension. Average time to surgery now ranges from 3 to 15 days after birth. New treatments including ECMO and permissive hypercapnia with gentle ventilation to minimize barotrauma have led to incremental increases in survival rates which now range from 78% to 94%. Other treatments such as partial liquid ventilation, inhaled nitric oxide, surfactant-replacement therapy, and maternal corticosteroid therapy prior to birth require additional study in patients with CDH.

Surgical repair in the child with delayed presentation. The timing of repair in patients who present with CDH beyond the neonatal period typically occurs within days of presentation, or earlier if symptoms are acute. The prognosis in late-presenting CDH is good. It does not depend on lung hypoplasia as in neonatal CDH, but relates to accurate diagnosis of the condition and immediate operative correction in symptomatic cases. Complications of delayed repair in the symptomatic patient include incarceration or strangulation of herniated bowel and cardio-respiratory arrest due to mediastinal compression by the herniated viscera.

SUGGESTED READINGS

1. Deprest JA, Nicolaides K, Gratacos E. Fetal surgery for congenital diaphragmatic hernia is back from never gone. *Fetal Diagn Ther.* 2011;29:6-17.
2. Fotter R, Schimpl G, Sorantin E, Fritz K, Landler U. Delayed presentation of congenital diaphragmatic hernia. *Pediatr Radiol.* 1992;22:187-191.

3. Berman L, Stringer D, Ein SH, Shandling B. The late-presenting pediatric Bochdalek hernia: a 20-year review. *J Pediatr Surg.* 1988;23:735-739.

4. Dott MM, Wong LY, Rasmussen SA. Population-based study of congenital diaphragmatic hernia: risk factors and survival in Metropolitan Atlanta, 1968-1999. *Birth Defects Res A Clin Mol Teratol.* 2003;67:261-267.

5. Mayer S, Klaritsch P, Petersen S, et al. The correlation between lung volume and liver herniation measurements by fetal MRI in isolated congenital diaphragmatic herni: a systematic review and meta-analysis of observation studies. *Prenatal Diag.* 2011;31:1086-1096.

6. Schaible T, Kohl T, Reinshagen K, et al. Right- versus left-sided congenital diaphragmatic hernia: postnatal outcome at a specialized tertiary care center. *Pediatr Crit Care Med.* 2012;13:66-71.

7. Skarsgard ED, Harrison MR. Congenital diaphragmatic hernia: the surgeon's perspective. *Pediatr Rev.* 1999;20:e71-e78.

8. Stevens TP, van Wijngaarden E, Ackerman KG, Lally PA, Lally KP for the Congenital Diaphragmatic Hernia Study Group. Timing of delivery and survival rates for infants with prenatal diagnoses of congenital diaphragmatic hernia. *Pediatrics.* 2009;123:494-502.

9. Stolar CJH, Dillon PW. Congenital diaphragmatic hernia and eventration. In: O'Neill JA Jr., Rowe MI, Grosfeld JL, Fonkalsrud EW, Coran AG, eds. *Pediatric Surgery.* 5th ed. St. Louis: Mosby; 1998:819-837.

10. Thibeault DW, Sigalet DL. Congenital diaphragmatic hernia from the womb to childhood. *Curr Probl Pediatr.* 1998;28:5-25.

CASE 1-3

Five-Week-Old Boy

DUSTIN R. HAFERBECKER

HISTORY OF PRESENT ILLNESS

A 5-week-old boy presented to the emergency department with a one-day history of fever and "wheezing." His visit to the hospital was prompted by a rectal temperature of 38.6°C. His respiratory difficulty seemed worse with feeding. There had been no emesis, diarrhea, rhinorrhea, cough, or cyanosis. He had been drinking approximately 4 ounces of a cow milk-based formula every 3 hours. His only ill contact was his mother who had cough and rhinorrhea for one week.

MEDICAL HISTORY

The boy was born by spontaneous vaginal delivery at 39 weeks gestation. His birth weight was 3900 g. The pregnancy, labor, and delivery were uncomplicated. Prenatal ultrasound revealed polyhydramnios but was otherwise normal. The mother's prenatal laboratory studies included a negative group B *Streptococcus* screen. Testing for antibodies to human immunodeficiency virus had not been performed. The infant had not previously been hospitalized.

PHYSICAL EXAMINATION

T 38.5°C; HR 180 bpm; RR 70/min; BP 62/40 mmHg; SpO$_2$ 96% in room air

Length 25th percentile; Weight 50th percentile

The infant was ill appearing with moderate respiratory distress. His anterior fontanelle was open and flat. There was no conjunctival injection or discharge. There was intermittent grunting and nasal flaring. Moderate intercostal and subcostal retractions were present. Breath sounds were diminished throughout the left chest. The right lung was clear to auscultation. There was no wheezing. The heart sounds were normal. The liver was palpable 1 cm below the right costal margin. The spleen was not palpable. The moro reflex, grasp, tone, and reflexes were normal. There were no rashes or petechiae.

DIAGNOSTIC STUDIES

Arterial blood gas revealed the following: pH, 7.40; PaCO$_2$, 40 mmHg; PaO$_2$, 214 mmHg; and bicarbonate, 26 mEq/L. Complete blood count demonstrated 37 900 white blood cells/mm^3 (3% band

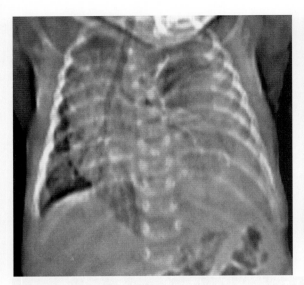

FIGURE 1-4. Chest radiograph.

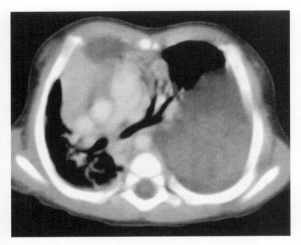

FIGURE 1-5. Chest CT scan.

forms; 67% segmented neutrophils; and 30% lymphocytes). The platelet count was 520000/mm³ and hemoglobin was 9.4 g/dL. Serum electrolytes, blood urea nitrogen, and creatinine were normal. There were no white blood cells, protein, or nitrites on urinalysis. A blood culture was obtained. Lumbar puncture was not performed because of the patient's respiratory distress. Chest radiograph demonstrated left lower lobe consolidation with an associated pleural effusion causing rightward shift of the mediastinal structures (Figure 1-4).

COURSE OF ILLNESS

The patient was diagnosed with bacterial pneumonia and treated with vancomycin and cefotaxime. The blood culture was subsequently negative. CT scan of the chest, performed to better delineate the pulmonary findings, suggested an alternate diagnosis (Figure 1-5).

DISCUSSION CASE 1-3

DIFFERENTIAL DIAGNOSIS

In this 5-week-old boy with respiratory distress and lobar consolidation, the most likely diagnosis

is bacterial pneumonia with pleural empyema. Etiologic organisms in this age group include group B *Streptococcus, Streptococcus pneumoniae, Listeria monocytogenes,* and Gram-negative enteric bacilli. The radiographic appearance of the lung suggests a congenital lung malformation, such as pulmonary sequestration, bronchogenic cyst, and congenital cystic adenomatoid malformation. Infantile lobar emphysema is unlikely because the lung, despite causing mediastinal shift, does not appear to be overinflated. Other congenital considerations include enterogenic cysts and congenital diaphragmatic hernia. Acquired causes include mediastinal neoplasms, such as neuroblastoma and chronic pulmonary infection distal to an aspirated foreign body or an area of bronchiectasis. Chronic pulmonary infection may result in neovascularization of the infected tissue by ingrowth of systemic arteries. Such acquired systemic vascularization typically consists of several small arteries rather than one or two large arteries that typically supply a pulmonary sequestration. It may be impossible to make the distinction between true pulmonary sequestration and the so-called pseudosequestration secondary to chronic infection preoperatively.

DIAGNOSIS

CT of the chest (Figure 1-5) revealed a large (6 cm × 5 cm × 8 cm) heterogeneously enhancing mass with disorganized vasculature in the posterior aspect of the left hemithorax. These findings were most consistent with an **extralobar pulmonary sequestration**.

INCIDENCE AND ANATOMY

The term pulmonary sequestration refers to a congenital malformation consisting of abnormally developed pulmonary parenchyma that is separate from the normal lung. The tissue is nonfunctioning, does not communicate with the tracheobronchial tree, and derives its blood supply from the aorta. There may be a single large anomalous artery but occasionally multiple small anomalous arteries from above or below the diaphragm supply the sequestered lobe. The venous drainage may be pulmonary or systemic (inferior vena cava, azygous vein, or portal vein). Drainage into systemic veins produces a left to right shunt. In this case, the vessels appeared to drain into the azygous and hemiazygous veins.

The overall incidence of pulmonary sequestration is not well defined, but sequestrations have been found in 1% to 2% of all resected pulmonary specimens. Pulmonary sequestration occurs when an accessory lung bud originates during embryonic development. If the bud originates early, the sequestration is considered intralobar because the normal and sequestered lung shares a common pleural covering. If the bud originates later, the sequestration is considered extralobar because the sequestered lung has its own pleura. About 75% of reported cases of pulmonary sequestration are intralobar; 1% have both an intra- and extralobar component.

Associated malformations occur in 60% of extralobar sequestrations and 10% of intralobar sequestrations. The most common associated malformations include duplications of the colon or terminal ileum, esophageal cysts or communications, vertebral or rib anomalies, diaphragmatic hernia, and congenital heart disease (Table 1-4). Pulmonary sequestration is left-sided in 90% of cases and bilateral in fewer than 0.5% of cases. Approximately two-thirds of all cases involve the left lower lobe.

CLINICAL PRESENTATION

Most children with extralobar pulmonary sequestration present during the first year of life. They may be discovered during the neonatal period

TABLE 1-4.	Anomalies associated with pulmonary sequestration.*
Duplications of the colon or terminal ileum Esophageal cysts or communications Vertebral or rib anomalies Diaphragmatic hernia Congenital heart disease	

*Anomalies are more common with extralobar (60% of patients) than with intralobar (10% of patients) pulmonary sequestration.

while undergoing evaluation for other congenital anomalies. In such cases, the associated congenital anomalies usually dominate the clinical picture. A few children with extralobar sequestration present with respiratory distress when the sequestered lobe impairs ventilation by impinging on the surrounding lung. Cases not diagnosed in the neonatal period may be detected incidentally on chest radiographs obtained during a respiratory illness. Infection of an extralobar sequestration is uncommon.

Intralobar pulmonary sequestration is rarely detected during infancy; two-thirds of cases present after 10 years of age. Common symptoms include productive cough, hemoptysis, recurrent pneumonia, fever, and chest pain. A few patients with large supplying arteries have worsening exercise tolerance or congestive heart failure because of a large systemic arterial-to-pulmonary venous shunt through the sequestration. Infection of the sequestration, usually because of a fistula between the sequestration and the respiratory or digestive tracts, occurs more commonly with intralobar as compared to extralobar sequestrations.

Physical examination reveals dullness to percussion and decreased breath sounds in the area of the sequestration. Digital clubbing and cyanosis may be present, depending on the presence and severity of shunting. Skeletal abnormalities such as pectus excavatum, thoracic asymmetry, and rib anomalies are noted in some patients. Rarely, an intrathoracic bruit is heard in the region of the sequestration.

DIAGNOSTIC APPROACH

Prenatal ultrasound. Pulmonary sequestration may be diagnosed during routine obstetric screening or during investigation of polyhydramnios, which is reported in many cases.

Chest radiograph. It is difficult to distinguish between intra- and extralobar sequestrations by chest radiograph alone. Both are typically found in the postero-medial aspect of the lower lobe and calcifications are occasionally present. Intralobar sequestrations more often appear cyst-like. Air-fluid levels indicate a pulmonary communication. Extralobar sequestrations appear as a solid mass.

Chest CT. CT enables differentiation of pulmonary sequestration from other lung abnormalities.

Magnetic resonance angiography (MRA) and computed tomography angiography (CTA). Both MRA and CTA have been shown to provide excellent anatomic details and are helpful in preparation for surgical resection.

Angiography. Angiography of the thoracic and abdominal aorta demonstrates both the systemic arterial blood supply and the venous drainage. This technique, however, is largely being replaced by less invasive methods as discussed above.

Nuclear scintigraphy. After intravenous injection, peak radioisotope activity occurs earlier in lung tissue with normal pulmonary blood supply than in the sequestration with systemic blood supply. Nuclear scintigraphy has been proposed as an alternative to traditional angiography.

Other studies. Magnetic resonance angiography is a less invasive study that may eventually replace traditional angiography in the evaluation of pulmonary sequestration. An upper gastrointestinal barium study should be considered to exclude the possibility of a communication with the gastrointestinal tract.

TREATMENT

Symptomatic intralobar and extralobar sequestrations require immediate resection. Asymptomatic sequestrations also require removal because of the risk of subsequent serious infection. Extralobar sequestrations because of their separate pleural covering can often be removed without disrupting the normal lung. Intralobar sequestrations require lobectomy for removal because of the inability to

separate the sequestration from the normal lung. In cases of acute infection, preoperative antibiotic coverage should be directed against common respiratory pathogens, *Staphylococcus aureus*, and anaerobes. Vancomycin or clindamycin in combination with third-generation cephalosporins (e.g., ceftriaxone, cefotaxime) provides appropriate empiric coverage. The resected tissue should be sent for aerobic and anaerobic bacterial cultures, mycobacterial cultures, and fungal cultures, as well as microscopic examination.

Intraoperative mortality is highest in those with associated congenital anomalies. Intraoperative complications are usually due to severance of a systemic artery. Postoperative complications include emphysema, hemothorax, and bronchopleural fistulae; the incidence of each is approximately 1%. The long-term prognosis in those without other debilitating congenital anomalies is excellent.

In this case, MR angiography was performed and the extralobar sequestration was removed without complications on the following day. Cultures of the resected sequestration were sterile. The patient recovered uneventfully.

SUGGESTED READINGS

1. Yu H, Li HM, Liu SY, et al. Diagnosis of arterial sequestration using multidetector CT angiography. *Eur J Radiol.* 2010;76:274-278.
2. Carter R. Pulmonary sequestration. *Ann Thorac Surg.* 1969;7:68-88.
3. Collin PP, Desjardins JG. Pulmonary sequestration. *J Pediatr Surg.* 1987;22:750-753.
4. Kravitz RM. Congenital malformation of the lung. *Pediatr Clin North Am.* 1994;41:453-472.
5. Lierl M. Congenital abnormalities. In: Hilman BC, ed. *Pediatric Respiratory Disease: Diagnosis and Treatment.* Philadelphia: W.B. Saunders; 1993:457-498.
6. Oliphant L, McFadden RG, Carr TJ, et al. Magnetic resonance imaging to diagnose intralobar pulmonary sequestration. *Chest.* 1987;91:500-502.
7. Savic B, Birtel FJ, Tholen W, et al. Lung sequestration: report of seven cases and review of 540 published cases. *Thorax.* 1979;34:96-101.
8. Stocker JT, Kagan-Hallet K. Extralobar pulmonary sequestration: analysis of 15 cases. *Am J Clin Pathol.* 1979;72:917-925.

CASE 1-4

Fifteen-Month-Old Girl

EVAN S. FIELDSTON

HISTORY OF PRESENT ILLNESS

A 15-month-old girl was hospitalized for respiratory distress. She was well until 3 days prior to admission when she began coughing during a meal. She had moderate respiratory distress initially, which improved gradually. On the day of admission she had a fever to 39.5°C and worsening tachypnea. She received albuterol with some improvement in her respiratory status.

MEDICAL HISTORY

The patient was born at term after an uncomplicated pregnancy and delivery. She was diagnosed with reactive airways disease in infancy after three hospitalizations for wheezing. She received albuterol and prednisone for 5 days during each of those episodes. She also has mild gastroesophageal reflux (GER) diagnosed by a pH probe study at 7 months of age. An upper gastrointestinal barium study performed at that time was normal. Her symptoms of chronic cough improved after starting ranitidine at 11 months of age. At 12 months of age, she was treated with intravenous antibiotics for a right middle lobe pneumonia. She receives ranitidine for gastroesophageal reflux. She also received albuterol for wheezing approximately twice per week. A distant relative had been diagnosed with cystic fibrosis a decade ago and had died during infancy. There is no family history of atopic disease or asthma.

PHYSICAL EXAMINATION

T 37.4°C; HR 110 bpm; RR 44/min; BP 103/65 mmHg; SpO$_2$ 96% in room air

Weight 16.5 kg (10th percentile); Height 105 cm (25th percentile)

Physical examination revealed a lean child in mild respiratory distress. There was no conjunctival injection. The sinuses demonstrated symmetric transillumination. The oropharynx was clear.

There was no cervical lymphadenopathy. There were mild intercostal retractions with good aeration and mild diffuse wheezing. Breath sounds were slightly diminished in the right lower lobe. Cardiac examination was normal. There were no rashes or skin lesions. The remainder of the examination, including neurologic examination, was normal.

DIAGNOSTIC STUDIES

The girl's white blood cell count was 18 300/mm^3 with 9% band forms, 78% segmented neutrophils, and 13% lymphocytes. Her hemoglobin and platelet counts were normal. A blood culture was obtained, which was subsequently negative. Chest radiograph revealed a right middle lobe density. There was no hyperinflation or peribronchial thickening. A repeat upper GI barium study suggested the diagnosis (Figure 1-6A).

DISCUSSION CASE 1-4

DIFFERENTIAL DIAGNOSIS

The most common cause of recurrent wheezing in infants and children is bronchospasm, including bronchiolitis, reactive airways disease, and asthma, triggered by viral infections. Gastroesophageal reflux (GER) with pulmonary aspiration is an important consideration. Beyond GER, other causes of recurrent aspiration include cricopharyngeal incoordination, submucosal cleft palate, seizures, neuromuscular disorders, and tracheoesophageal fistula (TEF). Esophageal obstruction due to webs or strictures may also predispose to recurrent aspiration.

Although bronchiolitis and poorly controlled reactive airways disease remain a consideration in this case, the frequency of wheezing episodes and recurrent pneumonia warrant further investigation. Cystic fibrosis should be excluded, particularly in light of the family history. The differential

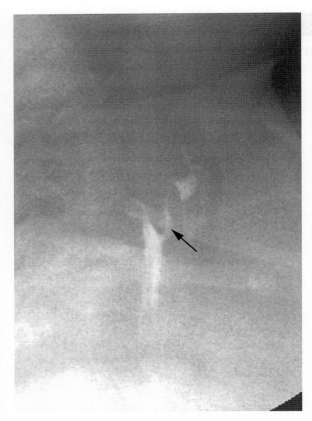

FIGURE 1-6A. Contrast esophagogram displays filling of the trachea through a small esophageal fistula (arrow), confirming presence of tracheoesophageal fistula without esophageal atresia, or H-type fistula.

diagnosis also includes extrinsic obstructing lesions, such as mediastinal lymphadenopathy, diaphragmatic hernia, and vascular rings. Intraluminal obstructing lesions can occur in this age group and include aspirated foreign body, bronchial papilloma or lipoma, and segmental bronchomalacia. The history of recurrent pneumonia may be a sign of underlying primary immunodeficiency, such as agammaglobulinemias, dysgammaglobulinemias, and phagocytic defects such as chronic granulomatous disease which, though typically inherited in an X-linked pattern, occasionally exhibits autosomal recessive inheritance. Infectious causes of recurrent or persistent pneumonia, such as *Coxiella burnetti*

(Q fever), *Histoplasma capsulatum*, and *Mycobacterium tuberculosis* are less likely in this age group.

DIAGNOSTIC TESTS

On direct questioning, her mother stated that the cough, although chronic, seemed worse when she drank liquids. This information, combined with a history of right middle lobe pneumonia, chronic cough, and recurrent wheezing, suggested chronic aspiration. The sweat test for cystic fibrosis was negative. The contrast esophagogram (Figure 1-6A) revealed filling of the trachea through a small esophageal fistula. **The diagnosis is tracheoesophageal fistula (TEF) without esophageal atresia (EA), otherwise known as H-type fistula.** In retrospect, her symptomatic improvement at 11 months of age coincided with her transition from a predominantly liquid to predominantly solid diet.

INCIDENCE AND ETIOLOGY

Esophageal atresia (EA) is characterized by incomplete formation of the esophagus and it is often associated with TEF, though not always (see Figure 1-6B for types of TEF with or without EA). TEF with or without EA occurs as a congenital abnormality in 1 per 3000 to 1 per 5000 live births. The most common form of TEF (proximal EA and distal TEF) occurs in 85% of cases. In this form, there is a blind esophageal pouch with fistula between the trachea and distal esophagus, with the fistula entering the trachea close to the carina. As the fetus tries to swallow amniotic fluid against a blind pouch, hypertrophy and dilatation occur. As a result, the trachea may be compressed, leading to tracheomalacia. The second most common variant is pure EA without a TEF (8% of cases). As the distal esophageal remnant is small, surgical repair is more challenging. H-type TEF (without EA) is the third most common variation (3%-5% of cases). It is most difficult to diagnose, especially when the fistula is long and/or oblique. Much rarer forms of EA with TEF (1% each) include EA with proximal TEF and EA with double TEF. In the former case, the esophagus connects to proximal trachea and the distal esophagus is underdeveloped. In the latter, the esophagus is noncontinuous, but each end forms a fistula to the trachea.

FIGURE 1-6B. Types of esophageal atresia (EA) and tracheoesophageal fistula (TEF). Types of esophageal atresia and tracheoesophageal fistula (incidence): **(A)** Type 1—esophageal atresia with distal tracheoesophageal fistula (87%); **(B)** Type 2, isolated esophageal atresia (8%); **(C)** Type 3, isolated tracheoesophageal fistula (4%); **(D)** Type 4, esophageal atresia with proximal and distal tracheoesophageal fistula (1%); and **(E)** Type 5, esophageal atresia with proximal tracheoesophageal fistula (1%). *(Reproduced with permission from Lalwani AK.* Current Diagnosis & Treatment in Otolaryngology: Head & Neck Surgery. *2nd ed. New York: McGraw-Hill; 2008.)*

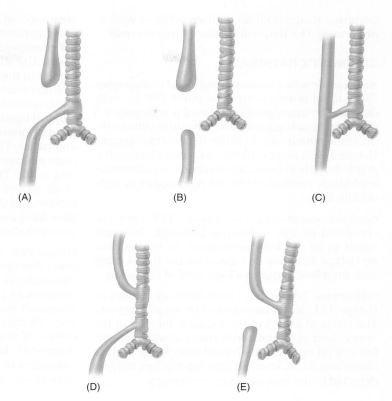

(A)   (B)   (C)

(D)   (E)

The anomalies arise from defective differentiation of the primitive foregut to the trachea and esophagus. The role of genetic factors is unclear; TEF has been described in siblings and identical twins. Autosomal dominant transmission has been reported in a few kindreds. Approximately 40% of infants with a TEF will have associated congenital anomalies, usually cardiac or gastrointestinal, including anal atresia, pyloric stenosis, duodenal obstruction, and malrotation. One cluster of congenital abnormalities, the VATER association (*V*ertebral anomalies, *A*nal anomalies, *T*racheo-esophageal fistula with *E*sophageal atresia, and *R*enal and *R*adial limb anomalies), is seen most often among infants of diabetic mothers.

TYPICAL PRESENTATION

Infants with an H-type TEF do not present in the neonatal period. Their symptoms are mild or moderate and persistent and include coughing, choking, and cyanosis with feedings. Because the tracheoesophageal connection is small, these symptoms usually occur with liquid or formula feeds. There is no dysphagia. Children with H-type TEF may have improvement of their symptoms when they transition from formula to more solid foods. Many children have recurrent episodes of pneumonia or pneumonitis due to aspiration of gastrointestinal contents through the fistula. On examination, abdominal distention occurs after crying as air traverses through the fistula into the stomach. Diffuse wheezing may be related to aspiration.

Unlike the patient in this case, infants with TEF and esophageal atresia are symptomatic from birth. They accumulate large amounts of oral secretions, which precipitate coughing, choking, emesis, and respiratory distress. Abdominal distention results from accumulation of intestinal air via the TEF. A flat, gasless abdomen suggests esophageal atresia either without a TEF or with an obliterated TEF that still requires surgical repair.

DIAGNOSTIC RATIONALE

Nasogastric tube placement and chest radiography. Esophageal atresia with or without TEF is easily detected by attempted passage of a radiopaque 5 or 8 French nasogastric tube. The tube coils in the proximal pouch and is visible on chest radiograph. H-type TEF is more difficult to detect. Chest radiograph may show evidence of recurrent pulmonary aspiration, particularly in the right upper or right middle lobe.

Contrast esophagogram. H-type TEF can be visualized by this technique, although the study needs to be carefully performed. As in this case, an H-type TEF may be missed on the initial study and, therefore, requires a high level of suspicion.

Endoscopy. Endoscopic visualization may reveal an H-type TEF not demonstrated by esophagogram. The tracheal aspect of the fistula is located in the upper third of the posterior tracheal wall, appearing as a pit or crescent-shaped hole. Dyes, such as methylene blue, instilled into the trachea may be detected in the esophagus by endoscopy.

TREATMENT

TEF with esophageal atresia. Esophageal atresia is treated with end-to-end or end-to-side anastomosis of the esophagus. A thoracoscopic approach has been proposed but requires further investigation. The timing of the operation and the choice of surgical approach depend on the infant's size and the presence or absence of comorbid conditions. Primary repair is preferred but a staged repair during the first several weeks or months of life is recommended for preterm infants as well as those with comorbid conditions, such as congenital heart disease. A tracheostomy should be performed if a staged repair is planned.

Immediate postoperative complications following TEF with esophageal atresia repair include leakage at the anastomotic site causing mediastinitis or sepsis. Strictures at the anastomotic site may develop at any time and require repeated esophageal dilatation. Tracheomalacia at the fistula site is common, resulting in brassy cough and impaired clearance of secretions. Esophageal dysmotility and gastroesophageal reflux are common.

Recurrence of the TEF occurs in 4% to 10% of cases. The manifestations of a recurrent TEF are similar to the presentation of children with H-type TEF. Recurrent tracheoesophageal fistulas do not close spontaneously and, therefore, also require surgical ligation. Survival rate is 95% in those with good respiratory function and no major congenital anomalies. The survival rate in infants with moderate pneumonia or congenital anomalies in addition to the TEF is approximately 70%. In a series of 82 patients with TEF and esophageal atresia, Holder and Ashcroft found that 79% of patients were alive and taking food by mouth 3 to 15 years postoperatively.

H-type TEF. An H-type TEF requires surgical ligation. Postoperative complications, such as tracheomalacia, strictures, and mediastinitis, are uncommon after repair of an H-type fistula. The prognosis in children with H-type fistulas is excellent. Morbidity and mortality are related to the extent of chronic pulmonary disease in infants diagnosed later in life. Infants with multiple anomalies or those with severe respiratory disease have greater morbidity.

SUGGESTED READINGS

1. Berseth CL. Disorders of the esophagus. In: Taeusch HW, Ballard RA, eds. *Avery's Diseases of the Newborn.* Philadelphia: W. B. Saunders Company; 1998:908-913.
2. Borruto FA, Impellizzeri P, Montalto AS, et al. Thoracoscopy versus thoracotomy for esophageal atresia and tracheoesophageal fistula repair: review of the literature and meta-analysis. *Eur J Pediatr Surg.* 2012 Nov 21 (published online ahead of print PMID 23172569).
3. Holder TM, Ashcraft KW. Developments in the care of patients with esophageal atresia and tracheoesophageal fistula. *Surg Clin North Am.* 1981;61:1051-1061.
4. Lierl M. Congenital abnormalities. In: Hilman BC, ed. *Pediatric Respiratory Disease: Diagnosis and Treatment.* Philadelphia: W. B. Saunders Company; 1993:457-498.
5. Quan L, Smith DW. The VATER association: vertebral defects, anal atresia, T-E fistula with esophageal atresia, radial and renal dysplasia, a spectrum of associated defects. *J Pediatr.* 1973;7:104-107.
6. Touloukian RJ, Pickett LK, Spackman T, Biancani P. Repair of esophageal atresia by end-to-side anastomosis and ligation of the tracheoesophageal fistula: a critical review of 18 cases. *J Pediatr Surg.* 1974;9:305-310.

CASE 1-5

Five-Week-Old Boy

EVAN S. FIELDSTON

HISTORY OF PRESENT ILLNESS

A 5-week-old Caucasian boy presented to the emergency department with worsening cough and respiratory difficulty. Two weeks prior to admission he was evaluated by his primary physician for poor weight gain and periodic emesis. His weight of 3050 g was the same as his birth weight. He had hemoccult positive stool and was diagnosed as being allergic to cow's milk protein. His formula was changed to a protein hydrolysate formula. One week prior to admission, his weight had increased to 3100 g. However, he began having more frequent episodes of emesis. Three days prior to admission he developed a cough, tachypnea, and audible wheezing. On being evaluated at a nearby hospital he was diagnosed with bronchiolitis, and treated with albuterol. His tachypnea has not improved despite receiving albuterol every 4 hours. His cough has increased in frequency. He is evaluated in the emergency department for worsening cough and continued tachypnea. His parents mention that the infant has always appeared dusky with crying but this color change has occurred more frequently during the past few days. He has also had numerous episodes of posttussive emesis. During the past three days he has taken only 2 ounces of formula every 4 hours. The parents deny ill contacts, diarrhea, and lethargy. Both parents smoke but only outside the home. There are no pets.

MEDICAL HISTORY

The boy was born at 37 weeks gestation after an uncomplicated pregnancy. The mother's group B *Streptococcus* colonization status was not known at the time of delivery so she received two doses of ampicillin prior to delivery. The infant's Apgar scores were 7 and 8 at 1 and 5 minutes, respectively. He had not previously required hospitalization.

PHYSICAL EXAMINATION

T 37.7°C; HR 160 bpm; RR 60/min; BP 78/37 mmHg; SpO$_2$ 88% in room air

Weight 3.0 kg (<5th percentile); Length 49 cm (<5th percentile)

Physical examination revealed a cyanotic infant in moderate respiratory distress. The anterior fontanelle was open and flat. There was no conjunctival injection or pallor. There were no oral mucosal ulcerations. Capillary refill was brisk. The heart sounds were normal. Femoral pulses were palpable and equal. There were intercostal retractions. There were rales and wheezes present diffusely. The liver edge was palpable 3 cm below the right costal margin. The remainder of the examination was normal.

DIAGNOSTIC STUDIES

Laboratory analysis revealed 10 200 white blood cells/mm^3 with 76% segmented neutrophils, 19% lymphocytes, and 3% monocytes. The hemoglobin was 13.0 g/dL and there were 350 000 platelets/mm^3. Hepatic function panel was as follows: total bilirubin, 0.3 mg/dL; alanine aminotransferase, 32 U/L; aspartate aminotransferase, 66 U/L. Prothrombin and partial thromboplastin times and fibrinogen split products were normal. Blood cultures were obtained. Chest radiograph revealed diffuse interstitial pulmonary edema but a normal cardiothymic silhouette.

COURSE OF ILLNESS

The patient was treated with ampicillin and cefotaxime for presumed bacterial sepsis. He also received albuterol. His respiratory status progressively worsened. An arterial blood gas revealed a pH 7.22; PCO$_2$ 65 mmHg; PO$_2$ 45 mmHg. The patient

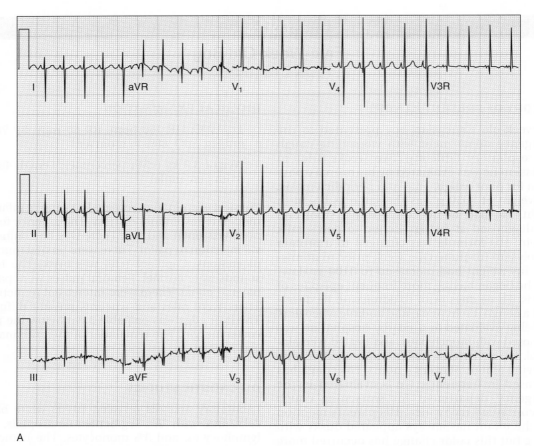

FIGURE 1-7A. Electrocardiogram with right axis deviation (QRS axis = 135°) and right ventricular hypertrophy.

required endotracheal intubation. Electrocardiogram suggested a possible diagnosis (Figure 1-7A).

DISCUSSION CASE 1-5

DIFFERENTIAL DIAGNOSIS

In an infant with cyanosis and respiratory distress, bacterial or viral sepsis must be considered. Children with either viral bronchiolitis or pertussis may present with cyanosis, respiratory symptoms, and rapid deterioration. In this child, the history of periodic cyanosis with crying since birth provided

a clue to the diagnosis being a congenital cardiac condition. The differential diagnosis includes a large ventricular septal defect (VSD), patent ductus arteriosus (PDA), truncus arteriosus, atrioventricular canal, single ventricle without pulmonary stenosis, and total anomalous pulmonary venous connection (TAPVC). This condition had been called total anomalous pulmonary venous return (TAPVR), but "connection" is deemed anatomically more appropriate for the range of findings. Unlike TAPVC, the other cardiac anomalies listed typically have electrocardiographic evidence of left atrial or left ventricular hypertrophy. Children with TAPVC have right ventricular hypertrophy.

DIAGNOSTIC TESTS

Electrocardiogram (Figure 1-7A) revealed right axis deviation (QRS axis = 135°) and right ventricular hypertrophy. Echocardiogram revealed a large and dilated right ventricle with a moderately hypoplastic left atrium and a patent foramen ovale. The pulmonary veins merged to form a common vein that drained into the portal venous system below the diaphragm. No pulmonary veins entered the left atrium. There were no other cardiac defects. **The echocardiogram findings confirmed the diagnosis of infradiaphragmatic total anomalous pulmonary venous connection (TAPVC)** (Figure 1-7B).

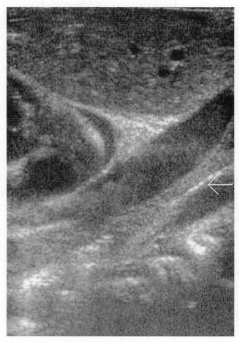

B

FIGURE 1-7B. Echocardiogram for infradiaphragmatic total anomalous pulmonary venous connection (TAPVC) shows large and dilated right ventricle with a moderately hypoplastic left atrium and a patent foramen ovale. The pulmonary veins merged to form a common vein that drained into the portal venous system below the diaphragm. No pulmonary veins entered the left atrium.

INCIDENCE AND ETIOLOGY

TAPVC defines an anomaly in which there is no direct connection between the pulmonary veins and the left atrium. Instead, the pulmonary veins merge to form a common pulmonary vein that connects either to one of the systemic veins or directly to the right atrium. During intrauterine life, the malformation does not compromise fetal circulation because pulmonary arterial resistance is high and some blood flows into the systemic circulation through the patent foramen ovale (PFO). The combined systemic and pulmonary blood flow to the lungs is only mildly elevated. After birth, as pulmonary resistance falls, a progressively larger proportion of the mixed venous blood flows to the lungs, causing massive pulmonary overcirculation.

Several classification schemes have been proposed based on physiologic or prognostic implications of the anomalous connections (Figure 1-7B). Generally, the connections are divided by whether the pulmonary veins merge with the coronary sinus of the right atrium (cardiac, 20% of cases) or with the systemic venous circulation above (supracardiac, 50% of cases) or below (infradiaphragmatic, 20% of cases) the diaphragm. Approximately 10% of cases are mixed.

In TAPVC, because all venous blood ultimately returns to the right atrium, a communication between the right and left sides of the heart is necessary to sustain life. It also explains why there is right ventricular hypertrophy. A patent foramen ovale or an atrial septal defect allows free communication between the two atria and, therefore, is considered part of the disorder. Without this connection, the anomaly would be fatal because of lack of systemic blood flow. Other intracardiac anomalies occur in up to one-third of cases and include common atrioventricular canal, transposition of the great arteries, tetralogy of Fallot, and hypoplastic left heart syndrome. Total anomalous pulmonary venous drainage directly into the right atrium occurs in patients with visceral heterotaxy and polysplenia.

The incidence of TAPVC is not clear. TAPVC occurred in 2% of cases in an autopsy series of 800 children with congenital cardiac disease who died in the first year of life. TAPVC also occurred in 41 (1.5%) of 2659 infants with cardiovascular malformations identified in the Baltimore-Washington

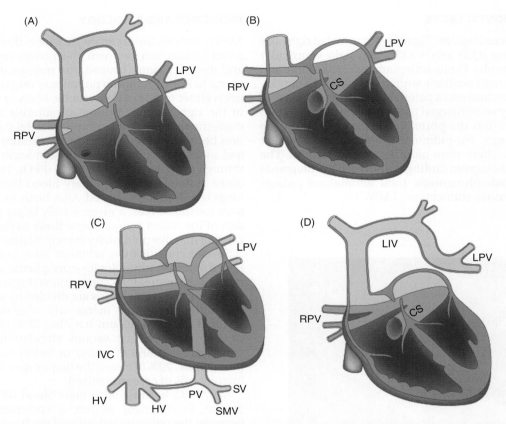

FIGURE 1-7C. Total anomalous pulmonary venous connection variants. Total anomalous pulmonary venous connection variants. **(A)** Supracardiac. Both right (RPV) and left (LPV) pulmonary veins join a common pulmonary venous confluence behind the heart that drains via a vertical vein to the undersurface of the left innominate vein and then to the right atrium. **(B)** Cardiac. The pulmonary venous confluence connects to the coronary sinus (CS) and then to the right atrium via the coronary sinus ostium. **(C)** Infradiaphragmatic. The pulmonary venous confluence drains inferiorly via a vertical vein to the portal vein (PV) or hepatic veins (HV) and then to the right atrium. **(D)** Mixed connections. Left pulmonary veins drain to the left innominate vein (LIV) and right pulmonary veins to the coronary sinus in this example. SV, splenic vein; SMV, superior mesenteric vein. *(Part C reproduced, with permission, from Fuster V et al. Hurst's The Heart. 13th ed. New York: McGraw-Hill, 2011.)*

Infant Study. There is no sex prevalence in TAPVC except for in infradiagphragmatic TAPVC, which is more prevalent in males than in females (3:1).

TYPICAL PRESENTATION

Clinical presentation of children with TAPVC depends on the presence or absence of pulmonary venous obstruction. Most children without obstruction present with tachypnea and failure to thrive with gradually worsening cyanosis and congestive heart failure. Approximately 50% of affected infants show symptoms in the first month of life and the remainder in the first year. Physical examination usually reveals cyanosis due to lack of left-sided flow of oxygenated blood, as well as tachpynea and dyspnea owing to pulmonary edema. Cyanosis may be minimal initially but increases as congestive heart failure progresses. Cyanosis occurs because the pulmonary veins carry oxygenated blood to the systemic venous circulation instead of to the left atrium. Congestive heart failure occurs because of increased pulmonary blood flow and pulmonary hypertension. Hepatomegaly and peripheral edema often accompany cardiac failure. There is typically no cardiac murmur, although there may be a systolic ejection murmur at the left upper sternal border. Cardiac examination may reveal right ventricular heave, fixed split S2, and an S3 gallop.

Obstruction is more common in children with infradiaphragmatic TAPVC because of venous compression as the common venous trunk passes through either the esophageal hiatus of the diaphragm or the portal venous circulation. Most children with infradiaphragmatic TAPVC and one-third of children with supracardiac TAPVC present with pulmonary venous obstruction. These infants are usually asymptomatic at birth but develop symptoms within the first few weeks of life. Infants with pulmonary venous obstruction present with rapidly progressive dyspnea, pulmonary edema, cyanosis, and congestive heart failure.

Alteration in the character of the cry ("neonatal dysphonia") occurs in one-fourth of infants with supracardiac TAPVC because of compression of the left recurrent laryngeal nerve as it passes the dilated common pulmonary vein. Infants with infradiaphragmatic TAPVC may have worsening cyanosis with swallowing, straining, and crying as a consequence of interference of pulmonary venous outflow by increased intraabdominal pressure or impingement of the esophagus on the common pulmonary vein as it exits through the esophageal hiatus. The child in the presented case did not have pulmonary venous obstruction despite having infradiaphragmatic TAPVC. His history of cyanosis with crying is consistent with infradiaphragmatic TAPVC.

DIAGNOSTIC RATIONALE

The diagnosis should be suspected on the basis of clinical presentation and workup should include the following studies.

Electrocardiogram. A tall peaked P wave in lead II or in the right precordial leads characterizes right atrial enlargement, a feature of TAPVC without obstruction. Right atrial enlargement is not usually present in TAPVC with obstruction because of fulminant presentation very early in life. Right ventricular hypertrophy is manifested by high voltages in the right precordial leads. Right axis deviation is always present because of right-sided hypertrophy (Figure 1-7A).

Chest radiograph. Lung fields reflect increased pulmonary blood flow. The cardiothymic silhouette may be normal, but may reveal cardiomegaly or "figure of 8" or "snowman" sign in supracardiac TAPVC, typically after 4 months of age.

Echocardiogram. Echocardiogram reveals signs of right ventricular volume overload. The right atrium is enlarged. The right ventricle is hypertrophied and dilated, compressing the intraventricular septum. The pulmonary arteries are dilated. The pulmonary veins are seen forming a common vein behind the heart. The size and orientation of the venous confluence are important for surgical planning. Associated intracardiac defects may be identified.

Cardiac catheterization. The accuracy of Doppler echocardiography precludes the routine need for diagnostic catheterization. Right ventricular pressures are usually equal to systemic pressures.

TREATMENT

While awaiting surgery, prostaglandin E1 (PGE1) should be administered to maintain patency of the ductus arteriosus. Complete surgical repair should be performed as early as possible. If there is obstruction, the repair should be done emergently. A large side-to-side anastomosis is created between the left atrium and the common pulmonary vein. The distal portion of the common pulmonary vein is occasionally ligated. The foramen ovale or atrial septal defect is also closed. A hypoplastic left atrium may require surgical enlargement.

Postoperative pulmonary venous obstruction complicates the course in approximately 17% of infants. This complication typically occurs within 6 months of the original repair and is associated with poor outcomes. Risk factors for death include earlier presentation after TAPVC repair, diffusely small pulmonary veins at presentation of postoperative pulmonary venous obstruction, and an increased number of lung segments affected by obstruction. Residual stenosis at the left atrial-venous anastomosis created at operative repair develops in 10% of children. This stenosis requires reintervention and patch plasty. Late atrial arrhythmias develop in a small number of patients.

SUGGESTED READINGS

1. Correa-Villasenor A, Ferencz C, Boughman JA, Neill CA. Total anomalous pulmonary venous return: familial and environmental factors: the Baltimore-Washington infant study group. *Teratology.* 1991;44:415-428.
2. Geva T, Van Praagh S. Anomalies of the pulmonary veins. In: Allen HD, Gutgesell HP, Clark EB, Driscol DJ, eds. *Moss and Adams' Heart Disease in Infants, Children, and Adolescents Including the Fetus and Young Adult.* 6th ed. Philadelphia: Lippincott Williams & Wilkins; 2001:736-772.
3. Hyde JA, Stumper O, Barth MJ, et al. Total anomalous pulmonary venous connection: outcome of surgical correction and management of recurrent venous obstruction. *Eur J Cardio-thorac.* 1999;15:735-740.
4. Michielon G, Di Donato RM, Pasquini L, et al. Total anomalous pulmonary venous connection: long-term appraisal with evolving technical solutions. *Eur J Cardio-thorac.* 2002;22:184-191.
5. Seale AN, Uemura H, Webber SA, et al; for the British Congenital Cardiac Association. Total anomalous pulmonary venous connection: outcome of postoperative pulmonary venous obstruction. *J Thorac Cardiovasc Surg.* 2012 Aug 11 (PMID 22892140) [epub ahead of print].
6. Shankargouda S, Krishnan U, Murali R, Shah MJ. Dysphonia: a frequently encountered symptom in the evaluation of infants with unobstructed supracardiac total anomalous pulmonary venous connection. *Pediatr Cardiol.* 2000;21:458-460.

CASE 1-6

Four-Month-Old Boy

TODD A. FLORIN

HISTORY OF PRESENT ILLNESS

A 4-month-old African-American boy was well until 9 days prior to admission when he developed fever to 38.9°C and a cough. Seven days prior to admission he was evaluated by his primary physician and treated with ranitidine for suspected gastroesophageal reflux. Four days prior to admission he developed tachypnea and grunting and received nebulized albuterol. On the day of admission he had continued fever and worsening cough. His oral intake was poor. He drank only 2-3 ounces of breast milk every 4 hours during the past day. His urine output was also decreased. Multiple family members had upper respiratory infections.

MEDICAL HISTORY

The boy was born at 40 weeks gestation after an uncomplicated pregnancy. He had received all of the appropriate immunizations for age, including the second dose of DTaP. There was no family history of asthma or sickle cell disease.

PHYSICAL EXAMINATION

T 37.0°C; P 120 bpm; RR 76/min; BP 102/72 mmHg; SpO_2 93% with 3 liters O_2 by nasal cannula

Weight 10-25th percentile; Length 10th percentile; Head circumference 10th percentile

The patient was awake and alert. The anterior fontanelle was open and flat. He had flaring of the alae nasi. There were moderate intercostal, subcostal, and supraclavicular retractions. Scattered rhonchi were present with diminished breath sounds at the bases bilaterally. There was no focal wheezing. The heart sounds were normal. The spleen was palpable just below the left costal margin. The remainder of the examination was normal.

DIAGNOSTIC STUDIES

The white blood cell count was 10 200/mm³ with 15% band forms, 68% segmented neutrophils, and 12% lymphocytes. The hemoglobin was 10.3 g/dL and the platelet count was 277 000/mm³. Arterial blood gas (ABG) revealed the following: pH, 7.42; $PaCO_2$, 30 mmHg; and PaO_2, 90 mmHg. Hepatic function panel revealed a total bilirubin of 0.3 mg/dL; alanine aminotransferase, 55 U/L; aspartate aminotransferase, 82 U/L; and lactate dehydrogenase, 3280 U/L. No antigens to respiratory syncytial virus, parainfluenza types 1, 2, and 3, influenza A and B, and adenovirus were detected by immunofluorescence of nasopharyngeal aspirate. Serum immunoglobulin results were as follows: IgG, 24 mg/dL (normal range, 27-73); IgM, 528 mg/dL (normal range, 37-124); and IgG, 650 mg/dL (normal range, 292-816).

COURSE OF ILLNESS

The patient was treated with nebulized albuterol and a racemic mixture of epinephrine without significant improvement in his respiratory status. An echocardiogram showed normal cardiac anatomy. The patient required endotracheal intubation for worsening respiratory distress. A chest radiograph suggested a diagnosis (Figure 1-8).

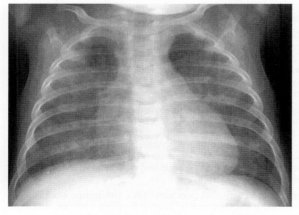

FIGURE 1-8. Chest radiograph of 4-month-old boy with fever and cough.

DISCUSSION CASE 1-6

DIFFERENTIAL DIAGNOSIS

The most common cause of progressive respiratory distress during infancy is bronchiolitis, most often caused by respiratory syncytial virus, adenovirus, human metapneumovirus, influenza viruses A and B, and parainfluenza viruses types 1, 2, and 3. The differential diagnosis of perihilar or diffuse infiltrates includes *Bordetella pertussis* or *Bordetella parapertussis*, *Chlamydia trachomatis*, and *Mycoplasma pneumoniae*. Herpes simplex virus and cytomegalovirus (CMV) may cause pneumonia in the young infant. CMV pneumonia is frequently associated with hepatosplenomegaly, thrombocytopenia, and lymphocytosis. *Pneumocystis jiroveci* (formerly *P. carinii*) pneumonitis (PCP) should be considered, particularly if there are maternal risk factors for human immunodeficiency virus (HIV) infection. The differential diagnosis of HIV-associated pneumonia is found in Table 1-5. Other conditions predisposing to PCP include primary B-cell defects, primary T-cell defects, and combined defects. The immune disorders most likely to present with PCP include severe combined immunodeficiency, DiGeorge anomaly or other 22q11 deletion syndromes (as a result of impaired thymus development), Wiskott-Aldrich syndrome, X-linked agammaglobulinemia, and hyper-IgM syndrome.

Noninfectious causes of pneumonia include gastroesophageal reflux associated with pulmonary aspiration, aspiration owing to foreign body or inhaled irritants, autoimmune diseases (e.g., sarcoidosis), and malignancies. Occasionally, an anatomic defect, such as tracheoesophageal fistula, may predispose to aspiration; of these, an H-type tracheoesophageal fistula is most likely to present after the neonatal period. Primary cardiac abnormalities (e.g., ventricular septal defect), pulmonary vascular abnormalities, and impaired lymphatic flow (e.g., congenital lymphangiectasia) may cause tachypnea and progressive respiratory distress in a 4-month-old child. Cystic fibrosis can masquerade as any of the above conditions.

DIAGNOSIS

Chest radiograph (Figure 1-8) revealed hazy ground-glass opacities bilaterally. There was no

TABLE 1-5. Differential diagnosis of pneumonia in patients with HIV infection.

Pneumonia Type	Organisms	Comments
Bacterial Pneumonia (NOTE: recurrent bacterial pneumonia is an AIDS-defining illness)	*Streptococcus pneumoniae, Haemophilus influenzae*	Most common etiologies; increased risk septicemia and bacteremia with low CD4 count; clinical presentation similar to non-HIV
	Legionella, Mycoplasma pneumoniae, Chlamydophila pneumoniae	Less common; rates similar to those without HIV
	Pseudomonas aeruginosa	More frequent in HIV; increased risk in patients with CD4 ≤ 50, underlying lung disease, neutropenia, corticosteroid use, malnutrition
	Staphylococcus aureus	More frequent in HIV; increased risk in patients with concomitant viral infection or injectable drug use
Tuberculosis	*Mycobacterium tuberculosis Mycobacterium bovis*	Increased risk of progressing from latent TB to active TB with HIV; occurs at any CD4 count; risk of extrapulmonary manifestations (lymph nodes, blood, CNS, bone, pericardium, peritoneum) increases with CD4 ≤ 200; more likely to have atypical findings (multilobar, diffuse infiltrates) in HIV; treatment similar in HIV and non-HIV, but must be cautious for drug interactions with HAART
Pneumocystis	*Pneumocystis jiroveci* (formerly *P. carinii*)	Most frequent AIDS-defining diagnosis; cannot be cultured; must be stained using Giemsa, Toluidine blue, silver, or monocolonal antibody stains; TMP-SMX is treatment of choice for prophylaxis and active disease; see text
Fungal Pneumonia	*Cryptococcus neoformans*	Encapsulated round/oval yeast; occurs with CD4 < 200, usually CD4 < 50; most frequently presents as meningitis or meningoencephalitis; up to 10% may present with acute respiratory failure; usually diffuse bilateral interstitial infiltrates on CXR (mimics PCP); diagnosis with culture or antigen testing; therapy with fluconazole in most cases, amphotericin B +/– flucytosine, if severe
	Histoplamsa capsulatum	Soil-dwelling fungus endemic to Ohio, Mississippi, and St. Lawrence River Valleys and Central and South America; most cases with CD4 < 150, though focal pneumonia may occur at CD4 250-500; usually presents with fever, fatigue, weight loss; many with normal CXR; diagnose using fungal cultures and *Histoplasma* polysaccharide antigen; amphotericin B followed by long-term itraconazole treatment of choice; consider itraconazole prophylaxis in adults with CD4 < 150 living in endemic areas, prophylaxis not recommended in children
	Coccidioides immitis	Soil-dwelling fungus endemic to southwestern US, northern Mexico, Central and South America; usually with CD4 < 100, though focal pneumonia may occur with CD4 > 250; fever, chills, night sweats, and weight loss common; diffuse reticulonodular infiltrates on CXR; no antigen test available, thus culture required for diagnosis; amphotericin B is first-line therapy; fluconazole or itraconazole can be used for focal pneumonia
Viral Pneumonia	*Cytomegalovirus*	Most frequent cause of viral pneumonia in HIV; most common congenitally transmitted infection; most disease is reactivation of latent infection; most cases with CD4 < 50; respiratory symptoms present for 2-4 weeks; variable CXR appearance—nodular or ground-glass opacities, alveolar infiltrates, nodular opacities; usually presents with disseminated disease; diagnosis requires identification of cytopathic inclusions and changes to the lung; treatment with ganciclovir or foscarnet
Parasitic Pneumonia	*Toxoplasma gondii*	Pulmonary involvement uncommon; occurs with CD4 < 100; nonproductive cough, dyspnea, fever; CXR with bilateral infiltrates; diagnose with serum *Toxoplasma* IgG antibody; Sulfadiazine plus pyrimethamine is first-line treatment

Source: Adapted from Huang L, Crothers KA. HIV-associated opportunistic pneumonias. *Respirology.* 2009;14:474-485.

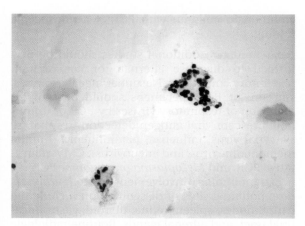

FIGURE 1-9. Gomori methenamine silver staining of a specimen obtained by bronchoalveolar lavage.

pleural effusion. **The diagnosis of *P. jiroveci* pneumonia was confirmed by Gomori methenamine silver staining of a specimen obtained by bronchoalveolar lavage** (BAL, Figure 1-9). The patient was treated with intravenous trimethoprim-sulfamethoxazole (TMP-SMX; 20 mg/kg/day trimethoprim component) and prednisone. He required ventilatory support for 5 days with gradual recovery. HIV DNA was detected in the patient's blood by polymerase chain reaction (PCR), confirming the underlying diagnosis of HIV.

INCIDENCE AND EPIDEMIOLOGY

Pneumocystis jiroveci is an opportunistic parasite with some features of protozoa, but greater genetic homology to fungi. Asymptomatic infection occurs early in life; up to 85% of immunocompetent children have antibodies by 4 years of age. Immunocompromised infants and children develop severe PCP as a result of primary infection.

The risk of PCP is related to the extent of T-cell deficiency or defect, immunosuppression and the use of chemoprophylaxis. PCP occurs in children with advanced HIV infection (25%-50%), primary immunodeficiencies (most notably severe combined immunodeficiency syndrome, 25%-50%), lymphoid malignancies such as acute lymphocytic leukemia (10%-20%), allogeneic bone marrow transplant (5%), and organ transplant (2%-10%) when no chemoprophylaxis is given. Patients with collagen vascular disorders, particularly Wegener's granulomatosis, are at risk for PCP if they are lymphopenic or receiving multiple immunosuppressive agents. Use of TMP-SMX prophylaxis reduces the PCP rate to less than 5% in HIV-infected children. Children receiving agents that impair cell-mediated immunity, including corticosteroids and cyclosporine, are at even higher risk of developing PCP. Patients with a history of PCP are at high risk for recurrence.

CLINICAL PRESENTATION

Severe PCP infection usually occurs in the first year of life in HIV-infected children not receiving TMP-SMX prophylaxis with the highest incidence between 3 and 6 months of life. A bronchiolitis-like illness occurs with gradually worsening tachypnea and accessory muscle use. Physical examination reveals the absence of fever and a paucity of findings on auscultation despite significant hypoxia. Rales and cyanosis develop as the illness progresses.

In older HIV-infected children, the spectrum of clinical manifestation varies. The classic symptom triad is fever, cough, and dyspnea. The symptoms may initially be mild and slowly progressive, delaying the diagnosis. High fevers are common. Findings on lung auscultation are often unimpressive compared to the degree of dyspnea, tachypnea (80-100/min), and hypoxia. Scattered rales, rhonchi, or wheezes may be heard as the illness resolves. Pneumothorax may occur in 2% to 4% of patients. In children with an underlying non-AIDS-associated PCP, the onset of symptoms occurs more abruptly over days rather than weeks as in HIV-infected children, but physical examination findings are similar.

DIAGNOSTIC APPROACH

PCP should be considered in any immunocompromised patient with respiratory symptoms, fever, and an abnormal chest radiograph. The diagnosis should also be considered in any patient with risk factors for HIV infection. If the patient does not have a known predisposing condition, testing to exclude HIV and congenital immune deficiencies should be performed.

Chest roentgenogram. Chest radiograph most commonly shows diffuse bilateral interstitial infiltrates, beginning in the perihilar region and progressing to the periphery. The lung apices are least affected. The infiltrates are classically described as granular, reticular, or ground-glass. Chest radiograph is normal in up to 40% of cases.

Examination of lower respiratory tract specimens. *Pneumocystis jiroveci* cannot be cultivated in culture, and thus identification of the organism in respiratory specimens, such as pulmonary parenchyma or lower respiratory tract secretions, is required for definitive diagnosis. Specimens can be stained using Gomori's methenamine silver, toluidine blue O, or Wright-Giemsa stains, or fluorescein-labeled monoclonal antibody stains. Monoclonal antibody stains are more sensitive than the general stains, and unlike many of the general stains, are able to stain both trophic and cystic forms of the organism. For these reasons, monoclonal antibodies have become the diagnostic "gold standard" at many institutions.

The diagnostic yield of various procedures follows: Induced sputum (children over 5 years of age), 20%-40%; BAL, 75%-95%; transbronchial biopsy, 75%-95%; and open lung biopsy, 90%-100%. The optimal procedure used to obtain a specimen depends on many factors, including the age and clinical status of the patient. The traditional algorithm involves examination of induced sputum in those over 5 years of age followed by BAL if the sputum sample is negative. Open lung biopsy is reserved for patients with a nondiagnostic BAL. Children less than 5 years should undergo BAL initially.

PCR, though still under investigation, may allow diagnosis with fewer invasive procedures. PCR assays seem to be more sensitive, but less specific, than traditional diagnostic methods, with PCR analysis of oral washes demonstrating a sensitivity of 80% compared to concomitantly obtained BAL. Sensitivity of PCR declines after initiation of treatment, and thus specimens should be collected before antibiotics.

Serum lactate dehydrogenase. Rising serum LDH reflects lung injury. Elevated serum LDH, while common in children with PCP, is a nonspecific finding.

Other studies. Additional studies should be performed to diagnose alternate or concomitant respiratory conditions. Nasopharyngeal aspirates, sputum, or BAL specimens should be sent for detection of respiratory viruses by PCR or immunofluorescent viral antigen detection (respiratory syncytial virus, influenza, parainfluenza, human metapneumovirus, and adenovirus), CMV quantitative PCR, and *Mycoplasma pneumoniae* PCR.

Extrapulmonary involvement due to *P. jiroveci* is rare; potential sites of dissemination include the lymph nodes, spleen, retina, thyroid, gastrointestinal tract, and adrenal glands. Routine radiologic imaging to exclude extrapulmonary manifestations of *P. jiroveci* is not necessary.

TREATMENT

TMP-SMX (15-20 mg/kg/day of TMP) remains the treatment of choice for PCP in children. The oral route can be used in mild cases if patients can reliably take and retain oral medication. Most children require treatment intravenously. The course of treatment is 14-21 days. If no improvement is demonstrated in 5-7 days, treatment should be changed to pentamidine. Pentamidine, atovaquone, or primaquine plus clindamycin may be used for children unable to tolerate TMP-SMX. Adjunctive therapy with corticosteroids within 72 hours of diagnosis reduces the occurrence of respiratory failure and improves oxygenation in moderately ill adults with PCP. Limited data in children suggest similar benefit.

Children with an episode of PCP require post-treatment prophylaxis with TMP-SMX (5 mg/kg/day of TMP) either daily or three times per week for the duration of risk (indefinitely for those with HIV). Chemoprophylaxis agents for those unable to tolerate TMP-SMX include oral atovaquone, aerosolized or intravenous pentamidine, or oral dapsone. Because of the high risk of acquiring PCP during the first year of life, all infants born to HIV-infected mothers require PCP prophylaxis from 4 weeks to 12 months of age, regardless of CD4+ lymphocyte counts; prophylaxis can be discontinued sooner if HIV infection had been excluded. After 12 months of age, prophylaxis is required if the CD4 percentage is less than 15% or if the CD4+ count is less than 500 cells/microliter (less than 200 cells/microliter in those over 5 years of age). Prophylaxis should also be considered in patients with AIDS-defining illnesses and oropharyngeal candidiasis. Patients in other high-risk groups including those with severe combined immune deficiency, lymphoproliferative malignancies, organ transplants, prolonged high-dose corticosteroid use, and those receiving intensified immuno-suppression with T-cell depleting therapies also require PCP prophylaxis.

SUGGESTED READINGS

1. Catherinot E, Lanternier F, Bougnoux ME, Lecuit M, Couderc LJ, Lortholary O. *Pneumocystis jirovecii* pneumonia. *Infect Dis Clin N Am.* 2010;24:107-138.

2. Centers for Disease Control and Prevention. Guidelines for the prevention and treatment of opportunistic infections among HIV-exposed and HIV-infected children. *MMWR.* 2009;58:1-166.

3. Grubman S, Simonds RJ. Preventing *Pneumocystis carinii* pneumonia in human immunodeficiency virus-infected children: new guidelines for prophylaxis. *Pediatr Infect Dis J.* 1996;15:165-168.

4. Huang L, Crothers KA. HIV-associated opportunistic pneumonias. *Respirology.* 2009;14:474-485.

5. Kovacs JA, Gill VJ, Meshnick S, Masur H. New insights into transmission, diagnosis, and drug treatment of *Pneumocystis carinii* pneumonia. *JAMA.* 2001;386:2450-2460.

6. Pyrgos V, Shoham S, Roilides E, Walsh TJ. *Pneumocystis* pneumonia in children. *Ped Resp Rev.* 2009;10:192-198.

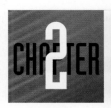

DECREASED ACTIVITY LEVEL

MATTHEW TEST

NATHAN TIMM

DEFINITION OF THE COMPLAINT

The term decreased activity level describes a wide spectrum of existence ranging from boredom to coma. The diagnostic evaluation focuses on encouraging parents to provide a detailed account, particularly with regard to the magnitude and time course of the changes. Clearly, the differential diagnosis of subtle behavioral changes developing during a period of several months differs from that of changes occurring during several hours.

COMPLAINT BY CAUSE AND FREQUENCY

The causes of decreased level of activity in children vary according to age (Table 2-1), and can be placed into several broad categories (Table 2-2). Additional issues to consider include whether there is depressed sensorium indicating an underlying central nervous system (CNS) disorder, weakness indicating a muscular disorder, or endurance problems suggesting a cardiac or pulmonary issue. Systemic illness may manifest with somnolence or lethargy.

CLARIFYING QUESTIONS

The patient who presents for evaluation of decreased level of activity represents a broad differential. Several important historical questions can help classify the underlying etiology:

- What is the time course of decreased level of activity?
  —Infectious etiologies typically present during a shorter time course than do other etiologies, such

as iron deficiency anemia or certain types of CNS malignancies.

- Is the patient febrile?
  —Fever, from an infectious etiology, can cause a decreased level of activity in children. However, hypothermia, particularly in neonates, can also result in decreased level of activity. In the neonate, hypothermia is a common manifestation of perinatally acquired herpes simplex virus infection and sepsis.

- Have the activities of daily living been impacted?
  —Cardiac or pulmonary disease may be reflected in decreased activity levels. In older children, this would be evidenced by poor physical play, whereas in infants, poor feeding. Secondary gain in an older child may play a role if school avoidance appears to be an issue.

- Is there a history of decreased oral intake or increased output?
  —Younger children are particularly sensitive to the metabolic demands of glucose utilization. Hypoglycemia can occur from increased losses from diarrhea and/or vomiting, and hyperglycemia from diabetes mellitus. In both instances, behavior changes can occur due to abnormal glucose levels.

- Has there been a change in behavior with friends or with school performance in the older child or adolescent?
  —Mental health causes, in particular depression, should always be investigated as potential culprit when behavior change impacts relationships and school. Drug and alcohol abuse should also be considered in adolescents.

TABLE 2-1.	Differential diagnosis of decreased activity by age.		
	Neonate/Infant	*School Age*	*Adolescent*
Common	Anemia	Anemia	Anemia
	Neonatal infections	Lack of sleep	Lack of sleep
	Hypoglycemia	Obesity	Obesity
	Ingestion	Hypoglycemia	Pregnancy
	Congenital heart defect	Ingestion	Infectious mononucleosis
		Boredom	Hypoglycemia
		Depression	Ingestion
			Boredom
			Depression
Uncommon	Intussusception	Intussusception	Adrenal insufficiency
	Polycythemia	CHF	Hypothyroidism
	Hypothyroidism	Pericarditis	CHF
	CHF	Uremia	Pericarditis
	Pericarditis	RTA	Uremia
	Uremia	JRA	RTA
	RTA		Myasthenia gravis
			Chronic fatigue syndrome
			Inflammatory bowel disease
			JRA

Abbreviations: CHF, congestive heart failure; RTA, renal tubular acidosis; JRA, juvenile rheumatoid arthritis

- Is there any history of trauma?
  —In the acute setting, head injury from mild traumatic brain injury to concussion to intracranial bleeds can result in abnormal level of activity.

- Is there any reason to suspect nonaccidental trauma?
  —Child abuse should always be taken into consideration in any child presenting with decreased level of activity. Physical, sexual, and neglect could all be demonstrated through a decreased level of activity. Any unusual injuries not consistent with

the child's age and mechanism of injury should also raise the clinician's concern for child abuse.

- Is there a history of ingestion?
  —Toxins frequently alter mental status in children. The mechanism may be through sedation (hypnotic agents, opiates, alcohols) or hypoglycemia (oral hypoglycemic agents or beta-blockers).

- Is there any history of abdominal pain or vomiting?
  —Intussusception can present with depressed mental status in a child between 6 months and 5 years of age.

CASE 2-1

Fifteen-Year-Old Girl

PHILLIP SPANDORFER

HISTORY OF PRESENT ILLNESS

A 15-year-old girl presented to the emergency department with a 3-month history of increasing fatigue. She gradually stopped participating in sports because of dizziness and palpitations. Her decreased level of activity has worsened to the point that as soon as she returns home from school in the afternoon she sleeps the rest of the day. She has had an 18-pound weight loss during this time period. Furthermore, for the past 5 days she has had a headache and occasional nonbloody, nonbilious

TABLE 2-2.	Differential diagnosis of decreased activity level by etiology.		
Diagnostic Category	*Disease*	*Diagnostic Category*	*Disease*
Infectious	Mononucleosis	**Pulmonary**	Asthma
	Hepatitis		Cystic fibrosis
	Human immunodeficiency virus		Sleep apnea
	Lyme disease		Primary pulmonary hypertension
	Cytomegalovirus	**Toxicologic**	Lead
	Meningitis		Hypoglycemic agents
	Encephalitis		Sedative/hypnotic agents
	Bacteremia		Antihistamines
	Histoplasmosis		Anticonvulsants
	Toxoplasmosis		Opiates
	Brucellosis	**Psychologic**	Depression
	Intestinal parasites	**Rheumatologic**	Systemic lupus erythematosus
Neurologic	Seizure		Juvenile rheumatoid arthritis
	Stroke		Sarcoidosis
	Intracranial injury		Dermatomyositis
	Vasculitis		Chronic fatigue syndrome
	Migraine		Fibromyalgia
Muscular	Myasthenia gravis	**Allergic**	Seasonal allergies
Cardiac	Congenital heart disease	**Endocrine**	Diabetes mellitus
	Congestive heart failure		Hypothyroidism
	Pericarditis		Hyperthyroidism
	Endocarditis		Adrenocortical insufficiency
	Cardiomyopathy		Cushing syndrome
			Primary aldosteronism
Hematologic	Anemia	**Metabolic**	Hypoglycemia
Gastrointestinal	Intussusception		Inborn errors of metabolism
	Inflammatory bowel disease	**Renal**	Uremia
	Liver disease		Renal tubular acidosis

emesis. For the past 4 days she has also had mild upper abdominal pain. The remainder of her history and review of systems were noncontributory.

MEDICAL HISTORY

She was the product of a full-term delivery and has had no major medical illnesses. She has not required any surgeries.

PHYSICAL EXAMINATION

T 37.2°C; HR 110 bpm; RR 16/min; BP 100/60 mmHg

Weight and Height 25th percentile

On examination she appeared pale and tired, but was nontoxic appearing. She answered questions appropriately. Her head and neck examination revealed pale conjunctiva. She did not have any papilledema. Her lungs were clear to auscultation. Cardiac examination revealed tachycardia, but there were no murmurs or other abnormal heart sounds. Her abdomen was soft with normal bowel sounds. There was no hepatosplenomegaly. Capillary refill was delayed at 3 seconds. Her neurologic examination was normal. Of particular interest is the fact that her cranial nerve examination and motor strength were also normal.

DIAGNOSTIC STUDIES

A complete blood count revealed a white blood cell count of 2100 cells/mm³ (3% bands, 45% segmented neutrophils, 51% lymphocytes), hemoglobin of 5.4 g/dL, and a platelet count of 173000/mm³.

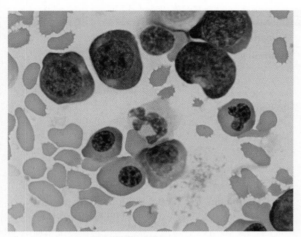

FIGURE 2-1. Peripheral blood smear. *(Photo courtesy of Marybeth Helfrich, MT, ASCP).*

The mean corpuscular volume (MCV) was elevated at 98.7 fL.

COURSE OF ILLNESS

The patient was hospitalized for evaluation of her severe anemia. The peripheral blood smear provided a clue to the diagnosis (Figure 2-1).

DISCUSSION CASE 2-1

DIFFERENTIAL DIAGNOSIS

The patient has a significant anemia. Anemia can be categorized on the basis of several etiologies. It could be because of nutritional deficiencies such as iron, folic acid, or vitamin B_{12}. It could also be because of hemoglobinopathy, such as sickle cell anemia or thalassemia. The anemia could be from a hemolytic process such as hereditary spherocytosis or glucose-6-phosphatedehydrogenase deficiency. Finally, anemia could be from a hypoplastic or aplastic crisis.

When evaluating anemia, it is easiest to arrive at the correct diagnosis by assessing the hematologic indices, specifically the MCV. If the MCV is low, anemia is a microcytic anemia and causes iron deficiency anemia, lead poisoning, anemia of chronic

disease, and thalassemias should be considered. If the MCV is normal, chronic disease, hypoplastic or aplastic crisis, malignancy, renal failure, acute hemorrhage, and hemolytic processes should be considered. Finally, if the MCV is high, the megaloblastic anemias should be evaluated, specifically folate deficiency, vitamin B_{12} deficiency, as well as some of the aplastic anemias.

DIAGNOSIS

Returning to our patient, we see that she had a macrocytic anemia as indicated by an elevated MCV of 98.7 fL. A hypersegmented neutrophil is located in the center of the peripheral blood smear (Figure 2-1). In the lower portion of the figure are several megaloblasts with a loose-appearing nuclear chromatin. Also noted are numerous misshapen mature erythrocytes, reflecting the mechanical fragility associated with megaloblastic anemias (Figure 2-1). The appropriate next step would be to measure the folate levels and vitamin B_{12} levels in her serum. Her folate levels returned at 8.2 ng/mL with normal in the range of 2-20 ng/mL. Her vitamin B_{12} level was less than 100 pg/mL with normal levels ranging from 200 to 1100 pg/mL. On further questioning, the patient stated that she has been a strict vegan for the past two years and has had no meat or animal-based products. Additionally, she did not take vitamin supplements and did not attempt to eat nonmeat-based foods containing vitamin B_{12}, such as fortified cereal and fortified meat analogues (e.g., wheat gluten, soy-products). **The diagnosis is dietary vitamin B_{12} deficiency.**

INCIDENCE AND EPIDEMIOLOGY

Dietary vitamin B_{12} must combine with a glycoprotein (intrinsic factor) that is secreted from the gastric fundus. The vitamin B_{12}-intrinsic factor complex is then absorbed at the terminal ileum via specific receptor mechanisms. Vitamin B_{12} is present in many foods and a pure dietary deficiency is rare. However, it may be seen in patients who do not drink any milk or eat eggs or animal products (vegans). Vitamin B_{12} deficiency can also result from lack of secretion of intrinsic factor in the stomach. When the cause of the lack of intrinsic factor is chronic atrophic gastritis, this condition is referred to as pernicious anemia. Other causes of vitamin B_{12} deficiency include surgical resection of the terminal ileum, regional enteritis of the terminal ileum, overgrowth of intestinal bacteria, disruption of the B_{12}-intrinsic factor complex, abnormalities/absence of the receptor site in the terminal ileum, or inborn errors of the metabolism of vitamin B_{12}.

CLINICAL PRESENTATION

Vitamin B_{12} plays an important role as a cofactor for two metabolic reactions, methylation of homocysteine to methionine and conversion of methylmalonyl coenzyme A to succinyl CoA. Vitamin B_{12} deficiency leads to accumulation of these precursors. Methionine is an important step in the synthesis of DNA. RNA production and cytoplasmic components are produced normally and the red blood cell production in the bone marrow yields large cells and hence a macrocytic anemia. Methionine is also converted to S-adenosylmethionine, which is used in methylation reactions in the central nervous system and hence CNS effects are seen with vitamin B_{12} deficiency. Neurologic manifestations in children include abnormalities, such as paresthesias, loss of developmental milestones, hypotonia, seizures, dementia, and depression. The neurologic changes are not always reversible.

DIAGNOSTIC APPROACH

Complete blood count and folic acid and vitamin B_{12} levels. The term megaloblastic anemia refers to a macrocytic anemia usually accompanied by a mild leukopenia or thrombocytopenia. The presence of a macrocytic anemia with normal folic acid levels and low vitamin B_{12} levels will diagnose most vitamin B_{12} deficiencies. However, reliance on abnormal hemoglobin may miss up to 30% of adult cases of vitamin B_{12} deficiency. On peripheral blood smear there are numerous schistocytes and misshapen mature red blood cells due to the increased mechanical red blood cell fragility associated with this condition. Erythroid precursors have loose appearing chromatin, giving them a characteristic appearance. Hypersegmented or multilobar neutrophils may also be noted. The appearance of at least one neutrophil with more

than six lobes or more than five neutrophils with more than five lobes is considered significant. To assist in the diagnosis of vitamin B_{12} deficiency, serum levels of homocysteine and methylmalonyl coenzyme A may be elevated. Levels of methylmalonic acid (MMA), a precursor to methylmalonyl coenzyme A, may be elevated as well.

Other studies. After the diagnosis of vitamin B_{12} deficiency has been made, further studies can be performed to identify the cause. Specifically, a comprehensive dietary assessment, evaluation for parasitic infections, Schilling test (measures ability to absorb orally ingested vitamin B_{12}), amino acid analysis, measurement of the unsaturated B_{12} binding capacity and transcobalamin II levels, genetic evaluation, and measurement of antibodies to parietal cells and intrinsic factor. Subspecialty consultation is often required to assist with the diagnosis.

TREATMENT

Treatment of vitamin B_{12} deficiency depends on the cause. Frequently, vitamin B_{12} administration is necessary. If the anemia is severe, treatment should be instituted slowly and in a monitored environment. For malabsorptive causes, long-term treatment will be indicated. The recommended treatment is monthly injections of 100 µg/d of vitamin B_{12}. Following the clinical response and laboratory values enables the clinician to titrate treatment to the patient's response. It is not known whether folic acid therapy in patients who have vitamin B_{12} deficiency will worsen the neurologic symptoms of the vitamin B_{12} deficiency and may mask the hematologic symptoms of the megaloblastic anemia. In this case, the patient received a vitamin B_{12} injection and then began oral multivitamin and vitamin B_{12} supplementation. She also received nutritional counseling to help her create a nutritionally balanced vegan diet.

SUGGESTED READINGS

1. O'Grady LF. The megaloblastic anemias. In: Keopke JA, ed. *Laboratory Hematology*. New York: Churchill Livingstone; 1984:71-83.
2. Rasmussen SA, Fernhoff PM, Scanlon KS. Vitamin B_{12} deficiency in children and adolescents. *J Pediatr.* 2001;138:10-17.

3. Snow CF. Laboratory diagnosis of vitamin B_{12} and folate deficiency: a guide for the primary care physician. *Arch Intern Med.* 1999;159:1289-1298.

4. Toh BH, van Driel IR, Gleeson PA. Pernicious anemia. *N Engl J Med.* 1997;337:1441-1448.

5. Whitehead VM, Rosenblatt DS, Cooper BA. Megaloblastic anemia. In: Nathan DG, Orkin SA, eds. *Nathan and Oski's Hematology of Infancy and Childhood.* 5th ed. Philadelphia: W.B. Saunders Company; 1998: 385-422.

CASE 2-2

Two-Week-Old Boy

MEGAN AYLOR

HISTORY OF PRESENT ILLNESS

A 16-day-old male presented to the emergency department with a 24-hour history of decreased level of activity and a choking episode with a feed. The infant has breastfed poorly since birth, worsening during the past several days. Two days prior to presentation, he was started on cow-milk-based formula supplementation; however, he continued to feed poorly. On the day of presentation, when the infant began to take a bottle, he gagged and choked and his eyes appeared to "roll into the back of his head" for approximately 2 seconds. Parents denied tonic-clonic, jerking activity, or color change, although he was less active after this episode. The infant has had decreased urine output, with only one wet diaper in the preceding 24 hours.

MEDICAL HISTORY

This was the fourth child born to a 28-year-old mother at 36 weeks gestation. The pregnancy was complicated by preterm labor and the mother received magnesium tocolysis. At 36 weeks gestation, the magnesium was stopped and labor was allowed to progress. Delivery was uncomplicated. Maternal prenatal labs and cultures were reportedly normal. The child was discharged from the hospital on the second day of life.

PHYSICAL EXAMINATION

T 37.5°C; HR 142 bpm; RR 32/min; BP 95/65 mmHg

Weight and Height 5th percentile

On examination he was observed as being thin appearing and awake, but only cried with stimulation. His anterior fontanel was sunken; his lips and mucous membranes were dry. He had decreased tear production. His lungs were clear. The cardiac examination revealed a normal rate and rhythm without any murmur or abnormal heart sounds. His abdomen was soft without any organomegaly. His extremities were cool with a 2-second capillary refill. Both testicles were descended. His neurologic examination was significant for symmetric hypotonia without any focal abnormalities.

DIAGNOSTIC STUDIES

The white blood cell count was 16 300 cells/mm³ (38% segmented neutrophils, 54% lymphocytes, and 6% monocytes). Hemoglobin level was 18.2 g/dL and platelet count was 658 000/mm³. The results of the basic metabolic panel revealed sodium level to be 115 mEq/L; potassium, 7.7 mEq/L; chloride, 81 mEq/L; bicarbonate, 16 mEq/L; blood urea nitrogen, 31 mg/dL; creatinine, 1.0 mg/dL; glucose, 89 mg/dL; and calcium, 10.7 mg/dL. A serum ammonia level was 39 µg/dL. Lumbar puncture revealed 1 white blood cell/mm³. The cerebrospinal fluid glucose and protein were normal. Cultures of cerebrospinal fluid, blood, and urine were obtained.

COURSE OF ILLNESS

Acutely, the infant received IV normal saline boluses for fluid resuscitation, as well as management to correct his hyperkalemia. He was empirically treated with intravenous hydrocortisone as well as ampicillin and cefotaxime owing to his ill appearance. He was admitted to the neonatal intensive care unit for further evaluation. Careful consideration of the laboratory studies suggested a diagnosis.

DISCUSSION CASE 2-2

DIFFERENTIAL DIAGNOSIS

Hyponatremia with hyperkalemia in a 2-week-old infant is most concerning for adrenal crisis due to congenital adrenal hyperplasia (CAH). Less common causes for adrenal crisis include adrenal hypoplasia congenita and bilateral adrenal hemorrhage. Other causes of electrolyte abnormalities in a young infant include water intoxication, inappropriate formula preparation, and gastroenteritis. Acute renal failure is uncommon in this age group, but can cause significant electrolyte disturbance. If an ill-appearing infant presents primarily with vomiting, pyloric stenosis and malrotation should be included in the differential diagnosis.

DIAGNOSIS

Additional laboratory evaluation revealed markedly elevated levels of 17-hydroxyprogesterone (>120000 ng/dL; normal 4-200 ng/dL), a precursor for 21-hydroxylase enzyme. Additionally, the ACTH level was markedly elevated at 541 pg/mL (reference range, 9-52 pg/mL). The laboratory pattern was consistent with a salt wasting form of congenital adrenal hyperplasia. **The diagnosis is 21-hydroxylase deficiency.**

INCIDENCE AND EPIDEMIOLOGY

The adrenal gland is responsible for the production of three categories of steroids; mineralcorticoids, glucocorticoids (cortisol), and androgens (dehydroepiandrosterone, androstenedione, 11-β-hydroxyandrostenedione, and testosterone). Congenital adrenal hyperplasia is a category of autosomal recessive enzyme disorders that result in a deficiency of cortisol synthesis. Cortisol deficiency results in hypersecretion of corticotropin-releasing hormone (CRH) and adrenocorticotropic

hormone (ACTH) and subsequent hyperplasia of the adrenal cortex. Depending on the location of the blockade, excesses or deficiencies of the mineralcorticoids and androgens can occur. The biochemical pathways of steroid synthesis are shown in Figure 2-2.

The incidence of CAH ranges from 1 in 5000 to 1 in 15000. Severity of illness depends on the severity of the genetic mutation. Although several enzyme deficiencies can result in CAH, 90%-95% are due to lack of 21-hydroxylase and 4% are due to 11β-hydroxylase deficiency. Other rare enzyme defects that have been described include 3β-hydroxysteroid dehydrogenase deficiency, 17α-hydroxylase deficiency, and cholesterol side chain cleavage enzyme deficiency, or lipoid CAH.

CLINICAL PRESENTATION

Clinical presentation of CAH depends on the gender of the patient as well as the enzyme deficiency. The key feature of classic 21-hydroxylase deficiency is androgen excess. Patients have inadequate production of glucocorticoids and mineralocorticoids and subsequent ACTH stimulation. Excess precursors are shunted to the androgen pathway, leading to androgen excess and virilization. In the female, there is usually some degree of clitoromegaly and labial fusion. CAH is the most common cause of ambiguous genitalia in genetic females. The female internal genital organs are normal. Androgen excess in male infants is often limited to subtle penile enlargement.

While 25% of patients with 21-hydroxylase deficiency present with virilization alone, approximately 75% of patients will also present with salt wasting. Mineralocorticoid deficiency results in an inability to exchange potassium for sodium in the distal tubule of the nephron and hence there is sodium loss in the urine and an inability to secrete potassium. This electrolyte abnormality is referred to as salt wasting. Patients with the salt wasting type of CAH become symptomatic shortly after birth. They have progressive weight loss, dehydration, and vomiting. If the condition is not recognized, adrenal crisis and death occur.

Virilized females are often diagnosed at birth due to the ambiguous genitalia, whereas male patients may be diagnosed at one to two weeks

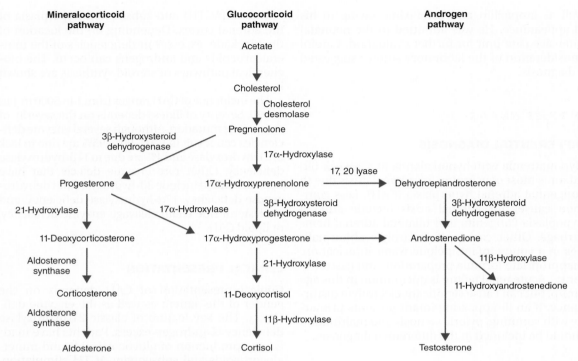

FIGURE 2-2. Adrenal steroid biosynthesis pathway.

of birth with a salt wasting CAH or in early child-hood when they present with premature develop-ment of secondary sexual characteristics. New-born screening for 21-hydroxylase deficiency is performed in most states in the United States of America.

The deficiency of 11β-hydroxylase results in both androgen and mineralocorticoid excess and therefore presents with virilization alone with-out salt wasting. Patients may have hypertension because of salt retention.

Other forms of CAH are extremely rare and may cause ambiguous genitalia in males. The 3β-hydroxysteroid dehydrogenase defect presents with salt wasting and virilization or ambiguous genitalia. The deficiency of 17α-hydroxylase may also cause hypertension and ambiguous genitalia. Lipoid CAH, while very rare, is often the most severe form, patients present with salt wasting and female phenotype.

DIAGNOSTIC APPROACH

There are several tests to assess for CAH.

Serum electrolytes. Hyponatremia, hyperkalemia, and hypoglycemia, while not diagnostic, are often the laboratory abnormalities that prompt further investigation.

Other studies. In classic 21-hydroxylase deficiency, serum levels of 17-hydroxyprogesterone are mark-edly elevated. Interpretation of 17-hydroxyproges-terone levels in neonates is difficult because this level may be elevated in sick or premature infants and in healthy infants during the first two days of life. Cortisol levels are typically low in patients with salt wasting variety and normal in patients with virilization.

In 11-hydroxylase deficiency, the levels of 11-deoxycorticosterone and 11-deoxycortisol are elevated. The 3β-hydroxysteroid dehydrogenase defect will cause levels of 17-hydroxypregneno-lone to be elevated as well as 17-hydroxyprogester-one and hence may be confused with 21-hydroxy-lase deficiency.

TREATMENT

Acutely, identification and management of adrenal crisis is critical. Aggressive fluid resuscitation and management of abnormal serum electrolytes as well as administration of stress dose IV hydrocortisone are paramount.

Long-term management of CAH includes administration of glucocorticoids to inhibit excessive production of androgens. The most frequently recommended glucocorticoid is hydrocortisone administered orally. Dosages should be individualized based on growth and hormone levels. The administration of exogenous glucocorticoids continues indefinitely. Children with CAH require higher doses of glucocorticoids during periods of stress, such as illness, infection, and surgery. In the long term, patients with 21-hydroxylase deficiency reach an adult height below their predicted height based on mid-parental target height; treatment with growth hormone alone or in combination with a luteinizing hormone releasing hormone analog.

If the patient also has salt wasting, then mineralocorticoid replacement and sodium supplementation are also required. Fludrocortisone (florinef) is the currently recommended mineralocorticoid.

In the neonate with ambiguous genitalia, determining the sex is important. Consultation with a pediatric urologist can assist in achieving a more normal appearance. Because CAH is autosomal recessive, it is important to test siblings of affected patients.

SUGGESTED READINGS

1. Laue L, Rennert OM. Congenital adrenal hyperplasia: molecular genetics and alternative approaches to treatment. *Adv Pediatr.* 1995;42:113-143.
2. Lim YJ, Batch JA, Warne GL. Adrenal 21-hydroxylase deficiency in childhood: 25 years' experience. *J Paediatr Child Health.* 1995;31:222-227.
3. White PC, New MI, Dupont B. Congenital adrenal hyperplasia (first of two parts). *N Engl J Med.* 1987;316: 1519-1524.
4. White, PC, New, MI, Dupont, B. Congenital adrenal hyperplasia (second of two parts). *N Engl J Med.* 1987;316:1580-1586.
5. Antal Z, Zhou P. Congenital adrenal hyperplasia: diagnosis, evaluation, and management. *Pediatr Rev.* 2009; 30(7):e49-e57.
6. Lin-Su K, Harbison MD, Lekarev O, Vogiatzi MG, New MI. Final adult height in children with congenital adrenal hyperplasia treated with growth hormone. *J Clin Endocrinol Metab.* 2011;96:1710-1717.

CASE 2-3

Three-Month-Old Girl

MEGAN AYLOR

HISTORY OF PRESENT ILLNESS

A 3-month-old female presented to the emergency department with several days of increasing fussiness and poor feeding. The infant has always breastfed well; however, three days prior to admission the infant developed a weak suck and difficulty breastfeeding. Although the number of wet diapers had not changed, they have been less saturated, and the baby has had no bowel movement during the previous four days. The parents related that the child's cry was not as loud as usual. The infant was evaluated by his pediatrician and referred to the emergency department. There has been no history of fever, vomiting, or diarrhea. There have been no ill contacts.

MEDICAL HISTORY

The infant has been healthy until this past week. Pregnancy and delivery were uncomplicated. There is a family history of pyloric stenosis in the father. A 2-year-old sibling is healthy.

PHYSICAL EXAMINATION

T 37.4°C; HR 156 bpm; RR 30/min; BP 100/80 mmHg

Weight and Height 50th percentile

On examination she was alert, but had a weak cry. Her head and neck examination was remarkable for bilateral ptosis and decreased facial expression. Cardiac and pulmonary examinations were normal. Her abdomen was distended but soft. On neurologic examination, she had a weak gag and poor tone. Her deep tendon reflexes were intact.

DIAGNOSTIC STUDIES

Laboratory testing revealed a white blood cell count of 10100 cells/mm³ (33% segmented neutrophils, 56% lymphocytes, 8% monocytes); hemoglobin, 11.7 g/dL; platelets, 490000/mm³; sodium, 139 mmol/L; potassium, 4.9 mmol/L; chloride, 106 mmol/L; carbon dioxide, 18 mmol/L; blood urea nitrogen, 12 mg/dL; creatinine, 0.3 mg/dL; and glucose, 58 mg/dL. A negative inspiratory force was measured at 20 cmH$_2$O.

COURSE OF ILLNESS

Intravenous glucose and normal saline were administered in the emergency department. The patient ultimately required endotracheal intubation due to inability to protect her airway. Her appearance combined with historical features suggested a diagnosis that was confirmed by additional testing.

DISCUSSION CASE 2-3

DIFFERENTIAL DIAGNOSIS

The diagnostic possibilities in this child with decreased activity and hypotonia include neurologic conditions that involve either the upper motor neuron (cerebral cortex and spinal cord) or lower motor neuron (anterior horn cell, peripheral

TABLE 2-3.	Causes of hypotonia in an infant.
Neurologic Disorders	
Upper motor neuron	Stroke
	Hemorrhage
	Transverse myelitis
	Mass effect
Lower motor neuron	Spinal muscular atrophy, type I
	Infant botulism
	Poliomyelitis
	Myasthenia gravis (neonatal or congenital)
	Myotonic dystrophy
	Congenital muscular dystrophy
	Guillain-Barré syndrome
	Heavy metal and organophosphate poisoning
Chromosomal Disorders	Trisomy 21
	Trisomy 13
	Prader-Willi syndrome
	Achondroplasia
	Familial dysautonomia
	Marfan syndrome
	Turner syndrome
Degenerative Disorders	Tay-Sachs disease
	Metachromatic leukodystrophy
Systemic Disease	Overwhelming sepsis
	Malnutrition
	Chronic illness
	Hypothyroidism
	Inborn errors of metabolism
	Ingestion

nerve, neuromuscular junction, or the muscle) (Table 2-3). Upper motor diseases, such as stroke, hemorrhage, and transverse myelitis, are possibilities. Lower motor diseases include poliomyelitis, spinal muscular atrophy, Guillain-Barré syndrome, congenital myasthenia gravis, botulism, and muscular dystrophies. Infectious etiologies such as overwhelming sepsis should be considered; however, lack of a fever makes these less likely. Ingestions can cause weakness, particularly barbiturates. Inborn errors of metabolism should be considered as well. Chromosomal disorders such as Down syndrome, Prader-Willi syndrome, achondroplasia, familial dysautonomia, and trisomy 13 may present with hypotonia as an early clinical feature; however, the acute onset in this case makes these diagnoses unlikely. The history of weakness, decreased feeding, weak cry, and constipation is a classic presentation of infant botulism.

DIAGNOSIS

The infant had significant hypotonia but was not tachycardic or hypotensive. An electromyogram (EMG) was obtained to assist with confirmation of the suspected diagnosis of infantile botulism. The EMG revealed a 56% incremental response that is consistent with a presynaptic neuromuscular junction disorder. The pattern is consistent with infantile botulism. Furthermore, stool studies isolated the botulinum toxin, type B. **The diagnosis of infant botulism was made.**

INCIDENCE AND EPIDEMIOLOGY

Up to 170 cases of botulism are reported in the United States annually, and the majority of cases are due to infant botulism. Although the disease has been reported in all 50 states, it is most common in California, Pennsylvania, and Utah. Unlike the adult form of botulism, which occurs after the ingestion of preformed toxin, infantile botulism occurs after the ingestion of *Clostridium botulinum* spores, found in soil and honey. Spores then germinate in the intestine, colonize the intestinal tract, and the organism produces toxin. The botulinal toxin, one of the most potent neurotoxins, irreversibly binds to the presynaptic cholinergic receptors and prevents the release of acetylcholine at the neuromuscular junction, leading to a descending flaccid paralysis.

CLINICAL PRESENTATION

The average age at onset is 10 weeks, with a range of 10 days to 7 months. Patients present subacutely with constipation and symptoms associated with cranial nerve palsies, including a weak suck, poor feeding, and subsequent irritability. As paralysis descends over subsequent days, patients develop head lag and generalized weakness. On physical examination, patients are hypotonic and hyporeflexic, with ptosis, poor head control, and diminished suck, gag, and respiratory effort. Mental status is not directly affected; however, infants are often irritable due to inability to feed well. Respiratory compromise is common; 70% of patients with infantile botulism will develop respiratory failure requiring mechanical ventilation. Patients may also have autonomic dysfunction manifested by decreased intestinal motility, distended urinary bladder, decreased tear production, decreased saliva production, periodic flushing and sweating, as well as fluctuations in their heart rate and blood pressure. Complications of therapy such as nosocomial infections may occur as a result of supportive care interventions.

DIAGNOSTIC APPROACH

Typically, the diagnosis is made on a clinical basis using the history and physical examination findings.

EMG. EMG can be helpful in making the diagnosis, particularly if an incremental response is found. Brief, small amplitude, overly abundant motor unit potentials suggest the diagnosis of infant botulism. If infant botulism is highly suspected and initial EMG testing is negative, repeat testing in 1-2 days is warranted.

Stool studies. Although results of stool testing are not immediately available, it is helpful to confirm the diagnosis by detection of botulinum toxin.

TREATMENT

Providing respiratory and nutritional supportive care, often in the ICU setting, is the mainstay of treatment. Because the disease is toxin mediated, antibiotics are not effective; in fact, aminoglycosides may worsen the paralysis by potentiating the neuromuscular blockade.

The development of human botulism immune globulin (BIG) has made a substantial impact on outcomes. When given within 3 days of hospitalization, BIG is shown to decrease duration of hospitalization, length of mechanical ventilation, ICU length of stay, and length of nasogastric tube feedings. The cost of hospitalization is reduced by half, offsetting the high cost of the therapy. Therefore, BIG should be initiated promptly when infant botulism is diagnosed clinically. Therapy should not be delayed while awaiting confirmatory stool studies.

Regeneration of the motor endplates takes weeks, often with waxing and waning clinical symptoms. However, patients generally survive with full neurologic recovery.

SUGGESTED READINGS

1. Frankovich TL, Arnon SS. Clinical trial of botulism immune globulin for infant botulism. *Western J Med.* 1991;154:103.

2. Long SS, Gajewski JL, Brown LW, Gilligan PH. Clinical, laboratory, and environmental features of infant botulism in Southeastern Pennsylvania. *Pediatrics.* 1985; 75:935-941.

3. Wigginton JM, Thill P. Infant botulism: a review of the literature. *Clin Pediatr.* 1993;32:669-674.

4. Cox N, Hinkle R. Infant botulism. *Am Fam Phys.* 2002; 65(7):1388-1392.

5. Underwood K, Rubin S, Deakers T, Newth C. Infant botulism: a 30-year experience spanning the introduction of botulism immune globulin intravenous in the intensive care unit at Children's Hospital Los Angeles. *Pediatrics.* 2007;120(6):e1380-e1385.

CASE 2-4

Eleven-Month-Old Boy

MATTHEW TEST

NATHAN TIMM

HISTORY OF PRESENT ILLNESS

An 11-month-old male was brought to the emergency department because of decreased activity level. He had a 3-day illness consisting of fever to 39°C and four episodes of nonbloody diarrhea each day. There was no history of emesis. On the day of presentation, despite drinking four 8-ounce bottles of an oral rehydration solution, he had decreased urine output. He also refused to play and instead wanted to lie down and rest. The mother called the paramedics when she felt that he was difficult to arouse.

MEDICAL HISTORY

The boy's prenatal and birth histories were normal. He had a history of wheezing with an upper respiratory infection at 3 months of age. He had no hospitalizations or surgeries. He was taking medications and had no allergies. His immunizations were current.

PHYSICAL EXAMINATION

T 40.3°C; HR 183; RR 46/min; BP 99/41 mmHg

Weight and Height 75th percentile

On examination, he was lethargic and minimally responsive to painful stimuli. The head and neck examination did not reveal any signs of external trauma. His gaze was disconjugate, but his pupils were reactive from 3 mm to 2 mm bilaterally. He had sunken eyes and dry mucous membranes. Respiratory examination revealed shallow, labored respirations with moderately increased work of breathing. He had intercostal and substernal retractions as well as abdominal breathing. Breath sounds were coarse to auscultation. Cardiac examination was significant for tachycardia without murmur or abnormal heart sounds. Abdominal examination revealed hypoactive bowel sounds but no tenderness, hepatosplenomegaly, or palpable masses. Rectal examination revealed gross blood. Neurologic examination was significant for overall hypotonia and unresponsiveness to voice or painful stimuli. His lower extremity deep tendon reflexes were 2+ and symmetric. He had an intact gag reflex and downgoing Babinski reflexes. The patient had a rash (Figure 2-3).

DIAGNOSTIC STUDIES

In the emergency department, blood, urine, and CSF studies and cultures were obtained. Additional laboratory studies revealed a white blood

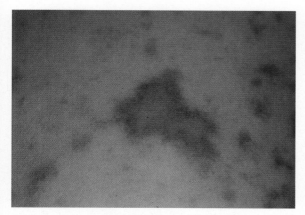

FIGURE 2-3. Photograph of a rash.

cell count of 13 400 cells/mm³, with 11% bands, 63% segmented neutrophils, 34% lymphocytes, and 2% monocytes. Hemoglobin was 6.6 g/dL; platelets, 195 000/mm³; sodium, 131 mmol/L; potassium, 5.8 mmol/L; chloride, 101 mmol/L; carbon dioxide, 18 mmol/L; blood urea nitrogen, 19 mg/dL; creatinine, 0.7 mg/dL; and glucose, 57 mg/dL. His prothrombin time (PT) was prolonged at 16.4 seconds (reference range, 10-12 seconds) and his activated partial thromboplastin time (PTT) is 29.1 seconds (reference range, 30-45 seconds). CSF studies revealed a gram stain significant for few white blood cells, a cell count of 100 WBCs/uL (65% neutrophils), glucose of 40 mg/dL, and protein 90 mg/dL. CT of the head was also normal. Serum and urine toxicology screens were negative.

COURSE OF ILLNESS

Patient was placed on 100% oxygen and provided with 40 mL/kg normal saline bolus and broad-spectrum antibiotics. A nasogastric tube was placed given the possibility of an upper GI bleed, and coffee-ground material was aspirated from the stomach. Given the findings of gross rectal blood, coffee-ground gastric contents, hypoactive bowel sounds, and low hemoglobin, the pediatric surgery staff was consulted in the emergency department on suspicion of an intraabdominal catastrophe, particularly intussusception or volvulus. He received

broad-spectrum antimicrobial agents and was immediately taken to the operating room for an exploratory laparotomy which did not reveal volvulus or intussusception. The patient's rash suggested a specific etiology (Figure 2-3).

DISCUSSION CASE 2-4

DIFFERENTIAL DIAGNOSIS

The differential diagnosis centers around two primary concerns. The first is an infectious etiology, including bacteremia, pneumonia, pyelonephritis, pyelonephrosis, or meningitis. In this particular case, the patient had blood, urine, and CSF studies performed to evaluate for infection and had broad spectrum antibiotics started. The low hemoglobin, hypoactive bowel sounds, and bright red blood from rectum make an abdominal process very concerning. This may include trauma (accidental or nonaccidental) or other causes of lower gastrointestinal bleeding (intussusception, malrotation with volvulus, meckel's diverticulum, henoch schönlein purpura, or some type of coagulopathy). In this particular case, the patient was taken into operating room for laparotomy to evaluate for a surgical abdominal emergency. However, the laparotomy was negative.

DIAGNOSIS

The patient's diffuse purpuric lesions suggested bacterial sepsis due to *Neisseria meningitidis* (Figure 2-3). His blood and CSF cultures ultimately grew *N. meningitidis*. **The diagnosis is meningococcal meningitis and sepsis.**

INCIDENCE AND EPIDEMIOLOGY

Neisseria meningitidis (meningococcus) is a Gramnegative diplococcus that causes bacteremia and meningitis. Meningococcus is a major burden worldwide, causing an estimated 170 000 deaths per year. There are 13 sero-groups; however, B, C, and Y are the three sero-groups most frequently implicated in the United States, each accounting for about 30% of systemic disease.

Neisseria meningitidis is a component of the normal flora of the upper respiratory tract, which is the only reservoir for the organism. Transmission occurs via the respiratory secretions and by person-to-person contact. Approximately 2.5% of children and 10% of the general population are asymptomatic carriers. Carriage rates have been shown to be higher in institutions, including universities, schools, prisons, and the military. In one study, 32.7% of persons between the ages of 20 and 24 years were asymptomatic carriers. Peak rates of infection occur between November and March. The incubation period is most commonly less than 4 days, but can be as long as 10 days. Fifty percent of cases of meningococcemia occur in children less than 2 years old. However, during epidemics, there is a shift in incidence toward older children, adolescents, and young adults. Factors associated with meningococcal infection include anatomic or functional asplenia and complement deficiency.

CLINICAL PRESENTATION

The disease caused by *N. meningitidis* varies from asymptomatic transient bacteremia to fulminant sepsis and death. Pathogenic *N. meningitidis* colonizes the respiratory tract and may invade the bloodstream. The patient becomes bacteremic and progressively sicker. The bacteremia may seed the meninges causing meningitis. Those patients who present with meningitis have a better prognosis than patients with bacteremia alone. Shortly after the administration of appropriate antibiotics, some patients have a marked clinical deterioration, ranging from hypotension to death. This deterioration is thought to be caused by stimulation of the host inflammatory pathway by endotoxin (a component of the gram negative bacterial cell wall). Meningococcal disease can lead to death in as few as 12 hours with 50% of deaths occurring within 24 hours of presentation. Invasive infection usually results in meningococcemia, meningitis, or both. However, it can infect any organ, including the myocardium, adrenals, lungs, and joint spaces. Approximately 55% of patients with meningococcal disease have meningitis. Additionally, 50% of patients have positive blood cultures.

A history of a preceding URI can often be elicited from patients with meningococcemia. The onset of illness is abrupt, with fever, lethargy, and rash. The rash is typically petechial and can progress rapidly to purpura due to a disseminated coagulopathy. Some patients develop fulminant meningococcemia with disseminated intravascular coagulopathy, shock, and myocardial dysfunction. Fulminant disease can be further complicated by adrenal hemorrhage (Waterhouse-Friderichsen syndrome), leading to rapidly progressive adrenocortical insufficiency and shock. There is a 20% mortality rate in cases of fulminant disease.

DIAGNOSTIC APPROACH

The prompt diagnosis of meningococcal disease requires a high index of clinical suspicion. Recovery of the organism from a normally sterile site provides the definitive diagnosis.

Appropriate cultures. The organism can be isolated from blood, CSF, and scrapings from the petechial rash. Blood cultures are positive in about 50% of patients with presumed meningococcal disease. Because the organism is a normal component of the nasopharynx, nasopharyngeal cultures are not helpful.

Other studies. PCR may be useful in the rapid diagnosis of meningococcal disease, particularly in patients who have been pretreated with antibiotics. Gram stain of the blood, CSF, or skin scrappings is also useful for the rapid detection of meningococci. Other laboratory studies that may affect management include serum electrolytes, prothrombin time, and partial thromboplastin times.

TREATMENT

Treatment of suspected cases of meningococcal infection should be administered as early as possible in the course of the disease, and antibiotic administration should not be delayed while waiting for a lumbar puncture. The initial antimicrobial coverage of meningococcal infections should be a third-generation cephalosporin, such as cefotaxime or ceftriaxone. Chloramphenicol, although rarely used, is appropriate for patients with anaphylactoid reactions to penicillins or cephalosporins. Although most isolates in the United States are sensitive to penicillin, penicillin-resistant isolates, first identified in Spain in 1987, are prevalent in Spain, Italy, and parts of Africa. In the United States, routine susceptibility testing is not indicated. Five to seven days of therapy is adequate for most cases of invasive meningococcal disease. Glucocorticoids have not been shown to be beneficial in the management of meningococcal disease. Treatment with heparin and other anticoagulants remain controversial. Aggressive fluid resuscitation and inotropic support are necessary for maintaining adequate perfusion in cases of septic shock.

Chemoprophylaxis is indicated for individuals who have been exposed to the index case within seven days prior to the onset of illness. Particularly, all household contacts, all daycare/nursery school contacts (children and adults), and health-care workers who had intimate exposure to secretions (mouth-to-mouth resuscitation, secretions that came in contact with the health-care worker's mucous membranes) should receive prophylaxis. Family members of the index case have a 400-800 times higher risk of invasive disease. If the index patient only received penicillin for therapy, then the patient should also be treated with chemoprophylaxis to eradicate the organism. School age classmates do not need chemoprophylaxis because they are not at an increased risk of disease. The drug of choice for chemoprophylaxis is rifampin. Ceftriaxone (intravenous or intramuscular) or a single-dose of ciprofloxacin are reasonable alternatives, although resistance to ciprofloxacin has been reported. Azithromycin has also been reported to be effective and can be used in areas with reported ciprofloxacin resistance. All cases require reporting to the local public health department.

A polysaccharide vaccine effective against serogroups A, C, Y, and W-135 was developed in the 1970s. More recently, a conjugate meningococcal vaccine against these four serotypes has been developed. Although the vaccine has been approved for individuals 9 months to 55 years of age, vaccination is recommended for routine administration in adolescents. Early administration is recommended for high-risk groups, including children who are functionally or anatomically asplenic or in those who have terminal complement deficiencies.

SUGGESTED READINGS

1. American Academy of Pediatrics. Meningococcal infections. In: Pickering LK, ed. *2012 Red Book: Report of the Committee on Infectious Diseases*. 29th ed. Elk Grove Village, IL: American Academy of Pediatrics; 2012: 500-509.
2. Anderson MS, Glode MP, Smith AL. Meningococcal disease. In: Feigin RD, Cherry JD, eds. *Textbook of Pediatric Infectious Diseases*. 6th ed. Philadelphia: W.B. Saunders Company; 2009:1350-1365.
3. Cohen J. Meningococcal disease as a model to evaluate novel anti-sepsis strategies. *Crit Care Med*. 2000;28:s 64-s67.
4. Gardner P. Prevention of meningococcal disease. *N Engl J Med*. 2006;355:1466-1473.
5. Hart CA, Thomson APJ. Meningococcal disease and its management in children. *BMJ*. 2006;333:685-690.
6. Panatto D, Amicizia D, Lai PL, Gasparini R. Neisseria meningitides B vaccines. *Expert Rev Vaccines*. 2011; 10(9):1337-1351.
7. Periappuram M, Taylor M, Keane C. Rapid detection of meningococci from petechiae in acute meningococcal infection. *J Infect*. 1995;31:201-203.
8. Rosenstein NE, Perkins BA, Stephens DS, Popovic T, Hughes JM. Meningococcal disease. *New Engl J Med*. 2001;344:1378-1388.
9. Stephens DS, Greenwood B, Brandtzaeg P. Epidemic meningitis, meningococcaemia, and Neisseria meningitides. *Lancet*. 2007;369:2196-2210.

CASE 2-5

Nine-Year-Old Boy

MATTHEW TEST

NATHAN TIMM

HISTORY OF PRESENT ILLNESS

A 9-year-old boy developed emesis about 5:00 p.m. one evening and thereafter went to sleep. A few hours later, the parents had a difficult time arousing him, and subsequently brought him to an emergency department. In the emergency department, the child was able to relate that he fell at school and hit his head against the wall. He did not lose consciousness at the time. He complained of a headache and had two additional episodes of emesis in the emergency department. He denied any potential ingestion.

MEDICAL HISTORY

The boy was a healthy child with no significant medical history. He did not take any medications and was not allergic to any medications. His immunizations were appropriate for age.

PHYSICAL EXAMINATION

T 37.5°C; HR 86 bpm; RR 26/min; BP 120/70 mmHg; SpO$_2$ 97% in room air

On examination he was asleep but was easily arousable. His head was atraumatic, but he had occipital pain with forward neck flexion. His occiput was diffusely tender, but no bony defects were palpated. Pupils were 4 mm and reactive to 2 mm. His tympanic membranes were normal in appearance. A fundoscopic examination was attempted, but was unsuccessful. Kernig's and Bruzinski's tests were negative. The remainder of his head and neck examination was normal. His lungs, cardiac, and abdominal examinations were normal as well. His neurologic examination revealed that his cranial nerves were intact. He was able to follow commands and respond appropriately.

DIAGNOSTIC STUDIES

A complete blood count and serum electrolytes were normal. Serum and urine toxicology screens were negative.

COURSE OF ILLNESS

The patient had a 5-minute generalized tonic-clonic seizure. He received phenytoin intravenously after the seizure activity ceased. Findings on the initial noncontrast head CT prompted a CT angiogram, which revealed the diagnosis (Figure 2-4).

DISCUSSION CASE 2-5

DIFFERENTIAL DIAGNOSIS

This case illustrates a patient who has an intracranial hemorrhage (ICH). The most common cause of ICH in children is from trauma (both accidental and nonaccidental). These traumatic hemorrhages most commonly occur in the extradural, subdural, or subarachnoid space. However, intraparenchymal hemorrhage can occur spontaneously, resulting from an arteriovenous malformation (AVM)

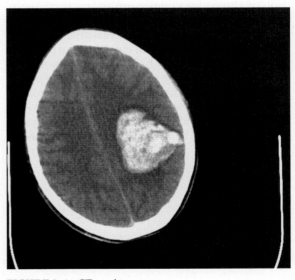

FIGURE 2-4. CT angiogram.

(50%), cavernous angioma, or aneurysm. Thrombocytopenia in a patient could also lead to ICH with minor head trauma as was reported in this patient.

DIAGNOSIS

The CT angiogram revealed a bilobed area of abnormal contrast accumulation in the posterior aspect of an intraparenchymal hemorrhage with concomitant intraventricular hemorrhage (Figure 2-4). **This patient had a ruptured segment of an arteriovenous malformation (AVM) with subsequent compression by the hematoma.** He subsequently underwent operative drainage of the hematoma and resection of the AVM.

INCIDENCE AND EPIDEMIOLOGY

Cerebral AVMs are a congenital vascular malformation. They most likely result from failed differentiation of the embryonic vessels into separate arterial and venous systems, which occurs between 3 and 12 weeks of fetal age. AVMs are arteriovenous shunts that consist of feeding arteries, a mass of coiled vessels (the nidus), and draining veins without a capillary network. Usually, there is no brain tissue between the two sides of the AVM, which allows a high-flow shunt from the arterial side to the venous side. The AVM, in essence, is stealing blood from the neighboring parts of the brain. Spontaneous thrombosis and subsequent recanalization may occur and may account for the change in size of an AVM over time. Ten percent of cerebral AVMs are in the posterior fossa, 10% in the midline, and the remainder in the cortex. They may be located superficially or deep. The incidence of cerebral AVMs is 1 per 100 000 persons. Fewer than 12% of cerebral AVMs are symptomatic. They are frequently diagnosed between the age of 20 and 40 years. About one-fifth of AVMs that become symptomatic do so before 15 years of age. Hemorrhage is the most frequent complication associated with AVMs, and it is more common in children than in adults. Besides hemorrhage of prematurity and early infancy, AVM is the most common cause of spontaneous hemorrhage in the pediatric population.

CLINICAL PRESENTATION

Intracranial hemorrhage is the initial manifestation in up to 80% of cases of cerebral AVMs and is associated with a 25% mortality rate in children. Seizures, which occur in about one-third of cases, may result from an acute hemorrhage, as a result of an epileptogenic focus from a previous hemorrhage, or as a result of chronic ischemia in tissue adjacent to the AVM due to poor perfusion secondary to steal phenomenon. Infants may present with congestive heart failure and hydrocephalus. Stroke and seizures are more commonly seen in older children. Intracranial hemorrhage may occur after an episode of trivial head trauma. Headache is a frequent symptom in patients with AVMs, although it is not a very specific clinical sign. Patients with untreated AVMs who have had previous hemorrhages are at a higher risk for re-bleeding. Other risks of hemorrhage include deep-seated or infratentorial AVM, deep venous drainage, female sex, and associated aneurysms. The presentation of the AVM varies with its location: superficial AVMs cause seizures more frequently, and deep AVMs tend to manifest with hemorrhage. AVMs generally continue to increase in size, increasing the risk of hemorrhage and ischemia, resulting in seizures, gliosis, and neurologic deficits. However, some AVMs may remain the same size and some may even regress.

DIAGNOSTIC APPROACH

Brain imaging. The diagnosis of an AVM can be made with CT, MRI, or cerebral angiography. CT is frequently obtained after the first hemorrhage and reveals only that a hemorrhage has occurred. If intravenous contrast is administered for the CT, the AVM nidus typically can be seen; however, the AVM is small, it may be missed on CT scanning. MRI is very helpful in diagnosing AVMs. Additionally, MRI is useful in the planning of the surgical correction of the AVM. MRI and magnetic resonance angiography (MRA) are also used to monitor patients after the AVM has been treated. Additionally, MRI is helpful in differentiating AVM from other hemorrhagic brain lesions, including malignancy and cavernous malformations. Angiography provides an excellent view of the vascular anatomy of the AVM and remains the gold standard for the diagnosis, treatment planning, and clinical follow-up.

TREATMENT

The aim of treatment is the complete removal of the AVM, because there is a high mortality from untreated AVMs. The options for removal include microsurgical excision, embolization of the AVM, and radiotherapy obliteration utilizing the gamma knife, proton beam, or linear accelerator. The therapeutic option most appropriate for the patient depends on the location and size of the AVM. If the location of the AVM is deep within the brain or on the motor cortex, excision might not be the best option. The effect of radiotherapy takes months or years, whereas surgical excision is immediately effective. Endovascular embolization alone is curative in less than 5% of lesions, but it remains an important adjuvant to surgical excision and radiotherapy.

Although the treatment of a ruptured AVM is widely accepted, the aggressive management of unruptured AVMs is more controversial, as it is important to note that these interventions are not without considerable risk. A meta-analysis of available studies concluded that intervention for an AVM is associated with a 5.1% to 7.4% median rate of permanent neurologic complications or death. Management decisions, including surgical intervention, radiotherapy, adjuvant endovascular embolization, or medical management, must be made on an individual basis and are best decided by a multidisciplinary approach involving the surgeon, endovascular neurosurgeon, and radiation oncologist.

SUGGESTED READINGS

1. Cahill AM, Nijs ELF. Pediatric vascular malformations: pathophysiology, diagnosis, and the role of interventional radiology. *Cardiovasc Intervent Radiol.* 2011;34:691-704.
2. Di Rocco C, Tamburrini G, Rollo M. Cerebral arteriovenous malformations in children. *Acta Neurochirurgica.* 2000;142:142-158.
3. Hofmeister C, Stapf C, Hartmann A, et al. Demographic, morphological, and clinical characteristics of 1289 patients with brain arteriovenous malformation. *Stroke.* 2000;31:1307-1310.
4. Menovsky T, van Overbeeke JJ. Cerebral arteriovenous malformations in childhood: state of the art with special reference to treatment. *Eur J Pediatr.* 1997;156:741-746.
5. Niazi TN, Klimo P, Anderson RCE, Raffel C. Diagnosis and management of arteriovenous malformations in children. *Neurosurg Clin N Am.* 2010;21:443-456.

CASE 2-6

Twenty-Month-Old Boy

MATTHEW TEST

NATHAN TIMM

HISTORY OF PRESENT ILLNESS

A 20-month-old boy was brought to the emergency department with decreased activity level. He had been vomiting for the previous 3 days with two or three episodes of nonbloody, nonbilious emesis per day. On the day of presentation, he had been acting listless all day and appeared pale to the family. There was no reported diarrhea. He had just recovered from hand-foot-mouth disease one week prior to developing these symptoms. The family denied any trauma or ingestions. There was no reported fever, rhinorrhea, or cough.

MEDICAL HISTORY

The patient had an elevated lead level (31 μg/dL; normal <5 μg/dL) one month prior to this presentation. His medical history was otherwise unremarkable. He had not undergone any surgical procedures. He was not taking any medications, was not allergic to any medications, and his immunization status was up to date.

PHYSICAL EXAMINATION

T 37.0°C; HR 75 bpm; RR 27/min; BP 100/68 mmHg

Weight 10th percentile; Height 50th percentile

On examination, he was somnolent but arousable. He fell asleep as soon as he was no longer being stimulated. His head was normocephalic and atraumatic. His tympanic membranes were pearly gray bilaterally, without hemotympanum. His mucous membranes were moist. His neck was supple, and there was full range of motion. His lung and cardiac examinations were normal. His abdomen was soft. There was no abdominal tenderness, masses, or organomegaly. His extremities were warm and well perfused. His neurologic examination revealed a Glasgow coma score of 13 but was otherwise normal.

DIAGNOSTIC STUDIES

A complete blood count revealed 12 100 WBCs/ mm^3 (86% segmented neutrophils, 9% lymphocytes, and 5% monocytes). Hemoglobin was 11.4 g/dL, and the platelet count was 851 000/mm^3. Samples were sent for a serum lead level determination. Serum electrolytes and transaminases were normal. A lumbar puncture revealed WBCs, 4/mm^3; RBCs, 4365/mm^3; glucose, 82 mg/dL; and protein, 31 mg/dL. A urine toxicology screen was negative. Additional laboratory evaluation revealed a PT of 13.0 seconds (reference range, 10-12 seconds) and a PTT of 36.6 seconds (reference range, 30-45 seconds).

COURSE OF ILLNESS

The child was hospitalized. During the next several days, he awakened and began to act normally. A head MRI performed at the time of admission suggested the diagnosis (Figure 2-5).

DISCUSSION CASE 2-6

DIFFERENTIAL DIAGNOSIS

Several diagnoses are possible for this child. Given the recent history of elevated lead levels, lead encephalopathy is a possibility. However, the presence of RBCs in the CSF and the expansion of the dural space on head MRI are suggestive of intracranial hemorrhage, which is not characteristic of lead encephalopathy. Causes of

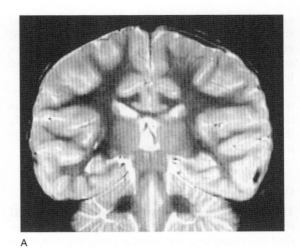

A

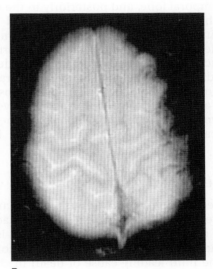

B

FIGURE 2-5. Head magnetic resonance images. **A.** Coronal view. **B.** Axial view.

intracranial bleeding must be considered. Head trauma, both accidental (e.g., motor vehicle accidents, substantial falls) and nonaccidental, are the most common causes of intracranial hemorrhage in children. Other causes include vascular abnormalities, such as arteriovenous malformations (AVMs), cavernous angiomas, and aneurysms, hematologic disorders such as von Willebrand disease, factor deficiencies, and thrombocytopenia, brain tumors, arachnoid cysts, cerebral infections, metabolic disorders such as glutaric aciduria and galactosemia, and hypernatremia.

Extradural, subdural, and subarachnoid hemorrhage are commonly due to trauma, whereas intraparenchymal hemorrhage is most commonly the result of vascular anomaly, hematologic abnormality, or brain malignancy.

DIAGNOSIS

The serum lead level was normal. Head MRI revealed extensive left subdural hemorrhage that extended over the frontal convexity, down to the temporal lobe, and posteriorly to the occipital lobe (Figures 2-5A and B). Dilated retinal examination performed by an ophthalmologist revealed multiple bilateral retinal hemorrhages. No fractures, either new or healing, were detected on radiographic skeletal survey (radiographs of all bones in his body). **The final diagnosis was child abuse.** Social services were involved and determined that a relative who lived in the house had caused the nonaccidental trauma in this child.

INCIDENCE AND EPIDEMIOLOGY

The recognition of child abuse is difficult and requires a high index of suspicion. The exact incidence of child abuse is not known, but it is more common than many may think. In 2007, homicide was the third leading cause of death in children age 1 to 4 years, with as many as 2500 children of all ages dying annually from inflicted injuries. Fortunately, from the early 1990 to 2009, there was a substantial decrease in physical and sexual abuse cases substantiated by child protective services. Nevertheless, child abuse remains a major problem in the United States of America, with an estimated 3.3 million reports and as many as 763 000 substantiated cases of child abuse in 2009 alone. Health-care providers play an essential role in the identification and reporting of suspected abuse, and in 2010, the American Board of Pediatrics designated a board certified specialty in child abuse pediatrics.

CLINICAL PRESENTATION

The presentation of child abuse varies according to the type of injury inflicted on the child, and medical personnel should be alert to any sign that may indicate abuse. The child may have been the victim of a one-time abuse or multiple previous episodes of abuse. It is estimated that an abused child has a 50% chance of further abuse. The abuse may be physical, sexual, emotional, or neglect. Physical abuse represents only 25% of the abuse cases in the United States. Victims of physical abuse may present with marks and bruises on the body, change in mental status, intracranial hemorrhage, or full arrest. In up to 40% of cases of abusive head injury, the child presents with no external signs of injury. The perpetrator may not have intended to harm the child, but may have over disciplined or punished the child, resulting in abuse.

Risk factors that place a child at increased risk for abuse include parental/caretaker factors, child factors, and situational factors. Caretaker factors that increase the risk of abuse occurring include caretakers who are not prepared to perform their role, have unrealistic expectations of the child, have a poor role model, use corporal punishment, have inconsistent discipline skills, have an unsupportive partner, have psychologic issue such as impulse disorder or depression, have been victims of abuse themselves, have a substance abuse problem, or who are not directly related to the child. Children who are handicapped, have developmental delays, or have behavioral problems are at increased risk. Sixty-seven percent of abused children are under 1 year of age and 80% are under 3 years of age. Economic difficulties, poor housing, crowding, illness, and unemployment are situations that increase the likelihood of abuse. Injuries that have occurred without any history, inconsistent histories, "magical" injuries, injuries that present with a delay in seeking care, and injuries that are inconsistent with the child's developmental age are concerning for abuse. Physical examination findings concerning for abuse include patterned marks (e.g., cigarette lighter burns, belt buckle bruises, immersion burns), multiple injuries, injuries at different stages of healing, and unexplained injuries. Figure 2-6 demonstrates retropharyngeal air secondary to inflicted trauma to the oropharynx. An accompanying liver laceration increased the suspicion of abuse in this patient.

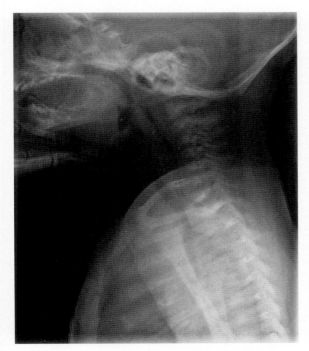

FIGURE 2-6. Lateral neck film demonstrating retropharyngeal air in a case of nonaccidental injury. The presumed mechanism was penetrating injury with a caregiver's finger. The infant also had a liver laceration identified on abdominal CT.

It is important to be able to determine what constitutes abuse and what does not. Being able to differentiate osteogenesis imperfecta from fractures due to child abuse, Mongolian spots from bruising, and ecthyma from a cigarette burn are important skills that health-care professionals should learn. Of note, one study found that 70% of parents of children with osteogenesis imperfecta experienced temporary loss of custody of their children for suspected child abuse. Bruising is the most common type of injury in physical abuse. However, normal bruising is common in children over 1 year of age and is typically on the lower extremities, not associated with petechiae, purpura, or mucosal bleeding. Suspicious sites of bruising include the butttocks, trunk, genitals, ears, back of hands, and neck. Nevertheless, it is often difficult to determine which injuries were sustained accidentally and which

were subsequent to nonaccidental trauma. When in doubt, a social services report should be filed.

DIAGNOSTIC APPROACH

There are a few studies that are frequently obtained on children who are suspected of being abused.

Radiographic skeletal survey. Radiographic skeletal survey (X-ray of all the bones in the child's body) is indicated in children under the age of 2 years. In patients with a high index of suspicion for abuse but a negative skeletal survey, a repeat skeletal survey should be performed after 2 weeks.

Radionuclide bone scan. A bone scan may also be helpful in detecting fractures that did not show up on the skeletal survey.

Dilated retinal examination. An ophthalmology consult is frequently helpful in detecting retinal hemorrhages.

Other studies. Laboratory studies are often indicated as well. A complete blood count and prothrombin and partial thromboplastin times should be obtained if the child presents with bruising. Liver function tests with amylase and lipase should be obtained if abdominal injury is suspected. Screening the urine and stool for blood is appropriate for abdominal trauma. Urinalysis may also be important for the detection of myoglobin if muscle injury has occurred. Screening for sexually transmitted diseases and semen may be appropriate if a child presents within 24 to 72 hours of a sexual assault. Toxicologic test are indicated if the child presents with altered mental status. Head CT or MRI may be indicated if the child has a large head or if there is reason to suspect intracranial injury; acute or chronic subdural hemorrhages may be identified. Testing for osteogenesis imperfecta should also be considered if fractures are a major component of the suspected abuse.

TREATMENT

The approach to the abused child is to first treat the medical emergencies. Anyone involved in the care of a child is a mandated reporter of suspected child abuse. It is not the job of the medical team to prove abuse and then report, but rather to report suspected abuse and allow the social services to perform further investigations. Occasionally, the physical examination findings alone are sufficient to trigger a social services report to be filed. Other times, it is the cumulative effect of the history, physical examination, laboratory results, and caretaker interactions that trigger the filing of a report. If the child is not safe to be discharged, hospitalization is warranted.

SUGGESTED READINGS

1. Christian CW. Child abuse. In: Zorc JJ, ed. *Schwartz's Clinical Handbook of Pediatrics*. 4th ed. Philadelphia: Williams & Wilkins; 2008:237-248.

2. Kemp AM. Investigating subdural haemorrhage in infants. *Arch Dis Child*. 2002;86:98-102.
3. Wood JN, Ludwig S. Child abuse. In: Fleisher GR, Ludwig S, eds. *Textbook of Pediatric Emergency Medicine*. 6th ed. Philadelphia: Lippincott Williams & Wilkins; 2010.
4. Preer G, Sorrentino D, Newton AW. Child abuse pediatrics: prevention, evaluation, and treatment. *Curr Opin Pediatr*. 2012;24:266-273.
5. van Rijn RR, Sieswerda-Hoogendoorn T. Imaging child abuse: the bare bones. *Eur J Pediatr*. 2012;171(2):215-224.
6. Vora A, Makris M. An approach to investigation of easy bruising. *Arch Dis Child*. 2001;84:488-491.

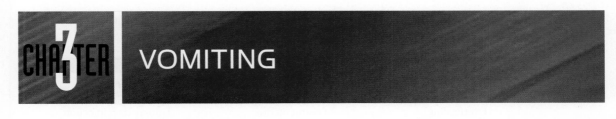

CHAPTER 3 VOMITING

PAUL L. ARONSON

DEFINITION OF THE COMPLAINT

Vomiting is defined as the forceful contraction of abdominal muscles and the diaphragm in a coordinated fashion expelling the gastric contents through an open gastric cardia into the esophagus and out through the mouth. The medullary vomiting center coordinates this process of vomiting via efferent pathways of the vagus and phrenic nerves. Stimulation of the medullary vomiting center occurs either directly or through the chemoreceptor trigger zone. Direct stimulation may occur through afferent vagal signals from the gastrointestinal tract or other sites including but not limited to the vestibular system, the cerebral cortex, or the hypothalamus. The chemoreceptor trigger zone in the area postrema of the fourth ventricle can be activated by noxious sights and smells or by chemical stimuli in the blood secondary to medications, metabolic abnormalities, and certain toxins.

Gastroesophageal reflux is not vomiting but rather regurgitation, and despite being projectile at times, is an effortless return of gastric contents into the mouth without nausea or coordinated muscular contractions.

COMPLAINTS BY CAUSE AND FREQUENCY

It is important to remember that vomiting is not a diagnosis but rather a symptom of an underlying pathologic process that requires a thorough evaluation. The causes of vomiting can be grouped based on age of presentation (Table 3-1) or etiology (Table 3-2).

QUESTIONS TO ASK AND WHY

Thorough history taking is imperative for formulating an accurate differential diagnosis and eventually discovering the correct etiology of vomiting. Consideration of the vomiting duration and pattern, the content of the emesis and associated symptoms provides a framework for creating a differential diagnosis. The following questions may help provide clues to the correct diagnosis:

- What is the duration of vomiting?
  —Acute episodes of vomiting carry a much different differential diagnosis than either chronic or cyclic vomiting. Acute vomiting is mostly due to infectious or metabolic conditions though it may also be caused by toxic ingestions or surgical emergencies, such as appendicitis and ovarian torsion. Chronic vomiting tends to have a gastrointestinal etiology and may be due to a partial mechanical obstruction as seen in hiatal hernia, or chronic gastrointestinal diseases, such as inflammatory bowel disease or celiac disease. Other conditions causing prolonged vomiting include peptic ulcers, dysmotility syndromes, increased intracranial pressure, psychogenic disturbance, pregnancy, and lead poisoning. Cyclic vomiting tends to be extraintestinal and is usually due to migraine or migraine equivalents, cardiac arrhythmias, or ureteral pelvic junction (UPJ) obstruction. Inborn errors of metabolism, while rare, are another cause of cyclic vomiting especially if associated with episodic neurologic symptoms.

TABLE 3-1.	Causes of vomiting and regurgitation in childhood by age.		
Disease Prevalence	**Newborn/Young Infant**	**Older Infant/Child**	**Adolescent**
Common	Gastroesophageal reflux	Gastroesophageal reflux	Gastroenteritis
	Overfeeding	Gastroenteritis	Urinary tract infection
	Gastroenteritis	Intussusception	Toxic ingestion
	Pyloric stenosis	Urinary tract infection	Medications
	Malrotation/midgut volvulus	Pulmonary infections	Inflammatory bowel disease
	Urinary tract infection	Toxic ingestion	Appendicitis
	Pulmonary infections	Medications	Pregnancy
	CNS infections		Ovarian torsion
	Sepsis		Ovarian cyst
			Pelvic inflammatory disease
			Migraine
Less Common	Increased ICP	Increased ICP	Increased ICP
	Other gastrointestinal obstructive lesions	Peptic ulcers	Peptic ulcer
	Obstructive uropathy	Pancreatitis	Pancreatitis
	Renal insufficiency	Hepatitis	Hepatitis
	Herpes simplex virus	Sepsis	Psychogenic
	Cow's milk protein allergy	CNS infection	Sepsis
		Foreign body	
Uncommon	Inborn errors of metabolism	Inborn error of metabolism	Adrenal insufficiency
	CAH	Reye syndrome	Cyclic vomiting
	Neonatal tetany	Adrenal insufficiency	Reye syndrome
	Kernicterus	Duodenal hematoma	Duodenal hematoma

Abbreviations: ICP, intracranial pressure; CNS, central nervous system; CAH, congenital adrenal hyperplasia

- Is there any timing pattern to the vomiting?
  —Episodes of vomiting that occur with a regular diurnal pattern are also helpful clues. Early morning vomiting can be very ominous due to increased intracranial pressure but could also occur secondary to morning sickness from pregnancy. Vomiting after eating specific foods may be due to a food allergy. Vomiting patterns may also become apparent if secondary gain is achieved, such as absence from school or tests, or it may be associated with school phobia. Vomiting that occurs shortly after eating is consistent with esophageal or gastric outlet obstructions or peptic ulcer disease, though may also be due to psychogenic vomiting.

- Is the vomiting effortless?
  —Gastroesophageal reflux occurs in almost all newborns, but by 6 months of age, less than 5% of children are symptomatic. It tends to be effortless, not associated with pain or morbidity. Rarely will reflux be severe enough to cause discomfort and arching, Sandifer syndrome (in which the reflux mimics seizure activity), or poor weight gain at which point medical therapy may be

necessary. True vomiting tends to be a more noxious event often causing pain and retching.

- Is there bilious emesis?
  —The presence of bilious emesis suggests an obstruction distal to the ampulla of Vater but may also be present in nonobstructed patients after prolonged episodes of vomiting due to a relaxed pylorus. Bilious vomiting in a neonate should be treated as a surgical emergency until proven otherwise. Neonates with bilious emesis may have intestinal obstruction associated with malrotation and midgut volvulus or less commonly, intestinal atresias. The absence of bilious emesis is also important, especially in neonates, because obstruction proximal to the ampulla of Vater (e.g., pyloric stenosis) may cause frequent nonbilious emesis.

- Is there any blood in the vomitus?
  —Either a Gastroccult or Hematest must first confirm the presence of blood in emesis. If blood is present then hematemesis must be distinguished from hemoptysis. The blood in hematemesis ranges

TABLE 3-2.	Causes of vomiting and regurgitation in childhood by etiology.		
Obstructive Gastrointestinal Disorders	Esophageal atresia or stenosis Hiatal hernia Congenital diaphragmatic hernia Pyloric stenosis Lactobezoar Malrotation Volvulus Intestinal atresia or stenosis Duplications Intussusception Adhesions Intramural hematoma Meconium ileus Meconium plug Meckel diverticulum Hirschsprung disease Imperforate anus Incarcerated hernia Annular pancreas Chronic intestinal pseudoobstruction Foreign body Ascariasis	**Metabolic**	Amino acid and organic acid defects Urea cycle defects Congenital adrenal hyperplasia Neonatal tetany Hypercalcemia Diabetic ketoacidosis Acidosis Galactosemia Fructosemia Phenylketonuria Adrenal insufficiency Reye syndrome Porphyria
		Renal	Urinary tract infections/pyelonephritis Obstructive uropathies Hydronephrosis Renal insufficiency Renal tubular acidosis Urinary calculi
Nonobstructive Gastrointestinal Disorders	Gastroesophageal reflux disease Achalasia Necrotizing enterocolitis Cow's milk protein allergy Eosinophilic gastropathy Inflammatory bowel disease Food poisoning Peptic or duodenal ulcer Celiac disease Superior mesenteric artery syndrome Viral gastroenteritis Bacterial enteritis Gastritis Pancreatitis Hepatitis Appendicitis Peritonitis	**Pulmonary**	Postnasal drip Asthma Pneumonia Foreign body aspiration Acute otitis media Labyrinthitis
		Toxicologic	Salicylate poisoning Acetaminophen overdose Theophylline toxicity Digoxin toxicity Iron ingestion Lead poisoning
		Miscellaneous	Pregnancy Ovarian torsion Ovarian cyst Pelvic inflammatory disease Testicular torsion Psychogenic Arrhythmias/cardiac abnormalities Cyclic vomiting Sepsis
Neurologic	Increased intracranial pressure Meningitis/encephalitis/abscess Seizure Migraine Hypertensive encephalopathy Motion sickness Concussion/postconcussive syndrome Kernicterus		

from bright red to coffee-ground depending on its length of time in contact with gastric contents, but tends to be darker red in color, acidic and associated with retching or gastrointestinal complaints. The blood in hemoptysis is bright red, frothy, alkaline, and associated with respiratory symptoms. Hematemesis may be due to peptic ulcers, Mallory-Weiss tears, esophagitis, esophageal varices, acute iron ingestion, gastritis, vascular malformations, or bleeding diatheses.

- Is undigested food present in the vomitus?
  —The presence of undigested food material is very common in children with gastroesophageal reflux who present with episodes of effortless postprandial regurgitation. Other conditions that predispose to undigested food in emesis include esophageal atresia or strictures, esophageal or pharyngeal (Zenker's) diverticulum, or achalasia. Old food present in the emesis may signify a gastric outlet obstruction or a gastric motility disorder.

- Is fecal material present in the emesis?
  —The presence of fecal material in the emesis is uncommon but when present suggests a distal intestinal obstruction such as Hirshsprung disease, peritonitis, gastrocolic fistula, or bacterial overgrowth in the stomach or small intestine.

- Is diarrhea occurring with the vomiting?
  —The presence of diarrhea and vomiting suggests a gastrointestinal disorder of which an infectious gastroenteritis is the most common, though if chronic in nature can be due to inflammatory bowel disease or celiac disease. Isolated vomiting tends to have a far greater differential involving many other organ systems. Isolated vomiting may occur in serious conditions, such as increased intracranial pressure, lower lobe pneumonia, intentional or unintentional medication or toxin ingestions, and diabetic ketoacidosis.

- Is there any abdominal pain?
  —When vomiting is accompanied by abdominal pain, the location of the abdominal pain, as well as the descriptive nature of the pain, can be clues as to the etiology. Pain in the right lower quadrant may be due to an acute appendicitis, whereas right upper quadrant pain is more likely to be gall bladder or hepatic in origin. Lower quadrant pain may also occur with ovarian torsion or pelvic inflammatory disease. The most common cause of diffuse abdominal pain with vomiting is gastroenteritis. Colicky pain tends to occur with an obstructed hollow viscous or urinary calculi, whereas well-localized sharp pain tends to occur when parietal peritoneum is inflamed. Flank or lateral pain signifies a renal etiology. Pain from peptic ulcer disease is often alleviated with vomiting, whereas pain secondary to pancreatitis or biliary tract disease is not improved with vomiting.

- Is fever present?
  —The presence of fever in a patient with vomiting is common. It may signify an infectious gastrointestinal process, such as acute viral gastroenteritis, bacterial enteritis, appendicitis, hepatitis, pancreatitis, peritonitis, or an acute extraintestinal infection, such as sepsis, meningitis, acute otitis media, pharyngitis, or urinary tract infections. Other causes of fever include inflammatory conditions, such as inflammatory bowel disease.

- Are there any other associated symptoms present?
  —Other information that may help in narrowing the differential includes the presence of weight loss, headache, lethargy, and poor school performance, as well as environmental and infectious exposures.

The following cases present less common causes of vomiting in children.

CASE 3-1

Seven-Week-Old Boy

TODD A. FLORIN

HISTORY OF PRESENT ILLNESS

The patient is a 7-week-old African-American boy who presents with a 2-day history of frequent vomiting. The vomiting is nonprojectile, nonbilious, and on one occasion, streaked with blood. Oral intake was poor. He had urinated once over an 18-hour period. On the day of admission he had profuse, watery diarrhea. No one in the family has had vomiting or diarrhea.

MEDICAL HISTORY

The patient was born at term weighing 3300 g. He was delivered via cesarean section due to arrested descent. Because of feeding difficulties in the nursery he was discharged home on a lactose-free formula. Since then his oral intake has been appropriate. He has not required previous hospitalization. He has received his first hepatitis B immunization.

PHYSICAL EXAMINATION

T 38.1°C; RR 50/min; HR 170 bpm; BP 86/38 mmHg; SpO$_2$ 88% in room air

Weight 10th percentile (4.0 kg); Length 25th percentile; Head circumference 10th percentile

Examination revealed an infant who was crying but consolable (Figure 3-1). The anterior fontanelle was open and slightly sunken. The mucous membranes were moist and the sclerae were non-icteric. The lungs were clear to auscultation and the cardiac examination was normal without any murmurs. The abdomen was soft and mildly distended without hepatomegaly or splenomegaly. The extremities were cool. He had no rashes, good tone, and a symmetric neurologic examination.

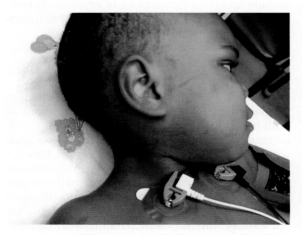

FIGURE 3-1. Photograph of a slightly older child with similar findings to the case patient.

DIAGNOSTIC STUDIES

Laboratory evaluation revealed 24 500 white blood cells/mm^3 with 9% band forms, 24% segmented neutrophils, 40% lymphocytes, 20% monocytes, and 5% atypical lymphocytes. The hemoglobin was 15.2 g/dL and the platelet count was 577 000 cells/mm^3. Red blood cell morphology noted mild anisocytosis, poikilocytosis, and burr cells. Serum chemistries were significant for a CO$_2$ of 10 mmol/L and cerebrospinal fluid cell counts, glucose and protein were normal; no bacteria were identified on Gram stain. His urine was dark yellow and turbid with a specific gravity of 1.038, a pH of 5.5, 3+ protein, and 5-10 granular casts without bacteria, nitrites, or white blood cells. On chest radiograph, the cardiac silhouette and lung fields were normal.

COURSE OF ILLNESS

The patient's oxygen saturation on pulse oximeter increased to 93% when oxygen was administered by nasal cannula. Four extremity blood pressures were obtained as follows: right arm, 90/32 mmHg; left arm, 88/42 mmHg; right leg, 80/40 mmHg; left leg, 76/35 mmHg. On arterial blood gas (ABG), the pH was 7.01; PaCO$_2$ 18 mmHg; PaO$_2$ 232 mmHg; bicarbonate level, 4.7 mEq/L; and base deficit, 24.7. The patient received multiple normal saline boluses and bicarbonate in an attempt to correct his metabolic acidosis. The appearance of the patient (Figure 3-1) in conjunction with the ABG suggested a diagnosis.

DISCUSSION CASE 3-1

DIFFERENTIAL DIAGNOSIS

Vomiting in early infancy can be a very worrisome symptom. The most common cause of emesis in this age group is gastroesophageal reflux, which can be physiologic or due to overfeeding. Anatomic obstruction should always be considered. Obstructive lesions include malrotation with a volvulus, esophageal or intestinal atresia, pyloric stenosis, meconium ileus, congenital adhesions or bands, incarcerated hernia, intussusception, and Hirschsprung disease. The level of the obstruction will determine whether the vomitus is bilious or the abdomen is distended. Infectious causes include gastroenteritis, sepsis, urinary tract infection, meningitis, pneumonia, and pericarditis. Neurologic causes, such as subdural hematoma, hydrocephalus, and mass lesions, should also be considered. Bloody streaks in the emesis could be due to a milk protein allergy, gastroenteritis, necrotizing enterocolitis, or achalasia.

Metabolic and endocrine disorders must be considered in this child who presents with vomiting and a significant metabolic acidosis. These disorders include congenital adrenal hyperplasia (CAH), adrenal hypoplasia, inborn errors of metabolism, including both amino acid and organic acid disorders, and galactosemia.

DIAGNOSIS

The patient was cyanotic, a feature best visualized with the contrast of his lips to the white portion of the blanket (Figure 3-1). An arterial blood gas (ABG) with co-oximetry measurements revealed acidosis with a pH of 7.01; $PaCO_2$, 18 mmHg; and PaO_2, 232 mmHg. **Co-oximetry readings revealed an oxyhemoglobin was 78.2%, methemoglobin 21.8%, and lactate level of 2.7 mmol/L confirming the diagnosis of methemoglobinemia.**

INCIDENCE AND EPIDEMIOLOGY OF METHEMOGLOBINEMIA

Although methemoglobinemia is a relatively uncommon condition in pediatrics, it may cause significant cyanosis and even death. Methemoglobin is a derivative of normal hemoglobin in which the iron component has been oxidized from the ferrous (Fe^{2+}) to the ferric (Fe^{3+}) state. The oxidized iron (Fe^{3+}) is unable to reversibly bind oxygen. Therefore, the oxidation of hemoglobin to methemoglobin produces a functional anemia by impairing the ability of the blood to transport oxygen. Methemoglobin occurs regularly in the body but rarely exceeds levels of 2% of the total hemoglobin because of antioxidant reactions in the body that reduce methemoglobin back to hemoglobin. The most important of these antioxidant reactions utilize either NADH-cytochrome b5 reductase or NADPH-methemoglobin reductase, although the latter system is largely inactive unless stimulated

by the presence of methylene blue as a cofactor. NAPDH-methemoglobin reductase reduces methylene blue, an action that has important therapeutic implications as described in the treatment section below.

Methemoglobin levels increase when there is a disturbance in the balance between the oxidation and reduction of heme iron. Infants are at an increased risk of methemoglobinemia for two main reasons: (1) an immature NADH-dependent enzyme system (cytochrome b5 and cytochrome b5 reductase) resulting in lower levels of these enzymes and (2) fetal hemoglobin is more easily oxidized than adult hemoglobin. Both of these concerns are heightened in a state of metabolic acidosis. Methemoglobinemia can be caused by exposure to oxidant drugs and chemicals, development of enteritis and/or acidosis, or inherited conditions (Table 3-3). The most common oxidizing agents in acquired methemoglobinemia include sulfonamides, aniline dyes, chlorates, quinones, benzocaine, lidocaine, metoclopramide, dapsone, and phenytoin. In young babies, topical anesthetics, such as topical benzocaine and lidocaine, are common causes of methemoglobinemia as a result of their use as remedies for circumcision and tooth eruption pain. Ingestion of well water nitrates can also cause methemoglobinemia. Gastroenteritis results in an oxidant stress as nitric oxide is released in the enteric endothelium, and can cause methemoglobinemia in infants. Less common causes include inherited deficiencies of erythrocyte methemoglobin reductase or the presence of M hemoglobin (congenital methemoglobinemia).

CLINICAL PRESENTATION

The clinical presentation of patients with methemoglobinemia depends on the concentrations of both hemoglobin and methemoglobin (Table 3-4). Increasing methemoglobin levels are associated with progressively more severe symptoms. Patients with lower hemoglobin percent concentrations are affected at lower percentage levels of methemoglobin. Patients with methemoglobin concentrations less than 10% rarely have symptoms unless they are already anemic. Most patients with concentrations between 10% and 25% will have cyanosis but few other symptoms. Levels from 30% to 50%

TABLE 3-3.	Agents typically implicated in methemoglobinemia

Local Anesthetics
  Benzocaine
  Lidocaine
  Prilocaine

Antimicrobials
  Chloroquine
  Dapsone
  Primaquine
  p-aminosalicylic acid
  Sulfonamides
  Trimethoprim

Analgesics
  Phenazopyridine
  Phenacetin

Nitrites and Nitrates
  Ammonium nitrate
  Amyl nitrate
  Butyl nitrite
  Isobutyl nitrite
  Nitroglycerin
  Nitric oxide
  Potassium nitrate
  Sodium nitrate

Miscellaneous
  Acetanilide
  Aminophenol
  Aniline dyes
  Benzene derivatives
  Bromates
  Chlorates
  4-Dimethyl amino phenolate
  Metoclopramide
  Naphthoquinone
  Nitrobenzene
  Nitroethane
  Paraquat
  Propanil
  Rasburicase

(Adapted from Blanc PD. Methemoglobinemia. In: Olson KR, ed. *Poisoning and Drug Overdose.* 5th ed. New York: McGraw-Hill/Lange; 2007.)

are associated with confusion, dizziness, fatigue, headache, tachypnea, and tachycardia. Levels greater than 50% are associated with severe acidosis, arrhythmias, seizures, lethargy, and coma. Lethal levels occur at around 70%.

DIAGNOSTIC APPROACH

Diagnosing a rare pediatric condition, such as methemoglobinemia, depends on having a high index of suspicion. Methemoglobinemia should be considered in cyanotic children without evidence of cardiac or pulmonary disease.

Bedside examination of blood. In a cyanotic patient, differentiating methemoglobin from deoxyhemoglobin is important. On white filter paper, blood containing a high level of methemoglobin turns chocolate brown, whereas blood containing deoxygenated hemoglobin appears dark red or purple initially but turns bright red on exposure to atmospheric oxygen.

Pulse oximetry. Oxygen saturation measured by pulse oximetry will be falsely elevated in the presence of high levels of methemoglobin. Most pulse oximeters use two wavelengths of light to determine "functional oxygen saturation," which is the ratio of oxyhemoglobin to all hemoglobin capable of carrying oxygen. Normally, all hemoglobin present can potentially carry oxygen so that *functional* and *true* oxygen saturation are equal. Because methemoglobin does not carry oxygen, it does not register as functional hemoglobin on the typical pulse oximeter. At normal methemoglobin levels (<2%), this exclusion is not important; however, at high methemoglobin levels (>10%) the functional and true oxygen saturations differ substantially resulting in unreliable pulse oximetry readings. Due to light absorption characteristics of methemoglobin,

TABLE 3-4.	Clinical symptoms of methemoglobinemia based on methemoglobin level.				
Methemoglobin Level	<15%	15%-20%	20%-45%	45%-70%	>70%
Clinical Symptoms	Asymptomatic	Cyanosis, mild symptoms	Marked cyanosis, confusion, dizziness, fatigue, headache, tachypnea, tachycardia	Severe cyanosis, severe acidosis, arrhythmias, seizures, lethargy, and coma	Typically lethal

the pulse oximetry readings will not drop below 82% unless accompanied by an increased level of deoxyhemoglobin. Newer generation pulse oximeters are available that use eight wavelengths of light and are able to accurately measure methemoglobin and carboxyhemoglobin continuously.

Arterial blood gas. Methemoglobinemia should be strongly suspected when there is a "saturation gap" in a cyanotic patient: a normal or elevated arterial partial pressure of oxygen (PaO_2) from an ABG with a low oxygen saturation on pulse oximetry.

Co-oximetry. Co-oximeters are spectrophotometers that measure light absorbance at different wavelengths, including the wavelengths for methemoglobin, oxyhemoglobin, deoxyhemoglobin, and carboxyhemoglobin. Co-oximeters accurately distinguish methemoglobin from oxyhemoglobin and provide a definitive diagnosis. Sulfhemoglobin and methylene blue (the treatment for methemoglobinemia) both produce erroneously elevated methemoglobin levels on routine co-oximetry. Therefore, co-oximetry generally should not be used to monitor response to methylene blue treatment. Newer generation co-oximeters are able to distinguish sulfhemoglobin and methemoglobin.

Potassium cyanide test. Elevated sulfhemoglobin levels can also cause a cyanotic appearance with a normal PaO_2, and can be mistaken for methemoglobin on some co-oximeters. If a newer generation co-oximeter that accurately detects sulfhemoglobin and methemoglobin is not available, the potassium cyanide test can be used to distinguish between these two hemoglobins. Methemoglobin reacts with cyanide to form cyanomethemoglobin. The formation of cyanomethemoglobin turns the blood from chocolate brown to bright red. Sulfhemoglobin appears dark brown initially and does not change color after the addition of potassium cyanide.

Additional studies. Although methemoglobinemia does not directly cause hemolysis, many of the agents that provoke methemoglobinemia can trigger hemolysis. Tests that evaluate for hemolysis (e.g., complete blood count, reticulocyte count, haptoglobin, and lactate dehydrogenase) and end-organ damage (e.g., electrolytes, liver function, creatinine, glucose) should be considered.

TREATMENT

Treatment depends on the methemoglobin level and the patient's symptoms. In all cases, the causative agent or process should be identified and eliminated or treated, if possible. Generally, consider administering specific therapy in symptomatic patients with methemoglobin levels greater than 20% or asymptomatic patients with methemoglobin levels greater than 30%. Consider treating patients with concurrent problems that impair oxygen delivery, such as anemia, cardiac disease, or pulmonary disease even if their methemoglobin levels are low. Symptomatic patients should receive proper airway management and supplemental oxygen as necessary. Intravenous methylene blue, after reduction to leukomethylene blue by NADPH-methemoglobin reductase, aids in the reduction of methemoglobin back to hemoglobin. It is the treatment of choice and should reduce methemoglobin levels significantly within 1 hour of administration. Exchange transfusions or hyperbaric oxygen may be necessary for those patients with extremely high levels that do not respond to methylene blue therapy or those patients with severe disease in whom methylene blue therapy is contraindicated (e.g., severe G6PD deficiency).

G6PD is the first enzyme in the hexose monophosphate shunt, which is the sole source of NADPH in the red blood cell. Patients with G6PD may not produce sufficient NADPH to reduce methylene blue to leukomethylene blue. As a result, methylene blue therapy may not be effective and may induce hemolysis in patients with G6PD deficiency, and is thus generally contraindicated in these patients.

SUGGESTED READINGS

1. Annabi EH, Barker SJ. Severe methemoglobinemia detected by pulse oximetry. *Anesth Analg.* 2009;108:898.
2. Barker SJ, Curry J, Redford D, Morgan S. Measurement of carboxyhemoglobin and methemoglobin by pulse oximetry: a human volunteer study. *Anesthesiology.* 2006;105:892.
3. Blanc PD. Methemoglobinemia. In: Olson KR, ed. *Poisoning and Drug Overdose.* New York: McGraw Hill; 2007: 262-264.

4. Osterhoudt KC. Methemoglobinemia. In: Erickson TB, Ahrens WR, Aks SE, et al., eds. *Pediatric Toxicology.* New York: McGraw Hill; 2010:492-500.

5. Pollack ES, Pollack CV. Incidence of subclinical methemoglobinemia in infants with diarrhea. *Ann Emerg Med.* 1994;24:652-656.

6. Umbreit J. Methemoglobin – it's not just blue: a concise review. *Am J Hematol.* 2007;82:134-144.

7. Wright RO, Lewander WJ, Woolf AD. Methemoglobinemia: etiology, pharmacology, and clinical management. *Ann Emerg Med.* 1999;34:646-656.

CASE 3-2

Nine-Month-Old Girl

PAUL L. ARONSON

HISTORY OF PRESENT ILLNESS

The patient is a 9-month-old girl who presents with a 12-day history of poor feeding, decreased activity, irritability, and frequent nonbloody, nonbilious emesis with feeds. Ten days ago she was diagnosed with viral gastroenteritis and 6 days prior to admission was treated with amoxicillin for an acute otitis media. Today she presents with continued emesis and decreased urine output having only two wet diapers in the previous 18 hours. The patient has a history of poor feeding and frequent episodic bouts of emesis lasting 2-3 days at a time. The parents deny any fever, diarrhea, cough, gagging with feeds, rash, bloody stools, ill contacts, recent travel, or animal exposure. Her diet consists of Nutramigen formula and various infant foods.

MEDICAL HISTORY

The patient is the full-term product of an uncomplicated pregnancy, labor, and delivery and was well until 3 months of age when she developed episodic vomiting. The emesis was nonbloody and nonbilious lasting 1-3 days and associated with decreased activity. It began while transitioning from breast milk to cow's milk-based formula at the age of 3 months and was therefore attributed to a "feeding intolerance." At 4 months she was changed to a soy-protein-based formula and then, finally, at 6 months Nutramigen was started without any relief in her symptoms. She was treated with ranitidine starting at 7 months for suspected gastroesophageal reflux. A sweat test performed at 8 months of age was normal.

PHYSICAL EXAMINATION

T 37.3°C; RR 50/min; BP 85/53 mmHg; HR tachycardic

Weight 6.5 kg (<5th percentile; 50th percentile for 5 month old); Length 66.5 cm (<5th percentile) and Head circumference 43.5 cm (25th percentile)

The patient was fussy but nontoxic appearing with scant nasal discharge and dry oral mucosa. She was tachypneic with clear lungs bilaterally. She had a soft systolic murmur at the lower left sternal border with a prominent S3 gallop. The liver edge was palpated 2 cm below the right costal margin and her spleen tip was also palpable. The extremities were warm and well perfused. There were no rashes and her neurologic examination was normal for age.

DIAGNOSTIC STUDIES

Laboratory analysis revealed 10 200 white blood cells/mm^3 with 41% segmented neutrophils, 53% lymphocytes, and 6% monocytes. The hemoglobin was 11 g/dL and the platelet count was 232 000 cells/mm^3. Serum electrolytes sodium 128 mmol/L, potassium 4.5 mmol/L, chloride 100 mmol/L, bicarbonate 20 mEq/L, blood urea nitrogen 19 mg/dL, creatinine 0.3 mg/dL, glucose 84 mg/dL, calcium 9.2 mg/dl. Her arterial blood gas showed a pH 7.43, PaCO$_2$ 31 mmHg, and PaO$_2$ 270 mmHg.

COURSE OF ILLNESS

A chest radiograph revealed mild cardiomegaly and a small right pleural effusion. An electrocardiogram (ECG) (Figure 3-2) was diagnostic.

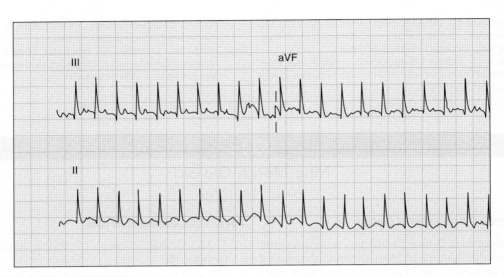

FIGURE 3-2. Patient's initial ECG.

DISCUSSION CASE 3-2

DIFFERENTIAL DIAGNOSIS

This patient presented with recurrent episodes of emesis with intermittent asymptomatic periods consistent with cyclic vomiting. Quantitative criteria for the diagnosis of cyclic vomiting include at least four episodes of vomiting per hour during the peak intensity and a frequency of no more than nine episodes per month. This is in contrast to chronic vomiting in which the patient has less frequent episodes of vomiting and less symptom-free days.

Cyclic vomiting frequently has a nongastrointestinal etiology. Causes include migraine headaches, abdominal migraines, and metabolic disorders including adrenal insufficiency, amino acidurias, and organic acidurias. Urea cycle defects may be present as episodic vomiting and neurologic symptoms due to hyperammonemia. Renal disorders such as ureteropelvic junction obstruction and renal calculi, as well as intermittent cardiac arrhythmias may also cause cyclic vomiting. Familial dysautonomia (Riley-Day syndrome) and Munchausen syndrome by proxy must also be considered. Gastrointestinal etiologies include pancreatitis, malrotation with intermittent volvulus, and intestinal duplications.

In patients with significant tachycardia and cyclic vomiting, an intermittent cardiac tachyarrhythmia must be strongly considered. The source of tachyarrhythmias include sinus, supraventricular, and ventricular. Differentiation of supraventricular tachycardia from sinus tachycardia may be difficult at times. Sinus tachycardia rarely exceeds 220 bpm in infants and 180 bpm in children and adolescents, has a normal P wave morphology and P wave axis, and varying heart rates due to changes in vagal and sympathetic tone.

Antidromic supraventricular tachycardia (SVT) due to an accessory pathway such as in Wolff-Parkinson-White (WPW) syndrome or SVT with a preceding bundle branch block (see later) may result in a widened QRS complex that resembles ventricular tachycardia. The absence of P waves and the presence of a wide QRS complex that is dissimilar to the QRS complex during sinus rhythm are more diagnostic of ventricular tachycardia (Figure 3-3).

DIAGNOSTIC TESTS

Diagnostic testing in the patient with cyclic vomiting is usually determined by the history and physical examination. The diagnosis of SVT was suspected in this patient by auscultation of a rapid heart rate or palpation of a pulse rate that was too

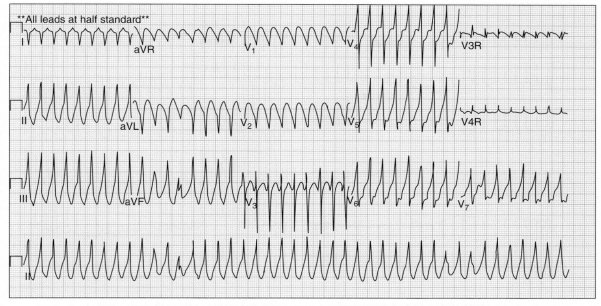

FIGURE 3-3. ECG demonstrates wide complex rhythm of ventricular tachycardia.

rapid to count. Confirmation of a diagnosis of SVT is made by an ECG demonstrating a narrow complex tachycardia with a heart rate above 220 bpm in infants or 180 bpm in children and adolescents, often without discernable P waves and a fixed rate (Figure 3-4). As discussed earlier, if an accessory pathway or bundle branch block is present, a wide complex supraventricular tachycardia may be present, although this is less common. Diagnosis may also be made after resolution of the tachycardia with vagal maneuvers or adenosine which do not resolve ventricular tachycardias (discussed further under Treatment).

DIAGNOSIS

The ECG in this patient revealed a narrow complex tachycardia of 270 bpm consistent with SVT (Figure 3-2). After applying ice to her face without success, she was cardioverted to a normal sinus rhythm with intravenous adenosine. An echocardiogram revealed mild left ventricular dilation, mild mitral valve regurgitation, and a small pericardial effusion but good cardiac function without

any structural defects. She was initially treated with digoxin and during the following 2 days and had normalization of her cardiac examination with resolution of her hepatomegaly. A repeat ECG prior to discharge showed mild right atrial enlargement and normal sinus rhythm without signs of preexcitation (i.e., no shortened PR interval or delta wave) (Figure 3-5). At discharge, she was transitioned to propranolol and after 2 months on therapy her weight had increased to the 25th percentile. In retrospect, her history of episodic feeding intolerance was likely due to episodes of supraventricular tachycardia.

INCIDENCE AND ETIOLOGY OF SUPRAVENTRICULAR TACHYCARDIA

SVT is a generic term encompassing a group of cardiac arrhythmias originating above the atrioventricular (AV) node. It is the most common sustained accelerated nonsinus tachyarrhythmia with an incidence of 1 per 250 to 1 per 1000 children. Two mechanisms account for virtually all cases of SVT: (1) an abnormal or enhanced normal

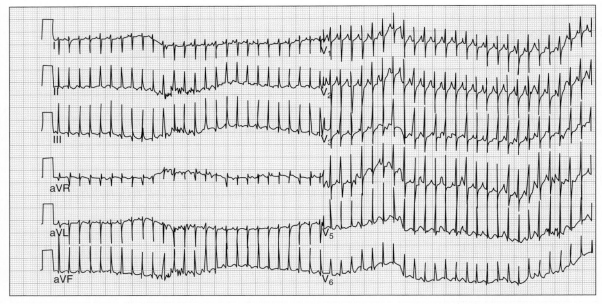

FIGURE 3-4. ECG demonstrates supraventricular tachycardia at the rate of 300 beats/min.

automatic rhythm and (2) a reentrant rhythm. Approximately 75% of patients with a reentrant rhythm will exhibit findings of preexcitation with a shortened PR interval and initial slurred upstroke of the QRS (delta wave) (Figure 3-6). Children less than 12 years are more likely to have an accessory atrioventricular connection while in adolescence, nodal reentry tachycardia increases in frequency.

Reentrant rhythms account for more than 90% of all cases of SVT. Two separate conducting pathways

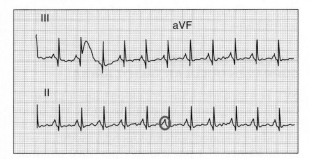

FIGURE 3-5. Patient's subsequent ECG with enlargement of P wave indicating atrial enlargement (circle).

must be present which lead to a cyclic pattern of excitation resulting in SVT. These pathways may be either within the atrium or atrioventricular. Atrial reentry rhythms may lead to either atrial fibrillation or atrial flutter.

Atrioventricular reentrant rhythms may be either through the AV node (nodal), or associated with an accessory atrioventricular pathway termed the bundle of Kent. Tachycardia may result from transmission of the impulse antegrade through the AV node and His-Purkinje system or through the accessory pathway with retrograde conduction through myocardium. The accessory pathway or AV node, respectively, then completes the circuit. This orthodromic reciprocating tachycardia (ORT) is the most common pattern seen in WPW syndrome and results in the typical narrow complex QRS tachycardia. Rarely the antegrade impulse travels via the accessory pathway and retrograde through the AV node and His-Purkinje system resulting in antidromic reciprocating tachycardia (ART).

Preexcitation occurs in 75% of those with accessory pathways. This implies that the accessory pathway can conduct the impulse in antegrade

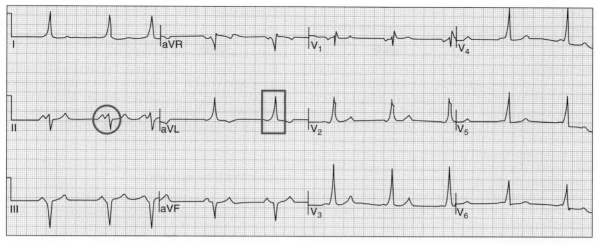

FIGURE 3-6. Shortened PR interval (circle) with delta wave (rectangle) as seen in preexcitation syndromes such as Wolff-Parkinson-White.

fashion from the atria to the ventricle. Bypassing the intrinsic delay of the AV node results in a shortened PR interval and a slurred upstroke of the QRS, the so-called delta wave (Figure 3-6). Twenty-five percent of accessory pathways will only transmit impulses in retrograde fashion from the ventricle to the atrium resulting in a normal (no evidence of preexcitation) resting ECG.

SVT secondary to increased automaticity or atrial and junctional ectopic tachycardias occurs more commonly in children with postoperative congenital heart disease or cardiomyopathies.

TYPICAL PRESENTATION

Approximately 50% of children present with their episode of SVT in the first year of life. Signs and symptoms of SVT depend on the age at presentation and the duration of the tachycardia. Episodes of SVT may last only a few seconds or may persist for hours. Many children tolerate these episodes extremely well, and it is unlikely that short paroxysms are dangerous. Infants with SVT exhibit nonspecific symptoms such as poor feeding and irritability, and will therefore often present with congestive heart failure because the tachycardia often goes unrecognized for a prolonged period. Episodes lasting more than 6-24 hours may result in an acutely ill child with evidence of cardiopulmonary distress resulting in

tachypnea, vomiting, lethargy, and ashen color. Physical findings in such cases include pallor, tachypnea, diaphoresis, hepatomegaly, and poor peripheral perfusion.

Older children may complain of lightheadedness, chest tightness, palpitations, and fatigue. Chest pain or discomfort is less common. The patient may become faint, dizzy, or even syncopal. If the rate is exceptionally rapid or if the attack is prolonged, heart failure may ensue.

DIAGNOSTIC RATIONALE

ECG. An ECG should be performed on any patient with tachycardia that is not felt to be due to normal sinus tachycardia. Patients with SVT have a very rapid and regular ventricular rate usually exceeding 220 bpm. The P waves are usually absent but when present have an abnormal axis and may precede or follow the QRS. Pending the results of the ECG, a chest radiograph or even echocardiogram may need to be performed.

TREATMENT

Treatment of SVT depends on the etiology and the duration of symptoms. Automatic rhythms are difficult to treat medically but respond well to ablation surgery.

Acute treatment of reentrant tachycardias depends on the age and stability of the patient. In hemodynamically stable children, vagotonic maneuvers should be attempted while obtaining intravenous access. Vagal maneuvers in the infant consist of placing ice over the mouth to stimulate the diving reflex or placing the infant's knees to the chest, while in older children should be asked to strain or breath hold. In patients who do not respond to simple vagal maneuvers, medical cardioversion should be attempted. Adenosine, a nucleoside derivative that blocks the orthodromic conduction at the AV node, is the medication of choice. Intravenous verapamil and propranolol can break SVT but are contraindicated in the acute setting for infants and children because of the risk of bradycardia, hypotension, and cardiac arrest. If these modalities fail or if the patient is hemodynamically unstable, synchronized electrical cardioversion should be performed immediately.

Once a patient has been successfully converted to a normal sinus rhythm, first line maintenance therapy is the β-blocker propranolol for most infants and older children, although digoxin is also used. Infants should be monitored for hypoglycemia after initiating propanolol, and are often able to be weaned off therapy as the SVT is usually self-limited. In children with evidence of preexcitation syndrome (e.g., Wolff-Parkinson-White), digoxin and calcium channel blockers are contraindicated and those patients are usually managed with β-blockers.

Radiofrequency ablation of the accessory pathway is one choice for definitive treatment. Success rates range from approximately 80% to 95%, depending on the location of the bypass tract or tracts. Surgical ablation of bypass tracts can also be successful in selected patients.

SUGGESTED READINGS

1. Rowe PC, Newman SL, Brusilow SW. Natural history of symptomatic partial ornithine transcarbamylase deficiency. *N Engl J Med.* 1986;314:541-547.
2. Losek JD, Endom E, Dietrich A, Stewart G, Zempsky W, Smith K. Adenosine and pediatric supraventricular tachycardia in the emergency department: multicenter study and review. *Ann Emerg Med.* 1999;33(2):185-191.
3. Salerno JC, Seslar SP. Supraventricular tachycardia. *Arch Pediatr Adolesc Med.* 2009;163(3):268-274.
4. Kleinman ME, de Caen AR, Chameides L, et al. Part 10: Pediatric Basic and Advanced Life Support: 2010 International Consensus on Cardiopulmonary Resuscitation and Emergency Cardiovascular Care Science With Treatment Recommendations. *Circulation.* 2010; 122:S466-S515.

CASE 3-3

Three-Year-Old Girl

AMY FELDMAN

HISTORY OF PRESENT ILLNESS

The patient is a 3-year-old Caucasian female presenting with a 1-year history of intermittent vomiting, increasing in frequency during the past 2 weeks. During the past year the patient has had nonbloody, nonbilious emesis approximately one time per day. The emesis is not associated with eating, nor does it occur at a specific time of the day. Occasionally, she wakes from sleep with emesis. She complains of photophobia and a sensation that there is a foreign body in her eyes. Her mother states that she seems to urinate more than other children. She denies abdominal pain, diarrhea, and rashes. Her mother denies noticing any lethargy, change in appetite, change in behavior, change in balance, or change in vision.

On the day prior to admission, her primary care physician began treatment with cefixime for presumed sinusitis after the patient had 3 days of cold symptoms and fever to 38.8°C.

MEDICAL HISTORY

The patient's medical history is significant for failure to thrive since birth. She has always been below the 5th percentile for weight and height. Her family history is significant for a mother with Graves disease and two maternal cousins on dialysis for unknown reasons.

PHYSICAL EXAMINATION

T 36.8°C; RR 24/min; HR 118/min; BP 98/55 mmHg

Weight 11.1 kg (<5th percentile); Height 86 cm (<5th percentile)

Physical examination revealed a thin pale female in no acute distress. She had moist mucous membranes and a small amount of clear nasal discharge. Her optic discs were not able to be visualized. Her neck was supple with full range of motion. Cardiovascular and pulmonary examinations were normal. Her abdomen was soft, nontender, and nondistended without any masses, hepatomegaly, or splenomegaly. She had no rashes, petechiae, or purpura. Cranial nerves 2-12 were intact. She had normal speech, gait, and reflexes.

DIAGNOSTIC STUDIES

Laboratory evaluation revealed a normal complete blood count. Serum chemistries were as follows: sodium, 128 mmol/L; potassium, 2.0 mmol/L; chloride, 105 mmol/L; bicarbonate, 21 mEq/L; blood urea nitrogen (BUN), 37 mg/dL; creatinine, 2.2 mg/dL; glucose, 89 mg/dL; calcium, 7.9 mg/dL; phosphorus, 3.1 mg/dL; and magnesium, 2.0 mg/dL. Liver function tests were normal. Urinalysis showed a specific gravity of 1.010, pH of 6.5, trace blood, 3+ protein, 1+ glucose, and hyaline casts. Urine electrolytes were as follows: sodium 38 mmol/L, potassium 22 mmol/L, and chloride 37 mmol/L. A chest radiograph was normal as was an ECG. A renal ultrasound displayed small echogenic kidneys. A brain MRI was normal.

COURSE OF ILLNESS

The patient received an intravenous bolus of normal saline and was admitted to the hospital with a diagnosis of renal failure of unknown etiology. Her electrolytes slowly normalized throughout hospitalization after IV and oral supplementations.

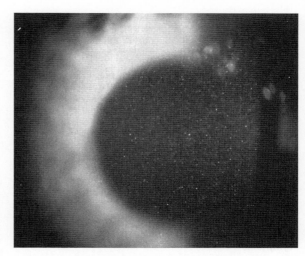

FIGURE 3-7. Retinal examination of patient with similar findings. *(Reproduced, with permission, from Oppenheim RA, Mathers WD. The eye in endocrinology. In: Becker KL, ed. Principles and Practice of Endocrinology and Metabolism. Philadelphia: Lippincott Williams and Wilkins; 2001:1968.)*

While in the hospital, she underwent an ophthalmologic slit-lamp evaluation which provided a diagnosis (see Figure 3-7).

DISCUSSION CASE 3-3

DIFFERENTIAL DIAGNOSIS

This patient displayed signs and symptoms of Fanconi syndrome (Table 3-5), a generalized dysfunction of the proximal renal tubule resulting in an excessive loss of amino acids, glucose, bicarbonate, uric acid, and phosphate into the urine. Fanconi syndrome can be hereditary or acquired. Hereditary causes of Fanconi syndrome include cystinosis, Lowe syndrome (oculocerebrorenal syndrome), galactosemia, hereditary fructose intolerance, tyrosinemia, Wilson disease, Dent disease, Fanconi-Bickel syndrome, glycogen storage disease, mitochondrial disorders, and Alport syndrome. Acquired causes of Fanconi syndrome include nephrotic syndrome, Sjögren syndrome,

TABLE 3-5.	Signs and symptoms of Fanconi syndrome.

Signs

Serum: Hyperchloremic metabolic acidosis with a
  normal anion gap
    Low sodium
    Low potassium
    Low phosphate
    Low uric acid

Urine: Increased amino acids
    Increased bicarbonate
    Increased low molecular weight proteins
    Increased glucose (1 to 2 plus)
    Increased albumin (1 to 2 plus)
    Increased potassium, sodium, magnesium, and
      phosphate
    High pH (>5.5)
    Specific gravity 1.01 to 1.015

Symptoms

Failure to thrive
Vomiting
Polydipsia and polyuria
Dehydration
Rickets, bowing deformities, osteomalacia

renal vein thrombosis, cancer, or damage from drugs (Azathioprine, Gentamycin, Tetracycline) or heavy metals (lead, mercury, and cadmium).

DIAGNOSTIC TESTS

The diagnosis of Fanconi syndrome is made by documenting excessive loss of amino acids, glucose, phosphate, and bicarbonate in the urine in the absence of high plasma concentrations. Once Fanconi syndrome has been diagnosed, further testing can be performed to determine the specific etiology. In a newborn or infant, testing should be done as clinically indicated for tyrosinemia (urine succinylacetone), galactosemia (erythrocyte galactose-1-phosphate uridyltransferase), hereditary fructose intolerance (urinary reducing substances), and Lowe syndrome. In a child with a history suspicious for heavy metal ingestion, serum levels can be obtained.

DIAGNOSIS

This patient had serum and urinary findings consistent with Fanconi syndrome. An ophthalmologic

evaluation revealed crystals in the cornea consistent with cystine deposits (Figure 3-7). Subsequently, an elevated leukocyte cystine level was obtained confirming the diagnosis of cystinosis.

INCIDENCE AND EPIDEMIOLOGY OF CYSTINOSIS

Cystinosis is a rare autosomal recessive lysosomal storage disorder that occurs in approximately 1 in 200 000 live births in North America. The carrier frequency is approximately 1 in 225 people. The disease predominately affects individuals of European descent; however, there have been reported cases in most ethnicities. Cystinosis results from a deletion or mutation of the *CTNS* gene on chromosome 17p13 which encodes for the cystine transport protein, cystinosin. As a result of this defect, intracellular cystine accumulates in almost all body cells and tissues.

CLINICAL PRESENTATION

Three forms of cystinosis exist and differ based on severity of symptoms and age of onset. Infantile or nephropathic cystinosis is the most common form and presents between 3 and 18 months of age. Patients develop symptoms of Fanconi syndrome including dehydration, electrolyte imbalance, failure to thrive, and rickets. With time, patients develop tubulointerstitial and glomerular disease leading to chronic renal failure. Infants with nephrogenic cystinosis are unable to sweat, and subsequently have frequent episodes of fever and flushing. Characteristic corneal crystals become evident by 1 year of age and may cause photophobia or eye irritation. Fifteen percent of patients develop corneal ulcerations; however, visual acuity is not usually affected until 10 years of age. Patients with infantile cystinosis may develop hypothyroidism in the first decade of life secondary to accumulation of cystine crystals in the thyroid follicles. Without therapy, all patients develop end-stage renal disease by 10 years of life.

The second type of cystinosis is juvenile cystinosis. Patients with this form of the disease present in adolescence with proteinuria and chronic renal failure but do not have Fanconi syndrome. These patients have slower progression to end-stage renal disease and do not display failure to thrive.

The third type of cystinosis is ocular nonnephropathic cystinosis. These patients present in adulthood with photophobia. They do not have Fanconi syndrome, nephropathy, or retinal depigmentation. Adults with this form of cystinosis have intracellular cystine levels that are only moderately increased (30-50 times normal), as compared to infants with cystinosis who have intracellular cystine levels that are 100-1000 times normal. In ocular cystinosis, cystine crystals only accumulate in the cornea, bone marrow, leukocytes, and skin fibroblasts.

DIAGNOSTIC APPROACH

Cystinosis should be considered in any infant presenting with Fanconi syndrome and failure to thrive.

Urine studies. Findings are consistent with Fanconi syndrome including proteinuria, glucosuria, aminoaciduria, and phosphaturia.

Leukocyte cystine content. Leukocytes from peripheral blood can be tested to evaluate for an elevated cystine level.

Ophthalmologic examination. Corneal crystals are usually apparent on ocular slit lamp examination in patients older than 1 year of age.

Skin biopsy. Skin fibroblasts can also be tested to evaluate for an elevated level of accumulated cystine. This test is usually unnecessary, as blood can be sent to obtain the same information.

Prenatal testing. Prenatal diagnosis can be established by demonstrating increased levels of cystine in cultured amniotic cells or in a chorionic villus sample.

TREATMENT

In the early stages of the disease, management is aimed at correcting electrolyte abnormalities resulting from Fanconi syndrome and improving growth. Patients often require oral supplementation of bicarbonate, potassium, phosphorus, and 1,25-dihydroxyvitamin D. They may also require enteral nutritional supplementation. As renal failure progresses, patients require a renal transplant. Fanconi syndrome does not recur in the transplanted kidney; however, cystine continues to accumulate in nonrenal tissues. As a result, patients may develop decreased visual acuity, corneal ulceration, retinal degeneration, pancreatic exocrine insufficiency, diabetes mellitus, hypothyroidism, delayed sexual maturation, infertility, and pulmonary disease. Patients who survive into late adulthood may develop progressive neurologic and muscular problems as cystine crystals accumulate in both the brain and muscle.

In addition to electrolyte replacement and renal transplant to manage the Fanconi syndrome, all patients should receive oral cysteamine therapy. Cysteamine enters the lysosome and reacts with cystine to form a compound that is able to be transported outside of the lysosome, thus reducing the amount of intracellular cystine. Oral cysteamine is helpful at any stage of the disease, but is most effective when initiated early. If cysteamine is started before 2 years of age, renal failure is slowed and growth is improved. Cysteamine should be continued even after renal transplant to help reduce cystine levels in nonrenal tissues. Cysteamine can be given in an intraocular topical formation to help prevent ocular complications.

SUGGESTED READINGS

1. Gahl WA, Thoene JG, Schneider JA. Cystinosis. *N Engl J Med*. 2002;347:111-121.
2. Gahl WA. Early oral cysteamine therapy for nephropathic cystinosis. *Eur J Pediatr*. 2003;162:S38-S41.
3. Greco M, Brugnara M, Zaffanello M, et al. Long-term outcome of nephropathic cystinosis: a 20-year single-center experience. *Pediatr Nephrol*. 2010;25:2459-2467.
4. Kalatzis V, Antignac C. New aspects of the pathogenesis of cystinosis. *Pediatr Nephrol*. 2003;18(3):207-215.
5. Markello TC, Bernardini IM, Gahl WA. Improved renal function in children with cystinosis treated with cysteamine. *New Engl J Med*. 1993;328:1157-1162.
6. Nesterova G, Gahl W. Nephropathic cystinosis: late complications of a multisystemic disease. *Pediatr Nephrol*. 2008;23:863-878.

CASE 3-4

Ten-Year-Old Girl

AMY FELDMAN

HISTORY OF PRESENT ILLNESS

The patient is a 10-year-old Caucasian female who presents with vomiting. She was in her usual state of health until 5 days ago when she developed nonbloody nonbilious emesis 5-7 times per day. She complains of a 2-day history of weakness, dizziness, and lethargy. She also admits to anorexia, decreased urine output, and a 5-pound weight loss during the past week. She denies fever, diarrhea, abdominal pain, rash, joint pain, or dysuria.

MEDICAL HISTORY

The patient has a history of mild intermittent asthma but has never required steroids or hospitalization. She uses albuterol intermittently but is not on any maintenance asthma medications. Her family history is negative for autoimmune diseases or gastrointestinal diseases.

PHYSICAL EXAMINATION

T 37.8°C; RR 28/min; HR 138/min; BP 108/53 mmHg

Weight (22.9 kg) 5th percentile; Height (150 cm) 95th percentile

Physical examination revealed a lean female in no acute distress. She had dry mucous membranes and there were numerous hyperpigmented macules scattered about the buccal surface of her mouth and on her tongue (see Figure 3-8). Her cardiovascular examination revealed tachycardia but she had normal rhythm and good peripheral pulses. Her pulmonary examination was normal. Her abdomen was soft, nontender, and nondistended without any hepatosplenomegaly or palpable masses. Neurologic examination was grossly normal. Her skin appeared slightly bronzed.

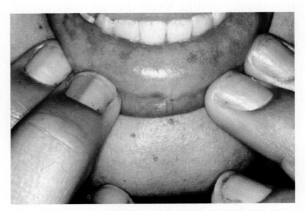

FIGURE 3-8. Skin and mucosal changes seen in primary adrenal insufficiency. *(Reproduced, with permission, from Strange GR, Ahrens WR, Schafermeyer RW, Wiebe RA, eds. Pediatric Emergency Medicine. 3rd ed. New York: McGraw-Hill; 2009.)*

DIAGNOSTIC STUDIES

Laboratory evaluation revealed a normal complete blood count. Serum chemistries were as follows: sodium, 123 mEq/L; potassium, 6.6 mEq/L; chloride, 95 mEq/L; bicarbonate, 14 mEq/L; blood urea nitrogen, 55 mg/dL; creatinine, 2.4 mg/dL; glucose, 40 mg/dL; calcium, 8.1 mg/dL; phosphorus, 5.2 mg/dL; and urinary sodium, 30 mEq/L. Urinalysis was notable for a specific gravity of 1.020 and three plus ketones. A venous blood gas had a pH of 7.25.

COURSE OF ILLNESS

The patient was admitted to the hospital and was given a normal saline bolus followed by an infusion of dextrose containing fluids. On further questioning, her mother reported that she had a 1-year history of salt craving and had recently developed dark spots on her body (see Figure 3-8). Based on the history, physical examination, and laboratory studies, she was given a presumptive diagnosis and was started on appropriate therapy.

DISCUSSION CASE 3-4

DIFFERENTIAL DIAGNOSIS

Patients who present with acute renal failure should first be categorized as having prerenal, renal, or postrenal azotemia. Prerenal azotemia is due to decreased renal perfusion secondary to hypovolemia, hypotension, hypoalbuminemia, or cardiac failure. Intrinsic acute renal failure is characterized by renal parenchymal damage and can be secondary to vascular dysfunction (renal vein thrombosis, hemolytic uremic syndrome, vasculitis), glomerular dysfunction (poststreptococcal, Henoch-Schönlein purpura, Lupus), or tubular dysfunction (acute tubular necrosis, interstitial nephritis, tumor lysis syndrome, drug-induced nephritis). Postrenal azotemia occurs secondary to obstruction of the urinary tract (posterior urethral valves, urolithiasis, hemorrhagic cystitis, tumor).

This patient's history of emesis and decreased oral intake, her physical examination of dry mucous membranes and weight loss, and her urinalysis with a high specific gravity and 3 plus ketones all suggest hypovolemic prerenal azotemia. Hypovolemia can occur from hemorrhage, vomiting and diarrhea, third spacing, or adrenal disease. Given the laboratory findings of hyperkalemia, hyponatremia, hypoglycemia, and high urine sodium, an adrenal etiology was suspected.

DIAGNOSTIC TESTS

Diagnosis of primary adrenal insufficiency begins with a basic metabolic panel that shows hypoglycemia, hyponatremia, and hyperkalemia. A 24-hour urine collection can be useful to look for high urinary excretion of sodium and low urinary excretion of potassium. The most definitive test for primary adrenal insufficiency is measurement of serum levels of cortisol before and after administration of ACTH. In primary adrenal insufficiency, resting levels of cortisol are low and do not increase normally after administration of ACTH.

DIAGNOSIS

This patient's histories of vomiting, anorexia, weight loss, salt craving, and hyperpigmentation were all suggestive of primary adrenal insufficiency

TABLE 3-6	Signs and symptoms of primary adrenal insufficiency.
Glucocorticoid Deficiency	
Hypoglycemia	
Increased insulin sensitivity	
Ketosis	
Decreased cardiac output, decreased vascular tone, hypotension	
Nausea, fatigue, headaches	
Hyperpigmentation	
Mineralocorticoid Deficiency	
Dehydration and weight loss	
Hypovolemia	
Hypotension	
Hyponatremia, hyperkalemia, acidosis	
Hyperreninemia	
Salt craving	
Androgen Deficiency	
Absence of secondary sexual characteristics	
Decreased pubic and axillary hair	
Decreased libido	

(see Table 3-6). Laboratory data of low serum sodium, glucose and bicarbonate, and elevated potassium and blood urea nitrogen were also consistent with the diagnosis. The patient underwent an ECG to ensure that her hyperkalemia was not causing cardiac abnormalities. The patient then underwent an ACTH stimulation test. Evaluation of the patient's blood obtained prior to administering ACTH revealed a low serum cortisol level and a high ACTH level. **After receiving ACTH, the patient failed to mount a cortisol response confirming the diagnosis of primary adrenal insufficiency.** She was started on appropriate glucocorticoid and mineralocorticoid IV replacement during hospitalization, which resulted in normalization of all of her labs. She was discharged home on oral hydrocortisone and Florinef.

INCIDENCE AND EPIDEMIOLOGY OF ADRENAL INSUFFICIENCY

Adrenal insufficiency can be primary or secondary in nature. In primary adrenal insufficiency (Addison disease), there is decreased or absent production of all three groups of adrenal steroid hormones. Primary adrenal insufficiency is uncommon and is estimated to affect 90 to 140 per

1 million people. Primary adrenal insufficiency can occur congenitally, or can develop later in life secondary to autoimmune destruction of the adrenal cortex, bilateral adrenal hemorrhage, adrenal degeneration (adrenoleukodystrophy), or adrenal injury from trauma, thrombosis, tumor, or infection (e.g., tuberculosis, meningococcemia).

The most likely etiology of primary adrenal insufficiency depends on the patient's age. At birth, the most common cause of adrenal insufficiency is adrenal hemorrhage from a perinatal event. In infants, congenital adrenal hyperplasia (CAH) is the most likely cause of adrenal insufficiency. In older children and adults living in developed countries, autoimmune destruction of the adrenal cortex is the most common cause of insufficiency. Forty-five percent of patients with autoimmune induced adrenal insufficiency have another autoimmune endocrinopathy or have autoimmune polyglandular syndrome. Type I autoimmune polyglandular syndrome is an autosomal recessive disorder resulting from mutation in the AIRE gene. It can result in chronic mucocutaneous candidiasis, ectodermal dysplasia, hypoparathyroidism, and Addison's disease. Type II autoimmune polyglandular syndrome can result in thyroid disease, Type I diabetes, and Addison disease.

Secondary adrenal insufficiency is more common and affects 150 to 280 per 1 million people. Secondary adrenal insufficiency is caused by lack of corticotropin-releasing hormone (CRH) or lack of adrenocorticotropic hormone (ACTH). These deficiencies may be the result of congenital abnormalities of the pituitary or hypothalamus, or may arise secondary to chronic steroid use or destruction of the pituitary/hypothalamus by infection, tumor, hemorrhage, or irradiation.

CLINICAL PRESENTATION

Primary adrenal insufficiency results in cortisol and aldosterone deficiency. As a result of these deficiencies, patients present with dehydration, hypoglycemia, hyperkalemia, ketosis, hypotension, and eventual shock.

The clinical presentation of a child with adrenal insufficiency depends on the age of the child and the etiology of the disease. Newborns and young infants often present in shock. They become ill during the course of a few days, and present with severe electrolyte abnormalities. Infants often will not have ketosis due to immature kidneys. In older children, adrenal insufficiency is often more insidious, taking several weeks or months to manifest. Older children present with muscle weakness, fatigue, anorexia, weight loss, emesis, and hypotension. Hyperkalemia may not be present initially.

Older children with primary adrenal insufficiency can develop hyperpigmentation, particularly on their skin, genitalia, and gingival and buccal mucosa. Hyperpigmentation results from cortisol deficiency. Without appropriate cortisol, there is decreased negative feedback on the hypothalamus and pituitary leading to increased secretion of ACTH and melanocyte-stimulating hormone. Infants usually do not display hyperpigmentation as this sign takes longer to develop.

The most worrisome presentation of primary adrenal insufficiency is the child who presents in adrenal crisis. These patients present in a shock-like state with labored breathing, hypotension, confusion, lethargy, and coma. Adrenal crisis is typically precipitated by an antecedent infection or bodily stress during which the body is unable to mount an adequate glucocorticoid response. This may occur in undiagnosed patients, or in previously diagnosed patients taking inadequate amounts of replacement therapy. In the absence of immediate and intensive therapy, the course can be rapidly fatal.

In patients with secondary adrenal insufficiency, there is no deficiency of mineralocorticoids. As a result, these patients present with fatigue, headaches, weakness, or hypotension but do not usually have electrolyte abnormalities. Hyperpigmentation does not occur because ACTH levels are not elevated.

DIAGNOSTIC RATIONALE

Diagnosing a patient with adrenal insufficiency depends on having a high index of suspicion as symptoms can be similar to those seen with gastroenteritis and other acute infections. Patients presenting with hyponatremia and hyperkalemia, especially in the setting of hyperpigmentation, should be considered to have adrenal insufficiency until proven otherwise.

Serum electrolytes. Hyponatremia, hypoglycemia, and hyperkalemia occur as described above.

Urinalysis. 24-hour urine collection shows high urinary excretion of sodium and chloride and decreased excretion of potassium.

Serum cortisol. The most definitive test for adrenal insufficiency is measurement of serum cortisol levels before and after administering ACTH. In a patient with primary adrenal insufficiency, resting cortisol levels are low and do not increase after administration of ACTH.

Other serum studies. Antiadrenal antibodies and other autoantibodies can be sent if an autoimmune etiology is suspected.

Abdominal CT scan. CT scan can be helpful in evaluating for calcifications, hemorrhage, or infiltration of the adrenal glands.

TREATMENT

Acute adrenal insufficiency is a life-threatening emergency that requires immediate treatment for shock and electrolyte abnormalities. After airway and breathing have been secured, intravenous or intraosseous access must be obtained immediately. Resuscitation continues with normal saline to correct hypotension and hyponatremia, and glucose to correct hypoglycemia. If hyperkalemia is severe, one must perform an ECG and consider therapies such as calcium carbonate, bicarbonate, insulin, or potassium-binding resins as necessary. Glucocorticoid therapy must be given when the diagnosis of adrenal insufficiency is entertained. Immediate management consists of 50-100 mg of hydrocortisone IV. If possible, blood levels of ACTH, cortisol, aldosterone, renin, 17-alpha-hydroxyprogesterone, and adrenal androgens should be obtained prior to giving hydrocortisone as steroids will change laboratory results. Mineralocorticoid therapy is not useful acutely because it takes several days for its sodium-retaining effects to occur. After the patient is stabilized, one must identify and treat the precipitating cause of the crisis if possible. Chronic therapy consists of daily replacement with hydrocortisone and fludrocortisone acetate (Florinef).

Patients with adrenal insufficiency need to be educated about their disease. Patients must understand the importance of increasing their hydrocortisone dose during periods of bodily stress. Every patient with primary adrenal insufficiency should wear a medical alert bracelet and carry stress dose steroids with them in case of an emergency.

SUGGESTED READINGS

1. Arlt W, Allolio B. Adrenal insufficiency. *Lancet.* 2003; 361:1881-1893.
2. Coursin DB, Wood KE. Corticosteroid supplementation for adrenal insufficiency. *JAMA.* 2002;287:236-240.
3. Laron Z. Hypoglycemia due to hormone deficiencies. *J Pediatr Endocrinol.* 1998;11:s117-s120.
4. Schatz DA, Winter DE. Autoimmune polyglandular syndrome: clinical syndrome and treatment. *Endocrinol Metabol Clin N Am.* 2002;31:339-352.
5. Shulman DI, Palmert MR, Kemp SF. Adrenal insufficiency: still a cause of morbidity and death in childhood. *Pediatrics.* 2007;119:e484-e494.
6. Ten S, New M, Maclaren N. Clinical review 130: Addison's disease. *J Clin Endocrinol Metab.* 2001;86:2909-2922.

CASE 3-5

Four-Year-Old Girl

AMY FELDMAN

HISTORY OF PRESENT ILLNESS

The patient is a 4-year-old female on interim maintenance chemotherapy for acute lymphoblastic leukemia (ALL) who presents to outpatient oncology clinic with emesis and bloody stools. She was doing well until 3 days prior to arrival when she developed decreased activity and anorexia. The following day she developed nonbloody, nonbilious emesis occurring about every 2 hours. The day before presentation, she had three bloody maroon colored stools. The morning before arrival to clinic, her emesis had increased to six times per hour and she had become listless at home. There was no history of fever, rash, abdominal pain, petechiae, or purpura. She had no sick contacts.

MEDICAL HISTORY

The patient was diagnosed with ALL 4 months ago. She last received chemotherapy 1 month ago. Her course has been uncomplicated except for one admission for pneumonia (1 month ago) and one admission for fever in the setting of a central line (1 week ago). During both admissions all of her blood cultures were negative.

PHYSICAL EXAMINATION

T 37.7°C; RR 28/min; HR 160 bpm; BP 100/60 mmHg

Weight 14.2 kg, 5th percentile (down from 16.6 kg 1 week ago); Height 150 cm, 95th percentile

General examination revealed a lethargic, disoriented child responding only to voice and painful stimuli. She had sunken eyes and dry mucous membranes without evidence of mucositis. Her cardiac examination revealed tachycardia but she had a regular rhythm with good peripheral perfusion. Her lung examination was normal. Her abdomen was distended but there was no tenderness, rebound, or guarding. Bowel sounds were hyperactive. There was a small amount of gross blood on rectal examination with no evidence of anal fissures or masses. Her cranial nerves were intact.

DIAGNOSTIC STUDIES

Laboratory evaluation revealed 10 200 white blood cells/mm³ with 6% band forms, 64% segmented neutrophils, 8% lymphocytes, and 20% monocytes. Her hemoglobin was 10 g/dL and her platelet count was 240 000 cells/mm³. Serum chemistries were as follows: sodium, 133 mmol/L; potassium, 3.2 mmol/L; chloride, 78 mmol/L; bicarbonate, 20 mEq/L; blood urea nitrogen, 105 mg/dL; creatinine, 1.4 mg/dL; glucose, 100 mg/dL; phosphorus, 7.2 mg/dL; uric acid, 20.6 mg/dL; bilirubin, 1.2 mg/dL; alanine aminotransferase, 342 U/L; aspartate aminotransferase, 96 U/L; lactate dehydrogenase, 1432 U/L; amylase, 36 U/L; lipase, 82 U/L; and ammonia, 24 µmol/L.

Abdominal radiographs showed multiple dilated loops of small bowel with no air in the distal large bowel. There was no visible free air in the abdominal cavity. Blood and urine cultures were drawn at the time of admission.

COURSE OF ILLNESS

The patient's altered mental status did not improve with fluid resuscitation. She was started on vancomycin and cefepime for broad-spectrum antibiotic coverage. She underwent a magnetic resonance imaging (MRI) of the head which was normal without signs of increased intracranial pressure or hemorrhage. A nasogastric tube was placed to decompress the abdomen. A CT scan of the abdomen was completed followed by a nuclear medicine imaging study which revealed the diagnosis (see Figure 3-9).

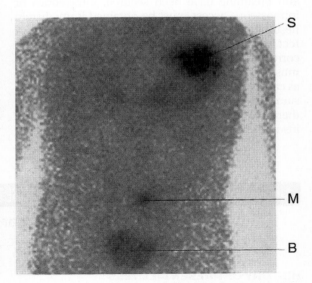

FIGURE 3-9. Meckel scan. *(Reproduced, with permission, from Sawin RS. Appendix and Meckel's diverticulum. In: Oldham KT, Colombani PM, Foglia RP, Skinner MA, eds. Principles and Practice of Pediatric Surgery. Philadelphia: Lippincott Williams & Wilkins; 2005:269-1282.)*

DISCUSSION CASE 3-5

DIFFERENTIAL DIAGNOSIS

The patient's abdominal radiograph with dilated loops of small bowel and a paucity of air in the large bowel suggested intestinal obstruction. The etiology of intestinal obstruction can be either intraluminal or extraluminal. In a 4-year-old child, causes of intraluminal obstruction include bezoars, fecal impaction, foreign bodies, intraluminal tumors, inflammatory bowel disease, parasites, or Hirschsprung disease. Extraluminal causes of obstruction in a child of this age include an incarcerated hernia, malrotation with volvulus, duplication system, extraluminal tumor or compressing lymph node, or adhesions from previous abdominal surgeries.

DIAGNOSTIC TESTS

In a child with suspected intestinal obstruction, blood tests are often normal early in the process. As vomiting and dehydration persist, the child may develop hemoconcentration, electrolyte abnormalities, and acidosis. Plain abdominal films in the upright and supine positions are helpful in evaluating the distribution of gas and fluid in the gastrointestinal tract. In complete obstruction, multiple air fluid levels and luminal dilation are seen proximally to the obstruction and the colon distal to the obstruction collapses. Perforation must be strongly considered if air is seen in the bowel wall, in the portal venous system, or within the peritoneal cavity. Contrast studies can be helpful in distinguishing ileus from obstruction. However, if perforation or colonic obstruction is suspected then barium should be avoided. Computed tomography can be helpful in localizing the obstruction and determining the etiology.

DIAGNOSIS

This patient had a CT scan that revealed a diverticulum with associated obstruction. A 99m-technetium(Tc)-pertechnetate scan was then performed which confirmed the presence of a Meckel diverticulum (see Figure 3-9). The patient was taken to the operating room where she was found to have a distal small bowel obstruction related to a Meckel diverticulum. The diverticulum was resected without any evidence of bowel wall infarction.

INCIDENCE AND EPIDEMIOLOGY OF A MECKEL DIVERTICULUM

A Meckel diverticulum is the most common congenital anomaly of the gastrointestinal tract, occurring in approximately 2% of the population. The diverticulum results from the incomplete obliteration of the vitelline duct, which connects the intestine to the yolk sac in the developing embryo. A Meckel diverticulum is usually 2 to 6 cm in length and is located on the antimesenteric border approximately 2 feet proximal to the ileocecal valve. Half of all Meckel diverticula will contain gastric, pancreatic, duodenal, or colonic ectopic tissue.

Meckel diverticula are more common in males, who also present more frequently with symptoms. They have been associated with other congenital anomalies including cardiac defects, cleft palate, and anorectal malformations.

CLINICAL PRESENTATION

Only 5% of all patients with a Meckel diverticulum will become symptomatic. Most frequently, symptomatic patients present within the first 3 years of life. The most common presentation is painless rectal bleeding, either bright red or maroon in color. Rectal bleeding is most often due to ectopic gastric tissue which produces acidic secretions that results in ulceration and bleeding. A Meckel diverticulum can also present with bowel obstruction resulting in abdominal pain, distension, and emesis. The most common reason for obstruction is when the diverticulum serves as a lead point for an intussusception. Obstruction can also result from intraperitoneal bands that connect the remnant vitelline duct to the ileum and umbilicus. Finally, a Meckel diverticulum can become inflamed (diverticulitis) resulting in severe right lower quadrant pain mimicking appendicitis. The inflamed diverticulum can perforate and result in peritonitis.

DIAGNOSTIC APPROACH

A Meckel diverticulum should be considered in any patient with painless rectal bleeding. Other causes of hematochezia are listed in Table 3-7. Plain abdominal radiographs and routine barium studies are not usually helpful in diagnosing a Meckel diverticulum.

TABLE 3-7.	Differential diagnosis for hematochezia.

Anal fissure
Hemorrhoid
Polyp
Arteriovenous malformation
Meckel diverticulum
Duplication system
Inflammatory bowel disease
Infectious colitis
Allergic proctitis

Meckel scan. The most useful study is a Meckel radionuclide scan which is performed after intravenous infusion of technetium-99m pertechnetate. The pertechnetate is taken up by gastric mucosa. In patients with ectopic gastric mucosa, there will be increased activity in the area of ectopic mucosa (usually the right lower quadrant). Uptake can be improved with administration of cimetidine, glucagon, or pentagastrin. In children, the Meckel scan has a sensitivity of 85% and a specificity of 95%. One must be aware of false positives and false negatives that may occur. False positives may arise from other sites of ectopic gastric mucosa, focal areas of small bowel pathology, vascular anomalies, bowel ulcerations, or bowel obstructions. False negatives may occur when the ectopic gastric tissue in the diverticulum is minimal or when the scintigraphic activity is diluted due to impaired vascular supply, brisk bleeding, or bowel hypersecretion.

Computerized axial tomography (CT scan). When the Meckel scan is nondiagnostic, a CT scan may be useful in detecting an inflamed or obstructing diverticulum.

LAPAROTOMY AND LAPAROSCOPY.

An inflamed Meckel diverticulum may be implicated as the cause of right lower quadrant abdominal pain or intestinal obstruction during surgical exploration. It may also be an incidental finding during abdominal surgery.

TREATMENT

Treatment starts with ensuring hemodynamic stability. Definitive therapy includes surgical resection of the Meckel diverticulum on an emergent or semi-elective basis. Associated intussusception usually requires surgical rather than hydrostatic reduction; partial bowel resection with primary anastomosis is occasionally required. The treatment of an asymptomatic Meckel diverticulum is less clear. Characteristics that may suggest an increased risk of developing complications, and thus a need for surgical removal, are younger age (<10 years), longer diverticulum (>2 cm), and a narrow base (<2 cm in diameter).

SUGGESTED READINGS

1. Bani-Hani K, Shatnawi N. Meckel's diverticulum: comparison of incidental and symptomatic cases. *World J Surg*. 2004;28:917-920.
2. Cullen JJ, Keith K, Moir C, Hodge D, Zinsmeister A, Melton J. Surgical management of Meckel's diverticulum. *Ann Surg*. 1994;220:564-569.
3. D'Agostino J. Common abdominal emergencies in children. *Emer Med Clin North Am*. 2002;20:139-153.
4. Sharma R, Jain V. Emergency surgery for Meckel's diverticulum. *World J Emerg Surg*. 2008;3:27.
5. Uppal K, Tubbs S, Matusz P, Shaffer K, Loukas M. Meckel's diverticulum: a review. *Clin Anat*. 2011;24:416-422.

CASE 3-6

Ten-Month-Old Girl

JOANNE N. WOOD

HISTORY OF PRESENT ILLNESS

The patient is a 10-month-old female who presents with a 1-day history of vomiting and fever to 38.3°C. The emesis is nonbloody and nonbilious.

She has a history of constipation and failure to thrive. She has had no recent changes in her stooling pattern of one hard bowel movement per week. Stooling is painful but is not associated with blood or mucous. Her mother uses prune juice, karo syrup, and laxatives to aid in bowel movements. The patient has had decreased oral intake for the past day with mild decreased urine output. Her mother also reports that the patient always has a distended abdomen.

MEDICAL HISTORY

She was born via spontaneous vaginal delivery at 39 weeks after an uncomplicated pregnancy. Her mother reports that the patient has been constipated since birth. She did not pass meconium prior to being discharged from the nursery on day 2 of life. She has a history of failure to thrive. She was growing at the 50th percentile until 4 months of age when her weight gain slowed and she began to cross percentiles on the growth curve. She also has a history of anemia, hypotonia, and developmental delay.

PHYSICAL EXAMINATION

T 38.7°C; RR 56/min; HR 150/min; BP 92/50 mmHg

Weight (6.2 kg); Length (66 cm); and Head circumference (40.5 cm), all significantly less than the 5th percentile for age

General examination revealed a pale, crying infant. Her heart and lungs were normal. Her abdomen was distended, tender with hypoactive bowel sounds, and a palpable mass in the right lower quadrant. There was no hepatomegaly or splenomegaly. Her neurologic examination was notable for general hypotonia.

DIAGNOSTIC STUDIES

Laboratory evaluation revealed 25 000 white blood cells/mm^3 with 81% segmented neutrophils, 10% lymphocytes, and 6% monocytes. The hemoglobin was 8.7 g/dL with hypochromia, occasional schistocytes, and burr cells. The MCV was 74.6 fL, the RDW was 23.2, and the reticulocyte count was 2.2%. The platelet count was 649 000 cells/mm^3. Serum chemistries were as follows: sodium, 137 mEq/L; potassium, 4.9 mEq/L; chloride, 115 mEq/L; bicarbonate, 18 mEq/L; blood urea nitrogen, 3 mg/dL; creatinine, 0.2 mg/dL; glucose, 98 mg/dL; alkaline phosphatase, 77 U/L; total bilirubin, 0.8 mg/dL; ALT, 98 U/L; and AST, 156 U/L.

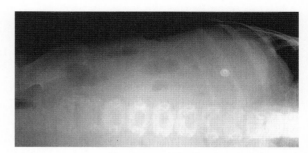

FIGURE 3-10. Abdominal radiograph.

COURSE OF ILLNESS

The chest radiograph was normal. An abdominal radiograph revealed findings that lead to an immediate therapeutic procedure (Figure 3-10).

DISCUSSION CASE 3-6

DIFFERENTIAL DIAGNOSIS

The abdominal radiograph revealed large pneumoperitoneum in this infant. Pneumoperitoneum on radiograph in a vomiting child with a distended, tender abdomen, and a palpable mass in the right lower quadrant, is a perforated hollow viscous until proven otherwise and requires immediate surgical exploration. Once the perforation is identified and repaired, the etiology of the perforation must be discovered and corrected.

In this case, the medical history of constipation since infancy suggests a potential underlying cause of the perforation. The differential diagnosis of constipation includes nonorganic or functional constipation, anatomic malformations (imperforate or anteriorly placed anus, stricture), abnormal abdominal musculature (prune-belly syndrome, gastroschisis, Down syndrome), intestinal nerve or muscle abnormalities (Hirschsprung disease, pseudo-obstruction secondary to visceral myopathies and neuropathies), metabolic/endocrine disorders (hypothyroidism, hypercalcemia, hypokalemia), spinal cord defects, drugs, intestinal disorders (celiac disease, inflammatory bowel disease, cystic fibrosis, cow's milk protein intolerance, tumor), connective tissue disorders, and botulism. Although in the majority of pediatric cases, constipation is attributed to nonorganic or functional constipation, there are features in this child's history that suggest an organic etiology. A history of hard stools that are passed only with difficulty in the neonatal period is suggestive of Hirschsprung disease, visceral myopathy, visceral neuropathy, or hypothyroidism. The delayed passage of meconium after 24 hours of life adds to the concern for Hirschsprung disease. In an infant with constipation and a history of delayed meconium cystic fibrosis should also be considered if an evaluation for Hirschsprung disease is negative. The history of failure to thrive and abdominal distention as well as the acute presentation with fever and vomiting also point to an organic etiology and are consistent with Hirschsprung disease.

DIAGNOSIS

The abdominal radiograph showed a moderate amount of free air in the abdomen suggesting bowel perforation (Figure 3-10). The patient was taken to the operating room where a large rush of air was felt upon entering the abdominal cavity. A massively dilated colon was discovered and an 18-cm segment of the colon was resected after a 3-mm perforation was found in the sigmoid colon. **Pathologic review of the resected segment confirmed the diagnosis of Hirschsprung disease.**

INCIDENCE AND EPIDEMIOLOGY OF HIRSCHSPRUNG DISEASE

Hirschsprung disease, the most common congenital cause of gut motility disorder, has an incidence of 1 in 5000 live births. Males are affected 2 to 4 times more often than females.

CLINICAL PRESENTATION

The clinical presentation of patients with Hirschsprung disease depends on the length of the aganglionic segment. In Hirschsprung disease, a failure in the craniocaudal migration of vagally derived neural crest cells in the hindgut during fetal development results in an aganglionic segment in the distal gut. The majority of cases (75%-80%) are classified as short-segment Hirschsprung disease because the aganglionosis is limited to the rectosigmoid area. In 20% of cases, long-segment Hirschsprung disease, aganglionosis extends proximal to the sigmoid. In less common variants of Hirschsprung disease the entire colon, the entire bowel, or only the distal rectum and anus are affected.

Most cases of Hirschsprung disease present in the neonatal period with failure to pass meconium within the first 24 hours of life and symptoms of intestinal obstruction including vomiting, abdominal distention, and refusal to feed. The passage of meconium occurs within the first 24 hours of life in more than 90% of normal neonates but in less than 10% of neonates with Hirschsprung disease. Some cases of short-segment Hirschsprung disease are detected later in infancy or childhood due to severe constipation with ribbon-like stools, persistent abdominal distention, vomiting, failure to thrive, and a rectum devoid of stool. Patients can also present with Hirschsprung's-associated enterocolitis which has a mortality of 20%. The signs and symptoms of HAEC may include fever, abdominal distension, foul-smelling stool, explosive diarrhea, vomiting, lethargy, rectal bleeding, and shock.

In the majority of cases Hirschsprung disease is an isolated disorder, but in 12% of cases it is associated with a chromosomal abnormality, and in 18% of cases it is associated with other congenital anomalies. Down syndrome is the most common chromosomal abnormality associated with Hirschsprung disease. Other syndromes associated with Hirschsprung disease include Smith-Lemli-Opitz syndrome, Waardenburg syndrome, Mowat-Wilson syndrome, congenital central hypoventilation syndrome, and Goldberg-Shprintzen syndrome.

DIAGNOSTIC APPROACH

A thorough history and physical examination should be performed in any child presenting with constipation. A history of delayed passage of meconium and signs of intestinal obstruction should prompt consideration of Hirschsprung disease. A history of ribbon-like stool, failure to thrive, and abdominal distention in an older child with severe constipation since birth should also lead to evaluation for Hirschsprung disease. The sudden onset of fever, abdominal distention, and foul-smelling explosive stool in a child with constipation raises concern for Hirschsprung's-associated enterocolitis.

A child with suspected Hirschsprung disease should be evaluated in a medical center with the facilities to perform the necessary diagnostic tests and the availability of pediatric gastroenterologists and pediatric surgeons. Evaluation should not be delayed as a delay in diagnosis and treatment increases the risk of Hirschsprung's-associated enterocolitis. There are multiple tests that may be helpful in diagnosing Hirschsprung disease, but rectal suction biopsy and anorectal manometry are the only tests that can reliably be used to exclude a diagnosis of Hirschsprung disease.

Abdominal radiographs. Plain abdominal radiographs in infants with Hirschsprung disease may show gaseous distention of the colon with a paucity of air in the rectum and a zone of transition in between.

Barium enema. In cases of Hirschsprung disease, a barium enema may show a zone of transition between a normally dilated proximal colon and the narrower aganglionic distal segment, irregular colonic contractions, irregular colonic mucosa, or an abnormal rectosigmoid index. A barium enema should not be used to diagnose Hirschsprung disease because of the risk of false negatives and false positives. Once a diagnosis of Hirschsprung disease is made, however, barium enema may be useful in determining the extent of the affected bowel. Also, barium enemas should not be performed if Hirschsprung's-associated enterocolitis is suspected due to the risk of perforation.

Anorectal manometry. The demonstration of a normal reflex relaxation of the internal anal sphincter in response to inflation of a balloon in the rectum can exclude a diagnosis of Hirschsprung disease. The test, however, can be difficult to perform and interpret in young infants.

Rectal biopsy. Rectal suction biopsy is the gold standard test for Hirschsprung disease. The presence of acetylcholinesteras positive nerve fibers and absence of ganglion is diagnostic for Hirschsprung disease. Occasionally, a full thickness rectal biopsy is needed if the suction biopsy is not diagnostic.

TREATMENT

Once a diagnosis of Hirschsprung disease is confirmed, plans for surgical management are necessary. In patients presenting acutely ill with Hirschsprung's-associated enterocolitis, fluid resuscitation, antibiotics, and rectal irrigation are indicated to stabilize the patient. Previously, patients underwent a multistage procedure. A temporary diverting ostomy was created first. Then when the child was older the aganglionic segment was resected and a coloanal anastamosis was performed. Some patients with enterocolitis, congenital anomalies, or other complications may still require an initial ostomy followed by a definitive repair at a later time. A laparoscopic single-stage endorectal pull-through procedure, however, is now the treatment of choice for most patients with Hirschsprung disease. Alternative approaches may be required for children with long-segment Hirschsprung disease and other less common forms of the disease.

SUGGESTED READINGS

1. Sreedharan R, Liacouras CA. Major symptoms and signs of digestive tract disorders. In: Kliegman RM, ed. *Nelson Textbook of Pediatrics.* 19th ed. Philadelphia: Saunders; 2011:1245-1247.
2. Constipation Guideline Committee of the North American Society for Pediatric Gastroenterology, Hepatology, and Nutrition. Evaluation and treatment of constipation in infants and children: recommendations of the North American Society for Pediatric Gastroenterology, Hepatology and Nutrition. *J Pediatr Gastroenterol Nutr.* Sep 2006; 43(3):e1-e13.
3. Kenny SE, Tam PKH, Garcia-Barcelo M. Hirschsprung's disease. *Semin Pediatr Surg.* 2010;19(3):194-200.
4. Amiel J, Sproat-Emison E, Garcia-Barcelo M, et al. Hirschsprung disease, associated syndromes and genetics: a review. *Journal of Medical Genetics.* January 1, 2008; 45(1):1-14.
5. Haricharan RN, Georgeson KE. Hirschsprung disease. *Seminars in Pediatric Surgery.* 2008;17(4):266-275.
6. Langer JC, Durrant AC, de la Torre L, et al. One-stage transanal soave pullthrough for Hirschsprung disease: a multicenter experience with 141 children. *Ann Surg.* October 2003;238(4):569-576.
7. Coran AG, Teitelbaum DH. Recent advances in the management of Hirschsprung's disease. *Am J Surg.* 2000; 180(5):382-387.
8. Jones KL. *Smith's Recognizable Patterns of Human Malformation.* 6th ed. Philadelphia, PA: Saunders; 2005.
9. Fiorino K, Liacouras CA. Congenital aganglionic megacolon (Hirschsprung disease). In: Kliegman RM, ed. *Nelson Textbook of Pediatrics.* 19th ed. Philadelphia: Saunders; 2011:1284-1287.

Two-Year-Old Boy

JOANNE N. WOOD

HISTORY OF PRESENT ILLNESS

The patient is a 2-year-old male who presents with a 2-day history of vomiting and abdominal pain. The emesis is bilious but nonbloody and the pain is periumbilical. He has had decreased urine output during the last day, although his oral intake has been good. His mother denies any history of fever or diarrhea.

MEDICAL HISTORY

The patient has been evaluated in the emergency department with nonbilious emesis three times in the past month. Each evaluation included normal electrolytes. A urinalysis performed at the last visit was within normal limits. The child was born at term by spontaneous vaginal delivery following an uncomplicated pregnancy. He has never been hospitalized nor had any surgeries. There is no family history of malignancy.

PHYSICAL EXAMINATION

T 37.8°C; RR 24/min; HR 88/min; BP 120/64 mmHg

Weight and Length are at the 75th percentile for age

The patient is resting comfortably and in no acute distress. His cardiac and pulmonary examinations are normal. His abdomen is soft, nontender with absent bowel sounds, and fullness in the left upper quadrant. There is no hepatomegaly or splenomegaly. His rectal examination reveals normal sphincter tone with hard guaiac negative stool in the rectal vault.

DIAGNOSTIC STUDIES

Laboratory evaluation revealed 23 000 white blood cells/mm³ with 1% band forms, 47% segmented neutrophils, 45% lymphocytes, and 7% monocytes. The hemoglobin was 12.2 g/dL and the platelet count was 300 000 cells/mm³. Serum electrolytes were normal.

COURSE OF ILLNESS

Abdominal radiographs show a left upper quadrant/flank mass displacing the bowel to the right. What are the most likely causes of an abdominal mass in this child?

DISCUSSION CASE 3-7

DIFFERENTIAL DIAGNOSIS

Vomiting associated with an abdominal mass is always an emergency and early imaging is imperative. The differential diagnosis of an abdominal mass in children includes organomegaly, malignant and nonmalignant tumors, congenital anomalies, and abscesses. The most likely etiology of an abdominal mass is dependent on the age of the child, location of the mass, and associated symptoms.

In young infants, the most common causes of abdominal masses are hydronephrosis and multicystic kidney which typically present as a flank mass. The most common cause of unilateral hydronephrosis is ureteropelvic junction obstruction, and posterior urethral valves (PUV) is the most common cause of bilateral hydronephrosis. Neonates with posterior urethral valves may also have a large palpable bladder. Hydronephrosis may also result from other causes of distal urinary tract obstruction and from renal vein thrombosis. Gastrointestinal duplications, gastrointestinal obstructions, ovarian cysts, and hydrometrocolpos can present as abdominal masses in neonates. Mesoblastic nephromas, which are usually benign tumors, can be seen in the neonatal period but are uncommon in older infants. Neuroblastoma is the most common malignant tumor in infants but Wilms tumor, extragonadal germ cell tumor, hepatoblastoma, and soft tissue sarcomas can also occur.

The likelihood of an abdominal mass being malignant is higher in older infants and children than in neonates. Neuroblastoma and Wilms tumor are the most common solid abdominal neoplasms in children but hepatocellular carcinoma, genitourinary tract rhabdomyosarcomas, teratomas, and ovarian germ cell tumors can also occur.

The location of the mass can provide clues regarding its likely origin (see Table 3-8). Right upper quadrant (RUQ) masses frequently arise from the liver. Nonmalignant hepatic masses include polycystic liver disease, benign hepatic tumors, vascular lesions, storage disease, abscesses, and hepatitis. Choledochal cysts and gall bladder obstruction may also present with RUQ masses while splenic lesions may present with LUQ masses. Flank and upper quadrant masses may be due to renal or adrenal etiologies. Right lower quadrant masses in a child with signs and symptoms of inflammation suggest an abscess from a ruptured appendix or inflammatory bowel disease.

In this patient, the location of the mass in the left upper quadrant to flank area is suggestive of a renal, adrenal, or splenic etiology. The history of decreased urinary output despite normal intake raises the possibility of an obstructive uropathy.

DIAGNOSIS

The patient was admitted to the hospital and underwent an abdominal sonogram that revealed a large cystic renal lesion. **Diuretic renography showed delayed emptying in an enlarged kidney with evidence of obstruction at the proximal ureter suggesting the diagnosis of ureteropelvic junction obstruction.** The diuretic renography also demonstrated decreased renal function. A nephrostomy tube was placed and the patient was discharged home with follow-up in 3 weeks for either pyeloplasty or nephrectomy if kidney function remained poor.

INCIDENCE AND EPIDEMIOLOGY OF URETEROPELVIC JUNCTION OBSTRUCTION

Ureteropelvic junction (UPJ) obstruction, the most common obstructive uropathy in children, has an annual incidence of 5 cases per 100 000.

There is a 2:1 male to female predominance. In the vast majority of cases (90%) only one kidney is affected with the left kidney being affected in 60% of cases.

CLINICAL PRESENTATION

Ureteropelvic junction obstruction is characterized by a blockage at the junction of the renal pelvis and the ureter that prevents urine from passing from the renal pelvis to the bladder. The blockage may be intrinsic or extrinsic in nature and can result from congenital or acquired conditions. The majority of cases of UPJ obstruction, however, are congenital and result from an intrinsic obstruction caused by an aperistaltic proximal segment of the ureter. Ureteral polyps, valvular mucosal folds, persistent fetal convolutions, and aberrant arteries are less common causes of congenital UPJ obstruction.

The majority of patients with congenital UPJ obstructions are now diagnosed prenatally on fetal ultrasound. Cases of congenital UPJ obstruction not detected on prenatal ultrasound may present in infancy with a painless palpable flank mass, poor feeding, or failure to thrive. Older children may present with episodes of colicky abdominal or flank pain accompanied by nausea and vomiting. Patients with UPJ obstruction may also present with hematuria after minor trauma or recurrent urinary tract infections.

DIAGNOSTIC APPROACH

Although the majority of cases of congenital UPJ obstruction are diagnosed prenatally, the diagnosis can be difficult to make in cases of asymptomatic infants with incidental renal pelvis dilation on prenatal ultrasound.

Renal and bladder ultrasonography. Ultrasonography is usually the preferred primary imaging study when an obstructive uropathy is suspected. A finding of dilated renal pelvis on fetal ultrasound should be evaluated with an ultrasound after birth. If possible, the ultrasound should be performed after the third day of life because of the oliguric state of newborns. If the ultrasonography is normal, it should be repeated in 1 month. Ultrasonography is also used to evaluate suspected cases of

Region	Organ	Malignant Disease	Nonmalignant Disease
Flank	Kidney	• Wilms tumor • Renal cell carcinoma • Lymphomatous nephromegaly • Clear cell carcinoma	• Hydronephrosis • Multicystic kidney disease • Polycystic kidney disease • Mesoblastic nephroma • Renal vein thrombosis
	Adrenal	• Carcinoma • Neuroblastoma • Pheochromocytoma	• Adenoma • Hemorrhage
	Retroperitoneal	• Neuroblastoma	
Right Upper Quadrant	Hepatic	• Hepatoblastoma • Hepatocellular carcinoma • Metastases • Mesenchymoma	• Focal nodular hyperplasia • Hemangioendothelioma • Hamartoma • Hepatitis • Storage disease • Abscess
	Biliary tree	• Leiomyosarcoma	• Obstruction • Hydrops • Choledochal cyst
	R. Adrenal	• See adrenal above	• See adrenal above
	R. Kidney	• See renal above	• See renal above
	Intestine		• Intussusception • Duplication
	Stomach		• Pyloric stenosis
Left Upper Quadrant	Spleen	• Leukemia • Lymphoma • Histiocytosis X	• Storage disease • Cysts • Mononucleosis • Congestive splenomegaly
	Intestine		• Intussusception
	L. Adrenal	• See adrenal above	• See adrenal above
	L. Kidney	• See kidney above	• See kidney above
Right Lower Quadrant	R. Ovary	• Germ cell tumor	• Cyst
	Intestine		• Abscess
	Lymphatic	• Lymphoma	• Lymphangioma
Left Lower Quadrant	L. Ovary	• Germ cell tumor	• Cyst
	Lymphatic	• Lymphoma	• Lymphangioma
	Intestine		• Stool
Pelvic	Bladder	• Rhabdomyosarcoma	• Obstruction
	Other	• Pelvic neuroblastoma	
	GU tract	• Rhabdomyosarcoma	• Hydrometrocolpos
Epigastric	Stomach		• Pyloric stenosis • Bezoar
	Pancreas	• Pancreatoblastoma	• Pseudocyst

TABLE 3-8. Malignant and nonmalignant etiologies of abdominal masses in children by location and organ.

This list includes many but not all of the etiologies of pediatric abdominal masses described in the literature.[3,4,6,14]

UPJ obstruction presenting in childhood. Ultrasonography can provide information on the laterality and severity of the hydronephrosis as well as changes to the renal parenchyma.

Voiding cystourethrography. Voiding cystourethrography (VCUG) is frequently performed in cases of hydronephrosis from UPJ obstruction to evaluate for associated vesicoureteral reflux (VUR).

Diuretic renography. In cases of congenital obstructive uropathy including UPJ obstruction, diuretic renography with 99m-Tc-mercaptoacetyltriglycine (MAG3) is considered the gold standard test for functional imaging. The uptake of the tracer during the diuretic renography provides a measure of the function of the kidney. The diuretic renography is also used to confirm the obstruction and assess the severity of the obstruction.

Magnetic resonance imaging. Magnetic resonance imaging has the potential to assess both anatomy and function but its use in cases of obstructive uropathy has not yet been fully validated.

TREATMENT

Historically open pyeloplasty was the treatment of choice for patients with congenital UPJ obstruction and was performed early with the goal of preserving renal function. More recently, however, selected cases of prenatally diagnosed congenital UPJ obstruction are undergoing conservative management. Infants with UPJ obstruction associated with an abdominal mass, bilateral severe hydronephrosis, a solitary kidney, or decreased renal function in the affected kidney still require prompt surgical intervention. Asymptomatic cases with good renal function, however, may be followed with serial renal ultrasounds and repeat diuretic renography. Indications for surgical intervention include symptoms related to UPJ obstruction, worsening renal function, stones, urinary tract infections, or hypertension. In select circumstances a percutaneous nephrostomy may be inserted to allow for drainage of the hydronephrotic kidney for a few weeks and then renal function is reassessed.

For patients who do require surgical interventions, less invasive procedures including percutaneous endopyelotomy, ureteroscopic endopyelotomy, and cautery wire balloon endopyelotomy have been developed in recent years as alternatives to open pyeloplasty. Unfortunately, the success rates with these techniques has been lower than with open pyeloplasty. Laparoscopic pyeloplasty, however, has been shown to have success rates similar to open pyeloplasty and is associated with reduced length of hospital stay and decreased morbidity. Laparoscopic pyeloplasty may not be universally available especially for pediatric patients. Robotic-assisted laparoscopic pyeloplasty techniques have also been developed but its advantages over regular laparoscopic pyeloplasty have not been clearly demonstrated.

SUGGESTED READINGS

1. Crane GL, Hernanz-Schulman M. Current imaging assessment of congenital abdominal masses in pediatric patients. *Semin Roentgenol.* 2012;47(1):32-44.
2. Mahaffey SM, Ryckman FC, Martin LW. Clinical aspects of abdominal masses in children. *Semin Roentgenol.* Jul 1988;23(3):161-174.
3. Chandler JC, Gauderer MW. The neonate with an abdominal mass. *Pediatr Clin North Am.* Aug 2004; 51(4):979-997, ix.
4. Brodeur AE, Brodeur GM. Abdominal masses in children: neuroblastoma, Wilms tumor, and other considerations. *Pediatr Rev.* January 1, 1991; 12(7):196-206.
5. Golden CB, Feusner JH. Malignant abdominal masses in children: quick guide to evaluation and diagnosis. *Pediatr Clin N Am.* 2002;49(6):1369-1392.
6. Zitelli BJ, McIntire SC, Nowalk AJ, eds. Zitelli and Davis' Atlas of Physical Diagnosis, 6th ed. Philadelphia: Saunders, 2012.
7. Canes D, Berger A, Gettman MT, Desai MM. Minimally invasive approaches to ureteropelvic junction obstruction. *Urol Clin N Am.* 2008;35(3):425-439.
8. Elder JS. Obstruction of the urinary tract. In: Kliegman RM, ed. *Nelson Textbook of Pediatrics.* 19th ed. Philadelphia: Saunders; 2011:1838-1847.
9. Peters CA, Chevalier RL. Congenital urinary obstruction: pathophysiology and clinical evaluation. In: Wein AJ, ed. *Campbell-Walsh Urology.* 10th ed. Philadelphia: Saunders; 2012:3028-3047.
10. Lam JS, Breda A, Schulam PG. Ureteropelvic junction obstruction. *J Urology.* 2007;177(5):1652-1658.
11. Schulam PG. Ureteropelvic junction obstruction. In: Litwin MS, Saigal CS, ed. *Urologic Diseases in America.* Washington DC: US Department of Health and Human Services, Public Health Service, National Institutes of Health, National Institute of Diabetes and Digestive and Kidney Diseases; 2012.
12. Nadu A, Mottrie A, Geavlete P. Ureteropelvic junction obstruction: which surgical approach? *Eur Urol Suppl.* 2009;8:778-781.
13. Braga LHP, Pace K, DeMaria J, Lorenzo AJ. Systematic review and meta-analysis of robotic-assisted versus conventional laparoscopic pyeloplasty for patients with ureteropelvic junction obstruction: effect on operative time, length of hospital stay, postoperative complications, and success rate. *Eur Urol.* 2009; 56(5):848-858.
14. Milla SS, Lee EY, Buonomo C, Bramson RT. Ultrasound evaluation of pediatric abdominal masses. *Ultrasound Clinics.* 2007;2(3):541-559.

CASE 3-8

Two-Year-Old Girl

KAMILLAH N. WOOD

HISTORY OF PRESENT ILLNESS

The patient is a 2-year-old African-American female who presents with vomiting for 1 week. The emesis is nonbloody and nonbilious occurring daily. After vomiting, the patient refuses to eat for the rest of the day. She has normal activity level and normal urine and stool output. The patient's mother feels that the child's face is swollen but denies any history of fever, diarrhea, and abdominal pain or weight loss.

MEDICAL HISTORY

She is a 36-week infant born via cesarean section secondary to fetal distress. She remained in the neonatal intensive care unit for 8 days, but has no residual problems. She has not required any surgery.

PHYSICAL EXAMINATION

T 36.5°C; RR 22/min; HR 111/min; BP 94/67 mmHg

Weight (14.8 kg) 75th percentile; Length (91 cm) 50th percentile

General examination reveals an alert child in no acute distress. Her cardiac and pulmonary examinations are normal. She has no hepatomegaly and no splenomegaly or costovertebral angle tenderness. Her examination was notable only for periorbital swelling and pitting edema of both lower extremities.

DIAGNOSTIC STUDIES

Laboratory evaluation revealed 14 600 white blood cells/mm^3 with 6% band forms, 34% segmented neutrophils, 55% lymphocytes, 6% eosinophils, and 5% monocytes. The hemoglobin was 14.7 g/dL and the platelet count was 383 000 cells/mm^3. Serum chemistries were as follows: sodium, 130 mmol/L; potassium, 3.5 mmol/L; chloride, 103 mmol/L; bicarbonate, 24 mEq/L; blood urea nitrogen,

9 mg/dL; creatinine, 0.4 mg/dL; glucose, 103 mg/dL; bilirubin, 0.1 mg/dL; ALT, 36 U/L; AST, 49 U/L; albumin, 1.4 g/dL; cholesterol, 122 mg/dL; ESR, 0 mm/h; and urinalysis negative (no protein). Chest and abdominal radiographs were normal.

COURSE OF ILLNESS

The patient was evaluated for a protein losing enteropathy because of hypoalbuminemia without proteinuria. An upper gastrointestinal contrast procedure and endoscopy were performed which confirmed the diagnosis (Figure 3-11).

DISCUSSION CASE 3-8

DIFFERENTIAL DIAGNOSIS

The patient was noted to have generalized edema associated with vomiting. Generalized edema may be caused by four mechanisms: (1) increased capillary permeability, (2) decreased oncotic pressures,

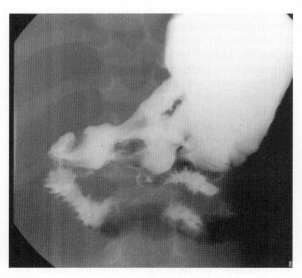

FIGURE 3-11. Upper gastrointestinal barium study.

TABLE 3-9.	Causes of hypoalbunemia.
Decreased Production	**Increased Loss (GI or Renal)**
Malnutrition	Impaired pancreatic
Liver cirrhosis	function
Viral hepatitis	Bacterial overgrowth in the
Autoimmune liver	small intestine
disease	Gastrointestinal infec-
Hepatic malignancy	tions (viral, bacterial, and
Metabolic disease	parasitic)
Budd Chiari leading to	Protein losing enteropathy
acute liver failure	Inflammatory bowel
Acetaminophen toxicity	disease
	Bowel resection
	Nephrotic syndrome
	Renal failure
	Renal amylodosis
	Cystic fibrosis
	Medications (neomycin)
	Severe burns (protein loss
	through exudation)

(3) increased hydrostatic pressures, or (4) impaired lymphatic drainage. Once cardiovascular disease has been ruled out as the cause of generalized edema it is usually secondary to hypoproteinemia of renal origin. This patient's generalized edema was attributed to decreased oncotic pressure from hypoproteinemia. Hypoproteinemia is due to either decreased production of proteins by the liver or increased renal or gastrointestinal losses. The causes of hypoalbunemia are summarized in Table 3-9. A negative urinalysis for protein and no evidence of hepatic disease makes a protein-losing enteropathy much more likely. Differential diagnosis of a protein-losing enteropathy includes celiac disease, Crohn disease, cystic fibrosis, intestinal lymphangiesctasia, gastritis, and eosinophillic gastritis, and Ménétrier disease.

DIAGNOSIS

After determining that the patient most likely had a protein-losing enteropathy, she underwent an upper gastrointestinal barium study that showed evidence of hypertrophic gastric folds (thumb printing and enlarged folds within the gastric antrum) (Figure 3-11). **The upper endoscopy performed the next day showed normal anatomy with histologic proof of Ménétrier disease including foveolar (pits) hyperplasia and marked oxyntic glandular loss with accompanying cystic changes.** Cytomegalovirus (CMV) serum IgM was positive and CMV was isolated from the urine by rapid shell vial testing.

INCIDENCE AND EPIDEMIOLOGY OF MÉNÉTRIER'S DISEASE

Ménétrier disease is an extremely rare condition with about 60 reported cases in the pediatric population. Initially described in 1888, it is characterized by a protein-losing gastropathy, gastric rugae hyperplasia, and hypoproteinemia. The gastric hyperplasia is a result of an increase of mucous cells with parietal cell atrophy, creating an altered gastric mucosa that secretes massive amounts of mucous. This results in low plasma protein levels with subsequent edema. Over a third of all pediatric cases show acute evidence of CMV infection, and some cases have been linked to *Helicobacter pylori* infection. The condition usually occurs in children under 10 years of age with a mean age of 5.6 years and a three to one male predominance. The etiology is felt to be due to an elevated transforming growth factor alpha (TGF-α) that triggers abnormal regulation of gastric epithelial growth factors.

TYPICAL PRESENTATION

The onset of clinical symptoms is abrupt, usually occurring 1 to 2 weeks after a viral prodrome. Gastrointestinal symptoms predominate with almost 80% having emesis, 50% with abdominal pain or anorexia, and 10% with frank upper gastrointestinal bleeding. Almost all patients present with generalized edema and a third with pleural effusions. Characteristic laboratory abnormalities include a low serum albumin and low total serum protein levels.

DIAGNOSTIC RATIONALE

Diagnosing Ménétrier disease when the clinical presentation is supportive depends on a combination of laboratory evaluation, radiographic findings, and endoscopic results.

Complete blood count. Laboratory findings are nonspecific and include a mild normochromic, normocytic anemia in 20% and eosinophilia in 60%.

Hepatic function panel. A low serum albumin, usually less than 2 g/dL, is supportive. Examination of the hepatic enzymes helps to discern whether a dysfunction of synthetic function is causing the hypoalbuminemia, but should be relatively normal in Ménétrier disease.

Upper gastrointestinal barium study. Contrast radiographs show swollen gastric rugae of the fundus and body with antral sparing which are pathonomonic for this disease. Diagnosis by ultrasonography has also been described.

Endoscopy. Endoscopy shows swollen convoluted rugae. Histologicfeatures include tortuous pits with cystic dilatations that may extend into the muscularis mucosae and submucosa, and an edematous lamina propria with increased numbers of eosinophils, lymphocytes, and round cells. Mucosal thickening, glandular atrophy, and hypochlorhydria occur. In addition, infectious studies can be obtained from the biopsy, including testing for *H. pylori*.

TREATMENT

Treatment for Ménétrier disease is mostly supportive including a high-protein diet, acid blockers to treat gastric inflammation, and diuretics to reduce edema. Appropriate therapy should be instituted in cases associated with *H. pylori*. The condition is self-limited usually resolving within weeks to months without recurrence or sequelae. Cases in adults tend to be more chronic, commonly requiring surgery and are also associated with an increased risk of gastric cancer.

SUGGESTED READINGS

1. Menetrier's Disease Feldman: *Sleisenger & Fordtran's Gastrointestinal and Liver Disease.* 6th ed. W. B. Philadelphia: Saunders Company; 1998:724-726.
2. Hassall E. Peptic diseases. In: Rudolph CD, Rudolph AM, eds. *Rudolph's Pediatrics.* 21st ed. New York: McGraw-Hill; 2003:1429-1435.
3. Meuwissen SG, Ridwan BU, Hasper HJ. Hypertrophic protein-losing gastropathy: a retrospective analysis of 40 cases in the Netherlands (The Dutch Menetrier Study Group). *Scan J Gastroenterol.* 1992;194:s1-s7.
4. Zenkl B, Zieger MM. Menetrier disease in a child of 18 months: diagnosis by ultrasonograph. *Eur J Pediatr.* 1988;147:330-331.
5. Fretzayas A, Moustaki M, Alexopoulou E, Nicolaidou P. Menetrier's disease associated with Helicobacter pylori: three cases with sonographic findings and a literature review. *Ann Trop Paediatr.* 2011;31(2):141-147.
6. Iwama I, Kagimoto S, Takano T, Sekijima T, Kishimoto H, Oba A. Case of pediatric Menetrier disease with cytomegalovirus and Helicobacter pylori co-infection. *Pediatr Int.* 2010;52(4):200-203.

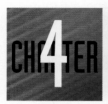

CHAPTER 4   COUGH

DEBRA BOYER
STEPHANIE ZANDIEH

DEFINITION OF THE COMPLAINT

Cough is one of the most common presenting complaints to pediatricians. Importantly, a cough is not a disease by itself, but rather a manifestation of an underlying pathology. A cough is a protective action, and can be initiated both voluntarily and via stimulation of cough receptors located throughout the respiratory tract (ear, sinuses, upper and lower airway to the level of the terminal bronchioles, pleura, pericardium, and diaphragm). A cough may serve to remove irritating substances, excessive/abnormal secretions, or may be secondary to intrinsic/extrinsic airway compression.

A cough is divided into four distinct phases: inspiratory, compressive, expiratory, and relaxation. These phases are characterized by deep inspiration, closure of the glottis, contraction of expiratory muscles with glottic opening, and relaxation of intercostal and abdominal muscles. Thus, one can see how selective patients with laryngeal or neuromuscular diseases may have ineffective coughs.

Classification should initially involve differentiating an acute from a chronic cough. A chronic cough is one which lasts longer than 3 weeks. Furthermore, the clinical description of the cough can often be helpful in suggesting an etiology: staccato (pertussis, chlamydia), barking (croup), grunting (asthma), or honking (psychogenic). Timing of the cough, relationship to daily activities, and age of the patient are important factors in further defining the etiology (Table 4-1).

COMPLAINT BY CAUSE AND FREQUENCY

Overall, some of the most common causes of chronic cough include viral upper respiratory tract infections and asthma (Table 4-2). Beyond these etiologies, age is very important in creating a differential diagnosis for the patient with a chronic cough (Table 4-3). Causes of cough may also be divided by diagnostic category including infectious, allergic/inflammatory, congenital malformations, irritants, aspiration, psychogenic, and other categories (Table 4-4).

CLARIFYING QUESTIONS

In most cases of a child who presents with a cough, the diagnosis is obtained with a thorough history and physical examination. The following questions may help to define the diagnosis:

* Did the cough begin with an upper respiratory tract infection?
  —The most common cause for a cough is a viral upper respiratory tract infection. This can occur with or without reactive airways disease/asthma. Without other significant generalized signs of illness or respiratory distress, often no significant initial evaluation or therapy is necessary. Many young children will have frequent (6–8) viral infections per year accompanied by a cough, giving the appearance of chronic cough.

* Are there systemic signs or symptoms that may suggest a particular etiology?

| TABLE 4-1. | History and physical examination for cough. | | | | | |

History

Age of onset	Time Frame	Triggers	Characteristics of Cough	Associated Symptoms	Environmental Influences	Response to Previous Therapy
Infant, Toddler, Adolescent	Acute < 3 weeks, Chronic > 3weeks	Activity; laughing or crying; exposure to cold air; changes in weather; recent upper or lower respiratory tract infection; recent choking episode	Dry vs. Moist Timing of cough (day, night, during sleep, with exercise, change of position, after liquids or solid) Type (croupy, brassy, staccato-like)	Fever Headache Weight loss Dysphagia Wheezing Dyspnea Hemoptysis Conjunctivitis	Exposure to cigarette smoke, wood stove, kerosene heater, dog or cat dander, dust or pollens	Over-the-counter medications, bronchodilators, oral or inhaled steroids, antibiotics

Physical Examination

Growth and Development	Nutritional Status	HEENT	Chest Examination	Heart Examination	Abdominal	Extremities	Skin
Height, Weight, and Head Circumference Appropriate Milestones	BMI	Allergic shinners, foreign body in ear, cobble-stoning of posterior pharynx sinus tenderness, nasal polyps	Increased anterior-posterior diameter of the chest, retractions, wheeze, crackles, hyper-resonance	Abnormal heart sounds	Hepato-and/or spleno-megaly	Digital clubbing	Eczema

—Fevers, sinus tenderness, and headaches can be present with sinusitis. Weight loss and night sweats may indicate tuberculosis or malignancy. Dysphagia suggests an esophageal foreign body, whereas dysphonia indicates laryngeal or glottic pathology.

| TABLE 4-2. | Most common causes of cough in children. |

Upper respiratory tract infections
Gastroesophageal reflux
Sinusitis
Croup
Asthma
Sinusitis
Bronchiolitis
Allergic rhinitis/postnasal drip

• In young infants, is there any history of conjunctivitis in association with a cough and tachypnea?
—Conjunctivitis and pneumonitis in a young infant may suggest infection due to *Chlamydia trachomatis.*

• Are there environmental stimuli that may irritate the airway?
—Passive smoke in infants and young children and active smoking in adolescents can trigger a chronic cough. Solvent fumes as well as recreational drug use can exacerbate a chronic cough.

• How is the cough related to time of day and to daily activities?
—A cough which is most prominent during or after eating is suggestive of aspiration or gastroesophageal reflux. If exposure to cold air and exercise precipitates the cough, reactive airway

TABLE 4-3.	Causes of cough in childhood by age.		
Disease Prevalence	*Infant*	*Preschool*	*School Age/Adolescent*
Common	Infectious -viral (RSV) -*Chlamydia trachomatis* -pertussis	Infectious -viral -*M. pneumoniae* -pertussis -bacterial	Infectious -viral -*M. pneumoniae* -pertussis
	Gastroesophageal reflux	Reactive airway disease/asthma	Reactive airway disease/asthma
		Foreign body aspiration	Psychogenic -habit cough -vocal cord dysfunction

Less Common	Congenital malformations
	-TE fistula
	-tracheobronchomalacia
	-vascular ring
	-lobar emphysema
	-bronchogenic cyst
	-pulmonary sequestration
	-laryngeal cleft
	-airway hemangiomas
	-congenital pulmonary airway
	  malformation (CPAM)
		Congenital malformations
		-TE fistula
		-tracheobronchomalacia
		-vascular ring
		-lobar emphysema
		-bronchogenic cyst
		-pulmonary sequestration
		-laryngeal cleft
		-airway hemangiomas
		-congenital pulmonary airway
		  malformation (CPAM)
			Infectious
			-bacterial pneumonia
			-HIV
			-measles
			-tuberculosis
			-fungal

	Infectious -bacterial pneumonia -HIV -measles -tuberculosis -fungal	Infectious -bacterial pneumonia -HIV -measles -tuberculosis -fungal	Allergic rhinitis/postnasal drip
	Cystic fibrosis	Cystic fibrosis	Cystic fibrosis
		Allergic rhinitis/postnasal drip	Sinusitis
		Sinusitis	Aspiration -GER -swallowing dysfunction
	Aspiration -GER -swallowing dysfunction	Aspiration -GER -swallowing dysfunction	Smoking
	Congestive Heart Failure	Croup	Foreign body aspiration
	Toxic exposure -passive smoke exposure -fume exposure	Toxic exposure -passive smoke exposure -fume exposure	
	Bronchopulmonary dysplasia		
Uncommon	Primary ciliary dyskinesia	Primary ciliary dyskinesia	Primary ciliary dyskinesia
	Interstitial pneumonitis	Hypersensitivity pneumonitis	Hypersensitivity pneumonitis
	Congenital immunodeficiency	Interstitial pneumonitis Congenital immunodeficiency Bronchiectasis Malignancy Airway papillomas Granulomatous disorders	Interstitial pneumonitis Congenital immunodeficiency Bronchiectasis Malignancy Airway papillomas Granulomatous disorders

TABLE 4-4.	Cause of cough in childhood by etiology.
Infectious	Viral Chlamydia species Pertussis Tuberculosis Fungal Sinusitis Human immunodeficiency virus Bacterial pneumonia Croup
Allergy/ Inflammatory	Allergic rhinitis/postnasal drip Reactive airway disease/asthma Hypersensitivity pneumonitis
Congenital Malformations	Tracheoesophageal fistula Tracheobronchomalacia Vascular rings Lobar emphysema Bronchogenic cysts Pulmonary sequestration Laryngeal cleft Congenital pulmonary airway malformation
Irritants	Active/passive smoking Fume exposure
Aspiration	Gastroesophageal reflux Neuromuscular diseases Foreign body aspiration
Psychogenic	Habit cough Vocal cord dysfunction
Miscellaneous	Cystic fibrosis Malignancy Bronchopulmonary dysplasia Congestive heart failure Interstitial pneumonitis Primary ciliary dyskinesia Granulomatous diseases

disease should be considered. Seasonal coughing suggests an allergic component. Similarly, a nighttime cough may indicate postnasal drip secondary to either allergies or sinusitis.

- Does the cough resolve with sleep?
  —Coughs which disappear when the patient is asleep or appear only when an adult is present may suggest a psychogenic cough.

- Is there a history of a choking episode?
  —Often, a significant choking episode occurs at the time of foreign body ingestion. For this reason, a thorough history is essential. Foreign body aspiration is most common in toddlers; however,

older siblings can often place inappropriate objects in the mouth of infants. If foreign body aspiration is suspected, one should obtain either lateral decubitus or inspiratory and expiratory chest roentgenograms.

- Is there a history of recurrent pneumonias or other infections?
  —Recurrent infections should cause one to consider immune dysfunction such as HIV and congenital immunodeficiencies. Recurrent pneumonias associated with sinusitis, multiple otitis medias, bronchiectasis, and situs inversus, suggest primary ciliary dyskinesia.

- How is the patient's growth?
  —Failure to thrive, steatorrhea, and recurrent pneumonias can occur with cystic fibrosis. Other features suggestive of cystic fibrosis are nasal polyps, recurrent sinusitis, and rectal prolapse.

- Is there any history of hemoptysis?

  —Hemoptysis can be seen with a viral or bacterial pneumonia. However, it is also present in many other conditions, including fungal disease, autoimmune diseases, granulomatous disorders, cystic fibrosis, congenital heart disease, tuberculosis, and pulmonary hemosiderosis.

GENERAL DIAGNOSTIC APPROACH

Commonly, cough is self-limited and rarely requires intervention. However, chronic cough (i.e., cough lasting longer than 3 weeks) suggests an underlying disease process requiring close investigation. A detailed history and physical examination will often lead to a diagnosis. However, adjunctive diagnostic tests, such as chest radiography and spirometry, may further aide this process. As discussed above, the patient's history will elucidate important information, such as age, circumstances present at onset of cough, nature of the cough, timing, triggers, and response to previous therapies. Medical, family, and medication histories will also provide important information regarding associated signs and symptoms. Physical examination will further validate a suspected diagnosis. Specifically, examination should pay particular attention to the presence and absence of the following: failure to thrive, signs of increased work of breathing (tachypnea, retractions, accessory muscle use, chest wall appearance, and airway sounds), allergic signs (shiners, boggy nasal turbinates, nasal polyps, halitosis, and pharyngeal cobblestoning), abnormal heart sounds, hepato- and/or splenomegaly, digital clubbing, cyanosis, and hypotonia. Chest radiography rarely provides a definitive diagnosis (except possibly in the case of foreign body aspiration) but will provide important information if subsequent diagnostic testing is required. Lastly, pulmonary function testing (when available), such as spirometry and lung volumes, will distinguish obstructive from restrictive processes. The differential diagnosis of chronic cough is broad, but with the appropriate approach, can be successfully diagnosed and treated.

SUGGESTED READINGS

1. Pasterkamp, H. The history and physical examination. In: Chernick V, Boat TF, eds. *Kendig's Disorders of the Respiratory Tract in Children*. Philadelphia, PA: W.B. Saunders Company; 1998:98-101.
2. Durbin WA. Cough. In: Hoekelman RA, Friedman SB, Nelson NM, Seidel HM, Weitzman ML, eds. *Primary Pediatric Care*. St. Louis, MO: Mosby; 1997:895-897.
3. Tunnessen WW. Cough. In: Tunnessen WW, ed. *Signs and Symptoms in Pediatrics*. Philadelphia, PA: Lippincott Williams & Wilkins; 1999:375-382.
4. Bachur R, Cough. In: Fleisher GR, Ludwig S, eds. *Textbook of Pediatric Emergency Medicine*. Philadelphia, PA: Lippincott Williams & Wilkins; 2000:183-186.
5. Morgan WJ, Taussig LM. The child with persistent cough. *Pediar Rev*. 1987;8:249-253.
6. Kamie RK. Chronic cough in children. *Pediatr Clin N Am*. 1991;38:593-605.
7. Chang AB. Cough. *Pediatr Clin N Am*. 2009;56:19-31, ix.
8. Goldsobel AB, Chipps BE. Cough in the pediatric population. *J Pediatr*. 2010;156:352-358.

The following cases represent less common causes of cough in childhood.

CASE 4-1

Sixteen-Year-Old Girl

DEBRA BOYER

TREGONY SIMONEAU

HISTORY OF PRESENT ILLNESS

The patient is a 16-year-old black female with a 2-week history of a dry cough. She described shortness of breath, which worsened while lying down. She had been sleeping on three pillows since her cough began. Her cough and shortness of breath were waking her at night and symptoms were somewhat relieved by sitting up. She had chest tightness with deep inspiration as well as pain when lying on her left side. She had intermittent fevers (38.0°C) during the last few weeks as well as drenching night sweats.

She was initially treated with albuterol for her cough without significant relief. One week into her illness she was seen by an allergist who noted decreased breath sounds on the left side. A chest roentgenogram was obtained and the patient admitted for further evaluation.

Review of systems revealed decreased appetite with early satiety. She had some weight loss during the last 12 months. She denied headaches, sore throat, or changes in her voice. She reported an episode of diffuse pruritis 2 months prior to admission.

MEDICAL HISTORY

The patient's history was remarkable for no prior significant illness and no hospitalizations. She had a fibroadenoma excised from her right breast 3 months prior to this admission. Her family history was significant for a maternal grandmother with uterine cancer, an aunt with breast cancer, and a maternal great-grandmother with thyroid cancer.

PHYSICAL EXAMINATION

T 38.1°C; P 127 bpm; RR 20/min; BP 139/73 mmHg

Weight 50th percentile; Height 95th percentile

Initial examination revealed an alert young woman, sitting forward, with noticeable shortness of breath and cough. Physical examination was remarkable for decreased breath sounds on the left, most significantly at the base. She had two small subcutaneous nodules on her left superior chest wall. The remainder of her physical examination was normal.

DIAGNOSTIC STUDIES

Laboratory analysis revealed a peripheral blood count with 21 200 WBC/mm³ with 94% segmented neutrophils, 3% lymphocytes, and 3% monocytes. Hemoglobin was 8.4 g/dL with an MCV of 63 fL. Platelets were 386 000/mm³. Electrolytes, blood urea nitrogen, creatinine, and liver function tests were normal. Erythrocyte sedimentation rate (ESR) was elevated at 60 mm/h.

COURSE OF ILLNESS

A chest computed tomography (CT) scan was obtained to further assess abnormalities on chest radiograph (Figure 4-1). The patient was admitted

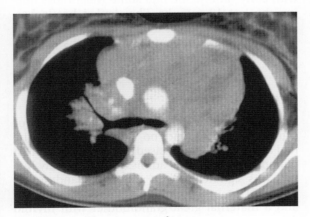

FIGURE 4-1. Chest computed tomogram.

to the intensive care unit with concerns of impending respiratory failure.

DISCUSSION CASE 4-1

DIFFERENTIAL DIAGNOSIS

The most common causes of cough in adolescents include infections and asthma. While viral infections are certainly the most common, other agents may include *Mycoplasma pneumoniae, Bordetella pertussis*, and bacterial infections. Less common infectious causes include HIV and related infections, measles, tuberculosis, and fungal infections. Patients with asthma would be most likely to have had a prior history of mild wheezing and possibly atopy. Other diagnoses that should be considered in an adolescent with a chronic cough include but are not limited to allergic rhinitis, sinusitis, gastroesophageal reflux, and smoking. Rare causes would include primary ciliary dyskinesia, interstitial pneumonitis, granulomatous disorders, and malignancies.

The concerning features of this case involve the patient's significant shortness of breath and orthopnea. These are not common complaints with simple viral infections or asthma exacerbations. Her persistent fevers and night sweats suggest a systemic disorder, such as tuberculosis or oncologic disease, and definitely warrant further investigation.

DIAGNOSIS

A chest roentgenogram revealed a large anterior mediastinal mass with rightward tracheal deviation. Chest CT revealed a large, bulky infiltrating anterior mediastinal mass that extended from above the level of the clavicle to near the level of the diaphragm (Figure 4-1).

It also extended posteriorly to involve the middle mediastinum. There was also bilateral axillary lymphadenopathy and a left pleural effusion. Chest tube placement yielded 1200 cc of pleural fluid with 3900 red blood cells/mm³, 772 white blood cells/mm³ (22% segmented neutrophils and 78% lymphocytes), pH 7.44, glucose 100 mg/dL, LDH 386 U/L, and amylase <30 U/L. A lymph node biopsy performed in the operating room revealed nodular sclerosing Hodgkin lymphoma. Bone marrow biopsy did not reveal hematologic involvement. With a negative abdominal CT scan, her lymphoma was considered Stage IIB and she commenced a course of chemotherapy.

INCIDENCE AND EPIDEMIOLOGY

Hodgkin disease is a malignancy of mature B cells. It has a bimodal age distribution in industrialized countries, with an early peak in 15-35 years old and a second peak after 50 years of age. There seem to be three separate forms of the disease: childhood (<14 years of age), young adults (15-34 years), and older adults (55-74 years). It is the most commonly diagnosed cancer for adolescents (15-19 years of age) and is rare among children less than 5 years of age. The incidence is slightly higher in males.

Hodgkin disease develops when a single transformed B cell is clonally expanded.

The malignant cells consist of Reed-Sternberg cells, lymphocytic and histiocytic cells. Interestingly, only 1% of the tumor consists of malignant cells. The greatest proportions of cells are inflammatory cells resulting from a significant cytokine release. Based on histology, there are four subtypes of Hodgkin disease: lymphocytic predominance, mixed cellularity, lymphocytic depletion, and nodular sclerosing. Nodular sclerosing is the most common type in adolescents, whereas mixed cellularity is more common in children with Hodgkin Lymphoma. Epstein-Barr virus (EBV) has been associated with some cases of Hodgkin disease with virus reactivation as a possible causative factor. This appears to be more common in younger children. Current 10-year survival rates are greater than 90% in patients diagnosed prior to the age of 45 years.

CLINICAL PRESENTATION

Often, a patient will present with firm but painless lymphadenopathy. Approximately 60% of patients may have mediastinal involvement as part of their initial presentation. It is rare to have primary disease present in subdiaphragmatic locations. Constitutional symptoms are common and include fatigue, weight loss, anorexia, fevers, and night sweats. Interestingly, as seen in this patient,

pruritis is often a complaint of patients with Hodgkin disease.

Abnormal laboratory findings may include leukocytosis, lymphopenia, eosinophilia, monocytosis, anemia, and thrombocytopenia. In contrast to many adults, most children have normal lymphocyte counts at diagnosis. Autoimmune disorders that can accompany Hodgkindisease include nephrotic syndrome and autoimmune hemolytic anemia, neutropenia, and thrombocytopenia. Nonspecific markers of inflammation such as the erythrocyte sedimentation rate and ferritin levels may be elevated.

DIAGNOSTIC APPROACH

A large pleural effusion and anterior mediastinal mass are concerning findings in this adolescent patient. Initial evaluation included a chest roentgenogram as well as aspiration of the pleural fluid.

Chest roentgenogram. Discovery of a large pleural effusion requires further diagnostic studies. Initially, lateral decubitus chest roentgenograms may be used to determine whether the fluid is free-flowing or loculated. Loculated pleural fluid suggests infection while free-flowing pleural fluid may be seen in many conditions. As in this patient, mediastinal masses, hilar lymphadenopathy, and pleural effusions may be noted in cases of malignancy.

Ultrasound. Chest ultrasound can facilitate management decisions by rapidly determining whether a pleural effusion is loculated or free-flowing.

Chest CT with intravenous contrast. CT of the chest may also be useful to analyze a pleural effusion for loculations. Chest CT is very useful to view the lung parenchyma in depth, revealing subtle lung disease not apparent on chest roentgenogram. Furthermore, a chest CT is able to further delineate masses, including mediastinal lesions and lymphadenopathy that may have been suggested on chest roentgenogram. With Hodgkin disease specifically, the most common extranodal disease sites include the lung parenchyma, chest wall, pleura, and pericardium.

Aspiration of pleural fluid. Ultimately, with a significant pleural effusion the pleural fluid should be aspirated. This is important from a diagnostic,

TABLE 4-5.	Pleural fluid analysis.	
Test	Transudate	Exudate
pH	7.4–7.5	<7.4
Protein (gm/dL)	<3.0	>3.0
LDH (IU)	<200	>200
Pleural/serum LDH	<0.6	>0.6
Glucose	Same as serum	Decreased
RBC (per mm³)	<5000	>5000
WBC (per mm³)	<1000	>1000

and in many cases, therapeutic, standpoint. Pleural fluid should be sent for pH, culture, gram stain, cell count with differential, glucose, protein, and LDH. These studies can help to divide pleural effusions into exudates and transudates (Table 4-5). Exudates are most common in parapneumonic effusions, neoplasms, and connective tissue disease, whereas transudates are more common in congestive heart failure, nephrotic syndrome, and cirrhosis. If the pleural fluid pH is greater than 7.4, it is unlikely to be an exudative process. Malignant pleural effusions, such as those from Hodgkin lymphoma, are exudative in nature and most often have quite reduced glucose levels. On occasions, malignant cells themselves are noted in the pleural fluid.

Tissue biopsy. The key to diagnosis of Hodgkin disease is pathologic confirmation of disease. This can be obtained from mass lesions as well as affected lymph nodes.

CT of neck/chest/abdomen and pelvis. Once the diagnosis of Hodgkin disease is established, these studies are performed in addition to a chest CT to stage the degree of disease.

MRI. In selected cases, MRI may be helpful in further delineating lymph node involvement and thus with staging of the disease.

Bone marrow biopsy. Useful for staging.

18-Fluorodeoxyglucose positron emission tomography (FDG-PET). PET scans are used to supplement initial staging and to monitor response to therapy. FGD-PET seems to be more sensitive than gallium scans in the detection of Hodgkin lymphoma.

TREATMENT

Determination of staging is essential in choosing the course of therapy for Hodgkin disease. Stages are based on the Ann Arbor staging classification and include:

- Stage I—Involvement of a single lymph node region or of a single extralymphatic organ or site.

- Stage II— Involvement of two or more lymph node regions on the same side of the diaphragm or localized involvement of an extralymphatic organ or site and one of more lymph node regions on the same side of the diaphragm.

- Stage III—Involvement of lymph node regions on both sides of the diaphragm.

- Stage IV—Diffuse or disseminated involvement of one or more extralymphatic organs or tissues with or without associated lymph node involvement.

Patients are stratified into low, intermediate, and high-risk categories on the basis of distribution of disease, bulk, and presence of B symptoms. Standard therapy for Hodgkin disease includes risk-adapted chemotherapy and involved-field radiation. Patients with favorable presentations (localized nodal involvement with no constitutional symptoms and without bulky disease) have been treated with fewer cycles of chemotherapy and lower radiation doses. In contrast, those patients with unfavorable presentations (constitutional symptoms, bulky mediastinal, or peripheral lymphadenopathy, and advanced Stage IIIB/IV disease) receive much more intense protocols.

SUGGESTED READINGS

1. Hudson MM, Onciu M, Donaldson SS. Hodgkin lymphoma. In: Pizzo PA, Poplack DG, eds. *Principles and Practice of Pediatric Oncology.* 5th ed. Philadelphia: Lippincott Williams & Wilkins; 2006:695-721.
2. Montgomery M. Air and liquid in the pleural space. In: Chernick V, Boat TF, eds. *Kendig's Disorders of the Respiratory Tract in Children.* 6th ed. Philadelphia: W.B. Saunders Company; 1998:389-411.
3. Punnet A, Tsang RW, Hodgson DC. Hodgkin lymphoma across the age spectrum: epidemiology, therapy, and late effects. *Semin Radiat Oncol.* 2010;20:30-44.

CASE 4-2

Seven-Week-Old Boy

DEBRA BOYER

LIANNE KOPEL

HISTORY OF PRESENT ILLNESS

The patient is a 7-week-old boy who was in good health until 3 weeks prior to presentation. At that time, he developed rhinorrhea, congestion, and cough. He had no history of fever. He was evaluated by his pediatrician. A chest roentgenogram demonstrated a left lower lobe infiltrate. He was then started on a 10-day course of erythromycin for treatment of pneumonia. On completion of this antibiotic course, his mother felt that his respiratory status had improved to some extent, but his work of breathing was still increased from his baseline. Furthermore, his cough was persistent in nature. One week later, a repeat chest roentgenogram revealed persistence of the left lower lobe infiltrate and he was referred for further evaluation. His review of symptoms revealed good oral intake and normal urine output.

MEDICAL HISTORY

He was born at 41 weeks gestation with a birth weight of 3000 g. There were no pregnancy or birth-related complications. He had no history of cyanosis or feeding difficulties. He was feeding on formula, taking two ounces every 2 hours. He has two older siblings who are both healthy.

PHYSICAL EXAMINATION

T 37.3°C; P 153 bpm; RR 54/min; BP RUE 93/59 mmHg, LUE 87/62 mmHg, RLE 94/63 mmHg; SpO_2 95% in room air

Weight 4.5 kg

Initial examination revealed a well-developed infant in moderate respiratory distress.

Physical examination was remarkable for nasal flaring, intercostal retractions, and intermittent grunting. He had good aeration and scattered rales at both lung bases. Cardiac examination revealed a normal S1 with a prominent P2. A II-III/VI systolic murmur was appreciated at the left sternal border. The liver edge was palpated 4 cm below the right costal margin. The remainder of the physical examination was normal.

DIAGNOSTIC STUDIES

Laboratory analysis revealed a peripheral blood count of 8400 white blood cells/mm^3 with 35% segmented neutrophils, 60% lymphocytes, and 5% eosinophils. The hemoglobin was 11.4 g/dL and there were 203 000 platelets/mm^3. Electrolytes, blood urea nitrogen, and creatinine were all within normal limits. Antigens of respiratory viruses were not detected by immunofluorescence of nasopharyngeal washings.

COURSE OF ILLNESS

An electrocardiogram was performed that suggested a diagnosis (Figure 4-2).

DISCUSSION CASE 4-2

DIFFERENTIAL DIAGNOSIS

The causes of persistent cough in infants are diverse, but the most common etiology are infections. Viral infections, including respiratory syncytial virus, parainfluenza, and influenza, are the most common. Normal children may develop up to eight viral respiratory infections per year, and if each infection lasts 7-14 days, recurrent infections can appear to cause a chronic cough. Bacterial infections may also cause prolonged cough. In infants with a history of conjunctivitis or maternal cervical infection, *Chlamydia trachomatis* should

FIGURE 4-2. *Left image:* Two-dimensional echocardiogram. *Right image:* Superimposed color Doppler flows, demonstrating systolic blood flow from left to right through the ventricular septal defect (in red-orange; normal aortic outflow shown in blue). *(From: Roger Breitbart, MD, Department of Cardiology, Children's Hospital Boston, with permission.)*

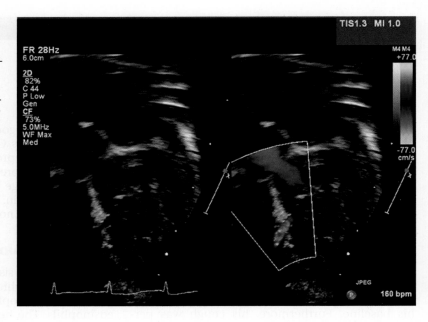

be considered. The staccato-like cough is the classic description associated with this infection. *Bordetella pertussis* can occur in infants and presents with a chronic cough, along with apneic pauses, gagging, cyanosis, and bradycardia. Most often, infants are unable to generate the force necessary for the classic "whoop." Certainly, other bacterial pneumonias should be considered with the lobar infiltrate noted on chest roentgenogram in the case above.

There are several noninfectious causes of persistent cough in infants. Asthma should always be considered, especially if there is associated wheezing and clinical response to bronchodilators. One should consider gastroesophageal reflux as a possible etiology for cough in infancy. Other less common causes of cough in this age group would include congenital malformations, including tracheoesophageal fistulas, tracheobronchomalacia, vascular rings, lobar emphysema, bronchogenic cyst, pulmonary sequestration, laryngeal cleft, and airway hemangiomas. Cystic fibrosis should be on the differential diagnosis, particularly if the patient has a history of meconium ileus, steatorrhea, failure to thrive, or a positive family history for this disease.

Congestive heart failure should always be considered, particularly if there are also feeding difficulties, poor growth, tachycardia, tachypnea, nasal flaring, intercostal retractions, grunting, murmur, and/or hepatomegaly. Etiologies in infancy may include volume overload (patent ductus arteriosus, truncus arteriosus, ventricular septal defect, common atrioventricular canal, total anomalous pulmonary venous return), myocardial dysfunction (myocarditis, anomalous left coronary artery), arrhythmias (supraventricular tachycardia), pressure overload (coarctation of the aorta, aortic stenosis), and secondary causes (hypertension, sepsis).

The features of this case that prompted additional evaluation were the presence of a heart murmur, a loud P2, bilateral rales, and hepatomegaly on the physical examination, as well as biventricular hypertrophy seen on the electrocardiogram. Additional suspicious features would have been the recognition of cardiomegaly and increased vascular markings on the chest roentgenogram.

DIAGNOSIS

Electrocardiogram revealed a ventricular rate of 150 bpm and biventricular hypertrophy. An echocardiogram revealed a large perimembranous ventricular septal defect (VSD) with left to right shunting. It also demonstrated moderately depressed biventricular function with a shortening fraction of 29%. **The diagnosis is a perimembranous VSD.**

INCIDENCE AND EPIDEMIOLOGY

Ventricular septal defects account for up to 40% of cardiac anomalies, making them the most common cardiac malformation seen in children. Studies have shown the incidence of VSD in newborns to be 5-50 per 1000 children with a slight female predominance. VSDs are the most common form of congenital heart disease associated with chromosomal disorders, although most patients with VSD do not have a chromosomal abnormality. Other types of genetic disorders that have recently been shown to be associated with VSD include single gene defects, such as mutations in *TBX5* and *GATA4*. Single gene defects account for only 3% of patients with congenital heart disease. VSD has also been associated with environmental factors such as maternal infection or teratogens.

VSDs may be classified into four types: perimembranous, also known as membranous or infracristal (most common, 80%); outlet, also known as subpulmonary, supracristal, conal, infundibular, or doubly committed subarterial (5%-7%); inlet (5%-8%); and muscular (5%-20%). A diagram of various types of VSD is depicted in Figure 4-3. Muscular defects have the greatest likelihood to undergo spontaneous closure. Approximately 75%-80% of small VSDs will close spontaneously, most often by 2 years of age.

CLINICAL PRESENTATION

The size of the VSD, the pulmonary vascular resistance, and the relative pressures in the right and left ventricles, are all important determinants of the extent of the left to right shunt. Small defects are known as restrictive, because flow across them is limited by virtue of their size. Small VSDs tend

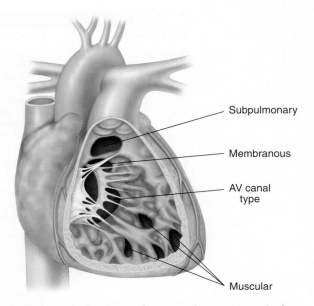

Subpulmonary

Membranous

AV canal type

Muscular

FIGURE 4-3. Anatomy of perimembranous ventricular septal defect. *(From the Multimedia Library of Congenital Heart Disease, Children's Hospital, Boston, MA, editor Robert Geggel, MD, www.childrenshospital.org/mml/cvp, with permission.)*

to have the loudest murmur and may also have a thrill. Most infants with small VSDs will have no significant symptoms and will thrive.

In contrast, the flow across larger, so-called non-restrictive defects is determined by the relative pulmonary to systemic vascular resistance. At birth, pulmonary vascular resistance is still elevated, resulting in a lack of shunt and the absence of a murmur on auscultation. As pulmonary vascular resistance declines over the next few weeks of life, the classic harsh, holosystolic murmur becomes apparent upon auscultation along the left sternal border. Most often, the murmur is heard around 1–6 weeks of age (see Table 4-6 for hints on physical examination that may suggest the type of VSD). With large defects, infants will often have a hyperactive precordium. In those infants with moderate or large VSDs, other symptoms can include tachypnea, irritability, diaphoresis or fatigue with feeding, and failure to thrive. These symptoms develop secondary to progressive heart failure and pulmonary edema. Not uncommonly, symptoms come

TABLE 4-6.	Physical examination that may suggest the type of VSD.
VSD Description	**Classic Physical Examination Findings**
Large VSD	Pansystolic murmur of constant quality (little variation with cardiac cycle) May have absence of systolic murmur Presence of diastolic rumble at apex (due to increased mitral flow) Absence of thrill Loud pulmonic component of second heart sound (elevated pulmonary pressure) Lateral displacement of precordial impulse (due to LV volume overload)
Small VSD	Louder pansystolic murmur Presence of thrill
Muscular VSD	Murmur best heard along left lower sternal border May have varying intensity throughout systole (due to change in size of defect with systolic contraction)
Perimembranous VSD	May have systolic click (due to tricuspid valve aneurysm)
Infundibular VSD	Murmur heard best along left upper sternal border
Eisenmenger Physiology	Cyanosis Digital clubbing Absence of systolic murmur Right ventricular heave Loud pulmonic component of second heart sound

VSD, ventricular septal defect; LV, left ventricle

to attention immediately following a respiratory infection, which stresses the infant's small reserve. The infant in the case above presented precisely in this manner, as evidenced by the left lower lobe infiltrate on chest roentgenogram consistent with probable pneumonia.

Patients with unrestricted left to right shunting experience an increase in pulmonary blood flow and increased pulmonary venous return, which may lead to left atrial and ventricular dilation and hypertrophy. The increased pulmonary blood flow can, over time, lead to elevated pulmonary artery pressure and reversal of the shunt across the VSD from right to left. This condition is known as Eisenmenger syndrome, with clinical features including cyanosis, desaturation, and erythrocytosis.

DIAGNOSTIC APPROACH

Chest roentgenogram. With small VSDs, the chest roentgenogram may be normal. In contrast, a large VSD may lead to significant cardiomegaly and increased vascular markings (see Figure 4-4). Later, as patients with untreated VSD develop increased pulmonary vascular resistance, there may be reduced vascular markings.

Electrocardiography. As with chest roentgenogram, the ECG may be normal with small VSDs. However, with moderate-sized VSDs, there will likely be left ventricular hypertrophy secondary to volume overload of the left ventricle and right ventricular hypertrophy secondary to pressure overload of the right ventricle. Importantly, these changes are not always evident in the ECG of infants with moderate-sized VSDs.

Echocardiography. Two-dimensional echocardiography with doppler is essential to pinpoint the size and location of a VSD. Ventricular, pulmonary artery, and interventricular pressure differences can be determined. Echocardiography also identifies associated cardiac defects and extracardiac vascular structures. Three-dimensional echocardiography, which has been studied more recently, may play a valuable role in characterizing the size and shape of the defect, as well as its spatial relationship to surrounding structures, prior to surgical or catheter-based closure of the defect.

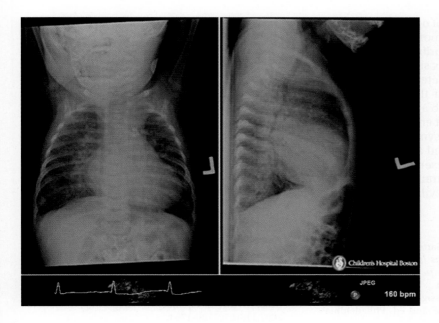

FIGURE 4-4. Four-month-old infant with large membranous ventricular septal defect. An anterior-posterior chest radiograph (*left panel*) shows situs solitus, moderate cardiomegaly, symmetrically increased pulmonary blood flow, and hyperinflation. (*From the Multimedia Library of Congenital Heart Disease, Children's Hospital, Boston, MA, editor Robert Geggel, MD,* www.childrenshospital.org/mml/cvp, *with permission.*)

Transesophageal echocardiography is used intraoperatively or when transthoracic echocardiography provides limited image quality.

MRI. Cardiac MRI can be used if echocardiography does not reveal sufficient detail. On occasion, MRI may be needed to evaluate extracardiac vascular anomalies.

Cardiac catheterization. Cardiac catheterization is necessary only for patients with complicated cardiovascular anatomy or physiology and need not be performed in all VSD patients. Pulmonary blood flow and vascular resistance may be evaluated in more detail than with Doppler echocardiography. This modality is also used for transcatheter closure of the VSD in certain patients with muscular defects.

TREATMENT

As mentioned, infants with small VSDs usually do not require any intervention.

They do require careful surveillance during the first 6 months of life, assessing growth and respiratory status. Many of these small VSDs will close spontaneously and require no further intervention.

Generally, those infants with moderate/large VSDs will develop some degree of congestive heart failure. Often, medical management is the initial therapy and may include diuretics and digoxin. On occasion, afterload reduction with angiotensin-converting-enzyme inhibitors is also required. In those patients with persistent failure to thrive, caloric augmentation may be required. If the patient's congestive heart failure and growth failure are not controlled with medical management, surgical intervention is required. Standard repair has been with patch closure via sternotomy and cardiopulmonary bypass. Significant postoperative morbidity is uncommon and surgical mortality is currently quite low.

In recent years, transcatheter VSD closure techniques have been developed, particularly for muscular VSDs. In addition, new hybrid techniques, which combine pediatric cardiac surgery, interventional pediatric cardiology, and transesophageal echocardiography, have been introduced.

Endocarditis prophylaxis guidelines were revised in 2007. For patients with uncomplicated VSDs, antibiotic prophylaxis prior to dental, gastrointestinal, and genitourinary procedures is no longer recommended as it may not be effective in preventing endocarditis. Patients should always be counseled that maintenance of optimal oral health and hygiene is advised, and is more likely to prevent endocarditis than antibiotics prior to dental procedures. However, prophylaxis is still recommended for 6 months following complete repair with prosthetic material, and for life if there is a residual defect at the site or adjacent to a prosthetic patch, since this scenario may inhibit endothelialization.

Patients with Eisenmenger syndrome are generally considered inoperable, and are offered symptomatic therapy for reduced exercise capacity and cyanosis. Partial exchange transfusion may be offered for symptomatic polycythemia.

SUGGESTED READINGS

1. Zitelli BJ. Chronic cough. In: Gartner JC, Zitelli BJ, eds. *Common & Chronic Symptoms in Pediatrics: A Companion to the Atlas of Pediatric Physical Diagnosis.* St. Louis: Mosby; 1997:189-200.
2. Shehab ZM. Pertussis. In: Taussig LM, Landau LI, eds. *Pediatric Respiratory Medicine.* 2nd ed. Philadelphia: Mosby/Elsevier; 2008:589-595.
3. Penny DJ, Vick GW. Ventricular septal defect. *Lancet.* 2011;377(9771):1103-1112.
4. McDaniel NL, Gutgesell HP. Ventricular septal defects. In: Moss AJ, Allen HD, eds. *Moss and Adams' Heart Disease in Infants, Children, and Adolescents: Including the Fetus and Young Adult.* 7th ed. Philadelphia: Wolters Kluwer/Lippincott Williams & Wilkins; 2008:667-682.
5. Minette MS, Sahn DJ. Ventricular septal defects. *Circulation.* 2006;114(20):2190-2197.
6. Chen FL, Hsiung MC, Hsieh KS, Li YC, Chou MC. Real time three-dimensional transthoracic echocardiography for guiding Amplatzer septal occluder device deployment in patients with atrial septal defect. *Echocardiography.* 2006;23(9):763-770.
7. Wilson W, Taubert KA, Gewitz M, et al. Prevention of infective endocarditis: guidelines from the American Heart Association: a guideline from the American Heart Association Rheumatic Fever, Endocarditis, and Kawasaki Disease Committee, Council on Cardiovascular Disease in the Young, and the Council on Clinical Cardiology, Council on Cardiovascular Surgery and Anesthesia, and the Quality of Care and Outcomes Research Interdisciplinary Working Group. *Circulation.* 2007;116(15):1736-1754.

CASE 4-3

Seven-Month-Old Girl

DEBRA BOYER

ALICIA CASEY

HISTORY OF PRESENT ILLNESS

The patient is a 7-month-old girl, who was well until 4 days prior to presentation. At that time, she developed a cough with fevers to 40.5°C. On the day of presentation, she developed wheezing and a rash on her trunk and face. This rash began on her chest and spread to her face. Over the preceding 4 days her cough had increased significantly. She received nebulized albuterol twice at home without relief. She had poor oral intake and urine output.

MEDICAL HISTORY

She was the full-term product of an uncomplicated vaginal delivery. She was brought to the emergency department three times for wheezing episodes. Her only medication was nebulized albuterol. At the time of presentation, the patient and her family were living in a shelter. A roommate at the shelter was recently hospitalized with a rash, fever, and pneumonia.

PHYSICAL EXAMINATION

T 40.6°C; P 168 bpm; RR 60/min; BP 102/55 mmHg; Oxygen saturation 99% in room air

Weight 50th percentile; Height 75th to 90th percentile

Initial examination revealed an alert baby, who was crying, but consolable. She appeared slightly pale. Physical examination was notable for an

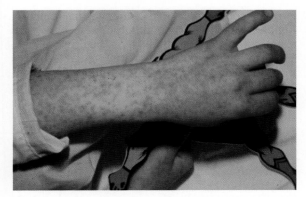

FIGURE 4-5. Example of a rash.

erythematous right tympanic membrane and bilaterally injected conjunctiva with yellow discharge. She had moderate rhinorrhea and some notable buccal thrush. Her oropharynx was mildly erythematous. Chest examination was remarkable for an elevated respiratory rate, but no retractions. She had fine expiratory wheezes bilaterally with decreased breath sounds at both bases. Her skin had a fine erythematous blanching maculopapular rash on her face and torso (Figure 4-5) and to a lesser degree on her extremities. Her palms and soles were spared. The rash appeared confluent in her perineal area and torso. The remainder of her physical examination was unremarkable.

DIAGNOSTIC STUDIES

Laboratory analysis revealed a peripheral blood count with 10900 white blood cells/mm³ with 41% segmented neutrophils, 50% lymphocytes, 8% monocytes, and no band forms. Her hemoglobin was 10.6 g/dL and there were 290000 platelets/mm³. A urinalysis was normal and a chest roentgenogram revealed mild hyperinflation, right middle lobe atelectasis, and some peribronchial cuffing.

COURSE OF ILLNESS

The patient received two nebulized albuterol treatments without significant change in her respiratory status. Blood and urine cultures were sent to the laboratory and revealed no growth. Her fever resolved during the next 2 days, her rash faded, and her respiratory status began to normalize. She was discharged after a 4-day hospitalization. Examination of the rash (Figure 4-5) suggested a diagnosis that was confirmed by blood work obtained during her hospitalization.

DISCUSSION CASE 4-3

DIFFERENTIAL DIAGNOSIS

Viral infections are the most common cause of a cough in infancy, with rhinovirus, coronavirus, respiratory syncytial virus, parainfluenzae, human metapneumovirus, and influenza among the leading agents. These viruses also commonly produce lower airway disease in infants, and thus, bronchiolitis often accompanies the cough. With bronchiolitis, infants frequently present with decreased aeration, diffuse crackles, and wheezing appreciated on auscultation. Fever and profuse rhinorrhea are common.

Other infectious etiologies are possible and should be considered in the differential diagnosis, including *C. trachomatis*, pertussis, and bacterial pneumonia. Less commonly, infants will present with pulmonary tuberculosis and fungal infections. Rarely, infectious entities such as measles or parasitic infections will present with cough.

While cough can be the presenting symptom with congenital malformations and underlying lung disease, this patient's presentation strongly suggested an infectious etiology. The features of this case that prompted additional evaluation included the rash and associated respiratory findings.

DIAGNOSIS

The rash was characteristic of measles (Figure 4-5). Antibody titers to measles were sent on admission and were negative. Repeat titers were sent prior to her discharge on hospital day 4. IgM antibodies specific for measles were found to be positive. **The diagnosis is measles.**

INCIDENCE AND EPIDEMIOLOGY

Measles is the infectious condition caused by the rubeola virus, an RNA virus of the family of paramyxoviridae. Measles remains endemic outside of North and South America. Prior to the introduction of the measles vaccine in 1963, 200 000-300 000 cases of measles were recorded each year in the United States. Since the measles vaccines usage, measles in the United States has dramatically decreased by 99%. By the year 2000, endemic transmission ended. Since then, there has been a median of 60 cases per year from 2001 to 2010. Unfortunately, there was a dramatic increase in the number of cases (222) and outbreaks (17) in 2011. Most recent cases of measles occurring in people born in the United States can be traced to imported exposure either from personal travel abroad or contact with individuals infected abroad. Exposures occurred most frequently in Europe or South East Asia. Of recent cases, most occurred in unvaccinated individuals. In the cases of unvaccinated children, many were ineligible for vaccination (too young or had a medical contraindication), the parents reported a religious or personal exemption or the patient was simply delayed in their vaccination schedule. Infrequently, cases of primary vaccine failure have been reported.

Measles is spread as an airborne virus, and thus persons become infected by direct contact with droplets from the respiratory secretions of infected patients. Measles is highly contagious and approximately 90% of susceptible people develop symptoms after exposure. The typical incubation period is 10 days (range 7-21 days). Generally, children are considered contagious from 3 days prior to the onset of the rash until 6 days after the onset of the rash. Mortality in the United States occurs about 1-2 per 1000 infections, and is more common in infants, children, and immunocompromised individuals. Hospitalization is frequently required and rates of hospitalization are highest among infants and children. Pneumonia is not uncommon and can be severe. Encephalitis is a rare, but still reported and devastating complication.

CLINICAL PRESENTATION

The prodromal phase begins with 3-5 days of malaise, fever, cough, coryza, and conjunctivitis. These symptoms increase over the course of the prodromal phase. Just prior to the development of the exanthem, Koplik spots are noted. These are bluish white spots on a red base and are found classically in the buccal mucosa, but may be found on the lips, palate,

gingiva, conjunctival folds, and vaginal mucosa. Koplik spots are pathognomonic of measles. The exantham begins as Koplik spots begin to slough. The rash begins typically on the face and then moves in a caudal direction. The rash is initially erythematous and maculopapular, but then becomes confluent. The rash generally lasts 5-7 days. The most persistent symptom is often the cough.

With typical measles, patients are generally ill for 7-10 days. Other manifestations can include pharyngitis, otitis media, lymphadenopathy, croup, bronchiolitis, sinusitis, diarrhea, vomiting, and dehydration. Febrile seizures can occur. However, more severe complications can occur and include pneumonia, bronchiolitis obliterans, tracheitis, mastoiditis, retropharyngeal abscess, appendicitis, acute encephalitis, myocarditis, pericarditis, hemorrhagic skin eruption, and keratitis. Measles during pregnancy is associated with increased maternal morbidity, fetal demise, and congenital malformations. Subacute sclerosing panencephalitis (SSPE) is a rare delayed neurologic complication of measles infection. This complication is fatal in most cases. SSPE consists of a degenerative CNS process that is associated with a persistent intracellular measles infection and can present years after infection.

DIAGNOSTIC APPROACH

The diagnosis of measles is generally based on clinical presentation and having a high index of suspicion for diagnosis. Often measles goes undiagnosed due to infrequent cases and confusion with other common illnesses presenting with rash and fever. Identification of cases is essential to limit spread and prevent outbreaks. For these reasons, all suspected cases should be confirmed. All known or suspected cases of measles should be reported to the State Health Department and the Center for Disease Control (CDC).

Serologic titers. Confirmation of measles infection can be made most conveniently by detecting measles-specific immunoglobulin M (IgM) in the serum. This is the most common method of diagnosis. Depending on the sensitivity of the assay, antibodies can be detected within 1-3 days after onset of rash. Measles IgM generally peaks 10 days after rash onset and usually remains 30-60 days after rash onset. The presence of measles-specific IgM antibodies will establish the diagnosis. Analysis of acute and convalescent titers of IgG can also be used.

Clinical specimen testing/collection. Measles infection can also be confirmed by the detection of measles virus RNA by nucleic acid amplication. This testing can be done on specimens such as nasopharyngeal/oropharyngeal swabs, nasal aspirates, throat washes, or urine. Virus isolation is best performed 1-3 days after onset of rash, but can be detected up to 7 days post. Clinical specimens can also be used to determine source of infection based on genetic sequence data.

TREATMENT

In uncomplicated measles, patients will only require supportive care, including antipyretics and fluids. Antibiotics are only necessary in cases of bacterial superinfection, particularly pneumonia. Typical organisms causing a superinfected bacterial pneumonia include *Streptococcus pneumoniae*, *Staphylococcus aureus*, *Haemophilus influenzae*, and *Streptococcus pyogenes*. Vitamin A deficiency has been associated with increased mortality and treatment with this has been shown to reduce mortality and complications. Treatment with vitamin A may be recommended for certain individuals.

PREVENTION

The measles, mumps, rubella (MMR) vaccination is administered at age 12-15 months with a second dose at 4-6 years. It is recommended that infants older than 6 months be administered the vaccine if international travel is planned. This vaccine is highly effective. Exposed susceptible individuals may be treated with vaccination and passive immune globulin.

SUGGESTED READINGS

1. Regamey N, et al. Viral etiology of acute respiratory infections with cough in infancy: a community-based birth cohort study. *Pediatr Infect Dis J.* 2008;27(2): 100-105.
2. Wilbert HM: Measles. In: Kliegman RM, Stanton BMD, St. Geme J, Schor N, Behrman R, eds. *Nelson Textbook of Pediatrics.* 19th ed. Philadelphia, PA: Saunders; 2011: 1069-1075.
3. Center for Disease Control and Prevention (CDC). Measles-United States, 2011. *MMWR Morb Mort Wkly Rep.* 2012;61:253-257.
4. Center for Disease Control and Prevention (CDC). Measles Homepage. http://www.cdc.gov/measles/. Accessed July 15, 2012.
5. Parker Fiebelkorn A, Redd SB, Gallagher K, et al. Measles in the United States during the postelimination era. *J Infect Dis.* 2010;202:1520-1528.
6. Watson JC, Hadler SC, Dykewicz CA, Reef S, Phillips L. Measles, mumps, and rubella-vaccine use and strategies for elimination of measles, rubella, and congenital rubella syndrome and control of mumps: recommendations of the Advisory Committee on Immunization Practices (ACIP). *MMWR Recommendations & Reports.* 1998;47(RR-8):1-57.

CASE 4-4

Three-Year-Old Boy

DEBRA BOYER

STEPHANIE ZANDIEH

HISTORY OF PRESENT ILLNESS

The patient is a 3-year-old boy with a history of asthma who presented with cough and chest pain. His illness began 2 weeks prior with left-sided chest pain with inspiration. The family had misplaced his baseline asthma medications. He was seen in the emergency department and felt to have musculoskeletal pain. His pain improved slightly, but he was brought back to the emergency department 8 days later with wheezing and rhinorrhea. He was described as having increased work of breathing and a significant cough. There was no fever. In the emergency department, he was felt to be in mild respiratory distress and was treated with prednisone and albuterol and then discharged. However, the following day, he developed blood streaked sputum evolving into a small volume of hemoptysis. He was brought back to the emergency department. There was no fever, chills, or weight loss.

MEDICAL HISTORY

The patient has a history of asthma for which he was hospitalized three times. His last admission was 3 years prior to this current presentation. His medications are albuterol which he receives twice a day and a fluticasone metered-dose inhaler that he has not received in several weeks.

PHYSICAL EXAMINATION

   T 37.2°C; P 70 bpm; RR 30/min; BP 108/52 mmHg; Oxygen saturation 99% in room air

In general, he was a well-appearing young boy in no acute distress. His physical examination was significant for a clear lung examination with no evidence of wheezes, rales, or rhonchi. The remainder of his physical examination was unremarkable.

DIAGNOSTIC STUDIES

Chest roentgenogram was obtained (Figure 4-6). Tuberculin skin test reaction was less than 5 mm.

COURSE OF ILLNESS

He was initially started on a course of azithromycin for a presumed *Mycoplasma pneumoniae* infection. His chest pain continued, but his hemoptysis had resolved. With concern for his chest roentgenogram findings, a further diagnostic test was performed which revealed the diagnosis.

DISCUSSION CASE 4-4

DIFFERENTIAL DIAGNOSIS

Considering the patient's medical history, the most common cause for his cough is likely to be

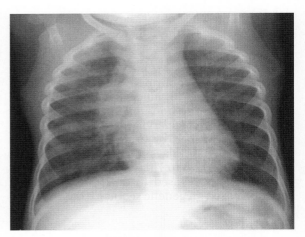

FIGURE 4-6. Chest radiograph.

asthma with a superimposed infectious process. His symptoms did appear to improve slightly with standard asthma therapy of bronchodilators and steroids. Allergic or sinus symptoms can also cause a significant cough in this age group. Similarly, one should inquire about a history of smoking or possible foreign body aspiration.

   The hemoptysis in this case is not unusual in many of the processes described. It is important to try and establish that this is true hemoptysis and not hematemesis or bleeding from the nasal passages (Table 4-7). With true hemoptysis, the most common etiologies include cystic fibrosis, pneumonia, bronchiectasis, congenital heart disease, and tracheobronchitis. Finally, the hilar adenopathy noted on chest roentgenogram should alert one to pursue a more thorough investigation, with consideration to mycobacterial infections and granulomatous disorders.

DIAGNOSIS

Chest radiograph revealed a right middle lobe infiltrate with right hilar adenopathy (Figure 4-6). Nasogastric aspirates were sent for acid fast bacilli (AFB) stain and cultures. AFB stain was negative but AFB culture revealed growth of mycobacterium avium-intracellulare. **The diagnosis is a pulmonary infection with mycobacterium avium-intracellulare.**

TABLE 4-7.	Hemoptysis versus hematemesis.			
	Color	*pH*	*Consistency*	*Symptoms*
Hemoptysis	Bright red, frothy	Alkaline	May be mixed with sputum	Accompanied by coughing, may be preceded by a gurgling noise
Hematemesis	Dark red or brown	Acidic	May contain food particles	May be proceeded by nausea

INCIDENCE AND EPIDEMIOLOGY

Nontuberculosis mycobacterium (NTM) are ubiquitous in the environment. They are found in soil, water, food, house dust, and domestic and wild animals. Human infection likely occurs with aspiration of aerosolized particles. Human-to-human transmission is not believed to occur.

It is difficult to determine the incidence of NTM infections as they are not a reportable disease to health authorities. Furthermore, symptoms are confused with *Mycobacterium tuberculosis* infections. It is also challenging to properly differentiate asymptomatic colonization from true infection. A positive culture for NTM does not always represent invasive disease. Moreover, interpretation of a single positive respiratory culture for MAI should take into account the possibility of environmental contamination.

The most common NTM organisms form the *Mycobacterium avium* complex (MAC) which consists of both *M. avium* and *Mycobacterium intracellulare*. Aside from patients with HIV, those with the greatest risk of becoming infected with pulmonary MAC are those patients with underlying lung disease. This includes patients with chronic obstructive pulmonary disease, chronic bronchitis, bronchiectasis, recurrent aspiration, and cystic fibrosis. However, reports of patients with no underlying lung disease and MAC infections have been reported. The southeastern part of the United States does appear to have a higher incidence of MAC infections.

Rarely, a patient will present with disseminated NTM infection. These patients should be investigated for an underlying immune deficiency, since patients with certain disorders such as IFN-γ receptor defects and IL-12 defects are highly susceptible to infections with NTM.

CLINICAL PRESENTATION

There are four major clinical syndromes of NTM infection that are most commonly seen in children: lymphadenitis, pulmonary infections, skin and soft tissue infections, and disseminated disease.

Pulmonary infections with NTM are rare in children, and are more often seen in the elderly. MAC is the most common NTM to cause pulmonary infections, but cases have been reported with *Mycobacterium kansasii* and *Mycobacterium fortuitum* as well. Symptoms are very similar to tuberculosis with a productive cough, fevers, and weight loss. Hemoptysis is less common, and is seen in less than 25% of patients with pulmonary MAC infections. It is rare for disease to disseminate beyond a pulmonary infection if the host is immunocompetent.

Wheezing is a common presenting symptom, and often hilar adenopathy leads to signs and symptoms of bronchial obstruction. It is common for these children to be evaluated for possible foreign body aspiration prior to the discovery of their NTM infection. On occasion, a child will have repeated illnesses with fever and cough and be diagnosed as having recurrent pneumonias.

DIAGNOSTIC APPROACH

NTM infections can only be diagnosed with a high degree of clinical suspicion. Diagnosis is based on isolating the organism in conjunction with appropriate clinical disease.

The following tests can be useful:

Blood tests. Complete blood counts, erythrocyte sedimentation rate, urinalysis, and serum chemistry tests are generally normal with NTM infections.

Sputum or gastric aspirate (mycobacterial culture and acid-fast stain.) Acid-fast stain of sputum and gastric aspirates are often negative in cases of NTM as the number of organisms may be quite small. Therefore, a negative AFB stain does not exclude the diagnosis of NTM infection. NTM can be grown from sputum and gastric aspirate culture, but results must be interpreted with caution, as asymptomatic patients may be colonized with NTM. Thus, clinical criteria have been developed requiring either radiographic evidence of disease with greater than one positive sputum samples, or reproducibility of positive cultures over the course of a year.

Purified protein derivation skin testing (PPD). Patients with MAC will generally have reactions of 0-10 mm. It is rare to see larger reactions. A positive PPD should never be considered diagnostic for NTM infection and a negative PPD should never eliminate the diagnosis.

Chest roentgenogram. This may reveal findings similar to infection with tuberculosis. Cavitary lesions are not uncommon, but are often smaller than with *M. tuberculosis*. Other radiographic presentations may include patchy, nodular infiltrates or even isolated pulmonary nodules. Hilar adenopathy may also be seen.

Bronchoscopy. Inadequate sputum samples are often obtained in children, and bronchoscopy may be indicated to obtain useful cultures. Adenopathy sufficiently large to cause bronchial obstruction can occur, and often bronchoscopy is performed in an attempt to rule out an anatomic etiology for the bronchial compression.

TREATMENT

As the majority of NTM organisms are resistant in vitro to single drug therapy, combination therapy is, therefore, generally the rule. Treatment will often include isoniazid, rifampin, rifabutin, ethambutol, streptomycin, amikacin, azithromycin, or clarithromycin. For many patients, treatment regimens may extend for 18-24 months and specifically for at least 12 months after sputum cultures have become negative. Many of these medications have significant side effects and patients should be monitored closely. Side effects include but are not limited to the following: rifampin (hepatitis), rifabutin (uveitis especially when used with macrolide, hepatitis, polyarthralgias), ethambutol (retrobulbar neuritis manifest by decreased visual acuity or red-green color discrimination), amikacin (ototoxicity, nephrotoxicity), azithromycin (reversible hearing loss, GI upset), and clarithromycin (GI upset).

SUGGESTED READINGS

1. Ferfie JE, Milligan TW, Henderson BM, Stafford WW. Intrathoracic *Mycobacterium avium* complex infection in immunocompetent children: case report and review. *Clin Infect Dis.* 1997;24:250-253.
2. Havlir DV, Ellner JJ. *Mycobacterium avium* complex. In: Mandell GL, Bennett JE, Dolin R, eds. *Mandell, Douglas, and Bennett's Principles and Practice of Infectious Diseases.* 5th ed. Philadelphia: Churchill Livingstone; 2000:2616-2630.
3. Osorio A, Kessler RM, Guruprasad H, Isaacson G. Isolated intrathoracic presentation of *Mycobacterium avium* complex in an immunocompetent child. *Pediatr Radiol.* 2001;31:848-851.
4. Starke JR. Nontuberculous mycobacterial infections in children. *Adv Pediatr Infect Dis.* 1992;7:123-159.
5. Starke JR, Correa AG. Management of mycobacterial infection and disease in children. *Pediatr Infect Dis J.* 1995;14:455-470.
6. Stone AB, Schelonka RL, Drehner DM, McMahon DP, Ascher DP. Disseminated *Mycobacterium avium* complex in non-human immunodeficiency virus-infected pediatric patients. *Pediatr Infect Dis J.* 1992;11:960-964.
7. Freeman AF, Olivier KN, Rubio TT, et al. Intrathoracic nontuberculous mycobacterial infections in otherwise healthy children. *Pediatr Pulmonol.* 2009;44:1051-1056.
8. Blyth CC, Best EJ, Jones CA, et al. Nontuberculous mycobacterial infection in children: a prospective national study. *Pediatr Infect Dis J.* 2009;28:801-805.

CASE 4-5

Two-Year-Old Girl

TODD A. FLORIN

HISTORY OF PRESENT ILLNESS

The patient is a 2-year-old girl who presented with a 1-month history of fevers and a nonproductive cough. Six weeks prior to presentation she developed fevers and a dry cough. Soon after, she was admitted to the hospital with the diagnosis of an otitis media and pneumonia. After a 2-day hospitalization, during which she received intravenous antibiotics, she was discharged home. Her parents felt that her symptoms had not improved. Her fevers continued and occurred every few days with maximum temperatures of 103-106°F. She was treated with nebulized albuterol without improvement in her cough.

She had a decreased appetite for the last month with a 2 kg weight loss. She also had nonbloody, nonbilious emesis occurring 3-4 times each day. Her parents reported 3-4 loose bowel movements each day. In her doctor's office, a stool sample was obtained and was tested positive for microscopic blood.

MEDICAL HISTORY

The patient was full term at birth with a birth weight of 2800 g. She has had four episodes of otitis media in the past and two episodes of sinusitis. Her only medication is albuterol as needed. Her family history is significant for having two aunts with asthma.

PHYSICAL EXAMINATION

T 40.0°C; P 140 bpm; RR 44/min; BP 98/60 mmHg; Oxygen saturation 90%-92% in room air; Weight 5th to 10th percentile

In general, she presented with very mild increase in her work of breathing. Her chest examination revealed good aeration throughout with bilateral end-expiratory wheezes present in the left upper lobe and right anterior lung field. No rales or rhonchi were noted. The remainder of her physical examination was within normal limits.

DIAGNOSTIC STUDIES

The complete blood count revealed a white blood cell count of 8800 cells/mm^3 with 66% segmented neutrophils, 27% lymphocytes, and 7% monocytes. Her hemoglobin was 12.2 gm/dL and her platelet count was 268 000/mm^3. Erythrocyte sedimentation rate was 24 mm/h. Electrolytes and liver function tests were within normal limits. Prothrombin and partial thromboplastin times were elevated at 15.1 seconds and 33.5 seconds, respectively. Blood and urine cultures did not reveal any growth.

COURSE OF ILLNESS

A chest roentgenogram was performed which revealed diffuse peribronchial thickening as well as subsegmental atelectasis in the right middle lobe. CT scan of her sinuses revealed extensive maxillary sinus disease with some ethmoidal opacification. A chest CT revealed subcarinal and hilar adenopathy.

Ultimately, a diagnostic procedure was performed which revealed the diagnosis.

DISCUSSION CASE 4-5

DIFFERENTIAL DIAGNOSIS

As with all other age groups, the most common etiology for a cough in the toddler is an infectious process. Viruses, *M. pneumoniae*, and pertussis should all be considered as possible infectious causes. Given her symptoms and the findings on chest radiograph, pneumonia, and bronchiolitis remain on the list of potential diagnoses. Almost equally as important in this age group is the possibility of a foreign body ingestion, which is often revealed during a thorough analysis of medical history. Another clue to foreign body ingestion is a focal finding on chest auscultation, as was seen in this patient, with localized wheezing. If there is a concern for a foreign body ingestion, inspiratory and expiratory chest roentgenograms may reveal the diagnosis. If the child is too young for these maneuvers, bilateral decubitus chest roentgenograms can be obtained. In the case of foreign body ingestion, these films may reveal persistent hyperinflation on the side where the foreign body has lodged.

Other concerning findings in this patient's history are her relatively poor growth, her diffuse sinus disease, and her history of frequent stooling. With this constellation of symptoms, one should include some rarer causes of cough in the differential diagnosis, including congenital immunodeficiencies, human immunodeficiency virus infection, and cystic fibrosis (CF).

DIAGNOSIS

Because of her poor growth, sinus disease, chronic cough, and frequent stooling, a sweat test was performed. **The results revealed sweat chloride levels of 96 mEq/L and 88 mEq/L (normal <40 mEq/L), thus revealing the diagnosis of cystic fibrosis.**

INCIDENCE AND EPIDEMIOLOGY

Cystic fibrosis is the most common lethal inherited disease in the Caucasian population. The incidence is approximately 1/2500 in Caucasians, 1/17 000 in African-Americans, and 1/90 000 in Asians. It is inherited in an autosomal recessive pattern with a carrier rate of 1/25. Life expectancy for patients with cystic fibrosis has improved dramatically during the last 50 years. In the 1950s, median survival was less than 5 years of age. The current predicted median age of survival for a person with CF is in the late 30s.

The gene for cystic fibrosis was discovered in 1989 and is located on chromosome 7. The gene product is a cyclic-AMP-activated chloride channel called the cystic fibrosis transmembrane conductance regulator (CFTR). CFTR is expressed in multiple organs including the pancreas, sweat glands, gastrointestinal tract, reproductive tract, and respiratory tract. Defective CFTR function results in dysfunctional electrolyte transport at the affected epithelial surfaces leading to dehydration of the luminal surfaces. This causes the development of

thick, viscid secretions that result in obstruction, inflammation, and progressive scarring of affected organs.

CLINICAL PRESENTATION

Given that CFTR gene expression is so diffuse, the clinical presentation of cystic fibrosis is quite diverse. The most common and life-threatening manifestations are related to respiratory disease, though extrapulmonary manifestations of cystic fibrosis are common (Table 4-8).

TABLE 4-8.	**Clinical manifestations of cystic fibrosis.**
Chronic sinus and/or pulmonary disease Persistent colonization and/or infection with CF pathogens (*Staphylococcus aureus*, nontypeable *Haemophilus influenzae*, *Pseudomonas aeruginosa*, *Stenotrophomonas maltophilia*, and *Burkholderia cepacia*) Chronic cough Persistent changes on chest radiograph Sinus changes, including recurrent sinusitis, nasal polyps Signs of airway obstruction, such as wheezing Digital clubbing	
Hepato-biliary Prolonged neonatal jaundice Biliary obstruction Biliary cirrhosis Portal hypertension Cholelithiasis	
Gastrointestinal Meconium ileus Distal intestinal obstruction syndrome Intussusception Rectal prolapse	
Pancreatic Pancreatic insufficiency Recurrent acute or chronic pancreatitis	
Genitourinary and renal Aspermia Acute salt depletion Chronic metabolic alkalosis	
Hematologic Bleeding diathesis	
Nutritional Failure to thrive Hypoproteinemia with associated edema Fat-soluble vitamin deficiencies	

Source: Adapted, with permission, from Farrell PM, Rosenstein BJ, White TB, et al. Guidelines for diagnosis of cystic fibrosis in newborns through older adults: Cystic Fibrosis Foundation consensus report. *J Pediatr.* 2008;153:S4-S14.

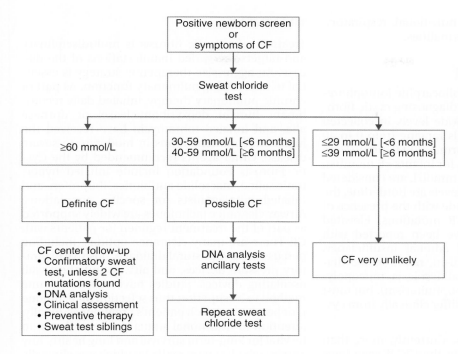

```
          Positive newborn screen
                    or
            symptoms of CF
                    |
                    v
            Sweat chloride
                test
                    |
    ------------------------------------------------
    |                         |                    |
  ≥60 mmol/L      30-59 mmol/L [<6 months]   ≤29 mmol/L [<6 months]
                 40-59 mmol/L [≥6 months]    ≤39 mmol/L [≥6 months]
    |                         |                    |
    v                         v                    v
 Definite CF             Possible CF          CF very unlikely
    |                         |
    v                         v
 CF center follow-up    DNA analysis
 • Confirmatory sweat   ancillary tests
   test, unless 2 CF         |
   mutations found           v
 • DNA analysis         Repeat sweat
 • Clinical assessment  chloride test
 • Preventive therapy
 • Sweat test siblings
```

FIGURE 4-7. Diagnostic approach to cystic fibrosis. *(Reproduced, with permission, from Farrell PM, Rosenstein BJ, White TB, et al. Guidelines for diagnosis of cystic fibrosis in newborns through older adults: Cystic Fibrosis Foundation consensus report. J Pediatr. 2008;153:S4-S14.)*

The initial presentation of cystic fibrosis can occur in a variety of ways. Increasing numbers of patients are being diagnosed before the onset of symptoms due to expanding newborn screening programs for CF (Figure 4-7). Symptoms present in infancy may include meconium ileus (present in 10%-15%), failure to thrive, rectal prolapse, and chronic cough. Failure to thrive due to intestinal malabsorption is the most common early manifestation of CF. Other presenting features in childhood can include nasal polyps, cough, frequent episodes of wheezing, frequent respiratory infections, liver disease, recurrent sinusitis and/or pancreatitis, and infertility.

The respiratory complications are the greatest cause of morbidity and mortality in CF. The classic pulmonary triad in CF is inflammation, impaired mucociliary clearance, and chronic airway infection. Recurrent acute pulmonary infections are common as a result of this triad, and may present similarly to recurrent viral infections or asthma. Common CF pathogens include *Staphylococcus aureus, Haemophilus influenzae, Pseudomonas aeruginosa, Stenotrophomonas maltophilia,* and *Burkholderia cepacia.* Eventually, the recurrent pulmonary infections will lead to lung tissue destruction and bronchiectasis. Complications in CF patients can include allergic bronchopulmonary aspergillosis (detected by chronic wheeze, lung function decline, chronic cough, and transient infiltrates on CXR), hemoptysis, and pneumothorax.

Gastrointestinal disease is also common in CF, and will often include pancreatic insufficiency. Therefore, failure to thrive is a common presentation, along with frequent bulky or malodorous stools indicative of fat malabsorption. Other gastrointestinal complications can include liver disease, CF-related diabetes, gastroesophageal reflux, and rectal prolapse. Thick mucoid impaction in the distal small bowel can result in distal intestinal obstruction syndrome (DIOS).

Fertility is commonly affected in both males and females with CF. Ninety percent of men with CF will have congenital bilateral absence of the vas deferens. Women will also have significantly decreased fertility due to nutritional, respiratory, and cervical mucous abnormalities.

DIAGNOSTIC APPROACH

Sweat test. Quantitative pilocarpine iontophoresis is the gold standard in diagnosing cystic fibrosis (Figure 4-7). The chloride levels in collected sweat are measured. Levels ranging from 0 to 40 mmol/L are considered normal, 40-60 mmol/L are borderline (30-59 mmol/L for infants <6 months), and levels greater than 60 mmol/L are considered positive. If sweat chloride levels are borderline, the diagnosis of CF can be made with the presence of two disease-causing CFTR mutations. Elevated sweat chloride levels have been reported with other entities (untreated adrenal insufficiency, malnutrition, hypothyroidism, nephrogenic diabetes insipidus, ectodermal dysplasia, mucopolysaccharidosis, and panhypopituitarism), but most of those other conditions differ clinically from cystic fibrosis.

Genetic mutation analysis. Currently, more than 1000 different mutations in the CFTR gene have been identified. Standard genetic testing will usually screen for around 20-70 mutations. Testing for a discrete group of approximately 40 of the most common disease-causing mutations will detect more than 90% of cases. Expanded sequence analysis of many more mutations is costly and may detect novel polymorphisms and mutations of unknown significance. Testing can be performed on blood or a buccal swab.

Chest roentgenogram. While a chest roentgenogram cannot be used to diagnose CF, it can certainly have suggestive features. These may include significant peribronchial thickening, hyperinflation, and bronchiectasis. Progressive pulmonary disease in patients with CF leads to nodular pulmonary infiltrates and apical cystic lesions that predispose to pneumothoraces.

Sputum culture. Initially, the majority of patients with cystic fibrosis are colonized with *Staphylococcus aureus* and *Haemophilus influenzae*. By young adulthood, nearly 80% of patients are colonized with *Pseudomonas aeruginosa*.

TREATMENT

Treatment for cystic fibrosis is multidisciplinary and targets the varied manifestations of the disease. An aggressive therapeutic strategy is essential to maximizing pulmonary function. As part of chronic pulmonary therapy, inhaled daily recombinant human deoxyribonuclease, or dornase alfa, and inhaled tobramycin have received the highest recommendations in moderate to severe disease. Other agents recommended by the Cystic Fibrosis Foundation include inhaled hypertonic saline, macrolide antibiotics, ibuprofen, and inhaled beta-agonists for specific populations. Airway clearance techniques are widely supported as part of the treatment regimen for patients with CF. There are many clearance options, including percussion and postural drainage, positive expiratory pressure devices, and airway and chest wall oscillating devices. Studies have not shown one method to be superior; thus selection of technique is dependent on each patient's preferences. Finally, attention to nutritional status has been shown to be vital for long-term survival and lung health. Any patient who has pancreatic insufficiency clinically or subclinically, as evidenced by low fecal elastase concentrations, should receive supplementation with pancreatic enzymes, in addition to fat-soluble vitamins.

Aggressively treating pulmonary exacerbations improves outcomes. Treatment includes antibiotics, increased airway clearance, and optimizing nutrition. Generally, antibiotic treatment should consist of combination therapy with 2-3 antibiotics with different mechanisms of action for approximately 14 days. Given the high prevalence of *Pseudomonas* in patients with CF, a combination of a beta-lactam and aminoglycoside can be considered appropriate.

For patients with end-stage pulmonary disease, lung transplantation is considered the final treatment option. The 5-year survival rate for children after transplant is approximately 50%, and success depends on a variety of factors. Ultimately, mutation-specific and gene therapies targeting the specific mutations and genes involved in CF are areas of current research that are still in the early stages of development.

SUGGESTED READINGS

1. Borowitz D, Robinson KA, Rosenfeld M, et al. Cystic Fibrosis Foundation evidence-based guidelines for management of infants with cystic fibrosis. *J Pediatr.* 2009;155:S73-S93.
2. Farrell PM, Rosenstein BJ, White TB, et al. Guidelines for diagnosis of cystic fibrosis in newborns through older adults: Cystic Fibrosis Foundation consensus report. *J Pediatr.* 2008;153:S4-S14.
3. McNally P. Cystic fibrosis. In: Florin TA, Ludwig S, eds. *Netter's Pediatrics.* Philadelphia: Elsevier; 2011: 246-249.
4. O'Sullivan BP, Freedman SD. Cystic fibrosis. *Lancet.* 2009;373:1891-1904.

CASE 4-6

Four-Month-Old Boy

DEBRA BOYER

PHUONG VO

HISTORY OF PRESENT ILLNESS

The patient is a 4-month-old boy who was a former 28-week premature baby who presented with a 1-week history of a cough. Over the next 4 days, his mother reported an increasing cough with no history of fever or rhinorrhea. He had decreased oral intake and decreased urine output. He had some posttussive emesis and no diarrhea. His uncle has been sick for the last 3 weeks with rhinorrhea and a cough.

MEDICAL HISTORY

The boy born at 28 weeks gestation and required endotracheal intubation for a short period of time after birth. While in the newborn intensive care unit, he did have a course of necrotizing enterocolitis that did not require surgery. He was ultimately discharged home with an apnea monitor and oral caffeine. However, recently his mother ran out of this medication and he had no longer been receiving it. He had two siblings who were healthy.

PHYSICAL EXAMINATION

T 37.2°C; P 138 bpm; RR 27-40/min; BP not obtained; Oxygen saturation 96% in room air and decreasing to 93% with feeds

Weight 25th percentile

On examination, he was alert with moderate respiratory distress and frequent episodes of coughing. His chest examination was significant for grunting with substernal, intercostals, and supraclavicular retractions. Rales were appreciated on the right with good aeration throughout. No wheezes were heard. The remainder of his physical examination was within normal limits.

DIAGNOSTIC STUDIES

The complete blood count revealed a white blood cell count of 25 400 cells/mm^3 with 51% lymphocytes, 17% atypical lymphocytes, 25% segmented neutrophils, and 6% monocytes. The hemoglobin was 12.3 gm/dL and the platelet count was 494 000/mm^3.

COURSE OF ILLNESS

The patient received an albuterol nebulizer treatment with no significant relief. While in the emergency department, he had frequent episodes of coughing with two episodes complicated by bradycardia to 60 bpm and desaturations to 80%. A chest radiograph was obtained (Figure 4-8). A presumptive diagnosis was made and the appropriate test sent for confirmation of the diagnosis.

DISCUSSION CASE 4-6

DIFFERENTIAL DIAGNOSIS

A cough in infancy is most likely related to an infectious process, with viral processes being the leading causes. Respiratory syncytial virus is a

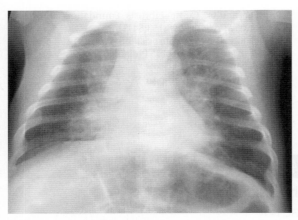

FIGURE 4-8. Chest radiograph.

also more likely to develop reactive airways disease in response to a viral infection.

DIAGNOSIS

Chest radiograph revealed bilateral perihilar infiltrates (Figure 4-8). Given the combination of the radiographic findings, worsening cough, dramatic leukocytosis, lymphocytosis with a substantial number of atypical lymphocytes, and contact with an adult with prolonged cough, a presumptive diagnosis of *B. pertussis* was made. A nasopharyngeal specimen was sent for *B. pertussis* PCR and was positive. **Thus, the diagnosis is infection with *B. pertussis.***

common cause of cough. However, other infectious etiologies should always be considered. Even with good adherence to vaccine regimens, bacterial infections such as *B. pertussis* are still possible in infants. While not commonly expected in this age group, *M. pneumoniae* infections rarely occur in infancy.

Reactive airway disease, most commonly secondary to viral infections, is also a common cause of cough in infancy. Gastroesophageal reflux should be considered as well, even with often few overt gastrointestinal symptoms.

Less common causes for cough in infancy include congenital malformations, such as tracheoesophageal fistula, tracheobronchomalacia, vascular rings, lobar emphysema, bronchogenic cysts, pulmonary sequestration, laryngeal cleft, and congenital pulmonary airway malformations. Furthermore, one should attempt to elicit a history for any possible swallowing disorder that might lead to recurrent aspiration.

Other less common causes of cough in infancy include cystic fibrosis, congestive heart failure, interstitial pneumonitis, and congenital immunodeficiencies.

This patient's history is suggestive of an infectious etiology, as he was in good health until approximately 1 week prior to presentation. However, his history of prematurity should add one more disease to the differential diagnosis in this patient, bronchopulmonary dysplasia. These patients are

INCIDENCE AND EPIDEMIOLOGY

Bordetella pertussis, a Gram-negative bacillus, is the causative organism for what is commonly referred to as whooping cough. A whooping cough syndrome can also be seen with *B. parapertussis*, *M. pneumoniae*, *C. trachomatis*, *C. pneumoniae*, and some adenoviruses.

Pertussis is considered one of the most highly communicable diseases, with transmission occurring via contact with respiratory tract secretions of an infected patient. With waning immunity from childhood vaccination, adults and adolescents are commonly the source of infection in infants and young children.

The true incidence is unknown as many cases in adolescents and adults are unrecognized. The World Health Organization estimates about 20 to 40 million cases of pertussis per year worldwide, with 90% of the cases occurring in developing countries and 295 000 reported deaths per year. The Centers for Disease Control and Prevention report that in the United States infants less than 1 year of age have the highest incidence with 55.2 cases per 100 000 population although adolescents and adults have the largest increase in incidence rates from 1980 to 2005. In general, the disease is endemic, but there are 3-5 year cycles of epidemics that occur in addition to the endemic levels. For unknown reasons, girls are affected at much higher rates and with higher morbidity than boys.

CLINICAL PRESENTATION

The incubation period is generally 1-3 weeks with the infectious period divided into three stages. The catarrhal stage begins with symptoms of a mild upper respiratory tract infection, and lasts a few days to 1 week. The paroxysmal stage then follows with the characteristic inspiratory whoop. Post-tussive emesis is common, and fever is infrequent. In infants, the whoop is generally absent, as they are unable to generate the force needed for this maneuver.

Increased intrathoracic and intraabdominal pressures during coughing may lead to conjunctival and scleral hemorrhages, petechiae on the upper body, epistaxis, and retinal hemorrhages. In infancy, apnea is a common complication with *B. pertussis* infections. Even young adults can suffer from episodes of laryngospasm. Seizures result from either hypoxia or hyponatremia from inappropriate secretion of antidiuretic hormone secretion.

In most cases, a pertussis infection lasts 6-10 weeks, but it is not uncommon for infants and children to have a persistent cough for 3-4 months following a pertussis infection. This chronic cough lasting for weeks to months characterizes the third stage of pertussis disease progression, the convalescent stage.

Respiratory distress between paroxysms of coughing suggests superinfection with various viruses (adenovirus, respiratory syncytial virus, cytomegalovirus) or bacteria (*Streptococcus pneumoniae* and *Staphylococcus aureus*). Other complications include pneumothorax, encephalopathy, and feeding difficulties in infancy. The disease is most severe in infants younger than 1 year of age, especially for premature infants.

DIAGNOSTIC APPROACH

Blood counts. Leukocytosis (white blood cell count >15000/mm³), usually due to an absolute lymphocytosis, is present in more than 75% of unvaccinated children during the late catarrhal and paroxysmal stages. The degree of lymphocytosis typically parallels the severity of illness. Lymphocytosis is less common and less extreme in previously vaccinated children who develop pertussis. Eosinophilia is uncommon.

Chest roentgenogram. Pulmonary infiltrates are often seen and are most commonly perihilar. Classically, a "shaggy" right heart border is seen but the finding is nonspecific. Peribronchial cuffing or atelectasis may also be observed. Consolidation if present is most likely from a secondary bacterial infection, rarely pertussis pneumonia. Pneumothorax or pneumomediastinum may also be seen as complications of pertussis infection. The chest radiograph should be performed to exclude other cases of cough or respiratory distress, such as pneumonia and congestive heart failure.

Bordetella pertussis culture. Growing the organism in culture is certainly the gold standard for diagnosis. The ability to grow the organism is highest during the catarrhal stage or early paroxysmal stage. A negative culture can be seen in patients who were previously vaccinated, have received pertussis therapy, or have been coughing far beyond the paroxysmal stage.

Direct immunofluorescent assay (DFA). This is performed on nasopharyngeal secretions and has variable sensitivity and low specificity. Furthermore, it requires a significant level of skill and is therefore not very reliable and reproducible.

Polymerase chain reaction (PCR). PCR has been used to document *B. pertussis* infections even after the organism will no longer grow in culture. Therefore, it is able to detect disease even in the late paroxysmal stage or after patients have received pertussis therapy. This is the preferred method to confirm the diagnosis of pertussis.

TREATMENT

As young infants with pertussis have a high risk for complications, there should be a low threshold for admitting these patients. Many of these infants will require intensive care unit admission to monitor for apneic episodes and neurologic sequelae.

Infants should be treated with a macrolide antibiotic, including erythromycin, azithromycin, and clarithromycin. Erythromycin is the most common choice. For infants less than 1 month of age, the AAP and CDC recommend the use of azithromycin. Erythromycin is the alternative; clarithromycin is not recommended. Azithromycin has fewer adverse side effects than erythromycin, which has been associated with the development of infantile hypertrophic pyloric stenosis. Trimethoprim-sulfamethoxazole is an alternative agent that can be used for children older than 2 months of age who cannot take macrolides for pertussis treatment or prophylaxis or who are infected with a macrolide-resistant strain.

The length of antimicrobial therapy is generally recommended to be 14 days. For the newer macrolides, azithromycin and clarithromycin, treatment course can be shorter (5-7 days). There is some controversy as to whether antibiotics administered during the catarrhal stage will decrease disease severity. However, antibiotics should still be administered, even in the paroxysmal stage, as this will limit the spread of the disease to others. Additionally, studies are underway assessing the efficacy of pertussis immune globulin as an adjunctive therapy in extremely ill infants.

Antibiotic prophylaxis is recommended for all household and close contacts and generally consists of 10-14 days of erythromycin. Azithromycin for 5 days or clarithromycin for 7 days can also be used for postexposure phrophylaxis. Certainly, prevention is essential to limit morbidity and mortality from pertussis. The acellular pertussis vaccine is currently the recommended form and is administered in combination with diphtheria and tetanus toxoids (DTaP). It is recommended that children receive five doses prior to school-entry.

SUGGESTED READINGS

1. American Academy of Pediatrics. Pertussis. In: Pickering LK, Baker CJ, Kimberlin MD, Long SS, eds. *2009 Red Book: Report on Infectious Diseases*. 28th ed. Elk Grove Village, IL: American Academy of Pediatrics; 2009:504.
2. Hewlett EL. *Bordetella* species. In: Mandell GL, Bennett JE, Dolin R, eds. *Mandell, Douglas, and Bennett's Principles and Practice of Infectious Diseases*. 5th ed. Philadelphia: Churchill Livingstone; 2000:2414-2419.
3. Hoppe JE. Neonatal pertussis. *Pediatr Infect Dis J*. 2000; 19:244-247.
4. Long SS, Edwards KM. Bordetella pertussis (pertussis) and other species. In: Long SS, Pickering LK, Prober CG, eds. *Principles and Practice of Pediatric Infectious Diseases*. 2nd ed. New York: Churchill Livingstone; 2003:880-888.
5. Senzilet LD, Halperin SA, Spika JS, et al. Pertussis is a frequent cause of prolonged cough illness in adults and adolescents. *Clin Infect Dis*. 2001;32:1691-1697.
6. Sprauer MA, Cochi SL, Zell ER, et al. Prevention of secondary transmission of pertussis in households with early use of erythromycin. *Am J Dis Child*. 1992; 146:177-181.

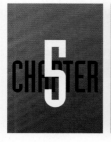

CHAPTER 5

BACK, JOINT, AND EXTREMITY PAIN

MEGAN AYLOR

DEFINITION OF THE COMPLAINT

Back, joint, and extremity pain are worrisome symptoms in children. Although benign musculoskeletal disease accounts for many cases, more sinister diagnoses should be ruled out. The inability of young children to clearly describe the location and nature of the pain contributes to diagnostic difficulties. Since the diverse complaints of back, extremity, and joint pain frequently share a common etiology, a uniform approach to such symptoms facilitates accurate diagnosis.

COMPLAINT BY CAUSE AND FREQUENCY

Back pain, or discomfort anywhere along the spinal and paraspinal area, reflects potential pathology in a wide range of organ systems, including musculoskeletal, central nervous system, pulmonary, vascular, and intraabdominal or retroperitoneal structures (Table 5-1). Young children who cannot accurately localize pain require indirect symptom assessment. For example, refusal to walk, irritability with repositioning, and reluctance to participate in specific activities often provide the earliest clues to identifying back pain.

Alteration in gait or changes in the use of a limb also suggest an underlying extremity or joint disorder (Table 5-2). Examining one joint above and below the site of the chief complaint can prevent missing a diagnosis in cases of referred pain. For example, knee pain may be the presenting symptom for hip pathology. Joint and extremity symptoms can also represent referred pain from a spinal or paraspinal process. The radicular symptoms of nerve root entrapment in the lumbar spine may present as foot pain.

Evaluation of back, extremity, and joint pain requires an understanding that extensive interplay of symptoms, findings, and etiologies exists among these diagnostic groups. Any patient with pain that interferes with activity, has associated neurologic symptoms (weakness, changes in reflexes, or bowel/bladder control), or has worrisome associated symptoms (weight loss, fever, worsening pain over time) should prompt a diagnostic evaluation.

CLARIFYING QUESTIONS

Routine inquiry into the onset, location, duration, character, radiation, and intensity of the pain may help clarify the diagnosis. Caretaker observations may supplement the history, especially in nonverbal patients. The timing of symptom onset relative to a traumatic injury can pose a particular diagnostic challenge. Many children with nontraumatic abnormalities will first notice a symptom following an insignificant injury. For example, a child with a spinal tumor may fall off a bicycle and complain of leg pain, when in fact the tumor was present for weeks, and the progressive paresis caused the child to fall from the bike. Incidental injuries are present in almost all children's recent history and may be associated with the underlying problem, but may not necessarily be the primary cause.

TABLE 5-1.	Causes of back pain in childhood by etiology.

Infectious/Inflammatory
Vertebral ostemyelitis
Spinal epidural abscess
Diskitis
Paraspinal pyomyositis
Pneumonia
Pyelonephritis

Orthopedic
Scheuermann (juvenile) kyphosis
Spondylolysis/spondylolisthesis
Scoliosis
Intravertebral disk herniation
Trauma
Muscle strain

Rheumatologic
Juvenile ankylosing spondylitis
Juvenile rheumatoid arthritis

Neoplastic
Osteoid osteoma
Neuroblastoma
Ganglioneuroma
Lymphoma
Leukemia
Eosinophilic granuloma

Miscellaneous
Sickle cell disease
Nephrolithiasis

TABLE 5-2.	Causes of joint or extremity pain in childhood by etiology.

Infectious/Inflammatory
Bacterial arthritis
Lyme arthritis
Disseminated *Neisseria gonorrhoeae*
Osteomyelitis
Pyomyositis
Acute rheumatic fever
Reactive/postinfectious arthritis
Immunization

Orthopedic
Trauma
Osteochondritis dessicans
Chondromalacia patella
Overuse syndromes
Osgood-Schlatter

Rheumatologic
Systemic juvenile idiopathic arthritis
Systemic lupus erythematosus
Dermatomyositis

Neoplastic
Leukemia
Lymphoma
Bone/soft tissue tumors
Metastatic malignancy

Hematologic
Sickle cell disease
Hemophilia

Miscellaneous
Kawasaki disease
Serum sickness
Behçet disease
Sarcoidosis
Henoch-Schönlein purpura
Guillain-Barré syndrome

Some particularly helpful questions are listed below:

• What is the age of the patient?
—In younger children, especially those under 5 years of age, back pain is often a manifestation of a serious underlying disorder. In contrast, older adolescents are more likely to have nonspecific musculoskeletal disorders similar to adults with back pain.

• What is the timing of the pain?
—Mechanical strains and stresses are often improved at night, and resolve within several weeks. However, spondylolysis, spondylolithesis, and Scheuermann disease may also improve with rest. Pain that worsens at night is more typical of neoplastic or infectious etiologies.

• Are there systemic symptoms?
—Fever, malaise, and weight loss are more suggestive of an inflammatory, neoplastic, or infectious etiology.

• Are there any neurologic findings?
—Bowel or bladder dysfunction, weakness, and changes on deep tendon reflexes are worrisome for spinal pathology such as syringomyelia, ruptured disc, or spinal cord tumor.

• Is there decreased range of motion of the back?
—Stiffness of the spine is an unusual finding in young children and may indicate infection, inflammation, or tumor. In adolescents, muscle spasm from overuse injuries limit the range of motion, but this finding resolves quickly.

• Is a deformity of the back noticeable?
—Deformity of the normal spinal curvature may represent primary spinal pathology, a

congenital or idiopathic process, or muscular abnormalities that contribute to progressive scoliosis or kyphosis. Splinting during acute pneumonia leads to transient abnormal lateral curvature of the thoracic spine. Midline skin lesions such as a hemangioma, sacral dimple, or hairy patch may be useful clues to underlying spinal dysraphism.

CASE 5-1

Two-Year-Old Boy

SANJEEV K. SWAMI

HISTORY OF PRESENT ILLNESS

A 2-year-old boy presented to the emergency department for evaluation of back pain. Three days prior to admission he began complaining of abdominal pain, refused to eat lunch that day, and spent most of the afternoon watching television rather than playing outside with his siblings. At that time, he was taken to a nearby hospital for evaluation. On examination, he had mild diffuse abdominal tenderness but no rebound tenderness or involuntary guarding. Abdominal radiographs showed significant stool in the rectum and distal colon. He was diagnosed with constipation, given a glycerin suppository, and discharged after producing a moderate amount of stool.

On the day of admission, he returned to the hospital with persistent abdominal pain and a new complaint of low back pain. His oral intake had been poor over the past few days. There had been minimal response to a glycerin suppository earlier that day. He also seemed particularly uncomfortable while his diaper was being changed. There was no fever, cough, hematemesis, hematochezia, dysuria, or urinary frequency. There were no ill contacts and no known trauma. The only pet was an elderly dog that had been euthanized earlier in the week.

MEDICAL HISTORY

Tympanostomy tubes had been placed at 15 months of age for recurrent otitis media. He had only one episode of otitis media after the tubes were placed. He did not have a prior history of constipation. He was not taking any medications on a regular basis. His family history was remarkable for a paternal uncle who had a myocardial infarction at 55 years of age.

PHYSICAL EXAMINATION

T 38.9°C; HR 130 bpm; RR 36/min; BP 115/55 mmHg; SpO_2 99% in room air

Weight 18.0 kg (>95th percentile)

The child appeared uncomfortable and refused to stand. The eyes, nose, and oropharynx were clear. The neck was supple. The abdomen was mildly distended and diffusely tender, particularly in the right lower quadrant. However, there was no rebound tenderness or involuntary guarding. There was no costovertebral angle tenderness. There was discomfort with passive flexion of the right hip. There was mild edema and tenderness to percussion along the right paraspinus muscle at the level of the L1 vertebrae. There was no kyphosis, scoliosis, or abnormal lordosis. There were no apparent sensory or motor neurologic deficits, though the degree of back and abdominal pain made assessment of muscle strength in the lower extremities difficult. There was no muscle atrophy. Rectal tone was normal. The deep tendon reflexes were symmetric and appropriately brisk. The remainder of the examination was normal.

DIAGNOSTIC STUDIES

Complete blood count revealed the following: 19700 white blood cells/mm³ (67% segmented neutrophils, 29% lymphocytes, and 3% monocytes); hemoglobin, 11.4 g/dL; and platelets, 390000/mm³.

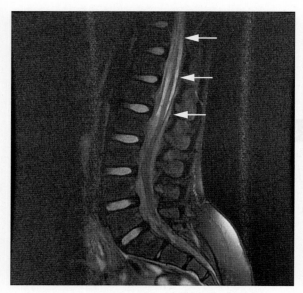

FIGURE 5-1. Magnetic resonance of the spine.

Serum electrolytes were remarkable for a bicarbonate level of 19 mEq/L and for blood urea nitrogen and creatinine levels of 7 mg/dL and 0.3 mg/dL, respectively. Urinalysis revealed a specific gravity of 1.020 and 3+ ketones but normal microscopy. Serum albumin and transaminases were normal. C-reactive protein (CRP) and erythrocyte sedimentation rate (ESR) were elevated at 7.9 mg/dL and 65 mm/h, respectively. Abdominal obstruction series revealed scattered air fluid levels and a small amount of stool in the rectum.

COURSE OF ILLNESS

Magnetic resonance imaging (MRI) of the spine localized the abnormality (Figure 5-1) and the definitive diagnosis was made by an interventional study.

DISCUSSION CASE 5-1

DIFFERENTIAL DIAGNOSIS

Back pain is a relatively common complaint among children though fewer than 2% of children with back pain require specific medical evaluation. In a young child, neoplastic, infectious, and inflammatory disorders should be considered. Traumatic injury is usually clear based on the history prior to presentation. Malignant causes may be primary or metastatic and include osteoid osteoma, neuroblastoma, Wilms tumor, and leukemia. Infectious or inflammatory causes include pyelonephritis, vertebral osteomyelitis, spinal epidural abscess, and pyomyositis. Diskitis in children usually involves the lower thoracic or lumbar spine. The presence of fever, if related to the back pain, makes diskitis less likely. Local tenderness and elevated CRP and ESR can be seen with many infectious and neoplastic causes. MRI of the spine readily differentiates diskitis, vertebral osteomyelitis, and spinal epidural abscess. Rheumatologic conditions include systemic juvenile rheumatoid arthritis and ankylosing spondylitis. Mechanical disorders, such as muscle strains and intervertebral disk herniation, are less likely in children, although spondylolysis and spondylolisthesis do present in this age group. The absence of neurologic findings, while reassuring, does not exclude any of the above entities.

DIAGNOSIS

MRI of the spine revealed an abnormal heterogeneous enhancing mass (Figure 5-1, arrows) in the epidural space at the L1-L3 vertebral level. There was associated compression of the thecal sac. Urine homovanillic acid and vanillylmandelic acid levels were normal, making neuroblastoma less likely. Gram-stain of purulent material drained during biopsy of the mass revealed many white blood cells and Gram-positive cocci. Group A *Streptococcus* subsequently grew from culture. **The diagnosis was spinal epidural abscess due to group A *Streptococcus*.** The demise of the pet dog did not appear to be related to this patient's diagnosis.

EPIDEMIOLOGY AND INCIDENCE

Spinal epidural abscesses occur rarely in children with one series reporting an incidence of 0.6 per 10 000 hospital admissions over a 15-year period at a free standing children's hospital. Most patients are previously healthy but predisposing risk factors include sickle cell disease (SCD), hematologic malignancy, and spinal surgery. Spinal epidural abscess occasionally complicates serial lumbar punctures and varicella infection. In adult patients, additional risk factors include trauma and invasive procedures (i.e., spinal aneasthesia). *Staphylococcus aureus* causes more than two-thirds of cases; additional pathogens have been reported (Table 5-3). With the emergence of community acquired methicillin-resistant *Staphylococcus aureus* (MRSA), the incidence of MRSA epidural infections has increased over recent years.

The infection is usually acquired by hematogenous spread and occasionally by direct extension from an adjacent site of infection. Associated osteomyelitis is present in approximately 50% of

TABLE 5-3.	Etiologies of epidural abscesses.
Pathogen	**Comments**
Staphylococcus aureus	Most common etiology
Group A *Streptococcus*	
Group B *Streptococcus*	Neonates or infants
Salmonella species	Patients with sickle cell disease; contact with reptiles or amphibians
Escherichia coli	Patients with inflammatory bowel disease Complication of a genitourinary tract infection
Pseudomonas aeruginosa	Patients with hematologic malignancies or neutropenia
Anaerobes	Patients with inflammatory bowel disease
Candida species	Rare; reported in immunocompromised patients and those with central venous catheters
Aspergillus flavus	Rare; reported in immunocompromised patients, particularly those with chronic granulomatous disease, and in patients with central venous catheters
Mycobacterium tuberculosis	More common in areas with a high prevalence of *M. tuberculosis*

cases. In one case series, 7 of 8 children with spinal epidural abscess had an associated psoas or paraspinal abscess.

CLINICAL PRESENTATION

Most children develop fever early during the course of infection. Common presenting complaints include back pain, limp, and refusal to walk. Hip pain is an unusual presenting complaint though it may be difficult to differentiate back from hip pain in an ill and irritable child. Depending on the level of involvement, progression of infection can cause spinal cord compression, muscle weakness, and bowel and bladder incontinence followed by paralysis. On examination, there may be tenderness over the vertebra or paraspinal tissues. Some children develop protective paraspinal muscle spasm. There may also be loss of normal curvature of the spine (usually decreased lumbar lordosis) and limited lumbosacral mobility. Abdominal pain is relatively common and can indicate radicular pain or associated psoas abscess.

DIAGNOSTIC APPROACH

Spinal epidural abscesses can present with a range of clinical and laboratory findings and a high level of suspicion is required to make the diagnosis early in the course of infection. Surgical aspiration should always be performed since identification of a specific pathogen permits optimal antibiotic selection. Other studies may increase the level of suspicion for spinal epidural abscess.

Complete blood count. The complete blood count typically reveals the nonspecific findings of acute infection. The peripheral white blood cell count is elevated in approximately 50% of cases. There may be a predominance of neutrophils or an increased percentage of immature polymorphonuclear cells. Thrombocytosis may be present.

CRP and ESR. These markers of inflammation are usually elevated, especially when there is an associated vertebral osteomyelitis. These markers of inflammation may also be elevated in noninfectious conditions such as malignancy. CRP and ESR have also been used to assess response to antibiotic therapy. The timing of their normalization has not been studied with epidural abscesses but likely parallels their trends in osteomyelitis where the CRP peaks within the first 2 days of treatment and returns to normal within 7-10 days and the ESR peaks within the first 5-7 days of treatment and returns to normal within 4 weeks.

Blood culture. Organisms are isolated from blood culture in approximately 10% of cases. When positive, the blood culture is invaluable in guiding specific antibiotic therapy.

Spine radiographs. Radiographs of the spine exclude other causes of back pain. Associated vertebral osteomyelitis may be evident in children with a prolonged duration of symptoms.

Spine MRI. MRI of the spine demonstrates the abscess, though definitive diagnosis requires biopsy. MRI reveals concomitant vertebral osteomyelitis in 20% to 50% of cases.

Tuberculin skin testing. Tuberculin skin testing should be performed if a bacterial organism has not been isolated from blood or abscess culture since *Mycobacterium tuberculosis* can cause spinal epidural abscesses.

Other studies. At the time of diagnostic biopsy, specimens should be sent for stains and cultures of aerobic and anaerobic bacteria, fungi, and mycobacteria. Radionuclide bone scans to detect osteomyelitis at sites distant from the abscess should be considered in cases where the abscess occurred as a consequence of hematogenous seeding. Cerebrospinal fluid (CSF) abnormalities are common with spinal epidural abscesses. In one case series, 33 (78%) of 42 children with spinal epidural abscess had findings consistent with meningeal infection (mild to moderate pleocytosis or hypoglycorachia). In 12%, elevated CSF protein was the only CSF abnormality. Examination of the CSF was completely normal in 10% of children with spinal epidural abscess. Lumbar puncture should not be performed when the abscess is located in the lumbar region.

TREATMENT

Standard management of epidural abscesses includes antibiotic therapy and surgical drainage.

Sporadic cases reported in the literature have been treated with antibiotics alone. Candidates for antibiotic therapy without surgical drainage may include patients without neurologic deficits and those with numerous abscesses that would be technically difficult to drain. In those children treated with antibiotics without surgical drainage, diagnostic surgical aspiration to identify the infecting organism should be strongly considered. This decision is usually made in consultation with infectious diseases and neurosurgical colleagues. The empiric antibiotic regimen should include agents with activity against *Staphylococcus aureus* such as oxacillin or vancomycin. Vancomycin should be the initial antibiotic when (1) MRSA accounts for more than 10% to 15% of local *S. aureus* isolates, (2) a household member works in a nursing home or other facility with high rates of MRSA colonization, and (3) the patient lives with someone known to be colonized with MRSA. Cefotaxime and metronidazole should be added if Gram-negative or anaerobic organisms are suspected. With increasing rates of Gram-negative resistance to third generation cephalosporins, many practitioners now recommend cefepime rather than cefotaxime. Ultimate antibiotic selection depends on results of blood and abscess culture. The duration of antibiotic treatment is usually determined by a combination of clinical (e.g., improved pain and function), laboratory (e.g., normalization of ESR and C-reactive protein levels), and radiologic imaging (e.g., resolved epidural fluid collection on MRI) improvement, but 6 weeks is usually the minimal duration of therapy.

Mortality rates for adults with spinal epidural abscesses range from 5% to 25%. Mortality rates are substantially lower in children. There were no deaths among the 34 children reviewed in one series. Approximately 75% to 85% of children treated for spinal epidural abscess will have normal neurologic function at the completion of therapy. Risk factors for persistent deficits include patients with multiple medical problems, previous spinal surgery, and severe neurologic deficit at presentation.

SUGGESTED READINGS

1. Auletta JJ, John CC. Spinal epidural abscesses in children: a 15-year experience and review of the literature. *Clin Infect Dis.* 2001;32:9-16.

2. Grewal S, Hocking G, Wildsmith JA. Epidural abscesses. *Bri J. Anaesth.* 2006;96:292-302.

3. Darouiche RO. Spinal epidural abscess. *N Engl J Med.* 2006;355:2012-2020.

4. Bair-Merritt MH, Chung C, Collier A. Spinal epidural abscess in a young child. *Pediatrics.* 2000;106:e39. (http://www.pediatrics.org/cgi/content/full/106/3/e39)

5. Yogev R. Focal suppurative infections of the central nervous system. In: Long SS, Pickering LK, Prober CG, eds. *Principles and Practice of Pediatric Infectious Diseases.* 3rd ed. Philadelphia: Churchill Livingstone; 2008:324-335.

6. Rubin G, Michowiz DS, Ashkenasi A, Tadmor R, Rappaport H. Spinal epidural abscess in the pediatric age group: case report and review of the literature. *Pediatr Infect Dis J.* 1993;12:1007-1011.

7. Tunkel AR. Subdural empyema, epidural abscess, and suppurative intracranial thrombophlebitis. In: Mandell GL, Bennett JE, Dolin R, eds. *Principles and Practice of Infectious Diseases.* 7th ed. Philadelphia: Churchill Livingstone; 2010:1279-1287.

CASE 5-2

Two-Year-Old Boy

MAYA A. JONES

HISTORY OF PRESENT ILLNESS

A 2-year-old boy presented with a 2-week history of difficulty walking. Initially, the parents noticed that he would no longer run while playing with his siblings. Then during the past week he began walking with a limp and refused to climb stairs. The patient has had no fever, cough, rhinorrhea, throat pain, diarrhea, trauma, and there are no sick contacts. The patient lives with his parents and siblings and they have one dog.

The parents brought the patient to his pediatrician who detected splenomegaly and tenderness over the right hip on physical examination. Therefore, hip radiographs and laboratory studies were obtained after which the patient was immediately referred to the emergency department.

MEDICAL HISTORY

The patient was born at term without complications. He had one hospitalization at 4 months of age for wheezing and had pneumonia at 12 months of age which was treated as an outpatient. He was not receiving any medications and had no allergies. Family history was remarkable for a maternal aunt with rheumatic heart disease.

PHYSICAL EXAMINATION

T 37.3°C; P 104 bpm; RR 34/min; BP 98/43 mmHg

Height and Weight both 25th percentile for age

On examination the child was pale and appeared tired. His sclerae were anicteric. The heart and lung sounds were normal. On abdominal examination, the spleen tip was palpable just below the left costal margin and the liver edge was palpable 3 cm below the right costal margin. There was mild discomfort with passive flexion of the right hip but he had full range of motion and there was no overlying erythema or warmth. The left hip was unremarkable. The testes were in normal position and were not enlarged, swollen, or tender. There were numerous petechiae scattered on his lower extremities bilaterally. There were multiple small lymph nodes palpable in the anterior cervical and inguinal regions.

DIAGNOSTIC STUDIES

Complete blood count revealed a white blood cell (WBC) count of 4300/mm³ with 3% band forms, 8% segmented neutrophils, and 85% lymphocytes, and an absolute neutrophil count of 473/mm³. The hemoglobin was 8.0 g/dL with a reticulocyte count of 1.3%, platelet count was 31000/mm³. C-reactive protein and erythrocyte sedimentation rate were 2.6 mg/dL and 60 mm/h, respectively. Serum lactate dehydrogenase (LDH), uric acid, transaminases, and electrolytes were normal. The hip radiographs performed earlier were reviewed (Figure 5-2A).

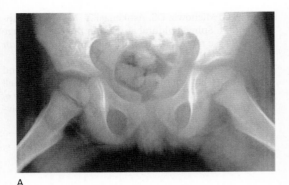

A

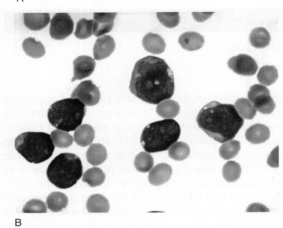

B

FIGURE 5-2. **A.** Hip radiograph. **B.** Peripheral blood smear.

COURSE OF ILLNESS

Results of the hip radiographs combined with results of the peripheral blood smear (Figure 5-2B) suggested a diagnosis.

DISCUSSION CASE 5-2

DIFFERENTIAL DIAGNOSIS

Infectious causes of hip pain in a young boy include septic arthritis of the hip, osteomyelitis of the femur or pelvis, and psoas abscess. The prolonged duration of symptoms with recent worsening in conjunction with an elevated C-reactive protein and erythrocyte sedimentation may indicate osteomyelitis of the femur with extension of infection into the hip joint. However, the mild rather than severe hip pain on examination and the subacute rather than acute nature makes septic arthritis of the hip unlikely. Children with pancytopenia in the context of osteomyelitis are usually critically ill. Toxic synovitis can cause hip pain in this age group. While pancytopenia can be caused by viral-mediated bone marrow suppression, the mild degree of pain is not consistent with joint effusion.

Causes of pancytopenia, hepatosplenomegaly, and bone pain include leukemia, epiphyseal tumors, neuroblastoma, infectious mononucleosis, hemophagocytic syndrome, and Gaucher disease. The normal uric acid and lactate dehydrogenase (LDH) do not exclude malignancy.

DIAGNOSIS

The hip radiographs revealed dense metaphyseal lines bilaterally with adjacent metaphyseal lucency, a finding suggestive of leukemia (Figure 5-2A). The peripheral blood smear revealed numerous cells with scant cytoplasm and finely dispersed to variably condensed chromatin morphologically consistent with lymphoblasts (Figure 5-2B). **Morphologic, cytochemical, and immunophenotypic features of the bone marrow aspirate were diagnostic of acute lymphocytic leukemia.** The child was initially treated with vincristine, dexamethasone, and intrathecal ara-C.

EPIDEMIOLOGY

Leukemia results from malignant transformation and clonal expansion of hematopoietic cells that have stopped at a particular stage of differentiation and are unable to progress to more mature forms. Leukemias are divided into acute and chronic subtypes and further classified on the basis of leukemic cell morphology into lymphocytic leukemias (lymphoid lineage cell proliferation) and nonlymphocytic leukemias (granulocyte, monocyte, erythrocyte, or platelet lineage cell proliferation). Acute leukemias constitute more than 95% of all childhood leukemias and are subdivided into acute lymphocytic leukemia (ALL) and acute nonlymphocytic leukemia, also known as acute myelogenous leukemia (AML). The following discussion focuses on ALL.

ALL, the most common pediatric malignancy, accounts for approximately 25% of all childhood cancers and 75% of all childhood leukemias. Most children are diagnosed between 2 and 5 years of age. In the United States, the incidence of ALL is higher in whites compared to blacks and in boys compared to girls. Genetic factors also affect the risk of ALL which occurs in siblings of children with ALL two to four times more often than in unrelated children. The concordance of ALL in monozygotic twins is approximately 25%. Children with chromosomal abnormalities, including trisomy 21, and syndromes characterized by chromosomal fragility, such as Bloom syndrome and Fanconi anemia, also have a substantially higher risk of leukemia.

CLINICAL PRESENTATION

The presenting signs and symptoms of children with ALL reflect both the degree of bone marrow infiltration with leukemic cells and the extent of extramedullary disease spread. Symptoms may be present for days or months and include fever, anorexia, fatigue, and pallor. Bone pain occurs with leukemic involvement of the periosteum and bone. Young children often develop a limp or refuse to walk. Headache, vomiting, and seizures suggest central nervous system (CNS) involvement. Rarely, children present with oliguria due to acute renal failure precipitated by hyperuricemia.

On examination, painless lymphadenopathy (50%) and hepatosplenomegaly (68%) result from extramedullary spread of the disease. Petechiae and purpura are more common but some children may also have subconjunctival and retinal hemorrhages. Children may also have focal bone tenderness. Testicular enlargement due to leukemic infiltration is present in 5% of boys. In addition to these physical examination findings, there are three life-threatening presentations of ALL, infection/neutropenia, tumor lysis syndrome, and hyperleukocytosis (summarized in Table 5-4) which require immediate attention and intervention.

TABLE 5-4.	Life-threatening presentations of ALL.	
Life-Threatening Presentation	Clinical Manifestations	Treatment
Infection or Neutropenia	Fever Sepsis Bacteremia Typhlitis: necrotizing enterocolitis occurring in profoundly neutropenic patients	Blood cultures Broad-spectrum antibiotics Pressor support
Tumor Lysis Syndrome	Rapid cell turnover leading to release of intracellular contents Hyperuricemia, hyperkalemia, hyperphosphatemia, hypocalcemia Renal failure	Aggressive hydration Alkanize urine (bicarbonate-containing IV fluids) Allopurinol/urate oxidase Frequent monitoring of electrolytes and renal function
Hyperleukocytosis	WBC> 100×10^3 Hyperviscosity, sludging CVA, renal insufficiency, pulmonary infarct	Exchange transfusion or leukapheresis Treat leukemia rapidly

Source: Reproduced, with permission, from Florin T, Ludwig S, et al. *Netter's Pediatrics*. Philadelphia: Saunders, 2011.

DIAGNOSTIC APPROACH

Complete blood count. The WBC is between $10\,000/mm^3$ and $50\,000/mm^3$ in 30% of children with ALL and greater than $50\,000/mm^3$ in approximately 20%. Neutropenia, defined as an absolute neutrophil count less than $500/mm^3$, is common at presentation. Other findings include moderate to severe anemia and an inappropriately low reticulocyte count. The platelet count is less than $100\,000/mm^3$ in approximately 75% of patients, however isolated thrombocytopenia rarely occurs. Leukemic cells may be noted on the peripheral blood smear, particularly if the WBC count is normal or high.

Bone marrow aspirate or biopsy. A bone marrow aspirate or biopsy definitively establishes the diagnosis of ALL since the morphology of blasts seen on peripheral smear may not reflect the true bone marrow morphology. Monoclonal antibody testing of the bone marrow for specific cell surface antigens identifies lymphocytes and granulocytes at different stages of development. When this immunophenotyping is combined with cytochemical staining and molecular genotyping, the diagnostic classification, treatment, and prognosis become more specific.

Other laboratory studies. Other laboratory abnormalities reflect either leukemic cell infiltration or excessive proliferation and destruction of leukemic cells. Serum transaminases may be mildly abnormal with liver infiltration but coagulation abnormalities are uncommon. Hypercalcemia results from leukemic infiltration of bone. Cell lysis leads to elevated phosphorus, LDH, and serum uric acid, reflecting increased purine catabolism.

Radiographs. Long bone radiograph abnormalities include transverse radiolucent metaphyseal growth arrest lines, periosteal elevation with reactive subperiosteal cortical thickening, and osteolytic lesions.

Computed tomography (CT). CT may reveal diffuse lymphadenopathy and hepatosplenomegaly. Approximately 5% to 10% of newly diagnosed patients have an anterior mediastinal mass detected on chest imaging.

TREATMENT

Although specific treatment strategies may vary between hospitals, all modern approaches treat leukemia, the complications of leukemia, and manage treatment-related complications. Acute management involves blood product transfusions and treatment of infection, hyperviscosity, compressive symptoms, and metabolic abnormalities. Tumor lysis syndrome describes the constellation of metabolic abnormalities resulting from spontaneous or treatment-induced tumor necrosis. Acute tumor cell destruction releases intracellular contents into circulation leading to hypocalcemia, hyperphosphatemia, hyperkalemia, and hyperuricemia. Management of tumor lysis syndrome includes

vigorous hydration, urine alkalinization, uric acid reduction, and diuretic therapy.

Specific therapy for ALL is instituted in three distinct phases. *Remission induction* therapy lasts approximately 4 weeks during which most children have a complete remission, defined as the absence of clinical signs and symptoms of disease, recovery of normal blood cell counts, and recovery of normocellular bone marrow. Agents currently used for remission induction include dexamethasone or prednisone, vincristine, and L-asparaginase. Other agents may be used if the patient is considered high-risk or has CNS involvement. *Consolidation therapy* aims to kill additional leukemic cells with further systemic therapy and prevent CNS relapse with intrathecal chemotherapy. *Maintenance therapy* continues remission achieved by the first two phases. It is required because shorter treatment protocols are associated with a high rate of relapse. Methotrexate and 6-mercaptopurine are often used for consolidation and maintenance therapy.

Children with high WBC counts ($>50000/mm^3$), younger than 2 years of age, or older than 10 years of age at the time of diagnosis have the worst prognosis. However, between 95% and 98% of children diagnosed with ALL achieve complete remission after induction therapy. Relapse occurs in 20% to 30% either during subsequent treatment or within the first 2 years after its completion. Relapse affects virtually any site of the body, though bone marrow relapse is most common. Since the introduction of effective CNS-directed therapy, the frequency of CNS relapse has decreased to approximately 5%. Isolated testicular relapse occurs in 1% of boys. Bone marrow relapse is often treated with intense chemotherapy combined with bone marrow transplantation. The event-free survival rate after relapse ranges from 30% to 60%.

Late sequelae of ALL therapy include second neoplasms, neuropsychologic effects, endocrine dysfunction, and other organ-specific complications. Second neoplasms occur in 2.5% of patients, CNS tumors being the most common. Children less than 5 years of age at ALL diagnosis and those who received cranial irradiation are at highest risk of second neoplasms. Short stature occurs due to cranial irradiation-induced growth hormone deficiency. Some late complications are related to specific chemotherapeutic agents such as cardiomyopathy from anthracycline or bladder fibrosis from cyclophosphamide therapy. Chemotherapy may also have long-term effects on the child's immune system. Recovery of the immune system usually occurs within 1-2 years after the completion of chemotherapy; however, some children may have low antibody titers of clinically significant viruses to which they have been previously immunized.

SUGGESTED READINGS

1. Hermiston ML, Mentzer WC. A practical approach to the evaluation of the anemic child. *Pediatr Clin N Am.* 2002;49:877-891.
2. Margolin JF, Poplack DG. Acute lymphoblastic leukemia. In: Pizzo PA, Poplack DG, eds. *Principles and Practice of Pediatric Oncology.* 3rd ed. Philadelphia: Lippincott-Raven Publishers; 1997:409-462.
3. Meister LA, Meadows AT. Late effects of childhood cancer therapy. *Curr Probl Pediatr.* 1993;23:102-131.
4. Neglia JP, Meadows AT, Robison LL, et al. Second neoplasms after acute lymphoblastic leukemia in childhood. *N Engl J Med.* 1991;325:1330-1336.
5. Pui CH, Crist WM. Biology and treatment of acute lymphoblastic leukemia. *J Pediatr.* 1994;124:491-503.
6. Rubnitz JE, Look AT. Molecular genetics of childhood leukemias. *J Pediatr Hematol Oncol.* 1998;20:1-11.
7. Sanders JE. Bone marrow transplantation for pediatric leukemia. *Pediatr Ann.* 1991;20:671-676.

CASE 5-3

Fourteen-Year-Old Boy

MEGAN AYLOR

HISTORY OF PRESENT ILLNESS

A 14-year-old boy presented to the emergency department complaining of left knee pain. Three days prior to this visit he noted left knee pain after playing basketball and began to limp. This knee pain improved over the next few days. However, on the day of presentation, he slipped and fell while walking across a wooden floor. As soon as he stood up, he again noted pain in his left knee that occasionally radiated to the left hip. There was no other bone pain. He did not strike his head and did not report headache, blurry vision, or loss of consciousness. There was no fever, weight loss, myalgias, or malaise.

MEDICAL HISTORY

The patient required overnight hospitalization at 8 years of age for disorientation following a car accident. His symptoms resolved fully. At the age of 10, he developed poststreptococcal glomerulonephritis and was treated with a short course of corticosteroids. He did not report taking any medications, currently. There was no family history of endocrine or autoimmune disorders.

PHYSICAL EXAMINATION

T 37.1°C; HR 105 bpm; RR 24/min; BP 125/80 mmHg

Weight 101 kg

Physical examination revealed an obese boy without visible evidence of head trauma. He was alert and cooperative. Heart and lung sounds were normal. The abdomen was soft without organomegaly. There was no deformity of either lower extremity. Passive flexion of the left hip accompanied by internal and external rotation significantly worsened the left knee pain. Internal rotation of the left hip was limited compared to the right hip. There was no tenderness, swelling, or erythema of the left knee. There was full range of motion of the left knee without discomfort when this joint was tested in isolation. There was no sign of knee ligament instability. The right lower extremity was normal. He had an antalgic gait and preferred not to place weight on the left leg due to pain.

DIAGNOSTIC STUDIES

The complete blood count revealed the following: 8600 white blood cells/mm³ (65% segmented

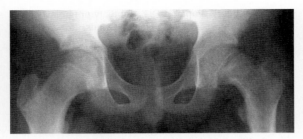

FIGURE 5-3. Antero-posterior (AP) radiographs of the hip.

neutrophils, 30% lymphocytes, and 5% mono-cytes); hemoglobin 13.1 g/dL; and 204 000 plate-lets/mm³. C-reactive protein was 0.7 mg/dL and the erythrocyte sedimentation rate (ESR) was 12 mm/h. Serum electrolytes and calcium were normal.

COURSE OF ILLNESS

Radiographs of the left knee were normal. Hip radiographs revealed the diagnosis (Figure 5-3).

DISCUSSION CASE 5-3

DIFFERENTIAL DIAGNOSIS

Diagnosing the cause of knee pain in an adoles-cent can be difficult. Since knee pain may actu-ally be pain referred from the hip via the obturator nerve, diagnostic considerations should include problems involving either the knee or the hip. In this case, although the patient was adamant in his complaint of pain localized to the knee, examina-tion of the knee was normal. The lack of physical findings localized to the knee makes septic arthri-tis of the knee and fracture of the distal femur, patella, proximal tibia, and fibula unlikely. Ante-cedent trauma raises the possibility of knee hyper-extension or patellar dislocation but the normal knee examination places these possibilities lower on the differential diagnosis. Osgood-Schlatter disease typically presents with localized tender-ness and swelling over the tibial tuberosity, find-ings that were absent in this case.

Hip disorders to consider in an adolescent boy include avascular necrosis of the femoral head, sep-tic arthritis of the hip, femoral or pelvic osteomyeli-tis, femoral neck fracture, chronic developmental

hip dysplasia, inguinal hernia, slipped capital femoral epiphysis, Ewing sarcoma, and osteo-genic sarcoma. Avascular necrosis of the femoral head can be caused by corticosteroid use and also occurs in children with sickle cell disease (SCD) and idiopathically (Legg-Calvé Perthes disease). The absence of fever combined with a normal C-reactive protein and ESR makes acute septic arthritis and osteomyelitis unlikely. In this case, radiographs of the hip narrowed the above differ-ential diagnosis even further.

DIAGNOSIS

Antero-posterior (AP) radiographs of the hip (Fig-ure 5-3) demonstrated inferior displacement of the left femoral head relative to the femoral neck. On the lateral frog leg view this displacement appeared posterior and medial relative to the fem-oral neck. **These findings confirmed the diagno-sis of slipped capital femoral epiphysis (SCFE).** The patient underwent percutaneous screw fixa-tion (Figure 5-4). Prophylactic screw fixation of the contralateral hip was also performed.

INCIDENCE AND EPIDEMIOLOGY

The term SCFE refers to displacement of the femo-ral head relative to the femoral neck through the physis (growth plate). This displacement results from either cumulative normal stresses acting on a weakened physis or by an acute traumatic event on a normal or previously weakened physis. SCFE occurs with an annual incidence of 2-3 cases per 100 000 persons. It typically develops during the adolescent growth spurt, occurring in boys 10-16 years of age and girls 10-13 years of age. The inci-dence is approximately 2.5 times greater in boys compared with girls. The incidence is also higher in African-Americans compared with Cauca-sians. Obesity is a predisposing factor. One-half to two-thirds of children with SCFE have weight-for-height profiles greater than the 95th percen-tile. Obesity may contribute by creating increased shear forces across the weakened physis during ambulation. Underlying endocrine or metabolic disorders that delay skeletal maturation, such as primary or secondary hypothyroidism, pan-hypopituitarism, and hypogonadism, should be

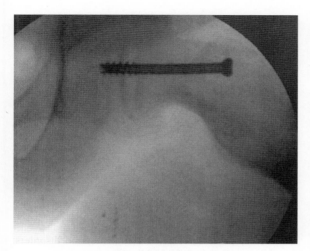

FIGURE 5-4. Percutaneous screw fixation.

suspected in children who fall outside the typical age or weight range for SCFE. In this case, corticosteroids the patient received at 10 years of age were not thought to be a contributing factor in the development of SCFE.

CLINICAL PRESENTATION

There are often considerable delays in the diagnosis of SCFE. Patients frequently complain of symptoms 3-4 months before diagnosis. Therefore, clinicians should have a high level of suspicion for the diagnosis of SCFE even in adolescents with vague complaints of hip, thigh, or knee pain.

Patients with SCFE usually complain of pain in the affected hip or groin. Pain perceived in the medial thigh and knee is due to referred hip pain along the sensory distribution of the femoral and obturator nerves. Isolated knee pain is the sole presenting feature in up to 15% of children diagnosed with SCFE. Early in the course, pain is usually associated with exercise, but as the slip progresses, the symptoms become more persistent and severe.

On physical examination, patients complain of pain with rotation of the hip. The pain is most prominent at the extremes of rotation. Internal rotation may be noticeably decreased. Furthermore, as the hip is flexed, the thigh rotates externally. This finding, when present, is nearly pathognomonic for SCFE in an obese adolescent. Thigh or gluteal muscle atrophy occurs with long-standing symptoms and disuse.

DIAGNOSTIC APPROACH

AP and frog leg lateral hip radiographs. On the AP view, a line drawn along the superior femoral neck (Klein's line) normally intersects a portion of the femoral head. In SCFE, the femoral head will be located below this line. On the frog leg lateral view, the femoral head is displaced posterior and medial to the femoral neck. In the early stages of SCFE, the only finding may be a widened and blurred physis. In chronic cases (symptoms present longer than 3 weeks), radiographs may reveal bony remodeling along the posterior and medial aspects of the femoral neck. Both hips should be examined since SCFE will be bilateral in 25% of cases. Approximately 20% to 50% of those with known unilateral involvement ultimately develop SCFE in the contralateral hip. Radiographs also allow exclusion of conditions with similar manifestations such as femoral neck fracture.

Additional imaging. Hip ultrasound, computed tomography, and magnetic resonance imaging have been used to confirm the diagnosis when hip radiographs are inconclusive.

Other studies. Consider evaluating thyroid and pituitary function in children outside the typical age or weight range for SCFE, as hypothyroidism and growth hormone deficiency also predispose to SCFE. Complete blood count, C-reactive protein, and ESR should be obtained when osteomyelitis or septic arthritis are diagnostic considerations.

TREATMENT

The goals of treatment are to prevent further slippage and restore function. The patient should not be allowed to bear weight on the affected extremity once the diagnosis has been confirmed. An untreated stable slip may progress to a more severe unstable slip, leading to increased morbidity. The most common surgical treatment involves percutaneous fixation of the displaced femoral head with one or more metallic pins or screws.

Prophylactic treatment of the asymptomatic contralateral hip is controversial. Complications of prophylactic pinning such as avascular necrosis, peri-implant femur fracture, and pain requiring hardware removal occur in approximately 5% of cases. However, the incidence of eventual bilateral involvement is relatively high, ranging from 15% to 40%. Among 133 patients with unilateral SCFE undergoing unilateral repair, 20 (15%) developed SCFE in the contralateral hip within 2 years. Therefore, some surgeons advocate for treatment of the contralateral hip at the time of initial surgery. Some orthopedic surgeons recommend fixation of an asymptomatic contralateral hip only in patients who are at highest risk of developing SCFE of the contralateral hip, such as those with known endocrine or metabolic disorders. The modified Oxford Bone Age Score may improve identification of children at greatest risk for contralateral SCFE who may benefit most from prophylactic pinning.

Outcome after repair is generally good but depends on the degree of abnormality prior to repair. Subsequent avascular necrosis of the femoral head complicates 15% of cases. Avascular necrosis is most often a consequence of vascular injury associated with initial femoral head displacement rather than a consequence of the repair. Patients with a moderate or severe degree of femoral head displacement at presentation are also more likely to develop associated osteoarthritis. Chondrolysis or destruction of cartilage may occur after pin placement but has also occurred in patients without any surgical therapy. Leg length discrepancy may result from incomplete reduction, avascular necrosis, or chondrolysis. Early recognition and treatment of SCFE prevents many of these complications.

SUGGESTED READINGS

1. Baghdadi YM, Larson AN, Sierra RJ, Peterson HA, Stans AA. The fate of hips that are not prophylactically pinned after unilateral slipped capital femoral epiphysis. *Clin Orthop Relat Res.* 2013 [Epub ahead of print, PMID 23283674].
2. Ledwith CA, Fleisher GR. Slipped capital femoral epiphysis without hip pain leads to missed diagnosis. *Pediatrics.* 1992;89:660-662.
3. Loder RT, Wittenberg B, DeSilva G. Slipped capital femoral epiphysis associated with endocrine disorders. *J Pediatr Orthop.* 1995;15:349-356.
4. Matava MJ, Patton CM, Luhmann S, Gordon JE, Schoenecker PL. Knee pain as the initial symptom of slipped capital femoral epiphysis: an analysis of initial presentation and treatment. *J Pediatr Orthop.* 1999;19:455-460.
5. Perron AD, Miller MD, Brady WJ. Orthopedic pitfalls in the ED: slipped capital femoral epiphysis. *Am J Emerg Med.* 2002;20:484-487.
6. Popejoy D, Emara K, Birch J. Prediction of contralateral slipped capital femoral epiphysis using the modified Oxford Bone Age Score. *J Pediatr Orthop.* 2012;32:290-294.
7. Sankar WN, Novais EN, Lee C, Al-Omari AA, Choi PD, Shore BJ. What are the risks of prophylactic pinning to prevent contralateral slipped capital femoral epiphysis? *Clin Orthop Relat Res.* 2012 [Epub ahead of print, PMID 23129473].

CASE 5-4

Sixteen-Year-Old Girl
MEGAN AYLOR

HISTORY OF PRESENT ILLNESS

A 16-year-old girl was admitted with joint pain and a 35 pound weight loss during the preceding 7 months. After completion of her gymnastics season 7 months prior to admission, the patient had noted decreased energy and stiff, slightly swollen peripheral joints bilaterally, including her elbows, wrists, knees, and ankles. She was diagnosed with juvenile rheumatoid arthritis and treated with naproxen, a nonsteroidal antiinflammatory drug (NSAID). Her pain improved slightly. Shortly after starting naproxen, she began having daily episodes of epistaxis that required 4-5 facial tissues to control the bleeding. Five months prior to admission she changed from naproxen to ibuprofen without significant change in the degree of joint pain.

Three months prior to admission she noticed a change in her bowel habits from two to three stools per week to daily stools that were frequently mixed with blood. One month prior to admission she developed intermittent cramping abdominal pain. She continued to have episodes of epistaxis and was treated with fluticasone nasal spray and an oral antihistamine for presumed allergic rhinosinusitis. Her weight decreased from 148 to 113 pounds. She complained of decreased appetite and activity level over the preceding few months. There were no fevers, flank tenderness, dysuria, urgency, or frequency. There was no change in mood or intentional weight loss. There was no change in her menstrual cycle. She had not traveled recently.

MEDICAL HISTORY

She had not previously required hospitalization. Menarche occurred at 11 years of age. Her periods were regular. There were no other medical problems. Her only medications were ibuprofen, fluticasone nasal spray, and oral antihistamines as previously mentioned. There was a family history of hypertension in older relatives.

PHYSICAL EXAMINATION

T 35.8°C; RR 18/min; HR 93 bpm; BP 123/66 mmHg

Weight 40 kg; Height 162 cm (50th percentile); Weight-for-height <5th percentile

Physical examination revealed a thin girl. Her palpebral conjunctivae were slightly pale. There were several superficial but actively bleeding erosions on the left medial nasal septum. There were no oral ulcers. Heart and lung sounds were normal. The abdomen was soft with mild right lower quadrant tenderness to palpation. There were no peritoneal signs. Bright red blood mixed with stool was detected on rectal examination. There was a small left knee effusion and bilateral ankle effusions. All joints had a normal range of motion.

DIAGNOSTIC STUDIES

Complete blood count revealed 8900 white blood cells/mm³; a hemoglobin of 9.6 mg/dL; and 463 000 platelets/mm³. Mean corpuscular volume was 70 fL. The reticulocyte count was 1.5%. Erythrocyte sedimentation rate (ESR) was 89 mm/h. Prothrombin time, partial thromboplastin time, and serum transaminases were normal. Serum albumin was 3.0 mg/dL. Urine pregnancy test was negative. There were no red blood cells or white blood cells on urinalysis. Stool was sent for bacterial culture, ova and parasite examination, and Clostridium difficile toxin detection. Abdominal radiograph revealed stool in the rectal vault.

COURSE OF ILLNESS

Upper gastrointestinal barium study with small bowel follow–through of contrast revealed the diagnosis (Figure 5-5).

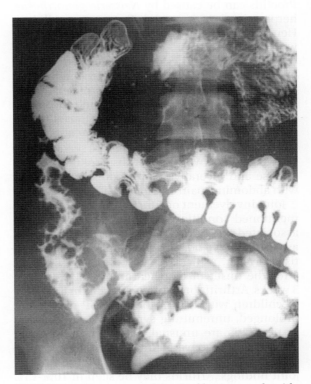

FIGURE 5-5. Upper gastrointestinal barium study with small bowel follow–through of contrast.

DISCUSSION CASE 5-4

DIFFERENTIAL DIAGNOSIS

In an adolescent, hematochezia with cramping abdominal pain has several potential causes. Patients with chronic NSAID use may develop gastrointestinal (GI) tract ulceration, though gastric and duodenal ulcers typically present with melena rather than bright red blood. Infectious enterocolitis may be caused by *Salmonella* species, *Shigella* species, *Campylobacter jejuni*, enteroinvasive and enterohemorrhagic *Escherichia coli* (including *E. coli* O157:H7), *Yersinia entrocolitica*, and *Clostridium difficile*. Parasitic causes include *Entamoeba histolytica*, *Cryptosporidium parvum*, *Schistosoma*, and *Strongyloides stercoralis*. Exposure to undercooked meat and clusters of patients with similar symptoms suggest a common infectious source. The absence of pertinent travel history makes some of the parasitic diseases less likely. Proctitis can be caused by *Neisseria gonorrhoeae*, herpes simplex virus, and *Treponema pallidum*. Henoch-Schönlein purpura (HSP) may present with bloody diarrhea. Vascular malformations of the GI tract often present with recurrent melena or hematochezia. Eosinophilic gastroenteropathy, a chronic, relapsing disorder characterized by eosinophilic inflammatory GI tract infiltrate, often manifests with abdominal pain and rectal bleeding. Abdominal complaints, including abdominal pain due to ileocecal ulcerations, are seen in up to 15% of patients with Behçet disease. Both Crohn disease and ulcerative colitis commonly present with abdominal pain and lower GI bleeding.

Joint involvement occurs in some of the above-mentioned conditions. Reactive arthritis can be associated with *Campylobacter* enteritis as well as with *Salmonella*, *Shigella*, and *Yersinia* enteritis. However, arthritis usually begins 1-6 weeks after the onset of diarrhea and resolves within 3 weeks. Arthritis or arthralgias occur in 65%-85% of children with HSP. Although HSP may recur, prolonged, unremitting symptoms without rash or nephritis are unusual. Children with Behçet disease usually have recurrent oral ulcers, genital ulcers, and iritis or uveitis in addition to the joint findings. Arthritis may be seen in 10%-15% of children with Crohn disease and ulcerative colitis.

DIAGNOSIS

During the GI barium study, contrast pursued a normal course through the duodenum, jejunum, and proximal ileum. However, only a thin line of barium connected the ileum to the cecum (Kantor string sign) indicating significant terminal ileal edema (Figure 5-5). Severe mucosal irregularity was noted in the distal ileum and ascending colon. **These radiologic findings combined with bloody stool, arthritis, nasal ulceration, anemia, and elevated ESR strongly suggested Crohn disease.** Colonoscopy revealed linear ulcerations and luminal edema in the ascending colon. She was treated with oral sulfasalazine, intravenous methylprednisolone, bowel rest, and parenteral nutrition support. Her symptoms improved during the course of 1 week. Three months later her weight had increased to 140 pounds.

INCIDENCE AND EPIDEMIOLOGY OF CROHN DISEASE

Crohn disease, a major form of inflammatory bowel disease (IBD), can segmentally involve any part of the GI tract from the esophagus to the colon. The inflammation involves the terminal portion of the ileum in approximately 90% of cases. Inflammation occurs in the ileum and colon together in 60% of cases, while the upper portion of the GI tract is involved in approximately 30% of cases. In contrast, inflammation in ulcerative colitis is continuous, beginning in the rectum and extending into the colon, while sparing more proximal portions of the GI tract. Isolated colonic involvement occurs in 10% of cases of Crohn disease, making distinction from ulcerative colitis difficult in some cases.

The prevalence of Crohn disease in North America ranges from 26 to 198 cases per 100 000 persons, with higher rates occurring in the northern latitudes. Crohn disease is most common among Caucasians and least common among Hispanics and Asian-Americans. Peak incidence occurs in young adulthood and a second smaller peak occurs during the sixth decade of life. Approximately 15% of patients with Crohn disease are diagnosed during childhood. The mean age of diagnosis in pediatric patients is 12.5 years. The etiology of Crohn disease, though not known, is likely a combination of environmental, genetic, and immunoregulatory factors. Up to 25% of patients with Crohn disease have a first-degree relative with IBD.

CLINICAL PRESENTATION

Approximately 80% of children present with abdominal pain, diarrhea, anorexia, and weight loss with or without extraintestinal manifestations. Recurrent oral ulcers are common. Abdominal pain in the right lower quadrant suggests ileocecal involvement, epigastric pain suggests gastroduodenal involvement, and periumbilical pain suggests generalized small bowel disease. Fifty percent of children will have gross or microscopic blood in the stool. Perirectal diseases such as fissures, fistulas, skin tags, and abscesses are present in up to 40% of patients.

Extraintestinal manifestations predominate in 8% to 10% of patients and are likely to be associated with diagnostic confusion and delay (Table 5-5). While more than 100 localized extraintestinal manifestions have been described, only the more common ones will be discussed. Joint

complaints, including arthritis, are the most frequent extraintestinal manifestation in children occurring in 15%-30% of cases. Approximately 50% of children with Crohn disease and peripheral arthritis develop ocular or skin findings (Table 5-5). Sclerosing cholangitis develops in 1% of children with Crohn disease. Symptoms of sclerosing cholangitis include jaundice, generalized pruritis, and abdominal pain. Pancreatitis can occur as both an extraintestinal manifestation of Crohn disease, and a complication of duodenal inflammation, sclerosing cholangitis, or drug therapy. Renal stones complicating Crohn disease may be due to calcium oxalate, calcium phosphate, or uric acid. Erythema nodosum tends to occur when intestinal disease is active but does not correlate with disease severity. Rashes due to trace mineral deficiencies may occur as a consequence of malabsorption.

DIAGNOSTIC APPROACH

Initial screening tests should include a complete blood count, ESR, liver function tests, and stool testing for blood, bacteria, and parasites. The results of the initial screening determine the need for further testing.

Complete blood count. Anemia is present in 40%-70% of cases. Mean corpuscular volume may be low due to the combination of iron deficiency and chronic inflammation. Vitamin B_{12} and folate deficiencies also contribute to anemia. The white blood cell count is typically normal. Thrombocytosis occurs in more than half the cases.

Acute phase reactants. C-reactive protein (CRP) and erythrocyte sedimentation rate (ESR) are elevated in most cases but a normal CRP or ESR does not preclude the diagnosis of Crohn disease.

Hepatic function tests. Serum transaminases and gamma-glutamyltransferase (GGT) may be mildly elevated in the absence of complications. Crohn-related complications, such as sclerosing cholangitis and chronic active hepatitis, lead to more significant elevation of the transaminases and GGT. Hypoalbuminemia reflects compromised nutritional status and diffuse inflammation.

Stool studies. Stool bacterial culture, ova, and parasite examination, and C. *difficile* detection

TABLE 5-5.	Extraintestinal manifestations of Crohn disease.
Site of Involvement	*Manifestation*
Eye	Uveitis Episcleritis Orbital myositis
Hepatobiliary System	Sclerosing cholangitis Chronic active hepatitis Cholelithiasis
Pancreas	Pancreatitis
Renal	Nephrolithiasis Entervesical fistula
Skin	Erythema nodosum Pyoderma gangrenosum
Vascular	Thrombophlebitis Vasculitis Deep vein thrombosis Pulmonary emboli Cerebrovascular disease
Bone and Joint	Arthritis—peripheral (knees, ankles, hips, wrists, elbows) Arthritis—axial (ankylosing spondylitis, sacroiliitis) Arthralgias Osteopenia Aseptic necrosis

should be performed in all children with bloody diarrhea and suspected Crohn disease to exclude other causes. Stool calprotectin and lactoferrin are nonspecific markers of inflammation that can help distinguish Crohn from noninflammatory illnesses such as irritable bowel syndrome.

Endoscopic evaluation. Endoscopic evaluation of the colon is the gold standard for diagnosis and should precede barium radiography in the presence of bloody diarrhea. Colonic mucosa biopsy, even if the mucosa appears normal, is required since microscopic inflammation with granuloma formation may be present. If possible, the examination should extend to the terminal ileum. Esophagogastroduodenoscopy may be required to assess upper GI tract symptoms. Video capsule endoscopy is increasingly being used to evaluate the small bowel of older children and adults. In a meta-analysis of adult patients with Crohn disease, the yield of capsule endoscopy was 63% compared with a yield of 46% for colonoscopy with ileoscopy, and 23% for small bowel barium radiography. Across all studies, the number needed to test with capsule endoscopy was three to yield one additional diagnosis of Crohn disease over small bowel barium radiography and seven to yield one additional diagnosis over colonoscopy with ileoscopy.

Upper GI tract barium study with small bowel follow through. This study is important early in the evaluation since the terminal ileum is involved in 90% of patients with Crohn disease. Features suggestive of Crohn include terminal ileal thickening (Kantor string sign), nodularity, ulcers, and fistulous connections.

Other studies. Serologic testing for inflammatory bowel disease may help differentiate Crohn disease from ulcerative colitis; however, these tests are not recommended as screening tests for inflammatory bowel disease. Serologic tests include anti-IgA and anti I-gG to *Saccharomyces cerevisiae* (Crohn disease) and perinuclear antineutrophil cytoplasmic antibody (p-ANCA; ulcerative colitis). Biomarkers such as fecal calprotectin show promise as screening tools. The following additional studies may be useful in assessing the patient's nutritional status: folic acid, vitamin B_{12}, fat-soluble vitamins (especially vitamin D), prothrombin time, partial thromboplastin time, zinc, iron, total iron-binding capacity, calcium, magnesium, phosphorus, and prealbumin.

TREATMENT

Therapeutic strategies include a combination of medical and surgical interventions. Medical therapy includes corticosteroids, 5-aminosalicylates, immunomodulators, and antibiotics. Corticosteroids are the mainstay of treatment for moderate to severe symptoms of Crohn disease. They exert antiinflammatory effects by decreasing cytokine release, capillary permeability, and neutrophil and monocyte function. Newer corticosteroids have a strong affinity for intestinal steroid receptors leading to high topical antiinflammatory potency. Since they are rapidly transformed into inactivated metabolites by the liver following absorption, they cause fewer systemic side effects. For example, budesonide binds to intestinal receptors 15 times more efficiently than prednisolone but undergoes rapid hepatic metabolism and hence systemic bioavailability is only 10% compared with 80% for prednisolone. Delayed-release (time- and pH-dependent) formulations of budesonide permit more effective delivery of the drug to the terminal ileum and proximal colon.

Oral sulfasalazine consists of 5-aminosalicylic acid (5-ASA) bound to sulfapyridine. The sulfa moiety functions as a carrier, facilitating delivery of the agent to the colon where it is cleaved by resident bacteria into therapeutically active 5-ASA. The 5-ASA decreases colon inflammation by inhibiting leukotriene synthesis via the lipoxygenase pathway of arachidonic acid metabolism. It also decreases neutrophil-mediated tissue damage by interfering with myeloperoxidase activity and scavenging reactive oxygen species. Newer oral 5-ASA analogues (e.g., mesalamine) function by either pH-dependent or timed-release mechanisms that allow the drug to be distributed throughout the small bowel.

Immunomodulators are becoming the standard of care in the management of Crohn disease. Azathioprine and 6-mercaptopurine interfere with purine synthesis and are used to maintain remission; however, their maximum effect is not realized for up to 6 months. Methotrexate is a second-line immunomodulator for refractory patients.

Biologic therapies are useful in the management of moderate to severe Crohn disease. Tumor necrosis factor-alpha (TNF-alpha), a cytokine, activates components of the immune system involved in Crohn disease. Infliximab, a chimeric (mouse-human) anti-TNF-alpha IgG antibody, binds to TNF-alpha and neutralizes its activity. Infliximab infusions administered at 4-12 week intervals induce remissions in patients with moderate to severe Crohn disease and facilitate healing of fistulas. Infliximab also permits significant reduction in steroid use in children.

Protein-calorie malnutrition is common. Nutritional support will help the patient maintain functional status and mitigate the loss of lean tissue. Elemental formula can itself help decrease bowel inflammation. The antibiotic metronidazole may reduce Crohn disease activity and is used to treat perianal fistulas and abscesses. Surgical intervention may be indicated for intractable disease, severe fistula formation, uncontrolled hemorrhage, and bowel perforation. More than 50% of children with Crohn's disease will require intestinal surgery within 10-15 years of diagnosis. The disease is not usually limited to one portion of the GI tract so surgery is not curative. Recurrent disease after bowel resection is common.

The course of Crohn disease is characterized by periods of symptom exacerbation and remission. Only 1% of children with well-documented Crohn disease will have no relapses after diagnosis and initial therapy. Many children with Crohn disease also suffer from medication- and central venous catheter-related complications. In the long term, impaired height velocity is common. Approximately 8% of patients with severe Crohn disease will develop colorectal cancer. Death from Crohn disease in childhood is rare; however, the risk of death is 1.5 times higher in affected adults compared with age-matched controls.

SUGGESTED READINGS

1. Di Nardo G, Alio M, Oliva S, Civitelli F, Casciani E, Cucchiara S. Investigation of the small bowel in pediatric Crohn's disease. *Inflamm Bowel Dis.* 2012;18:1760-1776.
2. Hyams JS. Inflammatory bowel disease. *Pediatr Rev.* 2000;21:291-295.
3. Hyams JS. Extraintestinal manifestations of inflammatory bowel disease in children. *J Pediatr Gastroenterol Nutr.* 1994;19:7-21.
4. Hyams JS. Inflammatory bowel disease. In: Altschuler SM, Liacouras CA, eds. *Clinical Pediatric Gastroenterology.* Philadelphia: Churchill Livingstone; 1998:213-221.
5. Mamula P, Telega GW, Markowitz JE, et al. Inflammatory bowel disease in children 5 years of age and younger. *Am J Gastroenterol.* 2002;97:2005-2010.
6. Stephens MC, Shepanski MA, Mamula P, Markowitz JE, Brown KA, Baldassano RN. Safety and steroid-sparing experience using infliximab for Crohn's disease at a pediatric inflammatory bowel disease center. *Am J Gastroenterol.* 2003;98:104-111.
7. Thomas DW, Sinatra FR. Screening laboratory tests for Crohn's disease. *West J Med.* 1989;150:163-164.
8. Triester SL, Leighton JA, Leontiadis GI, et al. A meta-analysis of the yield of capsule endoscopy compared to other diagnostic modalities in patients with non-stricturing small bowel Crohn's disease. *Am J Gastroenterol.* 2006;101:954-964.
9. Glick SR, Carvalho RS. Inflammatory bowel disease. *Pediatr Rev.* 2011;32:14-25.

CASE 5-5

Thirteen-Year-Old Boy

EVAN S. FIELDSTON

HISTORY OF PRESENT ILLNESS

A 13-year-old African-American male presented to the emergency department with a 2-day history of worsening back pain. The pain was located in his upper and lower back, and although he was uncomfortable in any position, standing upright made his back pain significantly worse. His pain was not relieved with cyclobenzaprine, a muscle relaxant. The patient had no history of trauma and he denied weakness, sensory loss, and bowel or bladder dysfunction as well as recent fevers, upper respiratory symptoms, cough, nausea, vomiting, weight loss, and night sweats.

MEDICAL HISTORY

The boy's medical history was remarkable for one previous episode of back pain 2 years earlier that required use of a wheelchair for 2 weeks. He received iron supplements for treatment of anemia that was discovered at that time. Additional details of that episode were not available. He had never been hospitalized and had no surgical problems. He was not sexually active and had no history of cigarette or drug use. Family history was significant for a sister with sickle cell trait.

PHYSICAL EXAMINATION

T 37.7°C; RR 24/min; HR 110 bpm; BP 105/70 mmHg; Weight 35 kg (<10th percentile)

The patient was a well-developed, well-nourished male crying in pain. Head, eyes, ears, nose, and throat were normal. There was no lymphadenopathy. There was no thoracic wall tenderness. The heart and lung sounds were normal. His abdomen was soft and nontender without hepatomegaly or splenomegaly. He had no point tenderness of his back; however, he complained of "inside pain" over his sacrum. Rectal examination revealed normal sphincter tone and no palpable masses. His extremities were warm with good peripheral pulses and full range of motion of all four extremities. His neurologic examination revealed normal strength, sensation, and 2+ reflexes.

DIAGNOSTIC STUDIES

Complete blood count revealed 8400 white blood cells/mm³ (81% segmented neutrophils, 17% lymphocytes, 2% basophils, 1% eosinophils, and no bands), hemoglobin of 10.4 g/dL; mean corpuscular volume (MCV) 72 fL; mean corpuscular hemoglobin content (MCHC) 23.4 g/dL; red cell distribution width (RDW) 15.1; and platelets 241 000 platelets/mm³, and a reticulocyte count of 3%. Blood smear showed anisocytosis, poikilocytosis, and polychromasia. Electrolytes, blood urea nitrogen, creatinine, and glucose were normal. Erythrocyte sedimentation rate was 20 mm/h. Urinalysis revealed small amounts of urobilinogen.

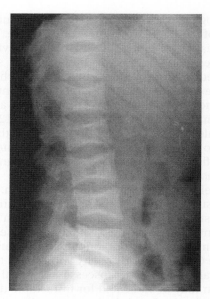

FIGURE 5-6. Plain radiograph of spine showing vertebral deossification due to marrow hyperplasia and flattened, widened vertebral bodies with biconcave depressions of the end plates known as "H-shaped" or "fish mouth" vertebrae.

COURSE OF ILLNESS

The patient was treated with morphine and ketorolac without much relief. He became febrile to 38.7°C and blood and urine cultures were obtained. The pain became localized to his sacral/coccygeal region, but he had no numbness or tingling and his reflexes remained normal. While abdominal radiograph did not reveal bowel obstruction, it suggested a likely underlying condition (Figure 5-6) that was later confirmed by specific testing. An MRI of the lumbosacral spine was negative for an abscess or a locally infiltrative process.

DISCUSSION CASE 5-5

DIFFERENTIAL DIAGNOSIS

Back pain is less common in children than in adults, but unlike adults, it usually is the result of a serious underlying pathology. In adolescents, traumatic or overuse injuries such as compression fractures, musculoskeletal strain, spondylolyis, spondylolith-esis, and lumbar disc herniation should be considered. Most of these injuries often present during the adolescent growth spurt and are associated with repeated lifting and back extension, especially in sports. Infections of the vertebral column that cause back pain include osteomyelitis and diskitis especially in toddlers and young children. Less common but serious causes include spinal epidural, paraspinal or psoas abscess, transverse myelitis, and pyomyositis. Urinary tract infections and pneumonia can cause back pain but these are less likely in the absence of urinary or respiratory symptoms. Neoplastic diseases like leukemia and lymphoma should be considered especially with progressive, indolent pain. Malignancies are usually accompanied by constitutional symptoms including weight loss, fatigue, fever, and loss of appetite. Rare causes of back pain include spinal hematoma, spinal tuberculosis (Pott disease), and brucellosis, a zoonotic infection transmitted from animals to man that causes flu-like symptoms including back pain. Back pain secondary to acute bone infarction often occurs in adolescents with sickle cell disease (SCD). Patients usually have normal or mildly elevated temperature and ESR. However, in some cases this condition is indistinguishable from acute osteomyelitis. SCD should be included in the differential diagnosis of an African-American child with back pain, anemia, and a family history of sickle cell trait. In this case, the acute fall in the patient's hemoglobin level, splenomegaly, vertebral abnormalities, and the persistence and severity of the patient's symptoms prompted further evaluation leading to the diagnosis. While most patients are diagnosed by newborn screening tests, some patients may inadvertently not be screened or may be lost to follow-up.

DIAGNOSTIC TESTS

Biconcave vertebral depressions, known as the "fish mouth" deformity, suggested the diagnosis of SCD (Figure 5-6), a group of conditions characterized by the presence of hemoglobin S in the absence of normal hemoglobin A or in a quantity greater than that of hemoglobin A. Hemoglobin electrophoresis confirmed the diagnosis of sickle-beta+ thalassemia (Sbeta+ thalassemia): HbA (18.4%),

HbS (63%), HbF (8.1%), HbA2 (7.7%). Sbeta+ thalassemia, a less severe form of SCD, results from inheritance of the sickle hemoglobin (HbS) and beta+ thalassemia genes. In Sbeta+ thalassemia, some normal beta-chains are produced and therefore some HbA is present. A similar hemoglobin profile may be seen in HbSS disease following transfusion. However, in this case, the patient never received a red blood cell transfusion. Therefore, his diagnosis was a vasoocclusive event secondary to underlying Sbeta+ thalassemia. In retrospect, the anemia diagnosed during his previous episode of back pain was likely due to SCD rather than isolated iron deficiency anemia.

INCIDENCE AND ETIOLOGY

SCD is an autosomal recessive genetic disorder characterized by the presence of sickle hemoglobin (HbS) in red blood cells. Approximately 8% of the African-American population carries sickle cell trait (heterozygote) and approximately 0.2% of African-American newborns have SCD (homozygote). More than 70 000 Americans have SCD. The most common forms of SCD are homozygous sickle cell disease (HbSS), sickle-hemoglobin C disease (HbSC), and two types of sickle beta-thalassemia: sickle-beta+ thalassemia and sickle-beta0 thalassemia (Table 5-6). Individuals who inherit the genes for both HbA and HbS have sickle cell trait, a generally benign and asymptomatic carrier state.

HbS results from an inherited abnormality of hemoglobin function caused by substitution of valine for glutamine at the sixth position of the beta-globin gene. Deoxygenated HbS polymerizes, distorting the shape of the red blood cell. Red

TABLE 5-6.	Genotypes of the four common types of sickle cell disease in the United States.	
Genotype	*Full Name*	*Frequency*
betaS/betaS	Sickle cell disease-SS	65%
betaS/betaC	Sickle cell disease-SC	25%
betaS/beta0 thalassemia	Sickle cell disease-S beta0 thalassemia	3%
betaS/beta+ thalassemia	Sickle cell disease-S beta+ thalassemia	7%

blood cell distortion leads to hemolysis and vaso-occlusion, the two dominant features of SCD. Beta-thalassemia generally results from single point mutations that result in decreased (beta+ thalassemia) or absent (beta0) synthesis of beta globin. This commonly results in microcytic and hypochromic anemia.

The occurrence of sickle cell-B thalassemia is determined by the distribution and prevalence of two abnormal genes. The sickle gene occurs in high frequency among populations in Equatorial Africa, Mediterranean, Middle East, and India; populations that were exposed during evolution to selection pressure from falciparum malaria. The distribution of beta-thalassemia tends to be sporadic with high frequencies in the Mediterranean and in South East Asia. The combination of beta thalassemia with the sickle mutation results in the combined heterozygous condition known as Hb S-beta thalassemia. The clinical problems are quite variable depending on the amount of Hb A produced. Sickle-beta0 thalassemia produces no normal beta-chains and therefore no Hb A. S-beta0 thalassemia resembles HbSS electrophoretically, hematologically, and clinically. In contrast, the spectrum of severity in Hb S-beta+ thalassemia varies ranging from very little Hb A production to near normal amounts depending on the beta thalassemia mutation.

TYPICAL PRESENTATION

Universal screening for SCD has been widely available in most states in the United States since 1986, and therefore most children with SCD are diagnosed as newborns. A few infants, even in states with universal screening, may not be screened and the diagnosis may be missed in others because of extreme prematurity, blood transfusions prior to screening, or inadequate follow-up after discharge. In some patients with sickle-beta+ thalassemia, the levels of Hb A are sufficiently high to impair polymerization of Hb S and reduce intravascular sickling of the red blood cells. The early clinical course in these patients is mild with significant symptoms appearing later in life.

Acute and chronic complications of SCD involve multiple organ systems (Table 5-7). Acute painful events are the most common cause of emergency

TABLE 5-7.	Complications of sickle cell disease by organ system.
Hematologic Anemia Aplastic anemia Recurrent infections Splenic infarcts Splenic sequestration Functional asplenia	**Skin** Chronic ulcers **Neurologic** Stroke Subarachnoid hemorrhage Coma Seizures
Pulmonary Increased intrapulmonary shunting Pleuritis Recurrent pulmonary infections Pulmonary infarcts	**Ocular** Vitreous hemorrhage Retinal infarcts Proliferative retinopathy Retinal detachment
Cardiovascular Congestive heart failure Cor pulmonale Pericarditis Myocardial infarction	**Gastrointestinal** Cholelithiasis (pigmented stones) Cholecystitis Hepatic infarcts Hepatic abscesses Hepatic fibrosis
Skeletal Synovitis Arthritis Aseptic necrosis of femoral head Small bone infarcts in hand and feet (dactylitis) Biconcave ("fishmouth") vertebrae Osteomyelitis	**Genitourinary** Hematuria Renal papillary necrosis Impaired renal concentrating ability (isosthenuria) Nephrotic syndrome Renal insufficiency Renal failure Priapism

room visits and hospitalizations among patients with SCD. These events may be precipitated by weather extremes or temperature changes, dehydration, infection, stress, and menstruation; however, the majority of painful events have no identifiable trigger. Painful episodes vary from mild to debilitating. Pain is usually self-limited, lasting from a few hours to a few days though inadequate treatment may prolong the episode for weeks. Bones and joints are major sites of pain in vasoocclusive events. Acute bone pain is caused by marrow ischemia resulting in necrosis and periosteal inflammation. Pain is widespread and migratory during the acute painful crisis. Local tenderness, warmth, swelling, and impaired motion occur with a severe pain episode as the generalized pain improves. In the finger and toes it is known as dactylitis. It is seen as early as 6 months of age, but usually stops by age 10 years due to the replacement of red marrow with fatty tissue. As seen in this patient, vertebral infarction may lead to collapse of the end plates known as "fish mouth" vertebra. No single clinical feature can reliably distinguish osteomyelitis from bone infarction. In the femoral head, aseptic necrosis of the femoral head occurs in 30% by 30 years.

Other manifestations of vasoocclusive events include acute chest syndrome, which occurs more often in children than in adults, but has higher mortality in adults than in children (4% vs. 2%). Stroke occurs more frequently in HbSS, in 8%-10% of patients by age 20 years, and is also more common in childhood with a high rate of recurrence (70%-90%). Priapism occurs in approximately 40% of males, including children. Leg sores and ulcers appear in 10% of patients, usually after the age of 10 years. Hepatomegaly is found in half of patients and cholelithiasis in 30%-70%. Over time, splenic infarcts lead to functional asplenia, which affects 14% of patients by 6 months and 94% of patients by age 5 years. Renal failure occurs in 5%-18% of patients with median onset of 23 years of age. Half of patients with SCD survey past the fifth decade, with many not having overt organ failure, but rather death from an acute episode of pain, chest syndrome, or stroke. Patients with more symptomatic disease and lower fetal hemoglobin levels had lower survival.

DIAGNOSTIC RATIONALE

Hemoglobin electrophoresis. This is the most common method in clinical laboratories used to determine hemoglobin phenotype.

Complete blood count with differential. At baseline, hemoglobin values in patients with S-beta+ thalassemia, reticulocyte, and white blood cell counts are close to normal with the major difference being a modestly low mean corpuscular volume (MCV) and mean corpuscular hemoglobin content (MCHC). This is in contrast to Hb SS disease where the steady-state WBC and reticulocyte counts are higher than in an unaffected person. The white blood count is often elevated with both bone infarcts and infection; however, a shift in the differential toward neutrophil predominance is more likely with osteomyelitis than with infarction.

Peripheral blood smear. Microcytosis, hypochromia, anisocytosis, and poikilocytosis characterize Hb S beta (+) thalassemia. Sickled cells are not always seen especially when high levels of non-S hemoglobin are present making the diagnosis less obvious in some cases.

Blood cultures. Blood cultures should be obtained before antibiotics are administered. Blood cultures are negative in bone infarction and frequently positive in osteomyelitis.

Sequential radionuclide bone marrow and bone scan. Diminished radionuclide uptake on the bone marrow scan is indicative of decreased blood flow in the bone marrow, and abnormal uptake on the bone scan at the site of pain are seen with bone infarction. In contrast, acute osteomyelitis results in normal activity on bone marrow scans and increased activity on bone scans.

Magnetic resonance imaging (MRI). MRI can replace bone scan in evaluation of bone pain in patients with sickle cell disease without exposure to ionizing radiation. MRI findings of cortical defects, adjacent fluid collections in soft tissue, and bone marrow enhancement suggest infection.

Plain radiography. Radiography is useful in monitoring the progression of established changes of infection, infarction, and osteomyelitis but not in diagnosing acute infections or infarctions. In older children and adolescents, plain radiographs may show deossification due to marrow hyperplasia and flattened, widened vertebral bodies with biconcave depressions of the end plates known as "H-shaped" or "fish mouth" vertebrae (Figure 5-6).

TREATMENT

Severe bone pain should be considered a medical emergency that prompts timely and aggressive management until the pain decreases to a tolerable level. Major barriers to effective management of pain are inadequate assessment of pain and biases against opioid use. Most of the time, these biases are based on clinician uncertainty regarding opioid tolerance and physical dependence, and confusion with addiction.

As previously mentioned, bone infarction resembles osteomyelitis. Fever in cases of bone infarction is due to necrosis and inflammation associated with marrow ischemia. Blood cultures must be obtained if empiric antibiotics are initiated. Appropriate antibiotics should cover *Salmonella* and *Staphylococcus aureus*, the most common causes of osteomyelitis in children with sickle cell disease.

Patients with signs of moderate to severe dehydration should receive 10-20 mL/kg of intravenous normal saline followed by intravenous fluid at or slightly above (1-1.5 times) the daily fluid requirement. It is important to assess the severity of pain at presentation and at frequent intervals using age-appropriate pain-measuring scales. Pain should be re-evaluated every 15 minutes until pain starts to decrease, then every 30-60 minutes as needed. Severe acute pain requires intravenous (IV) medication, such as morphine sulfate, hydrocodone, or fentanyl with or without nonsteroidal antiinflammatory drugs, such as ketorolac and ibuprofen. Patient-controlled analgesia (PCA) devices restore patient control over their pain and may be used for patients in severe pain. PCA pumps provide analgesic medication continuously at a low baseline rate and allow patients to self-administer an additional dose of opiod whenever they feel a need for more pain relief. Continuous epidural analgesia has been used in patients with pain below the fourth thoracic dermatome who failed IV PCA opioids, and nonopioid analgesics; however, not much information is available about its use in SCD patients.

Patient and parental preferences for pain medication should be considered since individual variations in drug metabolism determine dose-response to analgesia. The use of parental meperidine should be avoided because of CNS toxicity related to its metabolite normeperidine. Patients receiving opioids for more than 1 or 2 weeks should be weaned slowly over several days to prevent withdrawal symptoms. Side effects of opioids including respiratory depression and sedation should be monitored closely. Antiemetics like compazine or metachlorpropamide effectively treat symptoms of opioid-related nausea. Stool softeners to prevent constipation should be taken daily if patients remain on opioids for more than a few days.

Chronic treatment of SCD should be under the supervision of a hematologist and includes appropriate immunizations, penicillin prophylaxis in children, folic acid supplementation, and hydroxyurea to increase fetal hemoglobin production. Some patients may receive blood transfusions to decrease the risk of stroke.

SUGGESTED READINGS

1. Benjamin LJ, Dampier CD, Jacox AK, et al. *Guidelines for the Management of Acute and Chronic Pain in Sickle-Cell Disease.* APS Clinical Practice Guidelines Series, No. 1. Glenview, IL: American Pain Society, 1999.
2. Clarkson J. The ocular manifestations of sickle-cell disease: a prevalence and natural history study. *Trans Am Ophthalmol Soc.* 1992;90:481-504.
3. Ejindu VC, Hine AL, Mashayekhi M, Shorvon PJ, Misra RR. Musculoskeletal manifestations of sickle cell disease. *Radiographics.* 2007;27:1005-1021.
4. Embury SH, Hebbel RP, Mohandas N, Steinberg MH, eds. *Sickle Cell Disease: Basic Principles and Clinical Practice.* New York, NY: Raven Press; 1994.
5. Lane PA. Sickle cell disease. *Pediatr Clin N Am.* 1996; 43:639-664.
6. Moriarty B, Acheson, R, Condon P, Serjeant G. Patterns of visual loss in untreated sickle cell retinopathy. *Eye.* 1988;2:330-335.
7. Platt OS, Brambilla DJ, Rosse WF, et al. Mortality in sickle cell disease: life expectancy and risk factors for early death. *N Engl J Med.* 1994;33:1639-1644.
8. Serjeant GR, Sergeant BE. *Sickle Cell Disease.* 2nd ed. Oxford, England: Oxford University Press; 2001.
9. Yaster M, Kost-Byerly S, Maxwell LG. The management of pain in sickle cell disease. *Pediatr Clin N Am.* 2000;47:699-710.

Nine-Year-Old Boy

PAMELA A. MAZZEO

HISTORY OF PRESENT ILLNESS

A 9-year-old active young boy presented to his pediatrician with left ankle pain of approximately 5 days duration. The boy's mother reported that he had complained of various muscle injuries over the last month. Three weeks prior to presentation, he had begun limping, which he had attributed to having hurt his right hip while playing basketball. After a few days of "taking it easy," he reported complete resolution. Shortly thereafter, the boy had complained of left elbow pain, and his mother speculated that the injury had occurred while he was wrestling with his older brother. He received ibuprofen and after a few days of treatment was able to play video games without discomfort. Just over the past few days, the mother had noted the boy limping again, but he had denied any problems until the coach of his indoor soccer team sat him for the first time all season. The boy confessed that his left ankle had been hurting him, but he had not wanted to miss any games. The coach had called the boy's mother and told her he was not allowed back to practice until the doctor had checked him over.

The boy described the hip and elbow symptoms as vague pains, which worsened with movement of the specific limbs. He denied having had swelling or redness of the elbow or hip when they were bothering him, but he thought that his ankle was a "little puffy" now.

The mother reported that he had felt warm on occasion and that he had not been eating well. She felt that he had lost weight and she had found his sheets damp a few mornings when she woke him for school. The boy denied headache, rash, sore throat, nausea, vomiting, diarrhea, palpitations, or fatigue, and he asked if he could still make it to practice scheduled for later that day.

MEDICAL HISTORY

The patient had received all required immunizations and, aside from a broken nose from a stray softball 3 years earlier, he had no significant medical history. He had never required any regularly scheduled medications. He had no known medication allergies.

The boy's family history was significant for migraine headaches in his mother and maternal grandmother and Trisomy 21 in his youngest brother. There was no family history of arthritis or malignancy. His travel had been limited to 2 weeks at the New Jersey shore over the summer and 1 month of "sleep away" camp in northeastern Pennsylvania.

PHYSICAL EXAMINATION

T 38.6°C; HR 112 bpm; BP 112/60 mmHg; RR 18/min

The boy's weight was in the 60th percentile but was down 3 kg from his preparticipation physical examination 4 months earlier. His height was in the 75th percentile, up by 1 cm from earlier measurements.

The patient was a cooperative male in no acute distress. He was slender and his clothes hung loosely from his frame. Eyes, nose, ears, and oropharynx were not inflamed. His tonsils were 3+ and symmetric without erythema or exudates. His neck was supple with only shotty anterior cervical adenopathy. His thyroid was not enlarged. His lungs were clear with good aeration. His heart had a regular rhythm but was tachycardic with a soft systolic murmur at the apex, which was audible throughout systole. His abdomen was soft, nontender, and nondistended with no hepatosplenomegaly. The left ankle demonstrated a small effusion with increased warmth and mild erythema. There was exquisite pain with active and passive range of motion and with gentle palpation of the joint. All other joints were normal on examination. There was no rash.

DIAGNOSTIC STUDIES

A complete blood count revealed a white blood cell count of 12 200 cells/mm³ (74% neutrophils, 20%

lymphocytes, 5% monocytes, 1% eosinophils); a hemoglobin of 9.5 g/dL; and a platelet count of 556 000/mm³. A basic metabolic panel was normal, but inflammatory markers were elevated, with an erythrocyte sedimentation rate of 120 mm/h and a C-reactive protein of 8.3 mg/dL. A rapid streptococcal antigen test and culture of his throat were both negative. Radiographs of both ankles were normal.

COURSE OF ILLNESS

The patient was treated with doxycycline for presumed Lyme arthritis. He also received regularly scheduled naproxen with good symptomatic relief of his joint pain. Several days later, the Lyme antibody titers by Western blot were negative. An electrocardiogram (ECG) suggested another possible etiology (Figure 5-7). Additional testing confirmed the diagnosis, which mandated definitive ongoing treatment.

DISCUSSION CASE 5-6

DIFFERENTIAL DIAGNOSIS

This previously healthy young man presented with a 1-month history of joint pains, with true arthritis of the ankle demonstrated at the office visit. The arthritis involved relatively large joints affected in a nonsimultaneous sequence. This pattern is referred to as a migratory pattern, where new joint inflammation occurs after previous joint inflammation resolves.

The fever, weight loss, elevated inflammatory markers, and mild anemia were also noteworthy and suggested an infectious, rheumatologic, or malignant process.

Infectious etiologies of arthritis include primary infection of a joint space or infection of bone or soft tissue in close proximity to a joint, with or without direct communication of the infection with the joint. These are more likely to involve a single site, but multifocal infections can be seen with ongoing or intermittent bacteremia leading to multiple hematogenously seeded sites. When more than one joint is involved, postinfectious arthritis should be considered. These inflammatory joint reactions are sequelae of preceding infections, and are usually considered to be sterile and mediated through an immune response. Epstein-Barr and parvovirus B19 are among the common viral agents associated with this reaction, and meningococcus and Group A beta-hemolytic streptococcus are notorious bacterial causes for this phenomenon.

Arthritis characterizes late stage Lyme disease and develops 6-12 weeks after the tick bite. Large joints, especially the knees, are involved, and the recurrence of arthritis mimics a migratory pattern. Each bout of arthritis lasts 1-2 weeks but may become prolonged if left untreated. The involved joint often appears remarkably swollen, with little or no erythema, and ambulation is often maintained despite impressive effusion in the involved lower extremity joint. Carditis, presenting as heart block, can also complicate the picture but is more

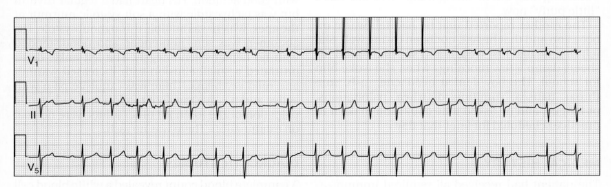

FIGURE 5-7. An electrocardiogram.

common in the early disseminated stage of the disease, which occurs a few weeks to months after infection.

The involvement of multiple joints and stigmata of acute inflammation make rheumatologic conditions an important consideration. Systemic-onset juvenile idiopathic arthritis can present initially with or without arthritis, but chronic arthritis of at least 6 weeks' duration is required for diagnosis. Systemic lupus erythematosus most often presents with joint involvement with constitutional complaints of fatigue, weight loss, fever, and a typical rash, and there is nearly always an elevation in the antinuclear antibody (ANA) titer. Progressive muscle weakness is characteristic of dermatomyositis, which may present with extremity complaints and, infrequently, true arthritis. Back pain eventually develops in ankylosing spondylitis, which is much more common in boys than in girls and is associated with HLA-B27 in 9 of 10 cases. Mixed connective tissue diseases may have overlapping features with many of these conditions, but the arthritis often involves small joints. Vasculitis syndromes may also present with arthritis, with Henoch-Schönlein purpura being the most common vasculitis of children. The characteristic palpable petechial or purpuric rash, especially evident in the lower extremities, in the absence of thrombocytopenia, is key in the diagnosis of this IgA-mediated vasculitis. Other inflammatory conditions, including Crohn disease, ulcerative colitis, Reiter syndrome, Behçet disease, or Sjögren syndrome, may also present with arthritis, constitutional symptoms, and elevated erythrocyte sedimentation rate, but other features of the illnesses are usually present, or eventually manifest themselves.

Joint or extremity pain, with fever and weight loss, can certainly raise the suspicion of a malignancy. True arthritis (joint effusion, warmth, erythema, and pain with range of motion) is not a typical presentation of musculoskeletal tumors but may be part of a paraneoplastic syndrome with reactive arthritis. Disseminated malignancies, such as neuroblastoma or leukemia, may also involve joints or the skeletal system through direct bony destruction in close proximity to a joint. Abnormalities may or may not be detected by plain radiographs of the involved limb.

DIAGNOSIS

The ECG revealed a ventricular rate of 110 bpm, sinus arrhythmia, first-degree atrioventricular block (P-R interval = 0.2 seconds), and a Mobitz II atrioventricular block (occasional atrial beats not conducted to the ventricle) (Figure 5-7). Echocardiogram revealed mild aortic insufficiency and moderate mitral regurgitation. The antinuclear antibody titers were less than 1:40. Anti-streptolysin-O titers and anti-DNase B titers were positive at 1:1955 and 1:680, respectively. **These findings confirmed the diagnosis of acute rheumatic fever (ARF).**

The negative Lyme serology and the elevated titers to streptococcal antigens make acute rheumatic fever (ARF) an important diagnostic consideration in this case. The Jones criteria are used to make the diagnosis (Table 5-8).

Two major or one major plus two minor criteria, along with evidence of preceding group A beta-hemolytic streptococcal (GABHS) infection, make the diagnosis of acute rheumatic fever (ARF) highly probable. This young boy demonstrated several features of this disease, including auscultatory evidence of valvular heart disease and a migratory polyarthritis (two major criteria), as well as fever, prologation of the PR interval on ECG, and elevated ESR and CRP (three minor criteria). Echocardiography revealed mild aortic valvular insufficiency and moderate mitral valve regurgitation with thickening of the mitral valve.

Response to aspirin and other NSAIDs is typical and, perhaps, a diagnostic clue. Children given aspirin for the arthritis of ARF have responded so

TABLE 5-8.	The Jones criteria for diagnosis of an initial attack of rheumatic fever.	
Major Criteria	*Minor Criteria*
Carditis	Fever
Arthritis	Arthralgia
Erythema marginatum	Elevated acute phase reactants (ESR, CRP)
Chorea	Prolonged PR-interval on an ECG
Subcutaneous nodules	

Plus evidence of a preceding group A streptococcal infection by culture, rapid antigen, or antistreptococcal antibody titers.

well as to go from bed-ridden to running down the halls within hours of the first dose. In the current day, the liberal use of ibuprofen for fever or analgesia may obscure the classic migratory pattern of arthritis in ARF due to the symptomatic relief this agent may provide.

INCIDENCE AND ETIOLOGY

Although ARF remains an important cause of cardiovascular disease worldwide, the incidence of ARF has been decreasing since the early 1900s in developed nations. Regional outbreaks occurred throughout the United States in the 1980s and 1990s, and this resurgence may have been related to the increased prevalence of strains of GABHS thought to be more "rheumatogenic."

Populations at greatest risk for ARF mirror the populations with increased incidence of GABHS pharyngitis: ages 5-15 years and older individuals in close living quarters, such as military recruits. In developing countries and in the United States in the early 1900s, poorer socioeconomic communities had higher rates of GABHS pharyngitis and ARF. However, more recent outbreaks of ARF in the United States occurred predominantly in suburban and rural middle-class communities, as well as among military recruits.

The pathogenesis of ARF is not completely understood; however, evidence increasingly points to the contribution of molecular mimicry, in which antibodies directed at GABHS cross-react with host antigens. Strains of GABHS that cause impetigo do not appear to be an important cause of ARF. Genetic susceptibility may also play a role in disease development. Recurrent disease with subsequent episodes of GABHS pharyngitis is common and, for this reason, secondary prevention is an important feature of disease management.

CLINICAL PRESENTATION

Acute rheumatic fever is a nonsuppurative sequela of GABHS pharyngitis. The symptoms begin approximately 2-4 weeks following throat infection; however, in many cases, a sore throat is not reported, even in retrospect. GABHS infections that do not include pharyngitis are not initiators of acute rheumatic fever.

Approximately 80% of patients present with arthritis, typically a migratory polyarthritis with predilection for large joints. In contrast to Lyme arthritis, the subjective pain of ARF arthritis often is much more severe than the objective findings visible to the examiner. Analysis of fluid from an acutely inflamed joint reveals an elevated white count in the range of 20 000-40 000 cells/mm^3 with a neutrophil predominance.

Carditis can involve any part of the heart, but the most typical is an endocardial process with particular affinity for the mitral and aortic valves. Acutely, the valves demonstrate insufficiency, but the lesions progress to stenosis over time. Involvement of the myocardium can be seen, especially with the more severe presentations of congestive heart failure. Pericarditis and epicarditis can also complicate the picture but rarely occur in isolation. Carditis develops in approximately half of patients but has been reported in up to 80% of patients in the more recent US outbreaks. Clinical signs accepted for evidence of carditis include appropriate murmurs, cardiomegaly, congestive heart failure, or pericardial friction rub. The most recent update of the Jones criteria (1992) does not consider echocardiographic evidence of valvulitis without auscultatory findings to be sufficient to establish the presence of carditis for ARF.

Erythema marginatum and subcutaneous nodules are seen infrequently. When erythema marginatum is fully developed, it has an indistinct serpiginous red border with central clearing and is nonpruritic. It is specific for ARF, but its usefulness is limited by the fact that the rash is evanescent and is present in less than 10% of patients. Subcutaneous nodules are usually a late finding of ARF and may correlate with more severe or prolonged carditis. The lesions are pea-sized, nontender, and tend to be located over extensor tendons at the elbows or knees or the Achilles tendon.

Sydenham chorea is a late manifestation of ARF and can present after resolution of the other features or in isolation if the other features were never clinically apparent. This movement disorder may start with subtle deteriorations of handwriting before evolving into the involuntary, uncontrollable, and purposeless choreiform movements. Due to the late onset of this feature, the presence of Sydenham chorea alone can be considered

TABLE 5-9.	Features associated with acute rheumatic fever.	
Symptoms	Signs	Laboratory Tests
Fatigue, malaise	Pallor	Anemia
Abdominal pain	Tachycardia out of proportion to fever	Thrombocytosis
Epistaxis		
Palpitations		

diagnostic of ARF if other causes of chorea have been excluded.

Some of the minor criteria for ARF overlap with some of the major criteria. Arthralgias, painful joints without objective findings of arthritis, should be considered only if arthritis is not used as a major criterion. However, PR prolongation by ECG can be considered in addition to auscultatory evidence of carditis. The ESR and CRP are significantly elevated with the acute illness, with ESR usually greater than 50 mm/h and often approaching or exceeding 100 mm/h. The fever has no characteristic pattern but usually resolves in 3 weeks, even without treatment.

Other clinical findings of ARF are less specific but are often part of the clinical picture (Table 5-9).

DIAGNOSIS

Establishing the diagnosis of ARF involves assessing for the presence of major and minor criteria, documenting a preceding GABHS infection, and excluding disorders that mimic ARF.

Jones criteria. The five major criteria have been discussed in the preceding section. Evaluation for the minor criteria includes clinical assessment (fever, arthralgias), laboratory assessment (ESR, CRP), and evidence of atrioventricular conduction delay by electrocardiogram (PR interval prolongation).

Evidence of preceding GABHS infection. This can be obtained by:

1. Throat swab yielding a positive antigen (rapid test) or culture for GABHS at the time of presentation or

documented in the preceding weeks. Most patients do not demonstrate a positive throat swab when presenting with ARF, having cleared the infection during the latent period. Furthermore, a positive throat swab at the time of ARF presentation may represent colonization, which does not necessarily indicate preceding GABHS pharyngitis.

2. History of scarlet fever in the preceding weeks. Scarlet fever does not occur during the presentation of ARF but is sufficiently specific for GABHS infection that it can serve as evidence of preceding infection.

3. Elevated serum GABHS antibodies (antistreptolysin O, antiDNAase B, antihyaluronidase, antistreptokinase). A commercial agglutination assay that tests for several streptococcal antigens is rapid and widely available but is less standardized and less reproducible than quantitative titers of specific antibodies. Quantitative ASO is positive in 80% of patients with ARF; when three antibodies are tested quantitatively, at least one will be elevated in 95% of ARF patients.

Excluding disorders that mimic ARF. When joint pain is the salient complaint, the differential diagnosis for ARF includes septic arthritis, juvenile rheumatoid arthritis, systemic lupus erythematosus, Lyme disease, postinfectious reactive arthritis, serum sickness, and malignancies. When carditis is the main manifestation, infective endocarditis and viral myocarditis/pericarditis should be considered.

TREATMENT AND PREVENTION

There are three distinct aspects to the treatment of ARF: eradication of the GABHS, secondary prophylaxis, and treatment of the ARF manifestations.

Eradication. At the time of ARF diagnosis, patients require treatment for acute streptococcal pharyngitis, regardless of the results of a throat culture or rapid antigen test. The treatment is not thought to alter the course of the active ARF illness but to remove the inciting agent. The recommended regimen is the same as that for streptococcal pharyngitis: 10 days of oral penicillin V or amoxicillin, or a single intramuscular dose of benzathine penicillin G. After completion of this therapeutic regimen, secondary prophylaxis is begun.

Secondary prophylaxis. Recurrence of ARF from a subsequent GABHS infection is a well-recognized phenomenon, and the degree of cardiac involvement increases with each episode of ARF. Asymptomatic as well as symptomatic GABHS throat infections can cause recurrences of ARF; therefore, prevention of these infections is vital, and continuous antibiotic prophylaxis is necessary for all patients with ARF. The American Heart Association (AHA) provides guidelines regarding choice of antibiotic, route and schedule of administration, and duration of prophylaxis. The risk for recurrence is greatest within the first 5 years after the initial attack; however, in some cases, lifelong prophylaxis may be indicated.

The AHA has also provided guidelines for which patients are at highest risk of bacterial endocarditis and should receive antibiotic prophylaxis against infective endocarditis (e.g., during dental procedures, cystoscopy, and intestinal surgery). Not all patients with rheumatic heart disease will warrant infective endocarditis prophylaxis, but those with certain conditions, as delineated in the guidelines, should be treated with a short course of additional antibiotics in accordance with the AHA's recommendations.

Treatment of the ARF manifestations. Antiinflammatory medications, such as aspirin, are effective in the treatment for the carditis and arthritis symptoms of ARF. Aspirin is highly effective for the symptomatic treatment of the arthritis of ARF, and failure to respond to this therapy should bring the diagnosis of ARF into question. Congestive heart failure is managed medically, with diuretics and inotropic support, or surgically, with valve repair or replacement, as indicated by the severity of the symptoms.

SUGGESTED READINGS

1. Special Writing Group of the Committee on Rheumatic Fever, Endocarditis, and Kawasaki Disease of the Council on Cardiovascular Disease in the Young of the American Heart Association. Guidelines for the Diagnosis of Rheumatic Fever: Jones Criteria, 1992 Update. *JAMA.* 1992;268:2069-2073.

2. Kliegman RM, Behrman RE, Jensen HB, Stanton, BF. *Nelson's Textbook of Pediatrics.* 18th ed. Philadelphia: WB Saunders Co; 2007.

3. Ruddy S, Harris ED, Sledge CB. *Kelley's Textbook of Rheumatology.* 6th ed. Philadelphia: WB Saunders Co; 2001.

4. Gerber MA, Baltimore RS, Eaton CB, et al: Prevention of rheumatic fever and diagnosis and treatment of acute Streptococcal pharyngitis : a Scientific Statement from the American Heart Association Rheumatic Fever, Endocarditis, and Kawasaki Disease Committee of the Council on Cardiovascular Disease in the Young, the Interdisciplinary Council on Functional Genomics and Translational Biology, and the Interdisciplinary Council on Quality of Care and Outcomes Research: Endorsed by the American Academy of Pediatrics. *Circulation.* 2009;119(11):1541-1551.

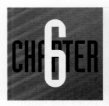

CHAPTER 6

POOR WEIGHT GAIN

STEPHEN LUDWIG

BRANDON C. KU

DEFINITION

Poor weight gain, growth failure, and failure to thrive (FTT) are conditions that involve a vast array of potential causes. The root of the problem may involve (1) inadequate caloric intake, (2) decreased ability to metabolize the ingested food, (3) increased caloric expenditure, or (4) abnormal caloric requirement. Whatever be the cause, a child's weight is a sensitive indicator of his or her general health. In the case of weight gain, health must be broadly defined and includes family, psychosocial, and socioeconomic causes as well as possible diseases and disorders.

Many cases of growth failure are diagnostically solved in the outpatient setting without the need for hospitalization. However, in some extreme cases, either because the growth delay is so significant or because the child is at a vulnerable age for long-term development, hospitalization is required. At times, the indication for hospitalization (Table 6-1) is a complex and/or obscure problem that requires a more intensive diagnostic evaluation.

CAUSE AND FREQUENCY

Growth failure is not a diagnosis on its own as it is a symptom of an underlying cause that must be identified to implement the appropriate intervention. The causes can be divided into broad categories of inadequate caloric intake, increased caloric wasting, increased caloric expenditure, and altered growth potential regulation (Table 6-2).

QUESTIONS TO ASK AND WHY

- What is the child's pattern of growth over time?
—This question helps establish timing of poor weight gain and whether it has existed for weeks or months. Reviewing past medical records including growth charts from the primary pediatrician can lead one to think about acute or chronic conditions.

- What aspects of growth have been affected?
—A comparison of weight, length, and head circumference may provide clues to the etiology as the sequence of events helps differentiate potential causes. With acquired conditions, the weight is affected first and most severely, followed by the length, and finally the head circumference. With congenital, genetic, or endocrine conditions, growth failure may be more symmetric across all three domains or have a recognizable pattern.

- Has the child developed any symptoms?
—Are there symptoms of gastrointestinal losses such as vomiting or diarrhea, indicating loss of nutritional intake? Are there symptoms of increased metabolic consumption such as cardiac or pulmonary disease, indicating increased caloric requirement? The history of such symptoms is vital in determining the etiology of growth failure and is often more revealing than laboratory tests.

- What has the child's diet and eating pattern been?
—A developmental sequence exists for the types of foods given to children and the manner in which they are presented. For example, children may be

TABLE 6-1.	Indications of hospitalization of children with failure to thrive.

Infants younger than 6 months of age
Below birth weight at 6 weeks
Head circumference falling below normal growth curve before 6 months of age
Signs of abuse
Signs of gross physical neglect
Persistent poor weight gain despite outpatient therapy
Underlying disease process being evaluated
Unsafe home environment
Caretaker deemed inappropriate

picky-eaters and may continually refuse food presented to them. Or they may want to eat table food and to manipulate food in their own mouths as they grow older. Parents who insist on offering the same types and amount of food instead of adapting to their children's development and changing needs may find their child resistant and failing to gain weight. In these situations, it may be beneficial to observe a meal to understand the process and identify any barriers that may exist.

- What is the state of the family unit and their lifestyle?

—This question explores the possible psychosocial and socioeconomic causes of growth failure? Is this family functioning in other ways? Are there support systems for the parents? Does the family have financial resources to purchase appropriate amounts of food for their growing children? Ascertaining a family's home environment assists the health-care professional in identifying causes that are not intrinsic to the patient.

SUGGESTED READINGS

1. Miller LA, Grunwald GK, Johnson SL, et al. Disease severity at time of referral for pediatric failure to thrive and obesity: time for a paradigm shift? *J Pediatr.* 2002;141:121-124.
2. Schwartz ID. Failure to thrive: an old nemesis in the new millennium. *Pediatr Rev.* 2000;21:257-264.
3. Shah MD. Failure to thrive in children. *J Clin Gastroenterology.* 2002;35:371-374.
4. Homer C, Ludwig S. Categorization of etiology for failure to thrive. *Amer J Dis Child.* 1981;135:848-851.
5. Zenel JA. Failure to thrive: a general pediatrician's perspective. *Pediatr Rev.* 1997;18:371-378.
6. Jaffe AC. Failure to thrive: current clinical concepts. *Pediatr Rev.* 2011;32:100-108.

CASE 6-1

Sixteen-Month-Old Boy

SANJEEV K. SWAMI

HISTORY OF PRESENT ILLNESS

The patient was a 16-month-old African-American male, admitted because of concerns for failure to thrive (FTT). He has also been noted by his parents to have lost some of his previously acquired developmental skills. During the week prior to admission, he has felt "warm"; his temperature was not measured. He was also having two to three loose stools per day. The stools were not bloody. He had no vomiting. He had a slight cough, but no rhinitis, rash, or ear pain. From a developmental standpoint, he was always delayed compared to his twin. He first rolled over at 10 months. He was not sitting or walking. He recently had been noted to be smiling less and interacting less. He receives early intervention services for occupational and physical therapy. The pediatrician prescribed nutritional supplements, but the family has not yet obtained them.

MEDICAL HISTORY

The boy was the first born of a twin pregnancy. His birth weight was 5 pounds and 10 ounces. He was delivered to a 20-year-old mother by Cesarean section for breech presentation. The baby has been bottle-fed and has had no previous hospitalizations. He had pneumonia at 7 months of age, which was treated in the outpatient setting. He was also treated for thrush at 9 months of age that responded promptly to oral

TABLE 6-2.	Causes of inadequate weight gain by etiology.

Inadequate Caloric Intake

Lack of appetite
  Chronic disease (e.g., central nervous system pathology, gastrointestinal disorders, chronic infections)
  Anemia (e.g., iron deficiency)
  Cardiopulmonary disease
  Psychosocial problems (e.g., anorexia, apathy, depression)

Difficulty with ingestion
  Feeding disorder
  Psychosocial problems (e.g., apathy, rumination)
  Neurologic disorders (e.g., cerebral palsy, hypertonia, hypotonia)
  Craniofacial anomalies (e.g., choanal atresia, cleft lip and palate, micro/retrognathia)
  Lack of suck/swallow coordination
  Generalized muscle weakness/pathology (e.g., myopathies)
  Tracheo-esophageal fistula
  Genetic syndromes
  Congenital syndromes (e.g., fetal alcohol syndrome)

Unavailability of food
  Inadequate maternal lactation
  Inappropriate feeding technique
  Insufficient/inadequate volume of food
  Inappropriate food for age
  Withholding of food (abuse, neglect)

Caloric Wasting (from inadequate absorption or increased losses)

Vomiting
  Central nervous system pathology (increased intracranial pressure)
  Intestinal tract obstruction (e.g., pyloric stenosis, malrotation)

Vomiting (*cont.*)
  Gastrointestinal reflux
  Metabolic disorders
  Drugs/toxins
Malabsorption
  Biliary atresia/cirrhosis
  Celiac disease
  Inflammatory bowel disease
  Enzymatic deficiencies (lactose intolerance, cystic fibrosis)
  Food or protein sensitivity/intolerance
  Infectious diarrhea
  Short bowel syndrome
Renal losses
  Diabetes
  Renal tubular acidosis

Increased Caloric Requirements

Increased metabolism/increased use of calories
  Congenital/acquired heart disease
  Chronic respiratory disease (e.g., bronchopulmonary dysplasia, cystic fibrosis)
  Malignancy
  Chronic/recurrent infection
  Endocrinopathies (e.g., hyperthyroidism, hyperaldosteronism)
  Chronic anemia
  Drugs/toxins (e.g., lead, levothyroxine)
Defective use of calories
  Metabolic disorders (e.g., aminoacideopathies, inborn errors of carbohydrate metabolism)
  Renal tubular acidosis

Altered Growth Potential Regulation

Prenatal insult
Chromosomal abnormality/genetic syndrome
Endocrinopathies

nystatin. Otitis media was recently diagnosed and treated at the clinic.

He has no allergies and receives no medication. He has not traveled outside the United States. The only pet was an older cat. One month ago the mother was hospitalized with a cerebrovascular accident. In the process of evaluation, she was found to be HIV-antibody positive.

PHYSICAL EXAMINATION

T 37.8°C; HR 130 bpm; RR 40/min; SpO$_2$ 100% in room air

Weight 7.94 kg (<5% for an 8-month-old); Height 75.5 cm (10th percentile; 50th percentile for an 11-month-old); Head circumference 47 cm (25th percentile)

In general, the child was apathetic and irritable, but consolable in his mother's arms. There was frontal prominence and bitemporal wasting. The tympanic membranes were normal in appearance and mobility. The oropharynx was clear; there was no thrush. Multiple small cervical, occipital, axillary, epitrochlear, and inguinal lymph nodes were palpable. The cardiac examination revealed a normal S1 and S2 with no murmurs, rubs, or gallops. The chest was clear to auscultation bilaterally. The abdomen was soft without tenderness or guarding. The liver edge was palpable 3 cm below the right costal margin while the spleen was palpable 2 cm below the left costal margin. The child was globally hypotonic but deep tendon reflexes were symmetrically increased. Plantar reflexes were down-going.

DIAGNOSTIC STUDIES

Complete blood count revealed the following: hemoglobin, 11.0 g/dL; white blood cell count, 37 900/mm³ (8% segmented neutrophils, 47% lymphocytes, 38% atypical lymphocytes); platelet count, 195 000/mm³. Serum electrolytes, blood urea nitrogen, and creatinine were normal. Additional laboratory studies included the following: lactate dehydrogenase, 1586; ALT, 98; AST, 139; alkaline phosphatase, 108; triglycerides, 212; and albumin, 3.4 mg/dL.

COURSE OF ILLNESS

HIV antibody testing was performed at the time of admission given the mother's recent diagnosis. The child's HIV antibodies were positive. Initial evaluation focused on determining this child's HIV status (in utero exposure vs. true infection) since maternal HIV antibodies may be present for the first 18 months of life. Additional testing by HIV polymerase chain reaction was positive confirming this child's diagnosis of HIV infection.

Given his HIV exposure, there was concern that his developmental regression could be secondary to HIV encephalopathy. A head CT scan, performed without contrast, revealed diffuse cerebral atrophy. Soon after hospitalization, the child began to have high fevers to 40.1°C, accompanied by tachycardia and tachypnea. His oxygenation remained adequate. After several days, he began to have persistent tachypnea with mild increased work of breathing, and occasional rales at the left lower lung field. A chest X-ray showed mild volume loss at the right upper lobe, as well as streaky atelectasis in the left lower lobe and right upper lobe. An abdominal ultrasound was obtained to look for increased retroperitoneal adenopathy, due to the possibility of disseminated *Mycobacterium avium* as a cause of his fevers. The abdominal ultrasound showed hepatomegaly with an increase in the echotexture of the liver, without focal masses

or abscess. There was no ductal dilatation or gallbladder wall thickening. There was also splenomegaly, without focal lesions within the spleen. Also noted were several enlarged nodes within the porta hepatis, as well as several enlarged retroperitoneal nodes in the paraortic area. The kidneys were normal.

What are the causes of fever and hepatosplenomegaly in an HIV-positive infant?

DISCUSSION CASE 6-1

DIFFERENTIAL DIAGNOSIS

There were many possible diagnoses to be considered in this case of FTT. The symptoms of diarrhea and fever were factors supporting an organic cause. However, the history of being noncompliant with obtaining the nutritional supplements and the situation of an over-stressed family with the mother having HIV and twins raised the consideration of some nonorganic factors. The possibility of mixed FTT was very high on the list.

As far as organic causes are concerned HIV is a well-known cause of FTT. Additional testing is required to differentiate between maternally transmitted antibodies and true infection in young infants. A positive PCR test confirmed true HIV infection as an explanation of the patient's FTT. Then, the onset of high spiking fevers prompted the evaluation for an opportunistic infection.

Diagnostic considerations in an HIV-infected child with fever are diverse (Table 6-3). A child who is HIV positive and who is febrile requires an exhaustive search to identify an organism. Initial evaluation should include a search for focal infection and a general assessment of severity of illness. The absence of specific localizing signs presents a greater diagnostic dilemma.

DIAGNOSIS

Toxoplasma IgM was negative, but IgG was positive, and the patient had a clinical picture consistent with disseminated toxoplasmosis. He had hepatitis, pneumonitis, and diffuse lymphadenopathy with an atypical lymphocytosis on peripheral blood smear. Ophthalmology was consulted to

TABLE 6-3.	Differential diagnosis of fever in an HIV positive child.

Viral Infections
  Hepatitis B
  Hepatitis C
  Herpes simplex virus
  Varicella zoster virus
  Cytomegalovirus
  Epstein-Barr virus

Focal Bacterial Infections
  Pneumonia
  Sinusitis
  Intra-abdominal abscess

Mycobacterial Infections
  Mycobacterium tuberculosis
  Mycobacterium avium complex

Fungal Infections
  Pneumocystis jirovecii pneumonia
  Cryptococcus neoformans

Parasites
  Toxoplasma gondii
  Cryptosporidium

Other
  Lymphoid interstitial pneumonia

evaluate for retinal changes. None were present. The patient was started on therapy for toxoplasmosis, including pyrimethamine, sulfadiazine, and leucovorin rescue. **The diagnosis is *Toxoplasmosis gondii*, an intracellular parasite.**

INCIDENCE, EPIDEMIOLOGY, AND LIFECYCLE

The organism is distributed widely and rates of infection vary greatly. Sixteen to forty percent of the population is estimated to be infected in the United States and the United Kingdom, while the rates of infection in Central and South America and continental Europe are between 50% and 80%. Human infection may be asymptomatic to severe, even fatal in individuals who are immunocompromised. Felines (cats) are the only definitive host.

The routes of transmission in humans include blood transfusion, organ transplantation, transplacental, and ingestion of chicken eggs, meat, milk, or oocysts in contaminated water or vegetables from feline fecal matter. The lifecycle of the parasite includes a sexual phase that occurs in

cats and an asexual phase that occurs in both cats and humans and other intermediate hosts (Figure 6-1). The incidence in cats, other animals, and in humans varies greatly by location and age of the population studied.

CLINICAL PRESENTATION

The clinical manifestations of toxoplasmosis vary depending on host factors and the timing of infection (Table 6-4). Approximately 70% to 90% of cases acquired postnatally are asymptomatic. For patients with an intact immune system the symptomatic cases most often involve lymphadenopathy with either tender or nontender nodes. These children may have a mononucleosis-like picture. In children who are immunocompromised, multiple organs may be involved. In AIDS patients, central nervous system involvement is common. Findings include headaches, hemiparesis, and visual disturbances. More severe presentations have included speech abnormalities, seizures, and the syndrome of inappropriate antidiuretic hormone secretion.

Congenital toxoplasmosis is often asymptomatic and bears no significant signs or symptoms, but 30%-40% of affected newborns will have some findings if evaluated closely. It is estimated that 1 in 3000 to 1 in 10 000 live births in the United States are afflicted by congenital toxoplasmosis. The affected newborns may have hydrocephalus, fevers, hepatosplenomegaly, prolonged hyperbilirubinemia, blindness, deafness, and other manifestations including diarrhea and feeding difficulties. Ocular toxoplasmosis may be a consequence of congenital infection or postnatally acquired infection.

Infection is lifelong with acute and chronic stages. Acute illness involves a period of parasitemia following the initial infection. With chronic infection, the parasite is encysted in the host tissue. Organisms may periodically break out of the cysts resulting in local reactivation of the disease. In immunocompromised hosts, the reactivation of disease may result in dissemination and systemic spread.

Long-term sequelae of congenital toxoplasmosis include developmental delay, seizures, spasticity, visual impairment, and deafness.

FIGURE 6-1. Lifecycle of *Toxoplasma gondii* (Courtesy of the Centers for Disease Control and Prevention, Division of Parasitic Diseases and Malaria—DPDx website: http://www.dpd.cdc.gov/dpdx/Default.htm).

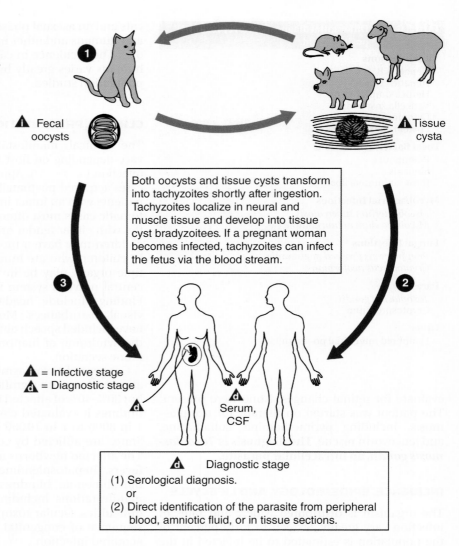

Both oocysts and tissue cysts transform into tachyzoites shortly after ingestion. Tachyzoites localize in neural and muscle tissue and develop into tissue cyst bradyzoitees. If a pregnant woman becomes infected, tachyzoites can infect the fetus via the blood stream.

▲ Fecal oocysts

▲ Tissue cysta

▲ = Infective stage
ⅾ = Diagnostic stage

Serum, CSF

ⅾ   Diagnostic stage
(1) Serological diagnosis.
    or
(2) Direct identification of the parasite from peripheral blood, amniotic fluid, or in tissue sections.

DIAGNOSTIC APPROACH

Toxoplasma gondii antibodies. Serologic tests are most commonly employed and measure the host antibody represented. *Toxoplasma gondii*-specific IgG serum antibody, at any titer, indicates a risk of active infection in an immunocompromised individual. Testing that shows seroconversion or a fourfold or greater rise in antibody titer in serum obtained 3-6 weeks apart can confirm the diagnosis. There are several toxoplasma serologic tests available; most experts use the Palo Alto Medical Foundation Toxoplasma Serology Laboratory (http://www.pamf.org/serology/) for complicated cases.

Other studies. The infection can also be confirmed by demonstration of the organism histologically or by identification of nucleic acid (polymerase chain reaction) in a site in which the encysted organism would not be present as part of a latent infection, such as cerebrospinal fluid or

TABLE 6-4.	Toxoplasmosis clinical syndromes.	
	Clinical Features	*Additional Factors*
Congenital	Wide clinical spectrum from subclinical disease to severely affected infants Intracranial calcifications, microcephaly, hydrocephalus, chorioretinitis, epilepsy, developmental delay, anemia, thrombocytopenia with petechiae Clinical features may be present at birth, or develop over time	Transmission lowest in first trimester, but associated with most severe form Disease transmitted in third trimester may be asymptomatic at time of delivery
Immunocompromised Host (patients with HIV/AIDS, solid organ transplant recipients, patients with hematologic malignancies, patients receiving immunosuppression with corticosteroids, cytotoxic drugs, or anti-TNF-α therapy)	Pneumonitis, encephalitis, chorioretinitis, and myocarditis are most common Untreated, disease often progresses to a disseminated form with high mortality	Disease can be from primary infection or reactivation of a latent infection Trimethoprim-sulfamethoxazole has some efficacy as a prophylactic agent Solid organ transplant recipients may be infected via the transplanted organ
Immunocompetent Host	Many infections are asymptomatic Often presents as cervical adenopathy Systemic illness similar to mononucleosis Can progress to a disseminated infection including myocarditis, pneumonitis, hepatitis, or encephalitis Chorioretinitis can be isolated or part of a systemic illness Can be a cause of fever of unknown origin	Usually self-limited
Ocular	Chorioretinitis and uveitis (posterior or panuveitis) Recurrences occur frequently	Can be due to acute infection or reactivation of latent disease Ocular disease can be from congenital or postnatal infection

bronchoalveolar fluid. When the diagnosis is made in an individual thought to be immunocompetent, HIV testing should be considered.

Lumbar puncture. The differential diagnosis of congenital toxoplasmosis is broad. Therefore, cerebrospinal fluid (CSF) testing should include cell count, protein, and glucose, and Gram stain and bacterial culture. Additionally, CSF testing should also be done for enteroviruses and herpes simplex virus by polymerase chain reaction and syphilis by CSF Venereal Diseases Research Laboratory (VDRL) testing.

Radiologic studies. A head ultrasound or CT may reveal diffuse intracranial calcifications. In contrast, intracranial calcifications in congenital cytomegalovirus infections are typically periventricular (Figure 6-2).

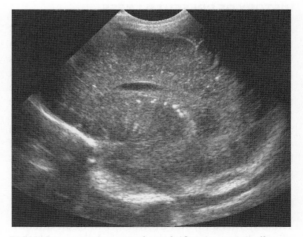

FIGURE 6-2. Periventricular calcifications typically found with congenital cytomegalovirus infection.

Ophthalmology consultation. Infants with congenital toxoplasmosis may have chorioretinitis and, less commonly, microophthalmia or cataracts. Chorioretinitis occurs in most infants with neurologic disease attributed to congenital toxoplasmosis and in almost two-thirds of infants with generalized toxoplasmosis. Chorioretinitis may also be present in congenital infections caused by cytomegalovirus, herpes simplex virus, rubella, and varicella zoster virus. Microophthalmia may also be present in congenital rubella, though this disease is rare in the United States.

TREATMENT

Combination therapy is recommended for treatment of toxoplasmosis. The primary medication is pyrimethamine, a folic acid antagonist. Leucovorin is administered with pyrimethamine to help counteract its bone marrow suppressive side effects. Sulfadiazine or clindamycin is recommended as an additional treatment agent. The combination of pyrimethamine with sulfadiazine acts synergistically.

Spiramycin is preferred in treating women during pregnancy. Trimethoprim-sulfamethoxazole also has efficacy in treating toxoplasmosis but is not considered to be a primary therapy. Other medications that have been used in combination with pyrimethamine include azithromycin, clarithromycin, atovaquone, and dapsone. HIV-infected patients with CD4+ T-lymphocyte counts less than 100-200/mm^3 may require continued suppressive antimicrobial therapy.

SUGGESTED READINGS

1. Hill D, Dubey JP. *Toxoplasma gondii*: transmission, diagnosis and prevention. *Clin Microbiol Infect.* 2002; 8:634-640.
2. Tamma P. Toxoplasmosis. *Pediatr Rev.* 2007;28:470-471.
3. Weiss LM, Dubey JP. Toxoplasmosis: a history of clinical observations. *Int J Parasitol.* 2009;39:895-901.
4. McAuley JB. Toxoplasmosis in children. *Pediatr Infect Dis J.* 2008;27:161-162.
5. Montoya JG. Laboratory diagnosis of *Toxoplasma gondii* infection and toxoplasmosis. *J Infect Dis.* 2002; 185:S73-S82.

CASE 6-2

Seven-Month-Old Boy

MAYA A. JONES

HISTORY OF PRESENT ILLNESS

A 7-month-old white male was admitted for evaluation of failure to thrive. The patient was a former twin B who was born at 37 weeks gestation. The mother's pregnancy was uncomplicated and the patient had been doing well until 3 months of age. At that time the patient had bilateral inguinal hernia repair. Since then his parents noticed that he has not been gaining weight. His stools were loose, foul smelling, and occurred 6-7 times per day. There was no history of fevers or vomiting and his appetite was described as greater than his twin brother who was thriving.

MEDICAL HISTORY

The boy was a former 37-week twin of an uncomplicated pregnancy, labor, and delivery. Mother denies having any sexually transmitted diseases.

He takes no medications and has no allergies. He received his immunizations during an office visit at 6 months of age. Family history was remarkable for a father with diabetes. The child lived with his mother, father, his twin, and 3-year-old sister. Both siblings were healthy. Developmentally, the child was unable to sit unassisted, had not rolled over, and still had some head lag on repeated testing.

PHYSICAL EXAMINATION

T 37.2°C; HR 110 bpm; RR 20/min; BP 78/50 mmHg

Height <5th percentile and Weight <5th percentile

In general, the child was emaciated but interactive. His head was normocephalic and pupils were equally round and reactive to light. The sclera was anicteric. The tympanic membranes were normal in appearance and mobility. The neck was supple with free range of motion. There was no lymph node enlargement or palpable masses. The chest was clear bilaterally. There were no murmurs, gallops, or rubs on cardiovascular examination. The abdomen was soft, nontender, and nondistended with positive bowel sounds. There was no hepatosplenomegaly or masses. The genitalia were normal. There was clinodactyly. Neurologic examination showed global weakness and head lag. The skin had a fine erythematous macular rash over the extremities.

DIAGNOSTIC STUDIES

Complete blood count revealed the following: hemoglobin, 2.2 g/dL; platelets, 180 000/mm³; and 1000 white blood cells/mm³ (2% band forms, 8% segmented neutrophils, 81% lymphocytes, and 9% monocytes). Serum electrolytes were as follows: sodium, 138 mEq/L; potassium, 3.6 mEq/L; chloride, 103 mEq/L; and bicarbonate, 22 mEq/L. The serum albumin was 4.2 mg/dL. Prothrombin and partial thromboplastin times were 12.5 and 31.0 seconds, respectively. A sweat test was normal.

COURSE OF ILLNESS

The patient was evaluated for malabsorptive stool pattern. He was shown to have increased fecal fat and evidence of pancreatic insufficiency. This finding in conjunction with findings on physical examination and complete blood count suggested a diagnosis.

DISCUSSION CASE 6-2

DIFFERENTIAL DIAGNOSIS

The differential diagnosis of growth failure due to malabsorption is a long one. Once the type of malabsorption is narrowed down to exocrine pancreatic dysfunction then the cause may be narrowed to hereditary and acquired causes. The hereditary causes include cystic fibrosis, Shwachman-Diamond syndrome, Johnson Rizzald syndrome,

TABLE 6-5.	Diagnostic studies in the evaluation of malabsorption.

Initial Screening Studies
Stool examination for occult blood, leukocytes, reducing substances, and pH
Stool examination for *Clostridium difficile* toxin, ova, and parasites
Stool cultures for infectious and viral pathogens
Serum electrolytes, albumin, and total protein
Urinalysis and culture

Quantitative and Qualitative Tests for Malabsorption
Breath H_2 studies
D-Xylose absorption for mucosal function
Fecal fat studies
Serum iron, vitamin B_{12} folate

Specific Diagnostic Studies
Sweat chloride test
Small intestinal biopsy for histology and mucosal enzyme
Contrast radiographic studies: upper gastrointestinal series with small-bowel follow-through and/or barium enema
Provocative pancreatic secretion testing
Ultrasound for biliary tree anomalies
Endoscopic retrograde cholangiopancreatograph (ERCP) for selective evaluation of biliary or pancreatic ducts

Source: Adapted from: Hill ID. Disorders of digestion and absorption. In: Rudolph CD, Rudolph AM, eds. *Rudolph's Pediatrics*, 21st ed. New York: McGraw-Hill; 2003.

Pearson's Pancreatitis and Bone Marrow syndrome, and isolated enzyme deficiency. Acquired causes result from chronic pancreatic and surgical causes.

Other causes of malabsorption are many and include defects in the luminal phase, the mucosal phase, or the transport phase of absorption and digestion. Table 6-5 shows tests that may be used to evaluate the different forms of malabsorption.

DIAGNOSIS

The presence of neutropenia and a skeletal abnormality (clinodactyly) in conjunction with pancreatic insufficiency suggested the diagnosis of Shwachman syndrome. The diagnosis is **Shwachman-Diamond syndrome, the second most common cause of hereditary pancreatic insufficiency; cystic fibrosis is the most common cause.** The stool pattern and growth pattern is similar to cystic fibrosis but patients with Shwachman syndrome will have other features. These are often short stature with a normal growth pattern. Skeletal deformities have been noted in the thorax and fingers. Some children will also manifest bone marrow dysfunction, more often causing neutropenia and frequent infections, but also anemia and thrombocytopenia.

INCIDENCE AND EPIDEMIOLOGY OF SHWACHMAN-DIAMOND SYNDROME

Shwachman-Diamond syndrome, an autosomal recessive disorder, results in exocrine pancreatic insufficiency, skeletal abnormalities (e.g., cinodactyly, syndactyly, supernumerary metatarsals), and bone marrow dysfunction, the latter of which predisposes to myelodysplastic syndrome and acute myeloid leukemia. The exact prevalence is unknown but estimates based on comparison cystic fibrosis data suggest a prevalence of approximately 1 per 75 000. There does not appear to be a racial or ethnic predisposition but males are more commonly affected than females.

Affected children have some degree of pancreatic insufficiency early in life. Thus, the diagnosis is typically suspected within the first year of life. The typical presentation includes malabsorption, steatorrhea, and failure to thrive. Symptoms related to deficiencies in fat-soluble vitamins (i.e., A, D, E, K) may also be present. Neutrophil migration defects and neutropenia predispose to recurrent bacterial infections, most commonly sino-pulmonary infections and, occasionally, skin and soft tissue infections and osteomyelitis. Bone marrow failure leads to anemia, easy bruising, and recurrent epistaxis. Defects in tooth enamel predispose to dental caries. Most patients have mild cognitive impairment. Children with Shwachman-Diamond syndrome are also at higher risk of hematologic malignancies.

DIAGNOSTIC APPROACH

The diagnostic approach is similar to that of a child with cystic fibrosis; yet the sweat test is normal but some of the other distinguishing features may be present. There is no single laboratory marker. Shwachman-Diamond syndrome is a clinical phenotype with central features of pancreatitis and bone marrow dysfunction. Other causes of pancreatic dysfunction must be eliminated.

Sweat test. The sweat test, performed to exclude cystic fibrosis as a cause of pancreatic insufficiency, reveals normal sweat chloride levels.

Complete blood count. The complete blood count typically reveals persistent or cyclic neutropenia, anemia, and, occasionally, thrombocytopenia.

Serum electrolytes. Serum bicarbonate may be low.

Hepatic transaminases. Hypoalbuminemia occurs as a consequence of malabsorption. Alanine and aspartate aminotransferases may be mildly elevated.

Fecal fat measurement. A 72-hour fecal fat measurement demonstrates an increase in fecal lipids and fatty acids, though the absence of steatorrhea does not exclude the possibility of Shwachman-Diamond syndrome.

Serum immunoglobulins. IgA and IgG levels may be low.

Bone marrow aspirate. Bone marrow may show hypoplasia with fibrosis. It may also reveal hematologic malignancy. Patients who have their first symptoms younger than 3 months of age, and those with low hematologic parameters at diagnosis and during follow-up are at highest risk for developing hematologic complications, both malignant and nonmalignant.

Radiologic evaluation. A skeletal survey may reveal osteopenia, metaphyseal chondrodysplasia (e.g., metaphyseal widening), costochondral thickening, and abnormal tubulation of the long bones. Abdominal MRI has been used to identify fatty replacement of the pancreas.

TREATMENT

Treatment includes enzyme replacement, nutritional support, infection prevention, and vigilance to detect hematologic malignancies. Careful attention should be paid to vitamin therapy of the fat-soluble vitamins and careful treatment for infections and other hematologic manifestations. The response to treatment is good in most cases. The patients may be prone to infections due to the neutropenia. Some patients may also develop acute myelogenous leukemia (AML).

SUGGESTED READINGS

1. Mark DR, Forstner GG, Wilchanski M, et al. Shwachman syndrome: exocrine pancreatic dysfunction and variable phenotypic expression. *Gastroenterology.* 1996;111: 1593-1602.
2. Baldassano R, Liacouras C. Chronic diarrhea: a practical approach for the pediatrician. *Pediatr Clin North Amer.* 1991;38:667-674.
3. Rothbaum R, Perrault J, Vlachos A, et al. Shwachman-Diamond syndrome: report from an international conference. *J Pediatr.* 2002;14:266-270.
4. Ruggiero A, Molinari F, Coccia P, et al. MRI findings in Shwachman-Diamond syndrome. *Pediatr Blood Cancer.* 2008;50:352-354.
5. Donadieu J, Fenneteau O, Beaupain B, et al. Classification of and risk factors for hematologic complications in a French national cohort of 102 patients with Shwachman-Diamond syndrome. *Haematologica.* 2012;97: 1312-1319.

CASE 6-3

Twenty-Day-Old Girl

STEPHEN LUDWIG

HISTORY OF PRESENT ILLNESS

This 20-day-old Caucasian female infant was referred to the emergency department by her primary care doctor for failure to thrive. She was at full-term gestation, 2.53 kg, born via spontaneous vaginal delivery with no complications during pregnancy. In the first 36 hours of life, she had poor feeding because of poor suck. She had normal bowel movements and normal urine output in the nursery. After 36 hours of life, she began to feed well, and was discharged with her mother. During the last 3 weeks, the baby had been seen several times by her primary physician for weight checks. She failed to regain her birth weight. She was feeding 2.5 to 3 ounces every 2-3 hours (approximately eight 3 ounce bottles per day). Formula was being made from powder and mixed appropriately. There was no emesis, arching, or irritability with feeds. She has had loose seedy stools for 2 days prior to admission. No blood was noted in the stool. There was nasal congestion but no fever. There were no ill contacts except that the mother had an illness with fever and headache one week prior to this visit.

MEDICAL HISTORY

The prenatal history was remarkable for maternal tobacco use (one-half pack per day) but no illicit drug use. Peripartum testing for group B *Streptococcus*,

hepatitis B, and HIV were negative. The prenatal ultrasound revealed normal fetal movements. The mother took prenatal vitamins but no other medications during pregnancy. The infant was born by vaginal delivery complicated only by the presence of meconium at delivery. The Apgar scores were not known.

There was no family history of still births or miscarriages. There were no known metabolic disorders, congenital heart disease, seizure disorders, or neurologic disease. There was no history of cystic fibrosis.

PHYSICAL EXAMINATION

T 36.9°C; HR 160 bpm; RR 40/min; BP 96/62 mmHg

Weight 2.42 kg (<5 percentile); Length 46 cm (<5 percentile); Head circumference 35 cm (10 percentile)

In general, the patient was cachetic but active. The anterior fontanel was open and flat. The posterior fontanel was approximately 1 cm wide. There were no dysmorphic facial features. The pupils were reactive bilaterally. The oropharynx was clear; specifically, there was no thrush. There was no lymphadenopathy. The heart and lung sounds were normal. The abdomen was soft. The liver edge was palpable 1 cm below the right costal margin. The skin was mottled and pale. A 1-cm hemangioma was located on the left parietal area. The neurologic examination was normal.

DIAGNOSTIC STUDIES

Serum sodium, 136 mEq/L; potassium, 5.5 mEq/L; chloride, 100 mEq/L; bicarbonate, 28 mEq/L; blood urea nitrogen, creatinine, glucose, calcium, magnesium, and phosphorus were normal.

COURSE OF ILLNESS

The 20-day-old infant with moderate malnutrition and failure to thrive was admitted for inpatient evaluation, including strict calorie counts and feeding observation. During the next 2 days, she had adequate caloric intake (as much as 180-200 kcal per kg per day) without documented weight gain. She was also noted to have increased stool output, with more output than intake. Her stools were positive for reducing substances. The stool pH was 5.5. All stools were heme negative.

DISCUSSION CASE 6-3

DIFFERENTIAL DIAGNOSIS

The differential diagnosis in this case was broad. When feeding the baby, a poor suck and swallow was noted. This difficulty with intake was questioned as to whether it was a primary problem (e.g., neuropathy, spinal-muscle atrophy) or secondary due to poor nutrition and weakness. When the child was fed, she gained more strength but still failed to gain weight. When no weight gain was noted despite adequate caloric intake, malabsorption was considered.

DIAGNOSIS

Sweat tests were obtained, which showed good sweat volumes over the collection time of 30 minutes. The sweat chloride was 95 and 105 at the two sites sampled (normal <40, borderline 40-60, abnormal >60). The sweat test was repeated and was again abnormal. The patient was diagnosed with cystic fibrosis (CF). Baseline chest X-ray was

normal. She was started on supplemental enzymes, as well as vitamin supplementation and nebulized albuterol and cromolyn. She did well with supplemental enzymes, documenting excellent catch-up growth while in the hospital. **The diagnosis of cystic fibrosis was considered when a normal, and eventually a supernormal, calorie intake was achieved and the infant failed to gain weight.** This clinical trial resulted in the suspicion of a malabsorption problem and cystic fibrosis was considered as the most common cause of malabsorption.

INCIDENCE AND EPIDEMIOLOGY OF CYSTIC FIBROSIS

The incidence of cystic fibrosis varies by population tested. Overall, it is the most common life-shortening inherited disease in North America. Cystic fibrosis is inherited as an autosomal recessive disease. Several gene sites have been recognized. The most important is the δF508 on the long arm of chromosome 7. In those of Northern European extraction, it occurs in 1 in every 2500 live births. Approximately 4% of whites are carriers of a cystic fibrosis gene. The manifestations of cystic fibrosis are very varied. Table 6-6 shows diagnostic criteria for cystic fibrosis.

CLINICAL PRESENTATION

The clinical presentation and age of presentation are varied. Manifestations may be evident at birth but in some cases have not become apparent until fertility evaluations in young adulthood have led to the diagnosis. All of the following systems may be involved: gastrointestinal, sweat glands, respiratory tract, reproductive, orthopedic, and endocrine/metabolic (hyperglycemia). Failure to thrive is one of the most frequent presenting signs. Table 6-7 shows the indications for sweat testing and also lists clinical findings in patients with cystic fibrosis.

DIAGNOSTIC APPROACH

Diagnostic approach is based on phenotypic presentation plus laboratory confirmation. The laboratory confirmation is usually based on a positive sweat test with a sweat concentration greater than

TABLE 6-6.	Diagnostic criteria for cystic fibrosis.[a]

Clinical/History
- One or more characteristic phenotypic features (chronic obstructive pulmonary disease, exocrine pancreatic insufficiency, sweat salt loss syndrome, male infertility)
- CF in a sibling or a positive newborn screen

Laboratory Evidence of Abnormal CFTR/CFTR Function
- A positive sweat test (a sweat chloride concentration > 60 meq/L on a sample of at least 100 mg, obtained after maximal stimulation by pilocarpine iontophoresis
- Identification of two CFTR mutations known to cause CF
- Diagnostic nasal potential difference

[a] Diagnosis requires at least one from each column.

TABLE 6-7.	Indications for sweat testing.

Gastrointestinal Tract
Chronic diarrhea
Steatorrhea
Meconium ileus
Meconium plug syndrome
Rectal prolapse
Cirrhosis/portal hypertension
Prolonged neonatal jaundice
Pancreatitis
Deficiency of fat-soluble vitamins
 (especially A, E, K)

Respiratory Tract
Upper
 Nasal polyps
 Pansinusitis on radiographs
Lower
 Chronic cough
 Recurrent bronchiolitis
 Recurrent wheezing
 Intractable "asthma"
 Recurrent or persistent atelectasis
 Obstructive pulmonary disease
 Staphylococcal pneumonia
 Pseudomonas aeruginosa (especially mucoid
 colony types) recovered from throat, sputum, or
 bronchoscopic cultures

Other
Digital clubbing
Family history of cystic fibrosis
Failure to thrive
Hyponatremic, hypochloremic alkalosis
Severe dehydration incompatible with
 clinical history
Heat prostration
"Tastes salty"
Male infertility

Source: Adapted from: Orenstein DM. Cystic fibrosis. In: Rudolph CD, Rudolph AM, eds. *Rudolph's Pediatrics.* 21st ed. New York: McGraw-Hill; 2003.

60 meq/L on a sweat sample of at least 100 mg. Genetic testing is also available (Table 6-6).

Tissue typing gives the indication for sweat testing which also shows the varied manifestations. Care must be taken because there may be causes of false positive and false negative testing. Indications for sweat testing are presented in Table 6-7.

Newborn screening. Earlier diagnosis of cystic fibrosis is possible in some cases since newborn infants with cystic fibrosis have elevated blood immunoreactive trypsinogen levels caused by obstructed pancreatic ductules. Infants with immunoreactive trypsinogen levels above the 99th percentile typically undergo confirmatory sweat testing and, in some cases, screening for the principal CF gene mutation (ΔF508).

TREATMENT

Treatment is best accomplished with a multidisciplinary team and involves treatment of the lungs, GI nutrition, and psychosocial aspects of the disease with the institution of care being delivered at specialized multidisciplinary center. While much research has been directed toward aggressively treating lung disease early in life to improve long-term pulmonary function and survival, recently the nutritional aspects of young children with cystic fibrosis have been stressed as important to outcomes. Konstan et al. demonstrated that nutritional status in children with cystic fibrosis at 3 years of age correlates with pulmonary symptoms later in life. In an observational study of 931 children with cystic fibrosis, they found that children with weight-for-age below the 5th percentile at age 3 years had lower pulmonary function at age 6 compared with those above the 75th percentile. Thus, poor growth and nutritional status, in addition to lung disease early in life, contribute to pulmonary function later in life.

The median survival rate has steadily increased from 14 years in 1969 to 32 years in 2000. Gene replacement therapy is under active investigation. Prenatal screening is being attempted and appears to have a high degree of patient satisfaction and understanding. Follow-up in a special cystic fibrosis center is important in order that multidisciplinary services be aimed at nutrition, pulmonary status, and avoidance of bacterial infections.

SUGGESTED READINGS

1. Collins F. Cystic fibrosis: molecular biology and therapeutic implications. *Science.* 1992;256:774-779.
2. Farrell PM, Fost N. Prenatal screening for cystic fibrosis: where are we now? *J Pediatr.* 2002;141:758-763.
3. Konstan MW, Butler SM, Wohl MEB, et al. Growth and nutritional indexes in early life predict pulmonary function in cystic fibrosis. *J Pediatr.* 2003;142:624-630.
4. Ratjen F, Doring G. Cystic fibrosis. *Lancet.* 2003;361: 681-689.
5. Amin R, Ratjen F. Cystic fibrosis: a review of pulmonary and nutritional therapies. *Adv Pediatr.* 2008;55:99-122.
6. McNally P. Cystic fibrosis. In: Florin TA, Ludwig S, eds. *Netter's Pediatrics.* Philadelphia: Saunders Elsevier; 2011.

CASE 6-4

Five-Day-Old Boy

KAMILLAH N. WOOD

HISTORY OF PRESENT ILLNESS

A 5-day-old Asian male was brought to his pediatrician for poor feeding. Compared to his siblings, his parents felt that he had been a poor feeder since birth. He was taking only 0.5 oz. every 2-3 hours. The mother had initially been breast feeding the baby but began to supplement with formula because of jaundice. In the clinic, the child was noted to have respiratory distress, and was felt to have a cardiac murmur. He was referred to the emergency department for further evaluation. In the review of symptoms there were no fevers or vomiting. The urine and stool patterns were normal. There was decreased activity but no diaphoresis with feeds, cyanosis, or abnormal movements. There was no rash. The infant had been in contact with a 2-year-old sibling with emesis and gastroenteritis.

MEDICAL HISTORY

There was good prenatal care and a prenatal ultrasound was normal. The infant was born by spontaneous vaginal delivery at 39 weeks gestation with a birth weight of 3100 g. The mother was positive for group B *Streptococcus* and received intrapartum penicillin. The infant received antibiotics empirically for the first 48 hours of life due to tachypnea but was discharged home with clinical improvement after cultures were negative. Family history was remarkable for leukemia in the maternal grandmother. The infant lived with her mother, father, and a 2-year-old sibling. The maternal grandfather died unexpectedly 2 days prior to admission.

PHYSICAL EXAMINATION

T 36.1°C; HR 168 bpm; RR 44/min; BP in the right arm 74/44 mmHg; left arm 85/53 mmHg; right leg 77/57 mmHg; left leg 77/53 mmHg; SpO_2 98% room air

Weight 2.9 kg

In general, the infant was awake, crying, and vigorous. The anterior fontanel was open and flat. There were no dysmorphic facial features. There were ecchymoses surrounding both eyes. The tympanic membranes were normal in appearance and mobility. There was no rhinorrhea. The mucosa was pink and moist and the oropharynx was clear. There were mild intercostals retractions but the lungs were clear to auscultation. An IV/VI systolic murmur was noted at the sternal border and radiated to the back. S1 and S2 were normal; however, an S3 gallop was also noted. The point of maximal impulse was displaced slightly to the left. The abdomen was soft and the liver edge was palpable 5 cm below the right costal margin. The spleen was not palpable. There were no palpable abdominal masses. The skin was jaundiced to the waist. Distal pulses were normal and symmetric. The neurologic examination was normal.

DIAGNOSTIC STUDIES

The chest radiograph revealed cardiomegaly and increased interstitial edema but no discrete infiltrates. The complete blood count demonstrated the following: 15500 white blood cells/mm³ (73% segmented neutrophils, 3% eosinophils, 13% lymphocytes, and 11% monocytes); hemoglobin, 21.5 g/dL; and 140000 platelets/mm³. Serum electrolytes were as follows: sodium, 140 mEq/L; potassium, 3.9 mEq/L; chloride, 105 mEq/L; and bicarbonate, 15 mEq/L. Tests of liver function were also abnormal: albumin, 3.0 mg/dL; total bilirubin, 17.5 mg/dL; alanine aminotransferase (ALT), 54 IU/L; aspartate aminotransferase, 163 IU/L; and gamma-glutamyl transferase (GGT), 700. The partial thromboplastin time was 28 seconds.

ECG showed diffuse T wave abnormalities but normal voltage. Echocardiography showed a diffusely dilated heart with a particularly large left ventricle. The shortening fraction was 22%. The heart was otherwise structurally normal. Lumbar puncture revealed the following: 17 white blood cells and 39 red blood cells per cubic millimeter. The protein and glucose were normal. No bacteria were seen on Gram stain of the cerebrospinal fluid (CSF). A herpes simplex virus polymerase chain reaction study from the CSF was negative.

COURSE OF ILLNESS

On admission, he was felt to have congestive heart failure and was treated with digoxin and furosemide. Initially, cardiomyopathy and myocarditis were considered most likely. Viral infections (coxsackie, enteroviruses, TORCH infections), bacterial infections, and metabolic storage diseases were all considered.

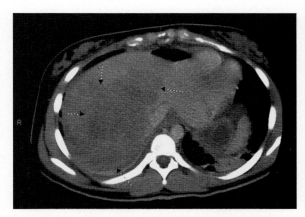

FIGURE 6-3. Abdominal CT revealing an enlarged liver with an ill-defined, lobulated, hypodense mass measuring approximately 13 cm × 9 cm × 7 cm.

The infant was initially treated with ampicillin, cefotaxime, and acyclovir until those studies returned negative. A head ultrasound was normal; specifically, no cerebral arteriovenous malformation was visualized. He continued to have mild elevation in his liver function tests. A CT of the abdomen suggested the diagnosis (Figure 6-3).

DISCUSSION CASE 6-4

DIFFERENTIAL DIAGNOSIS

The child presented with heart failure as the cause of his growth failure. The cause of heart failure may be cardiac or noncardiac (Table 6-8). The differential diagnosis of a liver mass in a child is also broad (Table 6-9). Although liver masses are uncommon solid tumors in children, it is important to understand the various types of masses that can present in children based on age and presentation. The most common liver neoplasm is from metastatic disease as it is in adults, with most primary liver masses being malignant. However, up to one-third of these masses are benign with the infantile hemangioendothelioma being the most common type.

DIAGNOSIS

Computed tomography of the abdomen revealed an enlarged liver with an ill-defined, lobulated,

TABLE 6-8.	Heart failure in the newborn.

A. Structural Heart Defects
1. At birth—Hypoplastic Left Heart Syndrome (HLHS)
   - severe tricuspid regurgitation
   - large systemic arteriovenous fistula
2. First week—Transposition of Great Arteries (TGA)
   - premature infant with large patent ductus arterious
   - total anomalous pulmonary venous return
3. 1-4 weeks
   - critical aortic stenosis or pulmonic stenosis
   - coarctation of the arteries

B. Noncardiac Causes
1. Birth asphyxia resulting in transient myocardial ischemia
2. Metabolic (acidosis, hypoglycemia, hypocalcemia)
3. Severe anemia (hydrops)
4. Overtransfusion or overhydration
5. Neonatal sepsis
6. Endocardial fibroelastosis (rare primary myocardial disease) causes congestive heart failure in infancy. Ninety percent of cases occur in the first 8 months of life.

hypodense mass (Figure 6-3). The hepatic artery was slightly dilated, which may have been the cause of the significant shunting into the lesion. Magnetic resonance imaging (MRI) of the liver was then performed for better detail of the liver process. On MRI, the patient was felt to have a mass lesion rather than an AVM. The patient underwent open biopsy of the liver mass which revealed a hemangioendothelioma. **The findings**

TABLE 6-9.	Differential diagnosis of a liver mass in a child.

Malignant Masses
Metastatic disease
Hepatoblastoma carcinoma
Hepatocellular carcinoma
Embyronal sarcoma
Angiosarcoma
Rhaboid tumor

Benign Masses
Hemangioendothelioma
Mesenchymal hamartoma
Focal nodular hyperplasia
Nodular regenerative hyperplasia
Hepatocellular adenoma

in this case were due to a large hemangioendothelioma or cavernous hemangioma. These lesions can cause congestive heart failure of the high output type.

INCIDENCE AND EPIDEMIOLOGY OF HEMANGIOENDOTHELIOMA

Liver tumors are rare in children and approximately 30% are benign (nonmalignant) (Table 6-10). Benign liver tumors may be classified into five groups: (1) tumor-like epithelial lesions (e.g., focal nodular hyperplasia); (2) epithelial tumors; (3) cysts and mesenchymal lesions (e.g., cystic mesenchymal hamartomas); (4) benign teratomas; and (5) mesenchymal tumors (e.g., hemangiomas, hemangioendotheliomas). Of these benign lesions, hemangioendothelioma is the most common. Hemangioendotheliomas are soft tissue tumors that demonstrate endothelial proliferation. Similar to cutaneous hemangiomas, these hepatic tumors increase in size during the first year of life and then undergo involution over a period of several months to years.

CLINICAL PRESENTATION

Most (90%) children present in the first 6 months of life, and are rarely discovered after 1 year of age. There is a slight female predominance, but no racial predilection. Before tumor involution, findings may include a palpable liver mass, jaundice, weight loss, anorexia, and fever. Life-threatening complications include rupture with hemorrhage, anemia, obstructive jaundice, or, as in this case, congestive heart failure. Many children have associated cutaneous hemangiomas, particularly if there are multiple hepatic lesions. Similar lesions may be found in the trachea, lungs, gastrointestinal tract, spleen, and pancreas. Although these lesions are benign, several serious complications can occur including high-output congestive heart failure due to large arteriovenous shunts. In addition, Kasabach-Merritt syndrome may be seen due to intratumoral platelet sequestration. Hypothyroidism may also be present secondary to high levels of type 3 iodothyronine deiodinase activity produced by the tumor.

TABLE 6-10.	Classification of liver tumors.		
Diagnosis	Age	Distribution of Lesions	AFP Level
Benign			
Hemangioendothelioma	<6 months	Single or multiple	Normal
Mesenchymal hamartoma	<2 years	Single	Normal
Inflammatory	Any	Single or multiple	Normal
UVC-related	Infant	Single	Normal
Malignant			
Hepatoblastoma	<3 years	Single	Elevated
Hepatocellular carcinoma	>3 years	Single or multiple	Elevated
Undifferentiated sarcoma	6-10 years	Single	Normal
Metastatic	Any	Single or multiple	Normal

DIAGNOSTIC APPROACH

Diagnostic approach is first based on ultrasound examination followed by CT or MRI with contrast. Measurement of alpha-fetoproteins (AFP) and liver enzymes will be helpful, and laboratory tests also frequently show anemia. A young child with multiple lesions and normal AFP most likely has hemangioendothelioma. An older child with elevated AFP most likely has hepatocellular carcinoma.

Complete blood count. Anemia is noted in 50% of patients. Thrombocytopenia, when present, may range from mild to severe.

Liver function tests. AST is frequently elevated. High bilirubin levels are usually due to obstructive jaundice.

Abdominal ultrasound. Hemangioendotheliomas are usually hypoechoic with well-defined margins. Doppler flow studies reveal high-flow velocity. Differentiation from arteriovenous malformations may be difficult by ultrasonography.

Abdominal CT. On CT, a low-attenuation mass with calcification is seen in approximately 40% of cases. Multifocal lesions are less likely to demonstrate calcification. These lesions usually have peripheral enhancement with central hypoattenuation due to central infarction or hemorrhage in larger lesions.

Abdominal MRI. On MRI, large lesions are heterogeneous with occasional high signal on T1-weighted imaging suggesting central hemorrhage.

Other studies. Biopsy is often required to distinguish these tumors from other hepatic masses.

TREATMENT

A hemangioendothelioma may be resected if singular and uncomplicated by thrombocytopenia. Nonoperative treatment with prednisone and/or interferon α is the treatment of choice. Cyclophosphamide has also been used for therapy, as has radiotherapy. Liver transplantation may be needed.

SUGGESTED READINGS

1. Reis-Filho JS, Paiva ME, Lopes JM. Congenital composite hemangioendothelioma: case report and reappraisal of the hemangioendothelioma spectrum. *J Cutaneous Pathol.* 2002;29:226-231.
2. Lu CC, Ko SF, Liang CD, et al. Infantile hepatic hemangioendothelioma presenting as early heart failure: report of two cases. *Chang Gun Med J.* 2002;25:405-410.
3. Zenge JP, Fenton L, Lovell MA, et al. Case report: infantile hemangioendothelioma. *Curr Opin Pediatr.* 2002; 14:99-102.
4. Ayling RM, Davenport M, Hadzic N, et al. Hepatic hemangioendothelioma associated with production of humoral thyrotropin-like factor. *J Pediatr.* 2001;138: 932-935.
5. Davenport M, Hansen L, Heaton ND, et al. Hemangioendothelioma of the liver in infants. *J Pediatr Surg.* 1995;30:44-48.
6. d'Annibale, Piovanello P, Carlini P, et al. Epithelioid hemangioendothelioma of the liver: case report and review of the literature. *Transplantation Proc.* 2002;34: 1248-1251.
7. Chung E, Cube R, Lewis R, Conran R. Pediatric live masses: radiologic-pathologic correlation, Part 1. Benign tumors. *Radiographics.* 2010;30:801-826.
8. Litten J, Tomilson G. Liver tumors in children. *The Oncologist.* 2008;13(7):812-820.

CASE 6-5

Three-Month-Old Girl

STEPHEN LUDWIG

BRANDON C. KU

HISTORY OF PRESENT ILLNESS

A 3-month-old female was referred by her pediatrician to the emergency department for failure to thrive (FTT). She has had problems gaining weight since 1-2 months of age and has been followed weekly for weight checks with poor weight gain. She was initially breast fed but had poor latching-on and was changed to Enfamil® with and then without Fe, Lactofree®, Prosobee®, and now is on Similac® with Fe. The family has tried thickening feeds with cereal and bananas with no improvement. She takes 4 ounces per feeding and is burped every 2 ounces. Intake is 28 ounces per day. She spits and vomits, sometimes forcefully, 1-2 oz per feed. The emesis was nonbloody, nonbilious, and occasionally projectile. The emesis has become worse over the last month. There has been no diarrhea. For the last 3 days, she has been less active than usual with glassy-appearing eyes. Urine output has decreased (only two wet diapers today compared to her usual 7-10 per day).

MEDICAL HISTORY

The infant was born to a 16-year-old mother. The mother had prenatal care since the second month of pregnancy. The child was born at term with a weight of 3440 g. There were no postnatal complications and she was discharged at 39 hours of age. Development had been normal. She rolled from front to back at 6 weeks of life. She received no medications. Her immunizations were current. The family history was unremarkable.

PHYSICAL EXAMINATION

T 37°C; HR 129 bpm; RR 18/min; BP 68/41 mmHg; Weight 3.89 kg (50th percentile for a 1-month-old child)

On examination, the child was crying but consolable. She had markedly decreased subcutaneous fat. The anterior fontanel was sunken. The pupils were reactive to light. There was no nasal discharge.

The heart and lungs were normal to auscultation. The abdomen was scaphoid with visible peristaltic waves. The spleen tip was palpable below the left costal margin. The extremities were slightly cool with 2-3 second capillary refill. The neurologic examination was normal.

DIAGNOSTIC STUDIES

White blood cells 8.800/mm^3 (1% band forms, 59% segmented neutrophils, and 30% lymphocytes, and 10% monocytes).

Hemoglobin, 12.9 mg/dL; platelets 195 000/mm^3; sodium, 129 mEq/L; potassium, 4.8 mEq/L; chloride, 65 mEq/L; bicarbonate, 53 mEq/L; blood urea nitrogen, 48 mg/dL; creatinine, 1.4 mg/dL; serum transaminases were normal; other studies included a cholesterol 206 and triglycerides 313.

COURSE OF ILLNESS

In the emergency department the patient received approximately 40 mL/kg of normal saline. She was admitted to the intensive care unit due to rapid but periodic breathing. An abdominal radiograph (Figure 6-4) revealed a markedly distended stomach with a paucity of bowel gas pattern beyond the stomach. Abdominal ultrasound (Figure 6-5) revealed the diagnosis.

DISCUSSION CASE 6-5

DIFFERENTIAL DIAGNOSIS

The differential diagnosis in this case included some form of upper bowel obstruction. There was a marked hypochloremic alkalosis to support this kind of loss along with the associated history. Severe gastroesophageal reflux, gastric outlet obstruction, pyloric stenosis, or some kind of duodenal anomaly

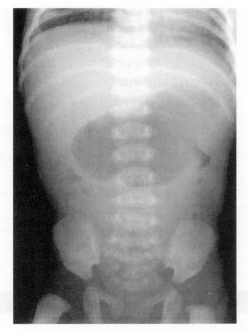

FIGURE 6-4. Abdominal radiograph.

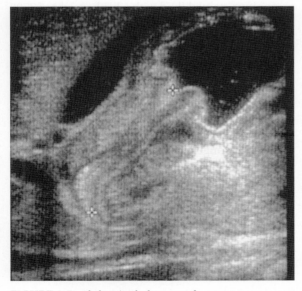

FIGURE 6-5. Abdominal ultrasound.

(e.g., duplication) was possible. The upper gastrointestinal radiograph delineated the lesion of pyloric stenosis. The electrolyte disturbance is characteristic of an upper bowel atresia with loss of sodium, chloride, and hydrogen ion.

DIAGNOSIS—PYLORIC STENOSIS

The abdominal ultrasound showed a thickened and elongated pylorus, with a maximal muscle length measuring 19 mm (Figure 6-5). The maximal muscle thickness was 5 mm. The gastric antrum was also imaged and there was evidence of significant fluid and debris from prior oral feeding. These findings were consistent with the diagnosis of pyloric stenosis. Once the patient's metabolic derangement was corrected, she was taken to the operating room for a pyloromyotomy. The postoperative course was uneventful. This case was unusual in terms of the late onset of pyloric stenosis. Most cases are identified in the first 3-6 weeks of life.

INCIDENCE AND EPIDEMIOLOGY OF PYLORIC STENOSIS

Pyloric stenosis occurs in males 1:200 and in females 1:1000. The mode of inheritance is polygenic and modified by sex. The findings are associated with smaller family size and higher socioeconomic status. It is more common in African-Americans and Asians.

CLINICAL PRESENTATION

The clinical presentation is based on vomiting (often projectile in nature), failure to gain weight, and constipation. There are no other associated symptoms. On examination, the hypertrophied pyloric muscle ("olive") is occasionally palpated in the right upper quadrant. This examination is best performed after the stomach has been emptied by means of a nasogastric tube. However, diagnosis rarely relies on clinical examination alone.

DIAGNOSTIC APPROACH

The palpation of the pyloric olive is often difficult and examiner dependent.

Serum electrolytes. Electrolytes reveal a hypochloremic metabolic alkalosis.

Abdominal ultrasound. Ultrasound typically reveals thickening of the pyloric muscle wall. When a broader differential diagnosis is being considered an upper gastrointestinal barium study should be considered. With the widespread availability of abdominal ultrasound, metabolic derangements at presentation are less common than in the past.

TREATMENT

The treatment is a simple pyloromyotomy, which opens the pyloric channel and allows the passage of food into the small bowel. This is a surgery that may be performed with laparoscopic technique. The symptoms resolve within a few days postoperatively.

There are no long-term complications and patients may be discharged postoperatively when they are able to tolerate feeding.

SUGGESTED READINGS

1. Garcia VF, Randolph JG. Pyloric stenosis: diagnosis and management. *Pediatr Rev.* 1990;11:292-296.
2. Letton RW Jr. Pyloric stenosis. *Pediatr Ann.* 2001;30:745-750.
3. Glatsein M, Carbell G, Boddu SK, et al. The changing clinical presentation of hypertrophic pyloric stenosis. *Clin Pediatr.* 2011;50:192-195.
4. Kumar R, Abel R. Infantile hypertrophic pyloric stenosis. *Surgery.* 2008;26:304-306.
5. Sola JE, Neville HL. Laparoscopic versus open pyloromyotomy: a systemic review and meta-analysis. *J Pediatr Surg.* 2009;44:1631-1637.

CASE 6-6

Twenty-One-Month-Old Boy

STEPHEN LUDWIG

BRANDON C. KU

HISTORY OF PRESENT ILLNESS

A 21-month-old boy presented with weight loss and crankiness. He was well until 5 months prior to admission when he developed otitis media. This was treated with amoxicillin. The otitis media seemed to recur 1 month later and he was treated with amoxicillin-clavulanate followed by cefuroxime. At the same time he began to develop 2-4 large, mushy, foul-smelling, pale, greasy bowel movements per day. He also seemed to have become a finicky eater with a very variable appetite. The patient also has developed intermittent vomiting and has now lost approximately three pounds and has not had linear growth in the past 3 months. Vomiting is often in the late day or evening, is nonbloody and nonbilious.

MEDICAL HISTORY

This was a former full-term infant born to a G1P1 mother. The pregnancy was complicated by preterm labor at 32 weeks gestation. He was born through meconium-stained fluid with a birth weight of 3700 g. He had been developing normally but recently was asking to be carried and not willing to walk for long periods of time. He tires easily but will not sleep. His only medication is a multivitamin. The mother is 29 years old and works as a nurse at a nearby university. The 30-year-old father works as a materials manager at a pharmaceutical company. The family history was remarkable for a maternal grandmother with ovarian cancer and a maternal grandfather with congestive heart failure and stroke. The family had been to Puerto Rico 5 months prior. The diet history revealed that the patient was initially breast fed, changed to Gerber formula with iron at 4.5 months; cereals were introduced at 6 months of age, followed by vegetables, fruits, and meats; he began to refuse meat at 1 year of age.

PHYSICAL EXAMINATION

Weight 8.77 kg (<5th percentile; 50th percentile for a 7-month-old); Height 80.5 cm (5th percentile; 50th percentile for a 13-month-old).

In general, the child was pale, wasted, and irritable. There were no oral or nasal ulcers. The neck was supple. There were many small cervical lymph nodes. The lungs were clear to auscultation. The abdomen was distended. There was no hepatosplenomegaly. There was a prominent vascular pattern on the abdomen as well as granular subcutaneous palpable patter. The genitourinary examination was normal. The remainder of the examination was normal.

DIAGNOSTIC STUDIES

White blood cells 9.300/mm³ (7% band forms, 28% segmented neutrophils, 52% lymphocytes, 4% atypical lymphocytes, and 9% monocytes).

Hemoglobin, 12.7 g/dL; platelets, 417000/mm³. The mean corpuscular volume was 83 fL; reticulocyte count was 1.3%; ESR, 2 mm/h; prothrombin time, 14.2 seconds; partial thromboplastin time, 31.5 seconds; creatinine, 0.5 mg/dL; albumin, 3.8 mg/dL; cholesterol, 142; triglycerides, 172; ALT, 134 IU/L; AST, 98 IU/L; LDH, 600; sweat test was normal.

COURSE OF ILLNESS

In the hospital, upper endoscopy revealed flat villous atrophy of duodenum and acute inflammation of lamina propria. What is the most likely diagnosis?

DISCUSSION CASE 6-6

DIFFERENTIAL DIAGNOSIS

The differential diagnosis of weight loss is very extensive and potentially involves almost every organ system. For this child, who had grown and developed somewhat normally, one would not expect a psychosocial cause unless there had been some recent change in the child's family constitution or living environment. The loss of weight and linear growth over a short period of time suggest an organic cause. The findings of pallor and abdominal distention would also suggest narrowing of the differential diagnosis to a disease-based cause.

DIAGNOSIS

The diagnosis is celiac disease. This is a genetically predisposing disease that manifests in children who eat gluten products or related peptides from other grains. Once exposed to gluten, there is an immunologically triggered reaction to the absorptive surface of the small bowel.

INCIDENCE AND EPIDEMIOLOGY OF CELIAC DISEASE

With newer diagnostic tests available the incidence of the disorder has increased. In people of European background, it has been identified in 1:250 of the general population. It has been identified all around the world.

CLINICAL PRESENTATION

The clinical presentations of celiac disease are many. The classic presentation is that of the case presented—weight loss and growth failure in the second year of life. Table 6-11 identifies other

TABLE 6-11.	**Clinical manifestations of celiac disease.**

"Classical" Gastrointestinal Form
  Age of onset under 2 years; diarrhea, failure to thrive, abdominal distension, proximal muscle wasting, irritability

Non-"classical" Gastrointestinal Form
  Age of onset childhood to adulthood; diarrhea, intermittent or mild, abdominal pain, bloating, nausea, vomiting, change in appetite, constipation

Nongastrointestinal Manifestations
  Musculoskeletal system: Short stature, rickets, osteoporosis, dental enamel defects, arthritis/arthralgia, myopathy
  Skin and mucous membranes: Dermatitis herpetiformis, atopic dermatitis, aphthous stomatitis
  Reproductive system: Delayed puberty, infertility, recurrent abortions, menstrual irregularities
  Hematologic system: Anemia (iron, folate, B_{12}), leukopenia, vitamin K deficiency, thrombocytopenia
  Central nervous system: Behavioral changes, epilepsy, dementia, cerebellar degeneration

Associated Conditions
  Autoimmune disorders: Type I diabetes mellitus, autoimmune thyroid disease, Sjögren syndrome, collagen vascular disease, liver disease (PBC), IgA glomerulonephritis
  Miscellaneous associations: Selective IgA deficiency, Down syndrome, hyposplenism, colitis

Asymptomatic Form
  Patients identified through screening studies

manifestations of the disease. Malabsorption prior to institution of a gluten-free diet may lead to nutritional deficiencies, including deficiency of iron, folic acid, and zinc.

DIAGNOSTIC APPROACH

The diagnosis has been made by biopsy of the small intestine. Biopsy is the time-proven method and should be made if there is a clinical suspicion despite enzyme test. The biopsy shows flat mucosa with villous atrophy and an increased number of lymphocytes.

Serologic testing. The serologic testing for the disease has improved to the point where serologic screening tests can be used to identify patients in whom intestinal biopsy is warranted. Antigliaden antibodies of both IgG and IgA are measured. Also measurable are antismooth muscle antibodies including antiendomysium and antireticular (IgA). The most recently used test shows IgA type antibody to tissue transglutaminase (tTG). The sensitivity of tTG antibodies is approximately 90% and the specificity is approximately 95% compared with intestinal biopsy. These values mean that most children with celiac disease will demonstrate antibodies to tTG and that false-positive results are relatively uncommon.

TREATMENT

The therapy involves a lifelong removal of gluten from the diet. This is a difficult challenge for children and their parents but is successful.

SUGGESTED READINGS

1. Farrell RJ, Kelly CP. Current concepts: celiac sprue. *N Engl J Med.* 2002;346:180-188.
2. Kolsteren MMP, Koopman HM, Schalekamp GMA, et al. Health-related quality of life in children with celiac disease. *J Pediatr.* 2001;138:593-595.
3. Scoglio R, Sorleti D, Magazzù G, et al. Celiac disease case finding in children in primary care. *J Pediatr.* 2002; 140:379-380.
4. Moore JK, West SRA, Robins G. Advances in celiac disease. *Curr Opin in Gastro.* 2011;27:112-118.
5. Setty M, Hormaza L, Guandalini S. Celiac disease: risk assessment, diagnosis and monitoring. *Mol Diagn Ther.* 2008;12:289-298.
6. Tursi A, Brandimarte G, Giorgetti GM. Prevalence of anti-tissue transglutaminase antibodies in different degrees of intestinal damage in celiac disease. *J Clin Gastroentrol.* 2003;36:219-221.

CASE 6-7

Eighteen-Month-Old Boy

STEPHEN LUDWIG

BRANDON C. KU

HISTORY OF PRESENT ILLNESS

This 18-month-old boy was brought to the emergency department for a chief complaint of draining ear. Once in the emergency department it was noted that he was markedly wasted. Vital signs included a body temperature below normal. Height, weight, and head circumference were below the 3rd percentile. Heart rate was 40 bpm with a respiratory rate of 26 per minute.

The examination of the ears showed bilateral draining otitis media. There was loss of hair that was brittle. There were multiple scabs on the body. The examination was very notable for loss of almost all-subcutaneous tissue (Figure 6-6). There was no reported weigh loss or diarrhea. The mother reported no other symptoms.

MEDICAL HISTORY

The child had been born in a healthy condition. The mother was married and living in a suburban community. The child had grown normally for several months but then the mother noted multiple food allergies and placed him on a restrictive diet. She had

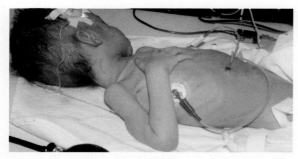

FIGURE 6-6. Picture of the patient with marked failure to thrive.

not sought regular care for the child but frequently sought advice from telephone hotlines and calls to multiple physicians' offices. The child had lost developmental milestones. The mother and father were both college graduates. There was no smoking or drinking in the house. Both parents admitted to using marijuana on a regular basis.

PHYSICAL EXAMINATION

T 35.9°C; HR 40 bpm; RR 16/min; Weight far below the 5th percentile; Height far below 5th percentile; Head circumference at 10th percentile

In general, the child was a weak-appearing and cachectic male with decreased movement and a weak cry. His hair was stubbled. He had a purulent draining otitis media. There was no adenopathy. The chest was clear. The heart rate was bradycardic with weak pulses. The abdomen was scaphoid with decreased bowel sounds. On the skin, there were multiple marks and scars and hyperpigmented macules in diaper area and diffusely. On neurologic examination, the child was dull, apathetic, and weak. He had decreased muscle mass and muscle tone.

DIAGNOSTIC STUDIES

Hemoglobin, 9.6 mg/dL; serum protein was below normal.

COURSE OF ILLNESS

The hospital course involved treating the ear infection and starting the child on nutritional support and iron. He responded with weight gain and improvement of his development. At the end of 2 weeks in the hospital, he had made tremendous strides in both growth and development. He ate large quantities of food.

DISCUSSION CASE 6-7

DIFFERENTIAL DIAGNOSIS

The severity of the child's condition prompted the consideration of a wide differential diagnosis. The parent's economic status and educational level prompted the medical care team to eliminate psychosocial causes. Yet, when confronted with the child's response to supportive care and feeding and normal laboratory pattern that he demonstrated, a nonorganic etiology for his life-threatening condition was revealed.

DIAGNOSIS

The final diagnosis was weight loss and developmental repression due to psychosocial causes. The diet that the mother selected for the child was too restrictive in content and calories. Her presenting complaint missed the obvious wasting and was a clue to her lack of perception and parenting ability. Parents underwent psychiatric testing and were felt to be unsuitable caretakers. The child recovered completely and was discharged to a foster home (Figure 6-7).

INCIDENCE AND EPIDEMIOLOGY OF PSYCHOSOCIAL CAUSES

The true incidence of psychosocial failure to thrive is not known. Many case series of children with failure to thrive (FTT) show that 40%-80% is due to psychosocial causes or a combination of psychosocial and medical causes (so-called mixed FTT). The epidemiology is varied and can result from postpartum depression, a lack of knowledge about parenting, or more overt child abuse and willful starvation. It is difficult to sort through the motivation of the parents, yet the results in the child are obvious and disturbing.

CLINICAL PRESENTATION

Clinical presentations are varied from children who have minor falling off on their growth parameters

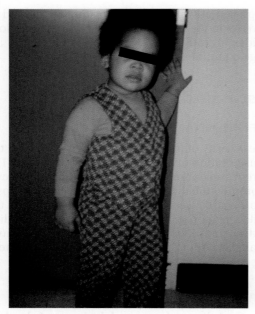

FIGURE 6-7. Picture of the child 16 months later.

to cases of death by starvation. Serial measures of length or height, weight, and head circumference are helpful in sorting through the causes and in differentiating psychosocial and medical etiology.

DIAGNOSTIC APPROACH

Diagnostic approach is best assessed by the signs and symptoms the child manifests. Without special symptoms, it is best to feed the child in a controlled setting and monitor the weight gain. There is no single battery of laboratory tests to be recommended. Some that may be helpful include CBC (iron-deficient anemia), urinalysis (UTI, RTA), and PPD for tuberculosis. HIV infection may also be a cause for failure to thrive. Skeletal survey for trauma may be indicated if there is suspicion of abuse.

TREATMENT

The treatment for nonorganic failure to thrive requires close follow-up and a multidisciplinary approach to meeting the needs of the child and the family. In some cases, the child will need to be removed from the care of the parents until a system of care and follow-up can be proposed. In this case, a foster home was used initially and then the child returned under close (weekly) supervision. Subsequently, a physical abuse episode caused long-term removal of the child. Usually nutritional recovery time will equal the length of time that the organic deprivation occurred.

SUGGESTED READINGS

1. Ludwig S. Failure-to-thrive and starvation. In: Ludwig S, Kornberg A, eds. *Child Abuse and Neglect: A Medical Reference.* 2nd ed. New York: Churchill-Livingstone; 1992.
2. Altemeier WA, O'Connor SM, Sherrod KB, et al. Prospective study of antecedents for nonorganic failure-to-thrive. *J Pediatr.* 1985;106:360.
3. Frank DA, Drotar D, Cook J, et al. Failure to thrive. In: Reece R, Ludwig S, eds. *Child Abuse: Medical Diagnosis and Management.* 2nd ed. Philadelphia: Lippincott Williams & Wilkins; 2001.

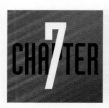

CHAPTER 7

ABDOMINAL PAIN

MARINA CATALLOZZI

DEFINITION OF THE COMPLAINT

Abdominal pain is a common complaint in pediatrics and has an extensive list of possible causes, not all gastrointestinal in etiology. Additionally, the etiology may be acute and life-threatening or more chronic in nature. The patient's clinical presentation, history, and physical examination along with directed testing usually elucidate the etiology and help clarify the treatment course.

Abdominal pain is usually stimulated by one of three pathways: visceral, somatic, or referred. Visceral pain is caused by a distended viscus (i.e., one of the organs of the body) that activates a local nerve and sends an impulse that travels through autonomic afferent fibers to the spinal tract and central nervous system. Precise localization of visceral pain is often difficult and frustrating because there are very few afferent nerves that travel from the viscera and the nerve fibers frequently overlap. Visceral pain is generally felt in the epigastric region, the periumbilical region, or the suprapubic area. Somatic pain, because it is carried by somatic nerves in the parietal peritoneum, muscle, or skin, is usually well localized and sharp. Referred pain, defined as abdominal pain perceived at a site remote from the actual affected viscera, can either be sharp and localized or diffuse. There is a great deal of individual variability in the experience of pain so that neuroanatomic, neurophysiologic, pathophysiologic, environmental, and psychosocial factors all play a part in the expression of pain. The frequency of the chief complaint of abdominal pain necessitates categorizing the presentation of abdominal pain into the following: acute abdominal pain and chronic abdominal pain.

In the case of acute abdominal pain, a patient or parent is usually able to pinpoint the onset of the pain to an event or time of day. If the pain is mild initially, it often becomes progressively worse and eventually interferes with sleep and normal activities. Other than intussusception (when one part of the intestine slips into itself), acute abdominal pain that requires surgical intervention does not recur and is not relieved without some intervention. Nausea, vomiting, diarrhea, fever, and anorexia often accompany acute abdominal pain. Patients most often appear acutely ill and position themselves to protect the abdomen from further examination. Chronic abdominal pain is defined as pain that lasts 2 or more weeks. Chronic abdominal pain does not usually require surgical intervention. Although formal definitions and guidelines exist, the definition basically includes any child who has abdominal pain with multiple episodes (minimum of three) over a long period (at least 3 months) without a known cause, for which the family seeks medical attention, and which interferes with the child's ability to function. In the past, the term recurrent abdominal pain was used as well, but in 2005 the American Academy of Pediatrics Subcommittee on Chronic Abdominal Pain suggested that the term be replaced with functional abdominal pain as it is thought to be the most common cause of chronic abdominal pain. Functional abdominal pain has no pathologic root. Because of the frustration for the family and child, as well as the extensive differential diagnosis for this problem, a consistent approach is vital. The approach must include a thorough history, arguably the most important component, physical examination, laboratory testing, imaging studies, and empiric interventions.

COMPLAINT BY CAUSE AND FREQUENCY

It is vital to remember that abdominal pain, although a frequent complaint, is not in itself a diagnosis, and a thorough evaluation of this symptom is required to determine the cause. The causes of abdominal pain in childhood vary by age (Table 7-1), can be based on whether the abdominal pain is acute or chronic in nature (Table 7-1), and can also be grouped by etiology (Table 7-2).

CLARIFYING QUESTIONS

Accurate diagnosis in a child with abdominal pain requires a thorough history and physical examination. There must be consideration of the type and location of pain to create a working differential to approach the individual patient with abdominal pain. The following questions may be helpful in arriving at a diagnosis:

- When did the pain begin and how long has it lasted?
  — The determination of acute or chronic pain is vital in considering the possible etiologies of the pain, identifying a patient who requires surgical intervention (i.e., intestinal obstruction, acute appendicitis, malrotation and midgut volvulus, Meckel diverticulum, incarcerated inguinal hernia, hypertrophic pyloric stenosis, trauma, Hirschsprung disease), and finally determining any other life-threatening causes of abdominal pain that do not require surgical intervention (i.e., intussusception, severe gastroenteritis, toxic overdose, sepsis, hemolytic uremic syndrome, diabetic ketoacidosis, myocarditis, peptic ulcer disease with perforation, fulminant hepatitis, ectopic pregnancy, pelvic inflammatory disease with tuboovarian abscess). Although gastroenteritis is the most common cause of acute pain and constipation considered the most common cause of chronic pain, other etiologies must be ruled out.
  While an infant will frequently display pain as a behavior change (i.e., poor oral intake, irritability, inconsolable crying), older children can verbalize

the character of the pain. For diagnoses such as irritable bowel syndrome, where the chronicity of the pain is an important feature of the diagnosis, the duration of pain is also vital. Additionally, with chronic pain, the timing of the pain is key. For example, pain that awakens a child from sleep suggests peptic disease whereas pain that occurs during dinner is often associated with constipation. Additionally, paroxysms of pain, where the child has 20-minute intervals of being well in between inconsolability, is classically seen with intussusception.

- What is the location of the pain?
  — Even when abdominal pain seems localized, a thorough examination must be performed to rule out other nongastrointestinal causes of the pain. Certain locations may herald specific disease processes. Perhaps, the most important of these is the association of appendicitis with acute pain in the right lower quadrant (even more specifically, tenderness over McBurney point). While appendicitis is the most common cause for emergency surgery (apart from trauma) in children, delayed diagnosis often occurs in children because a progressing disease process often results in the absence of the classic clinical findings. Acute appendicitis often does not have pain as the first symptom, but other surgical emergencies that are potentially life-threatening and catastrophic do (e.g., malrotation with volvulus, intussusception, ovarian torsion). The classic pattern associated with acute appendicitis of periumbilical visceral pain that travels to the right lower quadrant with subsequent nausea, vomiting, and anorexia is far less common in children younger than 12 than it is in adults. For infants, vomiting, pain, diarrhea, fever, irritability, grunting, and refusal to walk or limp are just a few of the nonlocalizing symptoms that lead to misdiagnosis and high rates of intestinal perforation. While the rates are low in children ages 2-5 years of age (<5%), the more classic signs and symptoms of right lower quadrant pain, vomiting, and fever are more common. As the incidence of appendicitis increases in school-aged children and adolescents, when the incidence peaks, so do the more common symptoms of vomiting, anorexia, and right lower quadrant pain.
  Right lower quadrant pain can also be associated with Crohn disease, mesenteric adenitis

TABLE 7-1.	Causes of abdominal pain by age.

Acute Abdominal Pain

Neonate/Infant	Colic Congential anomalies Electrolyte disturbance Hypertrophic pyloric stenosis Incarcerated hernias Infectious gastroenteritis Intestinal obstruction Intussusception Malrotation with or without volvulus Necrotizing enterocolitis Pyelonephritis/UTI Trauma/child abuse Tumors	**Toddler/ School Age (Cont.)**	Psoas abscess Pyelonephritis/UTI Sickle cell crisis Testicular torsion Trauma/child abuse Tumors Urolithiasis
Toddler/School Age	Acute appendicitis Acute glomerulonephritis Cholecystitis Cholelithiasis Dietary indiscretion Diabetic ketoacidosis Electrolyte disturbance Foreign body ingestion Hemolytic uremic syndrome Henoch-Schöenlein purpura Hepatitis Hirschsprung associated enterocolitis (HAEC) Infectious gastroenteritis Infectious mononucleosis Intestinal obstruction Intussusception Malrotation Meckel diverticulum Mesenteric adenitis Pancreatitis Peptic ulcer disease (+/− *H. pylori*) Pneumonia Porphyria	**Adolescents**	Acute appendicitis Cholecystitis Cholelithiasis Diabetic ketoacidosis Ectopic pregnancy Electrolyte disturbance Epididymitis Hepatitis Herpes zoster Infectious gastroenteritis Infectious mononucleosis Intestinal obstruction Meckel diverticulum Mesenteric adenitis Myocarditis Ovarian cyst Ovarian torsion Pancreatitis Pelvic inflammatory disease Pneumonia Porphyria Primary bacterial peritonitis Psoas abscess Pyelonephritis/UTI Sickle cell crisis Testicular torsion Trauma/child abuse Tumors Urolithiasis

Chronic Abdominal Pain

Neonate/Infant	Colic
	Disaccharidase deficiency/
	  malabsorptive syndromes
	Milk-protein allergy/eosinophilic
	  gastroenteritis
		Adolescents	Abdominal migraine
			Addison disease
			Aerophagia
			Carbohydrate malabsorption
			Collagen vascular disease
			Constipation
			Cystic fibrosis/meconium ileus
			  equivalent
			Dysmenorrhea
			Endometriosis
			Functional abdominal pain
			Gastritis
			Gastroesophageal reflux disease
			Heavy metal poisoning
			Hematocolpos
			Hiatal hernia
			Inflammatory bowel disease
			Irritable bowel syndrome
			Mittelschmerz
			Parasitic infection
			Peptic ulcer disease
			Recurrent pancreatitis
			Superior mesenteric artery
			  syndrome
			Wilson disease

Toddler/School Age	Abdominal migraine Addison disease Aerophagia Carbohydrate malabsorption Collagen vascular disease Constipation Cystic fibrosis/meconium ileus equivalent Functional abdominal pain Gastritis Gastroesophageal reflux disease Heavy metal poisoning Hiatal hernia Inflammatory bowel disease Irritable bowel syndrome Parasitic infection Peptic ulcer disease Recurrent pancreatitis Superior mesenteric artery syndrome Wilson disease		

TABLE 7-2.	Causes of abdominal pain in childhood by etiology.	

Infectious
Cat-scratch disease
Epididymitis
Gastroenteritis (viral or bacterial)
H. pylori gastritis
Hepatitis
Herpes zoster
Infectious mononucleosis
Mesenteric adenitis (frequently caused by group A
 streptococcus)
Necrotizing enterocolitis
Parasitic infections (i.e., giardia)
Pelvic inflammatory disease/Fitz-Hugh Curtis
 syndrome/tuboovarian abscess
Pneumonia
Psoas abscess
Subdiaphragmatic abscess
Tuberculosis of the spine
UTI

Toxicologic
Black widow spider bite
Heavy metals (i.e., lead)
Medications (i.e., anticholinergics, aspirin, and
 NSAIDS)

Metabolic
Addison disease
Diabetic ketoacidosis
Electrolyte disturbances (especially hypokalemia)
Hypoglycemia
Wilson disease

Tumor/Oncologic
Any benign or malignant tumor
Leukemia
Lymphoma
Spinal cord tumor
Testicular neoplasm
Wilm tumor

Traumatic
Child abuse
Duodenal hematoma
Splenic rupture

Congenital/Anatomic
Choledochal cyst
Cholelithiasis
Hematocolpos
Hiatal hernia
Incarcerated hernia

Intussusception
Intestinal obstruction (adhesions)
Malrotation with or without volvulus
Meckel diverticulum
Meconium ileus/meconium ileus equivalent
Ovarian torsion
Superior mesenteric artery syndrome
Testicular torsion
Urolithiasis/renal colic/stones

Allergic/Inflammatory
Acute rheumatic fever
Appendicitis
Cholecystitis
Diskitis
Gastritis
Glomerulonephritis
Henoch-Schöenlein purpura
Hemolytic-uremic syndrome
Inflammatory bowel disease
Milk-protein allergy/eosinophilic gastroenteritis
Pancreatitis
Peptic ulcer disease
Serositis associated with collagen vascular disease
Vasculitis

Functional and Other
Abdominal migraine
Aerophagia
Colic
Constipation
Dietary indiscretion
Disaccharidase deficiency
Dysmenorrhea
Ectopic pregnancy
Endometriosis
Familial Mediterranean fever
Functional dyspepsia
Functional abdominal pain syndrome
Gastroesophageal reflux disease
Hypertensive crisis
Irritable bowel syndrome
Malabsorptive syndromes
Mittelschmerz
Myocarditis
Nephrotic syndrome with ascites
Ovarian cyst
Pericarditis
Porphyria
Sickle cell crisis

associated with group A streptococcal pharyngitis, bacterial enterocolitis (particularly *Yersinia enterocolitica* and *Campylobacter jejuni*), Meckel diverticulitis, and intussusception. Right upper quadrant pain should prompt investigation for cholecystitis, cholelithiasis, Fitz-Hugh-Curtis syndrome, and right lower lobe pneumonia.

Left upper quadrant pain often indicates splenomegaly, hemolytic crisis, or splenic trauma. Epigastric pain may indicate peptic disease (such as peptic ulcer disease, esophagitis secondary to gastroesophageal reflux disease, gastritis), or pancreatitis. Suprapubic pain can suggest a urinary tract infection (UTI), menstrual disorders, or pelvic inflammatory disease. Some diagnoses commonly have radiation of pain and should always be investigated—back pain can be seen with pancreatitis or UTI, and gallstones frequently are associated with shoulder pain.

- Has there been a change in stool pattern, blood in the stool, or is the pain relieved with defecation? —Questions regarding stool pattern and consistency are important in both acute and chronic abdominal pain. In the acute setting, diarrhea early in the history can point toward an infectious etiology such as viral or bacterial gastroenteritis. Additionally, examination of the rectum and stool gives important diagnostic information. While bloody mucoid or currant jelly stools are seen late in the course of intussusception, hemoccult positivity can be seen earlier.

    For more chronic etiologies, such as constipation, irritable bowel syndrome, and inflammatory bowel disease, these questions can also clarify the diagnosis.

- Is there associated emesis? —While vomiting can occur with several of the etiologies of abdominal pain, vomiting in the absence of abdominal pain usually indicates upper intestinal tract disease. Bilious emesis heralds obstruction.

- Can the examination reveal the etiology of the abdominal pain? —When the diagnosis is unclear and surgical intervention remains a possibility, reassessment and reexamination by the same clinician is an important part of the evaluation. This is particularly important with diagnoses such as appendicitis where there is no definitive piece of historical examination or laboratory data that will make the diagnosis.

    Certain physical examination findings suggest the diagnosis—Cullen sign (discoloration of the umbilicus) or Grey Turner sign (discoloration of the flank) with hemorrhagic pancreatitis; Murphy sign (pain with deep palpation of the right upper quadrant) with gallbladder disease; and Rovsing sign (pain in the right lower quadrant with palpation of the contralateral side) in appendicitis.

- Is there an ingestion or toxin exposure? — Ingestion of certain medications or heavy metals (e.g., lead) can lead to chronic abdominal pain.

- Has there been a recent or preceding respiratory illness? — An upper respiratory infection frequently precedes intussusception as a mesenteric lymph node is thought to act as the lead point.

- Is there any significant family history? — This can be a key piece of history in diseases such as inflammatory bowel disease, familial Mediterranean fever, and cystic fibrosis.

- What is the child's weight and height? — Failure to thrive indicates a more chronic disease such as inflammatory bowel disease.

The following cases represent less common causes of abdominal pain in childhood.

CASE 7-1

Thirteen-Year-Old Boy

MARINA CATALLOZZI

HISTORY OF PRESENT ILLNESS

The patient was a 13-year-old male with a medical history significant for recurrent abdominal pain. The patient reported intermittent right upper quadrant pain during the last year. It occurred two to three times per week and lasted about 1 hour. It was sharp and stabbing in nature. It was not associated with eating or defecation and did not radiate.

He reported easy bruising, but denied any epistaxis, bloody or tarry stools, headache, and nausea or vomiting. He did report a 2-month history of tea-colored urine and a 5-pound weight loss.

MEDICAL HISTORY

His medical history was unremarkable. He was a full-term infant with no complications.

PHYSICAL EXAMINATION

T 37.3°C; RR 36/min; HR 80 bpm; BP 120/77 mmHg

Height 75th percentile; Weight 75th percentile

Initial examination revealed an alert and cooperative young man in no acute distress. Physical examination was remarkable for mild scleral icterus. There was good lung aeration bilaterally. On abdominal examination he had normoactive bowel sounds and tenderness to palpation in the right upper quadrant. Hepatosplenomegaly was present on abdominal examination with the liver 4 cm below the right costal margin (with a span of 10 cm) and the spleen 6 cm below the left costal margin. He was a Tanner stage IV male with normal genitalia and no evidence of trauma. The skin examination was significant for bruises on the lower extremities. His neurologic examination was normal.

DIAGNOSTIC STUDIES

Laboratory analysis revealed 3400 WBCs/mm^3 with 2% bands, 61% segmented neutrophils, 27% lymphocytes, and 3% monocytes. The hemoglobin was 12.8 g/dL and there were 51 000 platelets/mm^3. The erythrocyte sedimentation rate was slightly elevated at 12 mm/h. The hepatic function panel revealed a total bilirubin of 2.5 mg/dL; alkaline phosphatase, 450 U/L; albumin, 2.6 g/dL; and elevated transaminases with an aspartate aminotransferase, 266 U/L; alanine aminotransferase, 162 U/L; and a gamma-glutamyl transferase, 500 g/dL. Prothrombin (PT) and partial thromboplastin (PTT) times were 13 and 32 seconds, respectively. Fibrin split products, hepatitis A, B, C, and monospot testing were all negative. A urinalysis revealed small bilirubin, moderate blood (0-2 RBCs), and a urobilinogen of 2.0 mg.

COURSE OF ILLNESS

The patient was hospitalized and an emergent abdominal ultrasound was performed that showed portal venous thrombosis with evidence of portal hypertension, cirrhosis, cholelithiasis, and splenomegaly. There was no evidence of ascites. HIV ELISA was negative, ANCA was negative, and ANA was 1:80. Urine copper returned elevated at 296 µg/24 hours (normal range < 50 µg/24 hours), but the ceruloplasmin was within normal range at 53 mg/dL (range 25-63). A liver biopsy confirmed the diagnosis.

DISCUSSION CASE 7-1

DIFFERENTIAL DIAGNOSIS

The causes of liver disease, in particular hyperbilirubinemia and cirrhosis, in the pediatric population are diverse. Common causes include infectious diseases such as viral infections (hepatitis A, B, and C; cytomegalovirus; coxsackie virus; Epstein-Barr virus), bacterial infections, fungal infections, and parasitic infections. Inflammatory causes include ulcerative colitis, ascending cholangitis, and autoimmune hepatitis. Drugs and toxins are another important etiology to explore as common medications such as acetaminophen and acetylsalicylic acid and toxins like iron can cause liver damage. The differential diagnosis also includes causes of biliary obstruction, such as cholecystitis, cholelithiasis, biliary atresia, arteriohepatic dysplasia (Alagille syndrome), primary sclerosing cholangitis, fibrosing pancreatitis, and choledochal cysts. There is a long and important list of genetic and metabolic diseases that must be ruled out and includes cystic fibrosis, alpha-1-antitrypsin deficiency, Wilson disease, and several others.

DIAGNOSIS

Gross appearance of the liver in a patient with a similar condition revealed micronodular cirrhosis (Figure 7-1A). Histologic examination revealed micronodular cirrhosis with portal-portal bridging, chronic portal inflammation, and fatty change (Figure 7-1B). Rhodanine stain demonstrated copper (red-brown particulate material) within hepatocytes (Figure 7-1C). The patient was treated with penicillamine and pyridoxine. During the next several months, there were improvements in liver function and a stable platelet count of 65 000/mm^3. **The diagnosis is Wilson disease.**

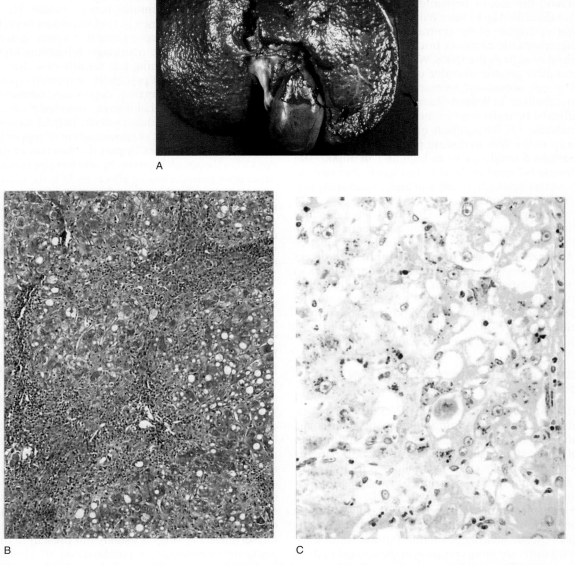

FIGURE 7-1. Histopathology demonstrating **A.** Gross appearance of the liver. **B.** Masson trichrome stain, 100×. **C.** Rhodanine stain, 400×. *(Photos courtesy of Dr. Bruce Pawel.)*

INCIDENCE AND PATHOPHYSIOLOGY OF WILSON DISEASE

Wilson disease, or hepatolenticular degeneration, was described by Kinnier Wilson in 1912 as a degenerative disease of the central nervous system with asymptomatic cirrhosis, but cases were first recognized as early as the 1880s. Wilson disease, the most common genetic disorder of copper metabolism, is a rare autosomal recessive disorder of copper metabolism. In Wilson disease, copper transport is affected by mutations in the ATP7B gene on chromosome 13. Recognition of more distinct mutations of the Wilson disease gene has increased the estimated incidence to as high as 1 in 30 000. The disease is found worldwide, but has higher rates in homogeneous, physically isolated, or culturally isolated populations.

Although copper is a vital trace element and coenzyme for several enzymatic systems, biliary excretion is important to keep the body's balance of copper. In Wilson disease, the inherited defect in the biliary system's excretion of copper leads to excess copper deposition in the brain, liver, and other organs. Copper's toxic effects include the generation of free radicals, lipid peroxidation of membranes and DNA, inhibition of protein synthesis, and altered levels of cellular antioxidants.

CLINICAL PRESENTATION OF WILSON DISEASE

The clinical presentation of Wilson disease is variable, with cases presenting with hepatic, neurologic, and psychiatric manifestations or a combination of these. Hemolysis is seen most often in patients who present with acute liver failure. Although clinical presentation is rare before 5 years of age, symptomatic cases have been reported. Because initial copper accumulation occurs in the liver, in the pediatric population hepatic manifestations usually precede neurologic manifestations. Neurologic symptoms are more common in the second to third decade of life.

Missed or delayed diagnosis of Wilson disease stems from the nonspecific array of clinical manifestations. Very young patients who are diagnosed either through family screening or through the incidental finding of Kayser-Fleisher rings on examination are said to be asymptomatic or presymptomatic. There is

even wide variability in the spectrum of liver disease seen ranging from asymptomatic with biochemical abnormalities to acute hepatitis, chronic active hepatitis, cirrhosis, and fulminant hepatic failure. There is a female predominance (4:1) of fulminant hepatic failure in Wilson disease. Central nervous system manifestations include neurologic symptoms (dystonia, tremors, dysarthria, gait disturbance, choreiform movements) and psychiatric symptoms (poor school performance, anxiety, depression, neuroses, psychoses). The ophthalmologic manifestation of the characteristic and diagnostically helpful Kayser-Fleisher rings is a result of accumulation of copper in the cornea and does not impact the function of the eye. Other tissues and systems in which copper deposition does have damaging effects include the endocrine, renal, skeletal, and cardiac systems. Coombs negative hemolytic anemia is a common complication of Wilson disease when there is acute liver failure and is thought to be secondary to hepatocellular necrosis with resulting release of copper ions in the circulation.

DIAGNOSTIC APPROACH TO WILSON DISEASE

The serious sequelae of a delayed diagnosis of Wilson disease indicate that the disease should be seriously considered and investigated in any patient between 3 and 55 years of age with any unexplained liver and neurologic disease. This is particularly important in children or adolescents with extrapyramidal or cerebellar motor disorders, atypical psychiatric disease, unexplained, hemolysis, and elevated transaminases either in the presence or absence of a family history of liver or neurologic disease. Additionally, individuals who are asymptomatic but whose family member has a confirmed or suspected case of Wilson disease should be investigated. Because the classic triad of hepatic disease, neurologic involvement, and Kayser-Fleisher rings is usually not present in the pediatric population, a combination of clinical findings, biochemical tests, and sometimes genetic testing is necessary to establish the diagnosis.

The American Association for the Study of Liver Diseases (AASLD) updated practice guidelines on Wilson disease in 2008. The AASLD also has a variety of algorithms to approach the diagnosis of the disease.

The AASLD recommends screening patients older than 3 years who have liver disease of unclear etiology, particularly those with accompanying neurologic manifestations. Screening should particularly focus on patients with autoimmune hepatitis, patients with hemolysis in the setting of acute hepatic failure, and any first-degree relatives of newly diagnosed patients.

Ophthalmology examination. Screening and diagnostic testing must include a slit-lamp examination. Ophthalmic slit-lamp of the cornea can demonstrate the characteristic golden-green granular deposits of Kayser-Fleischer rings in patients with concomitant neurologic manifestations. Given the presence of similar corneal rings in other diseases, and the frequent absence of Kayser-Fleischer rings in the pediatric population, their presence or absence neither confirms nor negates the presence of the disease. In the presence of neurologic disease, MRI of the brain can delineate the changes commonly seen in the basal ganglia.

Serum ceruloplasmin. Ceruloplasmin is a serum glycoprotein that is synthesized in the liver and contains six copper atoms. The gene affected in Wilson disease affects this transport system for copper and leads to decreased incorporation of copper into ceruloplasmin and decreased circulating levels of copper. Thus, in Wilson disease serum ceruloplasmin is decreased. Ceruloplasmin levels less than 50 mg/L support the diagnosis, but normal levels do not rule it out. Other diseases such as protein-losing enteropathy, nephrotic syndrome, and even heterozygotes for Wilson disease can have low ceruloplasmin levels. Additionally, it is an acute phase reactant and can be in the normal range in individuals with Wilson disease. Its production is also induced by hormonal contraceptives.

Urinary copper. Serum copper levels cannot be used in diagnosis of Wilson disease, but it is helpful in monitoring adherence and response to therapy. Urinary copper excretion is usually very high (> 100 μg/24 h) in symptomatic patients, but even greater than 40 μg/24 h is not normal and should be further worked up.

Liver biopsy. Liver copper concentration of more than 250 μg/g of dry tissue (five times the normal concentration) is diagnostic for the disease.

Brain imaging. MRI of the brain looking specifically for structural abnormalities of the basal ganglia can be performed for patients with neurologic manifestation of Wilson disease.

Genetic testing. Genetic studies, specifically mutation analysis by whole gene sequencing, are best reserved for patients in whom the other diagnostic studies have not established the diagnosis but for whom there is still a strong suspicion. Specific known mutation testing can be used to screen first-degree relatives of patients with Wilson disease.

TREATMENT

Immediately after confirmation of the disease, therapy should be initiated and continued for the remainder of the patient's life. The goal of therapy is to eliminate symptoms and prevent disease progression. The armamentarium of treatment includes dietary measures, pharmacologic therapy, and liver transplantation.

While a low-copper diet does not play a great role in the treatment of the disease, it is important for patients to avoid heavy copper-containing foods like shellfish, nuts, and chocolate.

Penicillamine, an orally administered copper chelator, decreases the body's pool of copper by increasing urinary copper excretion, and can effectively reduce or eliminate the effects of copper toxicity. The antipyridoxine effects of penicillamine necessitate the concomitant administration of pyridoxine three times a week. The dose can be increased if there is no clinical improvement or decrease in excretion of urinary copper. Adherence to therapy is followed with measurement of either urinary or serum copper, and serum ceruloplasmin levels. Side effects are more common with higher doses. Sensitivity reactions which include fever, rash, leukopenia, thrombocytopenia, and lymphadenopathy can often be overcome with gradual reinstitution of the medication. Penicillamine has consistently shown the successful results, with improvement in liver biopsy findings over time.

Trientine hydrochloride is an alternative chelating agent, particularly in patients with side effects such as nephrotoxicity and lupus-like syndrome from penicillamine. Although there is less urinary copper excretion with this agent, it appears to be equally effective clinically. Iron deficiency or sideroblastic anemia can be seen.

Zinc salts taken three times daily seems to protect hepatocytes by inducing metallothionein in enterocytes which blocks the intestinal absorption of copper. Other experimental chelators (tetrathiomolybdate) are available.

The indications for liver transplantation in patients with liver disease include acute hepatic failure (especially in association with hemolysis), advanced cirrhosis with decompensation, and hepatic insufficiency that progresses in the face of adequate treatment with chelation therapy. Liver transplantation in patients with only neurologic disease remains controversial. Patients receiving transplant display total reversal of the biochemical abnormalities they had previously.

Future directions of treatment include gene therapy, but presently early detection and chelation therapy are still the most important aspects of treatment.

SUGGESTED READINGS

1. Tunnessen WW. Jaundice. In: Tunnessen WW, ed. *Signs and Symptoms in Pediatrics*. 3rd ed. Philadelphia: Lippincott Williams & Wilkins; 1999:102-112.
2. Chitkara DK, Pleskow RG, Grand RJ. Wilson disease. In: Walker WA, Durie PR, Hamilton JR, Walker-Smith JA, Watkins JB, eds. *Pediatric Gastrointestinal Disease*. 3rd ed. Hamilton: B.C. Decker, Inc.; 2000:1171-1184.
3. Pearce JM. Wilson's disease. *J Neurol Neurosurg Psychiatry*. 1997;63:174.
4. Robertson WM. Wilson's disease. *Arch Neurol*. 2000;57:276-277.
5. Schilsky ML, Tavill AS. Wilson's disease. In: Schiff ER, Sorell MG, Maddrey WC, eds. *Schiff's Diseases of the Liver*. 10th ed. Philadelphia: Lippincott Williams & Wilkins; 2007.
6. Gaffney D, Fell GS, O'Reilly DS. ACP best practice no. 163 Wilson's disease: acute and presymptomatic laboratory diagnosis and monitoring. *J Clin Pathol*. 2000;53:807-812.
7. Sternlieb I. Wilson's disease. *Clin Liver Dis*. 2000;4:229-239.
8. Wilson DC, Phillips MJ, Cox DW, Roberts EA. Severe hepatic Wilson's disease in preschool-aged children. *J Pediatr*. 2000;137:719-722.
9. Balistreri WF, Carey RG. Wilson disease. In: Kleigman RM et al. eds. *Nelson's Textbook of Pediatrics*. 19th ed. Philadelphia: Elsevier Saunders; 2011.
10. Khanna A, Jain A, Eghtesad B, Rakela J. Liver transplantation for metabolic liver diseases. *Surg Clin North Am*. 1999;79:153-162.
11. Durand F, Bernuau J, Giostra E, et al. Wilson's disease with severe hepatic insufficiency: beneficial effects of early administration of D-penicillamine. *Gut*. 2001;48:849-852.
12. Roberts EA, Schilsky ML. American Association for Study of Liver Diseases (AASLD) diagnosis and treatment of Wilson disease: an update. *Hepatology*. 2008;47:2089-2111.
13. European Association for Study of Liver. EASL Clinical Practice Guidelines: Wilson's disease. *J Hepatol*. 2012;56:671.

CASE 7-2

Five-Year-Old Girl

MARINA CATALLOZZI

HISTORY OF PRESENT ILLNESS

A 5-year-old female was well until 2 days prior to presentation when she developed emesis and fever. On the day of presentation she had two bouts of nonbloody, nonbilious emesis and continued to have fever as high as 103°F. The patient pointed to the periumbilical area when describing her pain. Her parents also reported that she has had ear pain and a sore throat for the past 3 days. They deny cough, dysuria, and frequency.

She has had a good appetite and no weight loss. The parents reported that about six months ago the patient had an episode of abdominal pain. Her primary care physician reportedly felt stool in the abdomen and started her on prune juice which she stopped using regularly.

MEDICAL HISTORY

Birth history was normal with no complications at delivery or birth. She had mild asthma but no hospitalizations. Three years prior, she was exposed to tuberculosis and had a positive tuberculin skin test. She was treated with isoniazid for 9 months.

PHYSICAL EXAMINATION

T 39°C; RR 24/min; HR 119 bpm; BP 106/65 mmHg

Weight 22.9 kg, 70th percentile; Height 120 cm, 70th percentile

Physical examination revealed an alert, well nourished, and interactive child. There was no conjunctival pallor. The tonsils were 2+ bilaterally with mild erythema of the posterior pharynx. There was shotty cervical lymphadenopathy with enlarged superior cervical lymph nodes that were mobile and nontender. The lungs were clear and there was an I/IV systolic ejection murmur at the left lower sternal border. The abdominal examination revealed normal bowel sounds. On palpation, the abdomen was nontender, but a firm mass was felt in the periumbilical region and left upper quadrant. The mass had sharp borders, was approximately 6 cm × 4 cm, and was slightly mobile. Rectal examination revealed good rectal tone and the rectal vault was full of stool which was negative for occult blood. She was a Tanner I female with no inguinal lymphadenopathy. Her neurologic examination was normal.

DIAGNOSTIC STUDIES

Laboratory analysis revealed 11 500 WBCs/mm^3 with 2% band forms, 62% segmented neutrophils, 24% lymphocytes, and 9% monocytes. The hemoglobin was 14.3 g/dL and the platelet count was 251 000/mm^3. Electrolytes, blood urea nitrogen, creatinine, calcium, magnesium, and phosphorus were normal. Liver function tests were normal. The uric acid was 5.3 mg/dL and the lactate dehydrogenase, 747 U/L. The abdominal radiograph revealed a large amount of stool.

COURSE OF ILLNESS

A fleets enema was given with good results, but the mass was still palpable. Abdominal MRI suggested

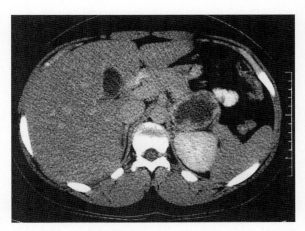

FIGURE 7-2. Abdominal MRI.

a diagnostic category (Figure 7-2). Biopsy of the mass confirmed the diagnosis.

DISCUSSION CASE 7-2

DIFFERENTIAL DIAGNOSIS

The finding of an abdominal mass in a child is an important one that can be attributed to causes as varied as bladder distention and life-threatening malignancies. The age of the patient, history, physical examination, and specific laboratory and imaging studies are crucial to arriving at the correct diagnosis. Children younger than 5 years are the group in which abdominal masses are most commonly identified, and the majority of abdominal masses that are identified in childhood by physical examination are secondary to organomegaly.

In neonates, retroperitoneal masses that arise from the genitourinary system are the most common and include hydronephrosis, multicystic-polycystic kidneys, mesoblastic nephroma, and renal vein thrombosis which is seen in infants of diabetic mothers or with severe hydration. Other possible etiologies include pelvic masses such as an ovarian cyst or hydrometrocolpos which presents with a suprapubic mass and vomiting as a result of hydronephrosis from obstruction of the ureters. Gastrointestinal etiologies include intestinal duplication, malrotation, and sacrococcygeal teratoma. Bladder distention, often as a consequence of posterior urethral valves, can also be common in the neonatal period. Hydronephrosis and multicystic-polycystic disease make up as much as a large percentage of the abdominal masses in neonates.

In infants, the most common malignant solid tumor is neuroblastoma. In childhood, Wilms tumor is the most common childhood abdominal malignancy. The classic presentation is that of an asymptomatic child whose parent notes an abdominal mass while bathing the child. Over half of Wilms tumor is seen before 5 years of age. Neuroblastomas that arise in the abdomen often cross the midline and more than half are seen within the first 2 years of life. The tumor can produce catecholamines and can therefore be clinically associated with tachycardia, hypertension, and skin flushing. The variability of the site of the primary tumor makes the clinical presentation variable, but constitutional symptoms such as fever and weight loss often occur. Other retroperitoneal masses seen in infants in children include rhabdomyosarcoma, lymphoma, Ewing sarcoma, and germ cell neoplasm. There are several liver lesions that can cause abdominal masses in this age group including benign solid tumors, malignant tumors, vascular lesions, and cystic hepatobiliary disease. There are also lesions of the stomach (carcinoma, leiomyosarcoma, fibrosarcoma), small bowel (duplication, Meckel, lymphoma), and colon (fecal mass also common in this age group), and omentum that can cause abdominal masses in this age group.

Adolescents can have many of the etiologies of abdominal masses that are seen in infants and children, but there are some diagnoses that are more common, pelvic masses in particular. Hematocolpos may not be clinically evident until menarche. Ovarian cystic lesions are common and the majority of these lesions are benign, with teratomas as the most common lesion of this type. Malignant ovarian lesions include germ cell tumors, dysgerminomas, choriocarcinomas, and gonadoblastomas. In the retroperitoneal region, renal cell carcinoma occurs most commonly at 14 years of age and presents with flank pain and hematuria.

Physical examination is the most important aspect of early detection of abdominal masses in children. Studies have shown that the majority of malignant abdominal masses in children could be palpated on initial examination.

DIAGNOSIS

MRI of the abdomen (Figure 7-2) revealed a 6 cm × 4.5 cm multiloculated mass arising from the left adrenal gland. There were no other retroperitoneal masses. During recovery, the biopsy of the tumor revealed ganglioneuroma. Metaiodobenzylguanidine (MIBG) scan was negative, confirming that the tumor was entirely a ganglioneuroma. The patient was started on a chemotherapy protocol to reduce the size of the mass before resection. **The diagnosis is abdominal ganglioneuroma.**

INCIDENCE AND EPIDEMIOLOGY OF GANGLIONEUROMAS

There is a spectrum of neuroblastoma tumors that includes ganglioneuromas, neuroblastomas, and ganglioneuroblastoma that arise from neural crest cells. Unlike neuroblastomas, ganglioneuromas are benign and differentiated tumors. Although the incidence of ganglioneuromas is not known, they are most common in children and young adults. They are usually found in the posterior mediastinum and retroperitoneum, and generally arise from the adrenal medulla. Much like pheochromocytomas, which are tumors of chromaffin cells of the adrenal medulla and adrenergic ganglia, adrenal ganglioneuromas can secrete epinephrine and norepinephrine giving rise to endocrinologic symptoms. There have been reports of malignant transformation of ganglioneuromas to neuroblastoma as well as mixed tumors with pheochromocytoma.

CLINICAL PRESENTATION

Ganglioneuromas are more commonly seen in children 5 years of age and older. Apart from the mass effect of any abdominal mass, ganglioneuromas can secrete catecholamines and present with the paraneoplastic syndrome seen with pheochromocytomas. Hypertension is the most concerning sign, and symptoms can include perspiration, tremor, nausea, vomiting, diarrhea, and other manifestations of Cushing syndrome. Because ganglioneuromas can be associated with neurofibromatosis type I or von Recklinghausen disease, clinical manifestations of this disease (such as axillary freckling and café au lait spots) may be noted.

DIAGNOSTIC APPROACH

Evaluation of an adrenal mass should include studies to detect ganglioneuroma, pheochromocytoma, and neuroblastoma.

Abdominal imaging. The initial study is usually an abdominal radiograph to exclude gastrointestinal obstruction. Some clinicians next obtain an ultrasound to determine the organ of origin and identify cysts, hemorrhage, and calcification. MRI may be used in lieu of ultrasound for clearer visualization of the adrenal gland. Additional imaging of the head, spine, or chest may be indicated to exclude metastatic disease.

Complete blood count. Pancytopenia indicates bone marrow involvement due to malignancy. Isolated anemia suggests either chronic illness or hemorrhage into the mass.

Electrolytes, calcium, phosphorus, uric acid, and lactate dehydrogenase. Abnormalities in these studies are seen with tumor lysis syndrome.

Urine HVA and VMA. In any patient with an adrenal mass, spot urine for homovanillic acid (HVA) and vanillylmandelic acid (VMA) should be obtained to detect neuroblastoma or pheochromocytoma.

Other studies. Plasma concentrations of normetanephrines or metanephrines (4-fold and 2.5-fold) above the upper reference limits indicate a pheochromocytoma with 100% specificity. MIBG scanning helps to rule out neuroblastoma.

TREATMENT

Treatment of abdominal ganglioneuroma is dependent on the patient's clinical manifestations. In general, resection is curative. If the patient has endocrinologic manifestations, these should be stabilized medically prior to surgical resection.

SUGGESTED READINGS

1. Squires RH. Abdominal masses. In: Walker WA, Durie PR, Hamilton JR, Walker-Smith JA, Watkins JB, eds. *Pediatric Gastrointestinal Disease.* 3rd ed. Hamilton: B.C. Decker, Inc; 2000:150-163.
2. Golden CB, Feusner JH. Malignant abdominal masses in children: quick guide to evaluation and diagnosis. *Pediatr Clin North Am.* 2002;49:1369-1392.
3. Waguespack SG, Bauer AJ, Huh W, Ying AK. Endocrine tumors. In: Pizzo PA, Poplack DG. eds. *Principles and Practices of Pediatric Oncology.* 6th ed. Philadelphia: Lippincott Williams & Wilkins; 2010.
4. Pacak K, Linehan WM, Eisenhoffer G, et al. Recent advances in genetics, diagnosis, localization, and treatment of pheochromocytoma. *Ann Internal Med.* 2001;134:315-329.
5. Celik V, Unal G, Ozgultekin R, et al. Adrenal ganglioneuroma. *Br J Surg.* 1996;83:263.
6. Meyer S, Reinhard H, Ziegler K, et al. Ganglianeuroma: radiological and metabolic features in 4 children. *Pediatr Hematol Oncol.* 2002;19(7):501.

CASE 7-3

Eleven-Year-Old Girl

MARINA CATALLOZZI

HISTORY OF PRESENT ILLNESS

The patient, an 11-year-old girl, was well until 1 year prior to presentation when she was diagnosed with streptococcal pharyngitis. At that time she had severe abdominal pain that caused her to double over in pain. Appendicitis had been considered, and an abdominal radiograph showed an enlarged loop of bowel. The patient was observed, but both the clinical picture and laboratories did not suggest appendicitis. No surgery was performed.

A streptococcal rapid antigen test was positive which promoted treatment with amoxicillin. Since that illness, the patient has had multiple illnesses and missed 42 days of school with episodes of headache and abdominal pain. The pain is described as noncrampy but sharp. The pain is described as generalized lower abdominal discomfort without radiation. She was diagnosed with three urinary tract infections during this time secondary to pyuria on urinalysis, but all cultures were negative. Symptoms have been particularly severe since she was diagnosed with mononucleosis 3 months ago. She has had a poor appetite and 10-pound weight loss with mononucleosis and lost 8 more pounds since then. At presentation, the patient had decreased intake secondary to a sore throat and difficulty swallowing secondary to pain. The patient just completed a full course of antibiotics for pharyngitis diagnosed clinically 3 weeks ago (cultures were negative). The patient has been missing half days of school for 2 months and has been sleeping in the afternoons. The week of presentation, the patient has complained of low-grade fevers (99.4°F-100°F), neck pain, diffuse abdominal pain, and frontal headache. On the day of admission the patient was noted to have hemoccult positive stool at the primary care provider's office after 3 days of diarrhea and loose stools. The primary care provider's work up-to-date has included a CT scan of the head and sinuses which was negative, stool for culture which was also negative, normal complete blood count, urinalysis, erythrocyte sedimentation rate, Lyme antibody testing, immunoglobulins, ANA, CXR, electrolytes, liver function tests, and thyroid testing.

MEDICAL HISTORY

The patient had reactive airways disease as a toddler which is no longer active. She also had a urinary tract infection at 5 years of age with a normal renal ultrasound. She sustained a concussion at day camp 2 years ago. She had no surgical history and was on no medication except for occasional albuterol with colds. Family history was significant for a maternal grandmother with diverticulitis, maternal grandfather with ulcers, and paternal grandmother with irritable bowel syndrome. There was no history of inflammatory bowel disease or childhood illnesses. The patient is in 5th grade and had done very well in school and been very involved in sports before this illness. The patient reports that she misses school and her friends.

PHYSICAL EXAMINATION

T 38.1°C; HR 124 bpm; RR 24 bpm; BP 105/71 mmHg

Weight 37 kg (75th percentile); Height 155 cm (90th percentile)

Physical examination revealed a thin female who appeared tired and anxious. There was erythema of the pharynx with enlarged tonsils and cobblestoning. There was no exudate and no asymmetry of the tonsillar crypts or soft palate. She had good dentition, halitosis, and cracked red lips. Her neck was supple with no adenopathy. Lungs were clear to auscultation and cardiac examination revealed no murmurs, rubs, or gallops. Abdominal examination revealed good bowel sounds in all four quadrants. There was diffuse tenderness, but no guarding, no rebound, and no hepatosplenomegaly. Rectal examination revealed no excoriation, skin tags, fissures, or hemorrhoids. She had good rectal tone without any palpable masses. She was Tanner II female and there were no obvious vaginal lesions. Neurologic examination was normal.

DIAGNOSTIC STUDIES

The complete blood count revealed a white blood count of 5800 cells/mm³. Hemoglobin and platelets were normal. Erythrocyte sedimentation rate was also normal at 14 mm. Electrolytes showed a sodium of 144 mEq/L; potassium, 4.2 mEq/L; chloride, 101 mEq/L; bicarbonate, 31 mEq/L; BUN, 7 mg/dL; and creatinine, 0.6 mg/dL. Urinalysis had a high specific gravity of 1.036 as well as 1+ protein, small bacteria, and large mucus. Rapid strep test was positive for Group A Streptococcal antigen. Amylase was 40 U/L and lipase 53 U/L. Stool cultures grew normal flora and Clostridium difficile testing was negative. Abdominal radiographs were normal except for scoliosis of the lumbar spine. There was no obstruction.

COURSE OF ILLNESS

An abdominal CT revealed the diagnosis (Figure 7-3).

DISCUSSION CASE 7-3

DIFFERENTIAL DIAGNOSIS

Weight loss in children is a concerning symptom that requires careful thought, especially when associated with abdominal pain. Oncologic processes should be considered and are frequently the biggest concern for parents. Acute and chronic

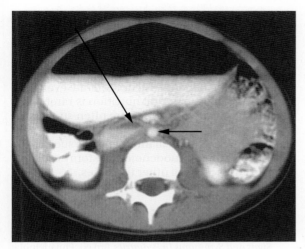

FIGURE 7-3. Abdominal CT. The large arrow indicates the duodenum and the small arrow indicates the aorta.

infections are probably the most common cause of weight loss in children. With acute infections like mononucleosis or pharyngitis, the child should regain the weight once the infection clears. This is one of the most concerning pieces of history in this case. In these cases more chronic, insidious infections like an abdominal abscess, chronic hepatitis, intestinal parasites, tuberculosis, urinary tract infection, or human immunodeficiency virus must be considered.

With associated abdominal pain gastrointestinal disorders such as chronic constipation, gastroesophageal reflux disease, inflammatory bowel disease (examining trends in growth parameters is key), pancreatitis, malabsorptive diseases such as celiac, or superior mesenteric artery syndrome must be considered.

Endocrinologic disorders associated with weight loss include Addison disease (abdominal pain and skin discoloration frequently seen), diabetes mellitus (with associated polyphagia, polydipsia, and polyuria), and hyperthyroidism. Cardiopulmonary disorders include asthma, chronic congestive heart failure, cystic fibrosis, and an untreated cardiac disease. Other causes include nutritional deficiencies (iron and zinc), neurologic diseases (increased intracranial disorders that lead to headache and neurodegenerative disorders), connective tissue diseases, and renal failure.

The most common causes of weight loss, particularly in adolescent girls, include dieting, increased physical activity, depression, anorexia nervosa, and bulimia nervosa. Although this patient's age and preceding illness made an eating disorder a possibility, it did not explain her associated abdominal pain.

DIAGNOSIS

Abdominal CT revealed abnormal dilation of the stomach and proximal duodenum with tapering of the second part of the duodenum to the level of the space between the superior mesenteric artery (SMA) and the aorta consistent with SMA syndrome (Figure 7-3). **The diagnosis is SMA syndrome.**

INCIDENCE AND EPIDEMIOLOGY OF SUPERIOR MESENTERIC ARTERY SYNDROME

SMA syndrome is an uncommon disorder and has also been referred to as cast syndrome, Wilkie syndrome, duodenal ileus, and arteriomesenteric duodenal compression syndrome. Extrinsic and acute, chronic, or intermittent duodenal obstruction is caused by compression of the transverse portion of the duodenum by the SMA anteriorly and the aorta and vertebral column posteriorly, that causes classic "megaduodenum" on upper GI. Although first described in 1861 by Von Rokitansky, many have disputed the existence of the syndrome and feel that it has been confused with other causes of megaduodenum such as diabetes, collagen vascular diseases, and other causes of chronic intestinal pseudoobstruction.

The syndrome is most common in older children and adolescents, is more common in females and in those that have risk factors for narrowing the angle between the aorta and the SMA and subsequently compressing the duodenum. These risk factors include height growth during the growth spurt that is not accompanied by weight gain, extreme lumbar lordosis, rapid weight loss that decreases the mesenteric fat pad, severe trauma, or surgery that requires prolonged bed rest, use of a body cast, and scoliosis surgery. Anatomic predisposition is present in persons with a short suspensory ligament of Treitz. Recently, there has been a connection with eating disorders in that it can clinically appear like an eating disorder and sometimes precipitate an eating disorder because of the development of food avoidance to avoid pain.

CLINICAL PRESENTATION

Presenting symptoms can be either acute or chronic (usually with exacerbations) and typically include epigastric and abdominal pain, bilious emesis, and pain after eating. Infrequently, patients present with small bowel obstruction. Severe cases that have gone undiagnosed may present with signs of malnutrition, dehydration with prostration, and electrolyte abnormalities.

DIAGNOSTIC APPROACH

Abdominal imaging. While plain abdominal radiographs are often normal, they can show gastric distention. The diagnosis is usually made by upper GI series which shows dilatation of the first two portions of the duodenum with a cutoff at the third potion of the duodenum. Hypotonic duodenography can also display the site of obstruction and CT can provide more detailed information about the aortomesenteric angle and anatomic issues that are creating the obstruction.

TREATMENT

Treatment should begin with stabilization of the patient. To avoid gastric perforation, nasogastric decompression with a nasogastric tube should be performed and intravenous fluids administered to correct electrolyte imbalances. The patient should be counseled to avoid positions which exacerbate the obstruction (the supine position) and either remain upright or in the left lateral decubitus position to open up the aortomesenteric angle. Although some patients will not tolerate even slow nasogastric feeds, parental nutrition is rarely warranted and nasojejunal feeds are often successful. The patient is treated conservatively until weight gain is achieved. Surgical interventions such as the Ladd procedure or duodenojejunostomy are indicated in cases that fail other therapies.

SUGGESTED READINGS

1. Tunnessen WW. Weight loss. In: Tunnessen WW, ed. *Signs and Symptoms in Pediatrics*. 3rd ed. Philadelphia: Lippincott Williams & Wilkins; 1999:36-40.
2. Wesson DE, Haddock G. The surgical abdomen. In: Walker WA, Durie PR, Hamilton JR, Walker-Smith JA, Watkins JB, eds. *Pediatric Gastrointestinal Disease*. 3rd ed. Hamilton: B.C. Decker, Inc.; 2000:435-444.
3. Shetty AK, Schmidt-Sommerfeld E, Haymon ML, Udall JN Jr. Radiological case of the month: superior mesenteric artery syndrome. *Arch Pediatr Adolesc Med*. 1999;153:303-304.
4. Jordaan GP, Muller A, Greeff M, Stein DJ. Eating disorder and superior mesenteric artery syndrome. *J Am Acad Child Adolesc Psychiatry*. 2000;39:1211.
5. Crowther MA, Webb PJ, Eyre-Brock IA. Superior mesenteric artery syndrome following surgery for scoliosis. *Spine*. 2002;27:e528-e533.
6. Biank V, Werlin S. Superior mesenteric artery syndrome in children: a 20-year experience. *J Pediatr Gastr Nutr*. 2006;42:522-525.

CASE 7-4

Nine-Year-Old Girl

MARINA CATALLOZZI

HISTORY OF PRESENT ILLNESS

A 9-year-old girl was well until 6 days prior to admission when she developed vomiting, abdominal pain, and lethargy. Four days prior to admission she was noted to have a fever to 102°F and cough. She received amoxicillin for a presumed lower lobe pneumonia with referred abdominal pain; chest radiograph was not performed. Over the next 2 days she had worsening of her abdominal pain and increased listlessness. Her mother reported that the whites of her eyes had looked yellow for the past 3 weeks.

MEDICAL HISTORY

The patient had no major illnesses or hospitalizations. She had four episodes of dizziness during the past 5 months that had been evaluated with an EEG and an ECG which were both normal. She was on no medication except for the amoxicillin for her diagnosis of pneumonia. Family history was significant only for several family members with diabetes mellitus. The mother required a splenectomy after blunt abdominal trauma.

PHYSICAL EXAMINATION

T 37.4°C; HR 118 bpm; RR 30 bpm; BP 91/50 mmHg; Oxygen saturation 94% on room air

Weight 27.9 kg (25th percentile)

The patient was responsive but withdrawn. There were mildly icteric sclera, no oral lesions, and no pharyngeal injection. The neck was supple with shotty lymphadenopathy. The lung examination was clear with equal breath sounds bilaterally. Cardiac examination revealed a normal precordium, mild tachycardia, normal S_1 and S_2, no gallop, and no murmur. The abdomen was soft and nontender with normal bowel sounds, and the liver was palpated 4 cm below the right costal margin and the spleen tip was palpable. The extremities were warm, but there were diminished pulses in both the upper and lower extremities. The neurologic examination was normal and the skin revealed no rash.

DIAGNOSTIC STUDIES

Complete blood count revealed a white blood count of 9600/mm³ with 72% segmented neutrophils and 23% lymphocytes. The hemoglobin and platelets were normal. Prothrombin time, partial thromboplastin time, electrolytes, blood urea nitrogen, and creatinine were all normal. A hepatic function panel revealed a bilirubin of 3.2 mg/dL; with an unconjugated bilirubin of 1.8 mg/dL; albumin, 3.8 gm/dL; alkaline phosphatase, 78 U/L; AST, 54 U/L; LDH, 237 U/L; and uric acid, 7.3 mg/dL. Lipase was 168 U/L and amylase 63 U/L. ECG revealed a sinus rhythm at 129 bpm, PR interval of 0.144 seconds, right axis deviation, normal voltage, and no ST segment changes. The chest radiograph was abnormal (Figure 7-4).

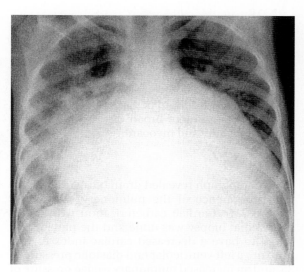

FIGURE 7-4. Chest radiograph.

COURSE OF ILLNESS

The patient had an ECHO which revealed a markedly dilated left ventricle to 5.4 cm, moderate to severe mitral regurgitation, and a markedly decreased shortening fraction of 10%-18%. The patient was started on furosemide and milrinone. Despite increasing doses, by the fourth hospital day the patient had distended neck veins, increasing dyspnea, cough, and lethargy. Repeat ECHO showed a decrease in the shortening fraction to less than 10% with a dilated and thin walled left ventricle, persistent severe mitral regurgitation, and moderate tricuspid regurgitation with a right ventricular pressure 30 mm greater than the right atrium.

DISCUSSION CASE 7-4

DIFFERENTIAL DIAGNOSIS

Myocarditis and other forms of heart disease are listed as possible etiologies for abdominal pain. Cardiomegaly on this patient's chest radiograph gave the first indication of heart disease and heart failure. Possible etiologies of this heart failure include congenital heart disease, particularly septal lesions, which must be ruled out in the pediatric population at any age. There are several possible causes of heart failure that include dilated cardiomyopathy, hypertrophic cardiomyopathy, restrictive cardiomyopathy, arrhythmogenic right ventricular dysplasia, obliterative cardiomyopathy, inflammatory cardiomyopathy (myocarditis), and giant cell myocarditis. In pediatrics, it is most helpful to make the more broad distinction between cardiomyopathy and myocarditis.

DIAGNOSIS

Chest radiograph revealed dramatic cardiomegaly and prominence of the pulmonary vasculature (Figure 7-4). Cardiac catheterization with endomyocardial biopsy was done and the patient was noted to have a decreased cardiac index of 1.47 mm/m^2, a left ventricular end diastolic pressure of 35, and an increased pulmonary wedge pressure of 38 and a right atrial pressure of 18. Biopsy revealed no inflammatory cells. The patient was diagnosed with idiopathic dilated cardiomyopathy and listed for cardiac transplant. **The diagnosis is idiopathic dilated cardiomyopathy.**

INCIDENCE AND EPIDEMIOLOGY OF DILATED CARDIOMYOPATHY

While heart failure represents a major problem in adult medicine, it is far less common in pediatrics. Excluding infancy when congenital heart disease is the most common indication for heart transplant, dilated cardiomyopathy is the primary indication for pediatric heart transplants throughout the world. The majority of cases of dilated cardiomyopathy have no definitive cause. Several genetic and molecular lesions have been identified, including mutations in the cytoskeleton, troponin, and other sarcomere protein genes. Autosomal dominant, autosomal recessive, and x-linked are some of the modes of inheritance of these genes that have been identified thus far. A relative with dilated cardiomyopathy is one of the diagnostic criteria for familial dilated cardiomyopathy. While it has long been known that the skeletal muscular dystrophies have skeletal involvement, familial dilated cardiomyopathy, although poorly understood, has been recognized more frequently.

The structural changes that occur in dilated cardiomyopathy include increased left ventricular mass, normal or reduced left ventricular wall thickness, and increased left ventricular cavity size. Histologic samples can show anything from focal myocyte death, increase in interstitial macrophage, and interstitial fibrosis.

Some new onset cardiomyopathy can be attributed to myocarditis. Survival rates can be as high as 80% and the infections can be either fulminant (usually with a better prognosis) or insidious. Arguably, insidious cases may be missed and later contribute to cases of idiopathic cardiomyopathy. Infectious agents (bacterial, spirochetal, fungal, protozoal, parasitic, rickettsial, and viral) have all been implicated. Worldwide, infections with *Trypanosoma cruzi* (Chagas disease) and *Corynebacterium diphtheriae* (diphtheria) are the most common causes of myocarditis while in the United States, viruses are more common. The two major viral etiologies are coxsackievirus B and adenovirus. Infections with hepatitis C, HIV, EBV, and CMV have also been implicated. Other causative etiologies of myocarditis include immune-mediated mechanisms, and toxins such as medications and heavy metals.

CLINICAL PRESENTATION OF DILATED CARDIOMYOPATHY

The clinical presentation of dilated cardiomyopathy encompasses that of clinical heart failure including fatigue, shortness of breath, cough, and abdominal pain. However, the clinical features are varied and can range from asymptomatic patients to those with fulminant cardiac failure. In myocarditis, there is frequently a history of a recent flu-like syndrome and sometimes arrhythmias secondary to the rapid ventricular dilatation.

DIAGNOSTIC APPROACH

The distinction between dilated cardiomyopathy and myocarditis is important, as it may alter the management that the child receives. Although clinical symptoms (clinical heart failure, recent flu-like syndrome accompanied by fever) and laboratory tests (leukocytosis, eosinophilia, elevated creatinine kinase, or troponin) can be helpful in supporting a diagnosis of myocarditis, they are not sufficient.

Echocardiogram. All patients should have an echocardiogram to rule out structural anomalies.

Myocardial biopsy. Although there are other non-invasive modalities that are important, myocardial biopsy is still the gold standard for diagnosis of myocarditis.

Other studies. Testing for infectious (e.g., coxsackie, adenovirus, echoviruses, RSV, CMV, EBV, HIV) and any other possible etiologies including autoimmune diseases (e.g., systemic lupus erythematosus) and mitochondrial diseases is warranted in all new cases of pediatric heart failure.

TREATMENT

Symptom counseling and management as well as supportive therapy are the mainstays of treatment. Although there is less evidence to support specific treatment of heart disease in the pediatric population, the therapy mirrors that of adult medicine and includes ACE inhibitors. Less frequently, beta blockers and digoxin are used. Although there is not strong literature and controversies persist, the standard is to treat cases of biopsy-proven myocarditis with immunomodulators (ranging from immunoglobulin therapy and steroids to cyclosporine and cytoxan) in an attempt to suppress the inflammation. Patients with progressively worsening heart failure may be candidates for mechanical-assist devices (i.e., LVAD or ECMO) which may provide stabilization until cardiac transplant can be achieved.

SUGGESTED READINGS

1. Davies MJ. The cardiomyopathies: an overview. *Heart*. 2000;83:469-474.
2. Burch M. Heart failure in the young. *Heart*. 2002;88: 198-202.
3. Batra AS, Lewis AB. Acute myocarditis. *Curr Opin Pediatr*. 2001;13:234-239.
4. Feldman AM, McNamara D. Myocarditis. *New Engl J Med*. 2000;343:1388-1398.
5. Luk A, Ahn E, Soor GS, Butany J. Dilated cardiomyopathy: a review. *J Clin Pathol*. 2009;62(3):219.

CASE 7-5

Eight-Year-Old Boy

MARINA CATALLOZZI

HISTORY OF PRESENT ILLNESS

The patient, an 8-year-old boy, was well until 4 hours prior to presentation. At that time he developed crampy periumbilical pain and bilious emesis. His family denied fever, diarrhea, or ill contacts. The pain was described as crampy and intermittent. He had six episodes of emesis prior to admission. His last bowel movement was 1 day prior to admission. His mother gave him an enema prior to presentation with no relief of symptoms.

MEDICAL HISTORY

The patient was a full-term infant without complications. His first episode of abdominal pain and bilious vomiting occurred about 3 years ago. During the past few years the pain and vomiting had been occurring about once every 4 months. The patient would have 2-3 days of emesis that was usually bilious and associated with abdominal pain. He had recently been treated with phenobarbital and atropine without good results. He also had a history of chronic constipation that responded to mineral oil. Three months prior to presentation he was admitted with similar symptoms and had a normal abdominal CT. The pain was never associated with eating and he never missed school. There was no family history of celiac disease, cystic fibrosis, or any gastrointestinal condition such as inflammatory bowel disease.

PHYSICAL EXAMINATION

T 36.5°C; HR 11 bpm; RR 24 bpm; BP 135/85 mmHg

Weight 26 kg

Physical examination revealed an alert child lying in bed crying in pain. There were no oral lesions. The neck was supple with no lymphadenopathy. The lungs were clear to auscultation and the cardiac examination reveals no murmurs, rubs, or gallops. On abdominal examination there were diminished bowel sounds and although soft there was intermittent guarding and a question of a mass in the left upper quadrant with no focal tenderness. There was no hepatosplenomegaly. Rectal examination revealed no fissures or skin tags; there was hard stool palpable in the rectal vault on digital examination. He was a Tanner I male. The neurologic examination was normal.

DIAGNOSTIC STUDIES

Complete blood count showed a white blood count of 14 500/mm³ with 80% segmented neutrophils, 3% band forms, 7% lymphocytes, and 2% eosinophils. The hemoglobin was 12 g/dL; hematocrit, 39.4%; and platelet count, 314 000/mm³. Serum bicarbonate was 18 mEq/L but the electrolytes, blood urea nitrogen, and creatinine were otherwise normal. Liver function tests, amylase, and lipase were also normal. Urinalysis was negative except for the presence of ketones.

COURSE OF ILLNESS

The patient had an abdominal radiograph that showed a paucity of bowel gas, stool in the rectum, and no free air. An upper GI series revealed the cause of the patient's cyclic vomiting (Figure 7-5).

DISCUSSION CASE 7-5

DIFFERENTIAL DIAGNOSIS

While the differential diagnosis of abdominal pain and vomiting is an important one, the key to the diagnosis in this patient was the cyclic nature of the vomiting. Cyclic vomiting syndrome is an idiopathic disorder characterized by severe episodic vomiting interspersed with periods of normal health. In a study of patients with cyclic vomiting syndrome, 12% were found to have potentially life-threatening disorders such as malrotation

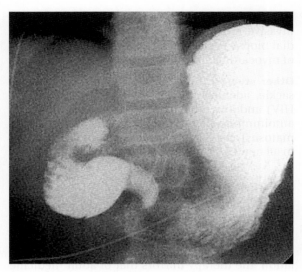

FIGURE 7-5. Upper GI series.

with volvulus, obstructive uropathy, or brain tumors. The most common cause of cyclic vomiting, accounting for as many as 50% of cases, is abdominal migraine. The family history is usually significant for migraines. The second most common cause is chronic sinusitis.

Apart from malrotation with intermittent volvulus, other gastrointestinal causes of cyclic vomiting include chronic idiopathic pseudoobstruction, intestinal duplication, pancreatitis or pancreatic pseudocyst, peptic ulcer disease, and superior mesenteric artery syndrome. Urinary tract etiologies include renal stones and intermittent ureteropelvic junction obstruction. There are also several endocrinologic and metabolic etiologies for cyclic vomiting including Addison disease, porphyria, ornithine transcarbamylase deficiency, methyl malonic acidemia, and hereditary fructose intolerance.

DIAGNOSIS

On the upper GI barium study, the ligament of Treitz was located at the midline in an abnormal position compatible with a midgut malrotation (Figure 7-5). The intraluminal contrast tapered in the proximal jejunum in an appearance compatible with the presence of a midgut volvulus. **The patient was diagnosed with malrotation.** Following the identification of malrotation on the upper GI, the patient underwent a Ladd procedure with appendectomy.

INCIDENCE AND EPIDEMIOLOGY OF MALROTATION

Understanding the underlying embryology that leads to malrotation is very important. At approximately 10 weeks' gestation, the intestines undergo counterclockwise rotation around the mesenteric artery and finally attach themselves to the posterior abdominal wall. The midgut then rotates 270 degrees around the superior mesenteric artery, with the duodenal-jejunal loop moving posterior to the superior mesenteric artery while the cecal-colic loop rotates anterior to the superior mesenteric artery. The duodenum and ascending colon can then attach to the posterior abdominal wall. This process of rotation and attachment helps to support normal GI tract motility as well as balanced gut to mesentery vascular supply.

With malrotation, the normal process is impeded and the cecum is in the right upper quadrant, near the duodenum, while the duodenal-jejunal loop remains to the right of midline. Because there is no mesenteric attachment, volvulus of the midgut is likely to occur with malrotation. The incidence of volvulus in association with malrotation is 44% in all age groups, but in neonates it is more likely to require bowel resection because of more significant damage to the bowel.

CLINICAL PRESENTATION OF MALROTATION

The clinical presentation of malrotation can vary widely. It is important to note that malrotation is commonly associated with other gastrointestinal anomalies, namely esophageal atresia, diaphragmatic hernia, jejunal atresia, duodenal atresia, omphalocele, gastroschisis, intussusception, prunebelly syndrome, and Hirschsprung disease. It has also been seen in association with heterotaxy and congenital heart disease.

Malrotation with midgut volvulus can occur at any age, but is most commonly seen in infancy. Acute volvulus presents with bilious emesis, abdominal distention, pain (constant rather than intermittent), and bright red blood per rectum (suggesting ischemia). It is a surgical emergency

and untreated ischemic bowel can lead to shock and sepsis with cardiovascular collapse.

A less commonly seen entity is malrotation with intermittent volvulus and usually presents with recurrent abdominal pain and vomiting and signs of failure to thrive.

DIAGNOSTIC APPROACH

Radiologic studies. Plain radiographs can reassure the clinician of the absence of intestinal perforation. CT is not recommended in children. Although both the barium enema and upper GI series can be used, the upper GI series is now preferred because of the possibility of cecal mobility on barium enema and its inability to show volvulus. An upper GI series that definitively shows malrotation includes one that reveals the corkscrew-like deformity of the duodenum, one that reveals the duodenum and jejunum in the right upper quadrant, or chronic obstruction of the duodenum.

TREATMENT

In neonates, any suggestion of volvulus indicates the possibility of ischemic gut and necessitates immediate surgical intervention. In older patients with rotational abnormalities definitive surgery is also performed. Timing depends on the presentation of the patient. If possible, patients should be prepared for surgery with nasogastric suction, fluid resuscitation, and prophylactic antibiotics to cover the possibility of bowel resection. The Ladd procedure allows definitive treatment with counterclockwise derotation of the midgut volvulus, lysis of bands, appendectomy, and placement of the duodenum in the right side of the abdomen and of the cecum in the left lower quadrant.

SUGGESTED READINGS

1. Tunnessen WW. Cyclic vomiting. In: Tunnesse WW, ed. *Signs and Symptoms in Pediatrics.* 3rd ed. Philadelphia: Lippincott William & Wilkins; 1999:503-507.
2. Olson AD, Li BU. The diagnostic evaluation of children with cyclic vomiting: a cost-effectiveness assessment. *J Pediatr.* 2002;141:724-728.
3. Little DC, Smith SC. Malrotation. In: Holder TM, Murphy, eds. *Ashcraft's Pediatric Surgery.* 5th ed. Philadelphia: Saunders Elsevier; 2010.

4. Liu PCF, Stringer DA. Radiography: contrast studies. In: Walker WA, Durie PR, Hamilton JR, Walker-Smith JA, Watkins JB, eds. *Pediatric Gastrointestinal Disease*. 3rd ed. Hamilton: B.C. Decker, Inc.; 2000:1555-1591.

5. Shuckett B. Cross-sectional imaging: ultrasonography, computed tomography, magnetic resonance imaging.

In: Walker WA, Durie PR, Hamilton JR, Walker-Smith JA, Watkins JB, eds. *Pediatric Gastrointestinal Disease*. 3rd ed. Hamilton: B.C. Decker, Inc.; 2000:1591-1633.

6. Nehra D, Goldstein AM. Intestinal malrotation: varied clinical presentation from infancy through adulthood. *Surgery*. 2011;149(3)386.

CASE 7-6

Two-Year-Old Girl

SANJEEV K. SWAMI

HISTORY OF PRESENT ILLNESS

The patient, a 2-year-old girl, was well until 1 month prior to admission, when she began to experience intermittent periods of abdominal pain. The pain was dull and diffused throughout the entire abdomen. It did not awaken her at night. One week prior to admission, the patient experienced mucousy, nonbloody diarrhea twice per day. URI symptoms developed 2 days prior to admission. A sibling had a "cold." The patient's family brought her to the primary medical doctor with complaints of fever and worsening abdominal pain. A three-pound weight loss history was elicited. There was a strong history of pica, specifically geophagy. The family has two cats and a new puppy.

MEDICAL HISTORY

History is significant for breath-holding spells (none recently) with an extensive work-up that included a normal EEG, a normal Holter monitor, and a normal ECG. Per her parents, growth was always "a concern." No other information was available with regard to her growth. She had no history of surgery and no drug allergies; her immunizations were up-to-date, and there was no significant family medical history.

PHYSICAL EXAMINATION

T 37.8°C; HR 120 bpm; RR 20/min; BP 92/62 mmHg

In general, the patient was an alert but pale child. The neck was supple. There was no prominent cervical adenopathy, and the trachea was midline. The lung fields were clear, and the cardiac examination was unremarkable, with no murmurs, rubs, or gallops. Abdominal examination revealed a soft and nontender abdomen with good bowel sounds, a palpable spleen tip, and a liver edge that was about 2 cm below the right costal margin. The patient was a Tanner I female, and the rectal examination revealed good tone, no tenderness on examination, no fissures, no masses, and a small amount of stool in the vault. Neurologic examination was normal.

DIAGNOSTIC STUDIES

Complete blood count revealed a white blood count of 39800/mm^3 with 1% band forms, 18% segmented neutrophils, 53% eosinophils, 17% lymphocytes, 3% basophils, the hemoglobin was 7.8 g/dL; hematocrit, 29.4% (MCV of 52.7 fL, MCHC of 29.7 pg, RDW of 19.5%), and platelets of 1000000/mm^3. Erythrocyte sedimentation rate was 20 mm/h.

COURSE OF ILLNESS

Chest and abdominal radiographs were normal, stool for ova and parasites as well as culture were pending. Serum immunoglobulins were elevated. Anti-A and anti-B isohemagglutinins were markedly elevated (A = 1:16,000, B = 1:512). ELISA was pending. The patient was discharged home after a normal ophthalmologic examination with outpatient follow-up to monitor the eosinophilia.

DISCUSSION CASE 7-6

DIFFERENTIAL DIAGNOSIS

Diseases that are transmitted from animals to humans are called zoonoses. The presence of pets in more than 50% of homes in the United States, and the acquisition of zoonoses via fecal-oral or direct contact puts children at higher risk for these infections. While this patient had a history of abdominal pain and diarrhea, the most important pieces of history were the family's pets and the patient's history of geophagia. Zoonotic diseases that are transmitted via the fecal-oral route and cause gastroenteritis in children include salmonellosis (*Salmonella* sp., approximately 5 million cases per year), campylobacteriosis (*C jejuni*), cryptosporidiosis (*Cryptosporidium parvum*), giardiasis (*Giardia* sp. found in 8% of children in US day care centers), dog tapeworm (*Dipylidium caninum*), and visceral larval migrans.

DIAGNOSIS

The clinical history along with laboratory abnormalities supported a diagnosis of visceral larva migrans.

INCIDENCE, EPIDEMIOLOGY, AND LIFE CYCLE

Visceral larva migrans or toxocariasis is caused by infection with dog ascarid (*Toxocara canis*) or cat ascarid (*Toxocara cati*). The reservoir for latent infection is usually female dogs. *Toxocara* eggs are passed in the feces of infected animals and require several weeks, depending on environmental conditions, to embryonate and become infective (Figure 7-6). Shedding rates vary from 13% to 75% for dogs and 21% to 55% for cats. Areas that usually harbor infectious ova include playgrounds and sandboxes where children might play. The disease in humans is primarily seen in children younger than 6 years, especially those with geophagus pica, who ingest soil that contain the larvae.

In the United States, children in kindergarten have been found to have antibody prevalence rates as high as 23% and a diagnosis of the disease is made in 3000 to 4000 patients per year. There are regional and socioeconomic variations with highest rates reported in the South and areas with higher rates of poverty.

CLINICAL PRESENTATION

The clinical spectrum of *Toxocara* infections varies from asymptomatic to primarily visceral to primarily ocular manifestations. Infectious eggs are ingested followed by penetration of gastric mucosa, incorporation into the portal circulatory system, and then spread into the systemic circulation. Damage from these traveling larvae and the marked eosinophilic response cause the clinical manifestations which can include fever, hepatosplenomegaly, abdominal pain, irritability, malaise, and pruritic rash. Pulmonary involvement can be seen in up to 86% of infected children and can be severe; it is often confused with asthma exacerbations, and visceral larva migrans may be an independent risk factor for asthma. Ocular complaints can occur alone and the subsequent strabismus, failing vision, uveitis, or endophthalmitis occur secondary to the local inflammatory response to the infection. The myocardium and central nervous system are also rarely affected.

DIAGNOSTIC RATIONALE

The age of the child, history of contact with dogs, and geophagus are all important historical clues to the diagnosis. Definitive diagnosis with biopsy of affected tissue is rarely warranted, and the yield is low. Additional clues include elevated serum gamma-globulins, a high white cell count with eosinophilia, and elevated titers of anti-A or anti-B isohemagglutinin (seen in 50% of patients). Serology is the laboratory test of choice and a titer of greater than 1:32 has good sensitivity and specificity.

TREATMENT

Treatment is controversial, and many children will improve without any specific therapy. Albendazole (10 mg/kg/day divided twice daily) has been used in the past but may lead to a more robust inflammatory response. Because of this, some experts recommend treatment with corticosteroids in addition to antiparasitic therapy if treatment is started. Prevention of repeat infection is crucial, and any affected pets should be treated promptly.

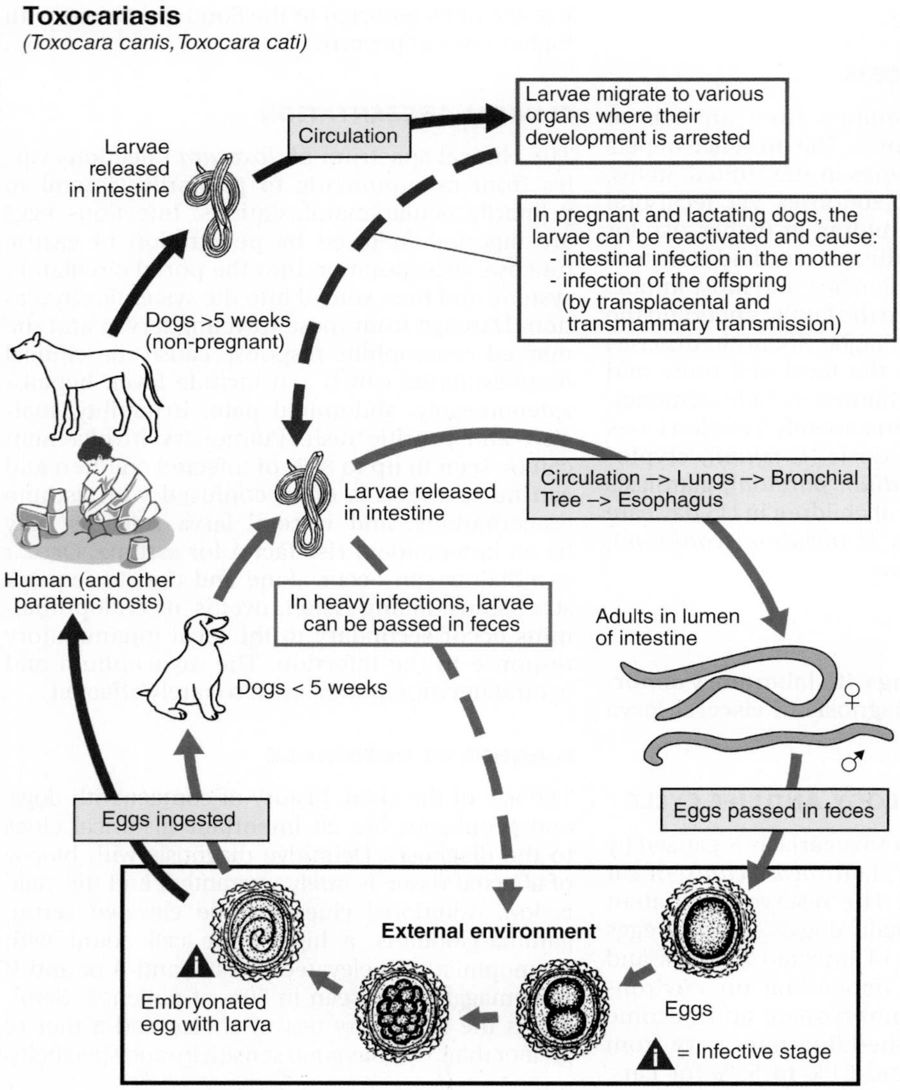

Toxocariasis
(Toxocara canis, Toxocara cati)

FIGURE 7-6. Lifecycle of *Toxocara canis* and *Toxocara cati*. *(Courtesy of the Centers for Disease Control and Prevention, Division of Parasitic Diseases and Malaria—DPDx website: http://www.dpd.cdc.gov/dpdx/Default.htm.)*

SUGGESTED READINGS

1. Tan JS. Human zoonotic infection transmitted by cats and dogs. *Arch Intern Med.* 1997;157:1933-1943.
2. Despommier D. Toxocariasis: clinical aspects, epidemiology, medical ecology, and molecular aspects. *Clin Microbiol Rev.* 2003;16:265-272.
3. Won KY, Kruszon-Moran D, Schantz PM, Jones JL. National seroprevalence and risk factors for zoonotic *Toxocara* spp. Infection *Am J Trop Med Hyg.* 2008;79:552-557.
4. Congdon P, Lloyd P. Toxocara infection in the United States: the relevance of poverty, geography and demography as risk factors, and implications for estimating county prevalence. *Int J Public Health.* 2011;56:15-24.
5. The Medical Letter on Drugs and Therapeutics. Drugs for Parasitic Infections. Mark Abramowicz, ed. New Rochelle (NY): The Medical Letter, Inc.; August 2004.

Three-Year-Old Girl

PAUL L. ARONSON

HISTORY OF PRESENT ILLNESS

The patient is a 3-year-old girl of Sri Lankan descent who was born in the United States. She presented to the emergency department with a fever of 105°F for the past 2 days. She complained of abdominal, knee, and elbow pain while febrile, but she was eating normally without a change in appetite and having no problems ambulating. She has had no complaint of headache, sore throat, rhinorrhea, cough, diarrhea, or vomiting. This has been a recurrent problem since 8 months prior when the family took a trip to one of the national parks. Upon returning from that trip she had her first episode of fever with a temperature to 104°F. That episode lasted 5 days. At that time she complained of a frontal headache, chills, rigors, and abdominal pain. She saw her regular pediatrician who diagnosed a viral syndrome. Her mother reports that the episodes occur at the end of every month. During her second febrile episode, she was told that the headache and abdominal pain were secondary to sinusitis with post-nasal drip and she was treated for clinical sinusitis with a 3-week course of antibiotics. She continued to have identical episodes every month. She had been treated a total of three times for acute sinusitis based on clinical diagnosis. Mom reports that she has not had any weight loss, rash, upper respiratory symptoms, cough, or joint swelling with these episodes. She has not traveled outside of the country or had any known tick bites. She has been seen by her regular doctor on multiple occasions during the episodes with normal examinations, multiple normal complete blood counts, and normal Lyme serology. She has had no tuberculosis exposure. She has had normal growth and development and is completely normal between episodes. Her mother does state that the doctor often tells her that her throat is "a little red," but all throat cultures have been negative.

MEDICAL HISTORY

The patient had a normal birth history. She has had no hospitalizations or surgeries and has allergic rhinitis. Her only medications are acetaminophen and ibuprofen during these febrile episodes. She was appropriately immunized and had a negative tuberculin skin test within the last 3 months. Her family history was negative for gastrointestinal disease, autoimmune disease, childhood illnesses, arthritis, cancer, or tuberculosis. She attended day care and the family has no pets.

PHYSICAL EXAMINATION

T 39.9°C; HR 112 bpm; RR 28 bpm; BP 106/73 mmHg

Weight 19.8 kg (95th percentile); Height 104 cm (90th percentile)

In general, the patient was talkative, pleasant, and in no acute distress. Her sclerae were anicteric, there was no conjunctival injection, and tympanic membranes were normal. The oropharynx was erythematous without tonsillar exudates, and there were no oral lesions noted. Neck examination revealed shotty cervical lymphadenopathy. Chest and heart examinations were normal. Abdominal examination revealed normoactive bowel sounds, diffuse tenderness without peritoneal signs, and no organomegaly. Neurologic examination was intact, and the skin showed no rashes or discoloration.

DIAGNOSTIC STUDIES

Complete blood count showed a WBC count of 15 800/mm³ with 64% segmented neutrophils, 22% lymphocytes, and 13% monocytes. The hemoglobin was 11.2 g/dL and platelets were 323 000/mm³. Liver function tests, basic metabolic panel, and immunoglobulin levels were all normal. Urinalysis, urine culture, blood culture, chest radiograph, rapid streptococcal antigen and throat culture, Lyme antibodies, Epstein-Barr virus and cytomegalovirus serologies, anti-nuclear antibody (ANA), stool culture, stool ova and parasites, malaria smear, CT scan of the head and sinuses, and gallium scan with triple phase bone scan were all negative. Erythrocyte sedimentation rate was elevated at 66 mm/h.

COURSE OF ILLNESS

Apart from the mild leukocytosis and elevated erythrocyte sedimentation rate, the patient's workup was negative. She became afebrile on hospital day 6 and was discharged home with close follow-up. Her complete blood count was checked two times a week for 2 months and her absolute neutrophil count was always normal. During the febrile episodes she always had an elevated white blood cell count and erythrocyte sedimentation rate that normalized when she was afebrile. The diagnosis was suggested by the constellation of symptoms including the recurrent fever and pharyngitis.

DISCUSSION CASE 7-7

DIFFERENTIAL DIAGNOSIS

Periodic or recurrent fever has several definitions in the literature. The most common features are that the fever is at least 38.4°C (some sources require higher fever of at least 39°C) and continues for 3-6 days, occurs at least three times over a 6-month period, has no identifiable etiology, is not accompanied by symptoms such as upper respiratory tract infection, and occurs at intervals that are separated by at least 1 week (and usually <4 weeks). The intervals without symptoms can be of variable duration or occur in a predictable pattern.

The causes of recurrent fever can be divided by category of diagnosis (Table 7-3) or whether the recurrences occur at irregular or regular intervals. There are several etiologies that could be attributed to recurrent fevers occurring at irregular intervals. These include infectious diseases that range from viral infections (i.e., Epstein-Barr virus, parvovirus B19, herpes simplex virus, repeated upper respiratory tract infections), bacterial infections (i.e., occult transient bacteremia, recurrent urinary tract infections, chronic meningococcemia, dental abscess, brucellosis, *Yersinia* infections, and mycobacterial infection), and parasitic infections (i.e., relapsing malaria with *Plasmodium vivax*

TABLE 7-3.	Etiologies of recurrent fever by diagnostic category.
Infectious Disorders	Recurrent upper respiratory tract infection Epstein-Barr virus Human herpes virus 6 Herpes simplex virus Parvovirus B19 Chronic meningococcemia *Borrelia* spp. Occult bacteremia (transient) Recurrent urinary tract infection Brucellosis *Yersinia enterocolitica* Atypical mycobacterium Malaria
Inflammatory Disorders	PFAPA (periodic fever, aphthous ulcers, pharyngitis, and adenopathy) Inflammatory bowel disease Behçet disease Systemic juvenile idiopathic arthritis Familial Mediterranean fever Hyper IgD syndrome Tumor necrosis factor receptor-associated periodic syndrome
Hematologic/ Oncologic	Cyclic neutropenia Leukemia Lymphoma
Miscellaneous	Drug fever Idiopathic/undiagnosed

or *ovale*, reactivation of *Plasmodium malariae*). Other etiologies of recurrent fevers that occur at irregular intervals include inflammatory diseases (i.e., inflammatory bowel disease, systemic juvenile idiopathic arthritis, Behçet disease), neoplasms such as lymphoma, and drug fevers. Viral infections and undiagnosed causes are the most common causes of recurrent fevers that occur with irregularity.

There are very few diseases that cause recurrent fevers at predictable and regular intervals. These causes include cyclic neutropenia, which usually recurs between 21 and 28 days, relapsing fever caused by *Borrelia* species, which recurs between 14 and 21 days, and PFAPA (periodic fever, aphthous ulcers, pharyngitis, and adenopathy) syndrome, which recurs between 21 and 28 days. There is also a group of hereditary causes of periodic fever that can occur at either regular or irregular intervals that should be considered. These include familial Mediterranean fever (FMF), hyper-IgD syndrome (HIDS), and tumor necrosis factor receptor-associated periodic syndrome (familial Hibernian fever or TRAPS). PFAPA and undiagnosed causes are the most common causes of recurrent fevers that occur at predictable intervals.

The clue to this patient's disease was the regularity of her febrile episodes and associated symptom of pharyngitis.

DIAGNOSTIC TESTS

Testing for recurrent fever is often extensive due to the broad differential diagnosis. As performed in our patient, testing usually includes complete blood counts which may demonstrate atypical lymphocytosis as seen in viral infections or neutropenia; erythrocyte sedimentation rate which may be nonspecifically elevated with infectious causes but may indicate inflammatory or rheumatologic conditions with significant elevations; serum viral and bacterial testing; specific testing for rheumatologic diseases such as ANA; and various imaging studies evaluating for occult infection or neoplasms such as lymphoma.

DIAGNOSIS

During one of the episodes of fever, the patient was found to have three aphthous mouth ulcers and an erythematous throat. **She was diagnosed with PFAPA syndrome (periodic fever, aphthous ulcers, pharyngitis, and adenopathy).**

INCIDENCE AND ETIOLOGY OF PFAPA

PFAPA syndrome is defined by recurrent and periodic episodes of fever (>39°C) that last between 3 and 6 days, occur approximately every 21-28 days, and are accompanied by certain clinical findings. There is a slight male predominance, and the disease usually manifests itself before 5 years of age. There seems to be no pattern of familial inheritance and no seasonal or geographic predilection. Although the etiology of PFAPA is not known, infectious and autoimmune causes have been implicated. PFAPA is considered the most common

cause of recurrent fever that occurs at regular and predictable intervals.

TYPICAL PRESENTATION

Children with PFAPA generally are well children in terms of growth and development who present with predictable patterns of fever described above. The three most common clinical findings are aphthous mouth ulcers, pharyngitis, and cervical adenopathy. The aphthous mouth ulcers are frequently missed because there are very small (<5 mm), few (usually two or three), painless, and resolve very quickly. These aphthous ulcers are in contrast to the large, painful ulcers that occur with herpes simplex virus gingivostomatitis (Figure 7-7). One case series of 94 patients found reports of associated aphthous mouth ulcers in only 70% of cases of PFAPA. Pharyngitis was found in only 72% of cases and is usually nonexudative. Cervical adenopathy is the most commonly seen sign in 88% of cases and is usually confined to the cervical region and relatively unremarkable (<5 mm nodes). While symptoms such as abdominal pain, nausea, and headache can sometimes be seen, upper respiratory symptoms are rare and usually indicate a viral upper respiratory infection. The most striking features of PFAPA are its predictable recurrence and overall wellness of the patient both during the episode and when the episode resolves.

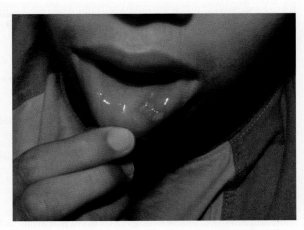

FIGURE 7-7. Herpes simplex virus gingivostomatitis.

DIAGNOSTIC RATIONALE

Diagnostic criteria that have been used are clinical in nature and include much of what has already been discussed: (1) regularly recurring fevers with early (<5 years old) age of onset; (2) constitutional symptoms without upper respiratory infection and either aphthous stomatitis, cervical lymphadenitis, or pharyngitis; (3) asymptomatic intervals between episodes; (4) normal growth and development; and (5) exclusion of cyclic neutropenia. Other fever syndromes also have characteristic features (Table 7-4).

Complete blood count. Included in the diagnostic criteria of PFAPA is the exclusion of the diagnosis of cyclic neutropenia. This distinction can be difficult as the two disorders have similar features. In cyclic neutropenia, neutropenia recurs approximately every 21 days. Although the fever in cyclic neutropenia usually occurs without accompanying infection, bacterial infection, in particular *Pseudomonas aeruginosa*, secondary to the neutropenia can occur. The best way to distinguish between the two is with a complete blood count. In PFAPA, complete blood count shows a mild leukocytosis during the episode. The white blood cell count normalizes in the absence of fever. To diagnose cyclic neutropenia, complete blood counts with differential must be checked regularly (at least twice per week for 2 consecutive months), as

the neutropenia does not always occur at the time of the fever. In cyclic neutropenia, an absolute neutrophil count of less than $500/mm^3$ is seen and it recovers on its own.

Other studies. Additional studies may be directed at other diseases in the differential diagnosis. Testing for mutation detection can be undertaken for patients with suspected TRAPS. The IgD levels are elevated in patients with hyper-IgD syndrome though several measurements may be required for confirmation. Genetic testing is also available for FMF.

TREATMENT

PFAPA usually persists for several years (>4 years) before spontaneous remission occurs. This remission begins with a period during which the episodes occur with decreasing frequency before resolving completely. During the years when the episodes occur, treatment includes supportive care and planning family events around the predictable fever. A single dose of corticosteroids at the beginning of the episode has been found to dramatically reduce the fever and should be the first line treatment. If this is not effective, prophylaxis with cimetidine can be attempted. Tonsillectomy has been found to effectively stop the episodes in some patients and can be

TABLE 7-4.	Features associated with some fever syndromes.			
Feature	*PFAPA*	*Hyper IgD*	*FMF*	*TRAPS*
Duration of fever	4-5 days	3-7 days	1-2 days	>7 days
Periodicity	26-30 days	14-28*	7-28*	None
Ancestry	None	Dutch, French	Jewish, Turkish, Arab, Armenian	Irish, Scottish
Associated symptoms	Stomatitis	Cervical lymphadenopathy	Peritonitis	Myalgias, arthralgias
	Pharyngitis	Diarrhea	Arthritis	Conjunctivitis
	Adenitis	Abdominal pain	Splenomegaly	Erythematous macules
				Edematous plaques

*Often unpredictable

Abbreviations: PFAPA, periodic fever, aphthous ulcers, pharyngitis, and adenopathy; FMF, familial Mediterranean fever; TRAPS, tumor necrosis factor receptor-associated periodic fever syndrome

considered if both corticosteroids and cimetidine are not effective. However, the risks of tonsillectomy must be weighed against the benign febrile episodes of PFAPA that usually resolve spontaneously over a period of years.

SUGGESTED READINGS

1. John CC, Gilsdorf JR. Recurrent fever in children. *Pediatr Infect Dis J*. 2002;21(11):1071-1077.

2. Long SS. Syndrome of periodic fever, aphthous stomatitis, pharyngitis, and adenitis (PFAPA)—what it isn't. What it is. *J Pediatr*. 1999;135:1-5.

3. Thomas KT, Feder HM, Lawton AR, Edwards KM. Periodic fever syndrome in children. *J Pediatr*. 1999;135(1):15-21.

4. Drenth JP, van der Meer JW. Hereditary periodic fever. *N Engl J Med*. 2001;345(24):1748-1757.

5. Burton MJ, Pollard AJ, Ramsden JD. Tonsillectomy for periodic fever, aphthous stomatitis, pharyngitis, and cervical adenitis syndrome (PFAPA). *Cochrane Database Syst Rev*. 2010;(24):CD008669.

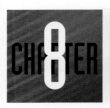

CHAPTER 8

ALTERED MENTAL STATUS

NATHAN TIMM

DEFINITION OF THE COMPLAINT

Altered mental status is a broad, nonspecific term that includes dysfunction of cognition, attention, awareness, or consciousness. Although not a defined disease, altered mental status is a symptom of an underlying disease process. The Glasgow Coma Scale provides a structured system for categorizing a child's mental status based on eye opening, verbal, and motor response. The simpler AVPU (alert, verbal, pain, unresponsive) provides rapid classification of a child's mental status. The onset of altered mental status is generally acute, chronic, or progressive and may be obvious or subtle in its presentation. This chapter will focus on the causes of acute altered mental status in children.

Although all disease processes that manifest themselves as an altered mental status are serious, life-threatening disorders must be recognized early and treated appropriately. The brain's reticulated activating system mediates wakefulness and disruption of these neurons results in an altered mental status. Infection, toxin-mediated, metabolic, and traumatic injury are the most common life-threatening disorders affecting the reticulated activating system. Unfortunately, the presentation of even the life-threatening disorders can be subtle and a high index of suspicion is necessary for proper diagnosis.

COMPLAINT BY CAUSE AND FREQUENCY

Altered mental status does not constitute a diagnosis, but it is a symptom of an underlying disease process that requires a thorough investigation.

The causes of altered mental status in childhood vary by age (Table 8-1) and may also be grouped based on the following etiologies (Table 8-2).

CLARIFYING QUESTIONS

A thorough history is necessary in any child presenting with an altered mental status. Precipitating factors and associated clinical features provide a useful framework for creating a differential diagnosis. The following questions may help provide clues to the diagnosis:

- Was there a preceding illness or fever?
  —Meningitis is a life-threatening cause of altered mental status and efforts should be made to immediately address this possibility. Toxic appearance, fever, and nuchal rigidity should prompt aggressive use of antibiotics pending cerebrospinal fluid (CSF) cultures. Rashes characteristic of varicella, *Mycoplasma pneumoniae* and Rocky Mountain spotted fever should be explored as possible causes of encephalitis. Shigatoxin release accompanying *Shigella* gastroenteritis and cerebellitis following varicella and other viral infections may result in an altered mental status.

- Is there a history of ingestion or toxin exposure?
  —Drug ingestion of only one tablet can be life threatening to a little toddler. Examples include clonidine, Beta-blockers, and calcium antagonists. Attention should be placed on defining the medications present in the home that the child has the potential to ingest. Furthermore, illness among other family members should prompt concerns of carbon monoxide. It is also important

TABLE 8-1.	Causes of altered mental status in childhood by age.		
Disease Prevalence	*Neonate/Infant*	*Toddler/School Age*	*Adolescent*
Common	Infection –meningitis –sepsis Hypoxia Hypothermia Metabolic –acidosis –hypoglycemia –hyper- or hyponatremia –hypocalcemia Trauma –birth –nonaccidental	Infection –meningitis –encephalitis –postinfectious Accidental ingestion Hypoglycemia Trauma –accidental –nonaccidental	Infection –meningitis –encephalitis –postinfectious Ingestion Hypoglycemia Trauma –accidental –nonaccidental Psychiatric
Less Common	Cardiac anomalies –decreased perfusion Seizure Metabolic disorders –hyperammonemia Hydrocephalus	Intussusception Seizure Carbon monoxide Hypertension Neoplasm Heavy metal poisoning	Carbon monoxide Neoplasm Hypertension
Uncommon	Stroke Kernicterus	Stroke Absence seizure Wernicke Subacute sclerosing Panencephalitis Central venous thrombosis	Stroke Pseudotumor cerebri Wernicke

TABLE 8-2.	Causes of altered mental status by etiology.		
Vascular	Cerebral infarction Arterial venous malformation Central venous thrombosis Hypertensive encephalopathy Decreased cerebral perfusion –congenital heart disease –anemia –hypovolemia	Metabolic	Hypoglycemia Hyper- or hyponatremia Hypoxia Hyperammonemia Diabetic ketoacidosis Uremia
		Gastrointestinal	Intussusception
Infection	Meningitis Encephalitis Sepsis Brain abscess Postinfectious Gastroenteritis (Shigellosis)	Oncologic	Primary brain tumor Metastatic CNS disease
		Psychiatric	Depression Psychosis Schizophrenia Autism
Trauma	Intracranial hemorrhage Concussion	Neurologic	Seizure Postictal Temporal lobe epilepsy Hydrocephalus Shunt malfunction Pseudotumor cerebrii
Toxins	Ethanol Carbon monoxide Anticonvulsants Methemaglobinemia Tricyclic antidepressants Heavy metals		

to remember that toxicologic screens do not test for a number of potentially harmful toxins including clonidine, organophosphates, and LSD.

- Is there a history of head trauma?
  —Head trauma at any age can present as an altered mental status. It is also important to remember that intracranial injury can present greater than 24 hours after the initial injury. Evidence of increased intracranial pressure, vomiting, severe headache, or focal neurologic examination should prompt emergent neuroimaging to rule out intracranial hemorrhage.

CASE 8-1

Three-Year-Old Boy

NATHAN TIMM

HISTORY OF PRESENT ILLNESS

The patient is a 3-year-old African-American boy who, according to his father, became unresponsive soon after he began "acting strange." The father reports that over the course of the afternoon his son complained of a headache and seemed to be sleepier. The boy regained consciousness after his father took him outside into the cold fall air. He was well prior to that afternoon and did not have any other illness. There was no witnessed ingestion. There were no sick contacts at home; however, that afternoon, both the mother and father developed nausea, headaches, and dizziness as well. The family had spent the day inside cleaning the attic, starting the furnace, and organizing the kitchen. An 8-month-old sister was taking a nap at home and did not appear to have any symptoms.

MEDICAL HISTORY

The boy had a febrile seizure at 1 year of age. He had an inguinal hernia repaired at 3 months of age. His medical history was otherwise unremarkable.

PHYSICAL EXAMINATION

T 37.5°C; RR 23/min; HR 100 bpm; BP 111/51 mmHg

Weight 50-75th percentile

Physical examination revealed an alert and playful child in no apparent distress.

There were no oral lesions. There was no lymphadenopathy. The lungs were clear and the heart sounds were normal. His neurologic examination was intact, and the remainder of his examination was also normal.

DIAGNOSTIC STUDIES

During the initial evaluation, the father revealed a key piece of history prompting a simple blood test that revealed the diagnosis.

DISCUSSION CASE 8-1

DIFFERENTIAL DIAGNOSIS

The etiology of central nervous system depression in a 3-year-old is diverse. Common causes include accidental toxin exposures including opiates, carbon monoxide, iron, sedative-hypnotics, clonidine, antihistamines, and alcohol. Metabolic disorders such as hypoglycemia, hyper/hyponatremia, and hypocalcemia should also be considered. Infectious causes such as food poisoning or postviral syndromes may cause multiple family members to experience similar symptoms. Less likely infectious causes are encephalitis and meningitis. Complex partial seizures with a brief postictal period should also be considered. The features of this case that are remarkable are the central nervous system depression that rapidly resolved when the child was taken outside and the similar symptoms present in other family members.

DIAGNOSIS

The father reported that he had turned on the furnace earlier in the day for the first time that fall. The child's carboxyhemoglobin (HbCO) value was 16.9%. **The diagnosis is carbon monoxide poisoning.**

INCIDENCE AND PHYSIOLOGY OF CARBON MONOXIDE POISONING

Accidental carbon monoxide poisoning accounts for nearly 500 deaths each year. House fires are responsible for the majority of these deaths; however, tobacco smoke, automobile exhaust, and faulty heating equipment causing incomplete combustion release carbon monoxide and contribute to accidental exposure. The gas is odorless and colorless and binds to hemoglobin with an affinity 200-300 times that of oxygen leading to tissue hypoxia (Figure 8-1). Increased minute ventilation and the presence of fetal hemoglobin make young children particularly susceptible to the effects of carbon monoxide.

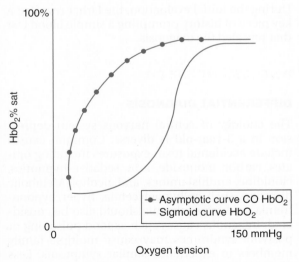

FIGURE 8-1. Oxygen/carbon monoxide dissociation curve. *(Tintinalli JE, Stapczynski JS, Ma OJ, Cline DM, Cydulka RK, Meckler GD: Tintinalli's Emergency Medicine: A Comprehensive Study Guide, 7th Edition: http://www.accessmedicine.com. Copyright © The Mc-Graw-Hill Companies, Inc. All rights reserved.)*

CLINICAL PRESENTATION

A high index of suspicion for carbon monoxide poisoning should be given to any child who is a fire victim or exposed to other devices that cause incomplete combustion. Clinical symptoms can be categorized into mild, moderate, or severe. Mild symptoms include headache, exercise-induced dyspnea, and confusion. Moderate poisoning causes nausea, vomiting, drowsiness, and incoordination. Severe intoxication leads to coma, convulsions, hypotension, and death. The classic "cherry red" skin color is rarely seen at any level of exposure.

DIAGNOSTIC APPROACH

Carboxyhemoglobin level. Carboxyhemoglobin level is the diagnostic and often prognostic test for carbon monoxide poisoning. Spectrophotometric detection methods using co-oximetry are most useful clinically because they distinguish between HbCO and oxygenated hemoglobin. HbCO levels may help stratify patients into mild, moderate, or severe intoxication; however, blood HbCO levels will fall rapidly over time and may not correlate with persistent cellular dysfunction. Mild symptoms develop with HbCO levels of 20%. HbCO levels 20%-60% present with moderate symptoms, while levels greater than 70% are often fatal.

Other studies. Anemia, myoglobinuria, and metabolic acidosis are other significant complications from carbon monoxide poisoning; therefore, complete blood count, urinalysis, electrolytes, electrocardiogram, and arterial blood gas should be obtained. Pulse oximetry is likely to be normal since it does not discriminate between the forms of hemoglobin.

TREATMENT

The antidote for carbon monoxide poisoning is oxygen. The half-life of carboxyhemoglobin is approximately 4 hours in a patient breathing room air at sea level. If that same patient is placed on 100% oxygen, the half-life of HbCO drops to 1 hour. The goal is to administer 100% oxygen until the HbCO level is less than 5%. Hyperbaric oxygen at 2-3 atmospheres further reduces the half-life of HbCO to 30 minutes; however, its routine use is still controversial. Risks from hyperbaric oxygen treatment include pneumothorax, oxygen toxicity, tympanic membrane rupture, and decompression sickness. Nevertheless, indications for hyperbaric oxygen include victims who are neonates, pregnant, or have history of coma, seizures, or arrhythmias secondary to intoxication and consultation with a hyperbaric center early on should be considered. Other management issues include correction of anemia if Hb is less than 10 g/dL to maximize oxygen-carrying capacity, decrease patient activity level with bed rest, and maintain urine output of more than 1 cc/kg/h if myoglobinuria is present, and monitoring acid-base status and treating metabolic acidosis with sodium bicarbonate if pH is less than 7.15.

Neurologic injuries such as impairment of concentration, attention, memory, and motor function occur in 25%-50% of patients with loss of consciousness or carboxyhemoglobin levels greater than 25%. These deficits may appear soon after exposure to carbon monoxide or up to 3 weeks later. These symptoms can last for 1 month or more in the most severe cases.

SUGGESTED READINGS

1. Baum CR. Environmental emergencies. In: Fleisher GR, Ludwig S, eds. *Textbook of Pediatric Emergency Medicine*. 4th ed. Philadelphia: Lippincott Williams & Wilkins; 2000:949-951.
2. Ellenhorn M, ed. *Ellenhorn's Medical Toxicology*. 2nd ed. Baltimore: Williams & Wilkins; 1997:1465-1475.
3. Morgan I. Carbon Monoxide Poisoning. In: Bates N, ed. *Paediatric Toxicology*. New York: Stockton Press; 1997:321-325.
4. Weaver LK, Hopkins RO, Chan KJ, et al. Hyperbaric oxygen for acute carbon monoxide poisoning. *N Engl J Med*. 2002;347:1057-1067.

CASE 8-2

Twenty-Month-Old Boy

NATHAN TIMM

HISTORY OF PRESENT ILLNESS

The patient was a 20-month-old African-American male who arrived by flight squad from another emergency department. The mother was on her way to the hospital and was not available; however, the squad relayed the history from the previous emergency department. The mother reported that her son had a week-long upper respiratory infection and developed a fever yesterday. Today he had four episodes of emesis and was more tired than usual. Several children in his day care have had bronchiolitis. There was a pet hamster at home.

MEDICAL HISTORY

There was no personal or family history of sickle cell disease. The child is otherwise healthy.

PHYSICAL EXAMINATION

T 37.5°C; RR 28/min; HR 140 bpm; BP 80/60 mmHg; SpO_2 85% in room air

Height 50th percentile; Weight 50th percentile

Initial examination revealed a pale appearing, lethargic child who was responsive to painful stimulation. Head and neck examination was significant for pale conjunctivae and scleral icterus. Mucous membranes were moist, and there was no meningismus or lymphadenopathy. Mild subcostal retractions were present but the lungs were clear to auscultation. The cardiac examination revealed tachycardia and a III/VI systolic ejection murmur at the left upper sternal border. There were no gallops or rubs. Capillary refill was

2 seconds and he had strong peripheral pulses. The abdomen was nondistended and soft. There was no hepatomegaly; however, a mildly tender spleen tip was palpable. The rectal examination was normal. There were no rashes, bruises, or petechiae noted on skin examination.

DIAGNOSTIC STUDIES

Laboratory analysis revealed 30 800 WBCs/mm³ with 77% segmented neutrophils, 14% lymphocytes, 7% monocytes, and 8% nucleated RBCs. The hemoglobin was 3.1 g/dL and there were 608 000 platelets/mm³. The mean corpuscular volume was 90 fL and the reticulocyte distribution width was 21. The reticulocyte count was 10.5%. The blood type was O+ with a negative direct Coombs test. Electrolytes were significant for a blood urea nitrogen of 22 mg/dL. The remainder of the electrolytes was normal. The child's glucose was 117 mg/dL and liver function tests were significant for a lactic dehydrogenase of 1250 U/L and total bilirubin of 5.2 mg/dL (direct fraction, 0.4 mg/dL). A chest radiograph showed no cardiomegaly. The urine was tea colored and urinalysis tested positive for hemoglobin. Blood and urine cultures were subsequently negative.

COURSE OF ILLNESS

The child was placed on 100% nonrebreather face mask and intravenous access was obtained. The child received 10 cc/kg normal saline. With these interventions the child's comfort level and vital signs improved with a pulse oximeter reading of 96%, heart rate of 110 bpm, and respiratory rate of 22 breaths per minutes. The results of the peripheral blood smear suggested the cause of his severe anemia (Figure 8-2). The mother arrived and provided an additional piece of information that confirmed the suspected diagnosis.

DISCUSSION CASE 8-2

DIFFERENTIAL DIAGNOSIS

The physical examination (pallor, scleral icterus, spenomegaly) and laboratory tests (anemia, elevated unconjugated bilirubin, elevated reticulocyte count) point toward the diagnosis of a

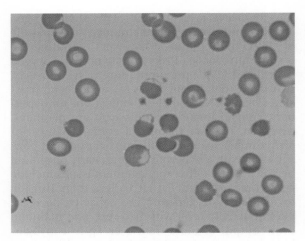

FIGURE 8-2. Peripheral blood smear.

hemolytic anemia. Hemolytic anemias can be classified into red blood cell intrinsic abnormalities or extrinsic forces acting on the red blood cell. Membrane (spherocytosis) and metabolic (glucose 6-phosphatase deficiency, pyruvate kinase deficiency) deficiencies in addition to the hemoglobinopathies (sickle cell and thalassemias) make up the intrinsic abnormalities of red blood cells that lead to hemolysis. The extrinsic causes are autoimmune hemolytic anemia, physical trauma on the red blood cell (prosthetic valve), infection (malaria) and drug/toxin (G6PD deficiency).

DIAGNOSIS

The mother provided additional information when she arrived. The child had been seen at an emergency department 4 days earlier when she found a mothball in his mouth. His hemoglobin at that time was 10 g/dL. The present blood smear showed schistocytes, blister cells, bite cells, 3+ anisocytosis, and 4+ poikilocytosis, consistent with red blood cell hemolysis (Figure 8-2). **The diagnosis of napthalene ingestion in a child with glucose-6-phosphatase dehydrogenase deficiency was confirmed.**

INCIDENCE AND EPIDEMIOLOGY

Glucose-6-phosphatase dehydrogenase (G6PD) deficiency is an X-linked enzyme disorder that affects nearly 200 million people worldwide. Kurdish Jews (60%), Saudi Arabian descent (13%), and African-Americans (11%) are most affected. The female heterozygote carrier state provides a survival advantage against malaria.

The enzyme G6PD is present in all cells in the body; however, red blood cells are most severely affected by its absence. G6PD aids in the biochemical pathway that replenishes glutathione, the chemical responsible for breaking down oxygen free radicals and peroxide. Therefore, the enzyme deficient patient is at particular risk when confronted with stressors leading to an "oxidative challenge." Fava beans, infection, and drugs such as antimalarials, sulfonamides, nitrofurantion, and naphthalene (mothballs) are the most notorious culprits leading to red blood cell damage in patients with G6PD deficiency.

CLINICAL PRESENTATION

Acute hemolytic anemia results in a child with G6PD deficiency after napthalene ingestion. Hemolytic anemia can develop as early as 1 day after naphthalene exposure. The oxidative metabolite, alpha-naphthol, causes a depletion of glutathione. The G6PD deficient red blood cell is unable to replenish the glutathione leading to hemoglobin and protein oxidation. Hemoglobin and proteins are denatured into Heinz bodies, and the red blood cell membrane is lysed. The spleen removes the Heinz body containing RBCs leading to splenomegaly and "bite cells" in peripheral smear. The destruction of the red blood cells leads to a normocytic anemia, increase in unconjugated bilirubin, increased reticulocyte production, and hemoglobinuria. The clinical features include nausea, emesis, dark urine, icterus, abdominal pain, pallor, and lethargy.

DIAGNOSTIC APPROACH

History and physical examination findings are the mainstay of the diagnosis. Additional laboratory test to help differentiate the hemolytic anemias include the following:

Complete blood count and peripheral smear. Peripheral blood smear reveals anisocytosis, poikilocytosis, schistocytes, bite cells, and occasional Heinz bodies.

Reticulocyte count. The reticulocyte count is usually elevated after hemolysis to compensate for increased red blood cell destruction.

Coombs test. Direct and indirect Coombs tests are negative in G6PD but should be performed to exclude autoimmune hemolytic anemia.

Serum haptoglobin. Binds to free hemoglobin and is decreased with hemolysis.

Hepatic function panel. Plasma indirect bilirubin, aspartate aminotransferase, and lactate dehydrogenase are elevated due to the release of intracellular enzymes during hemolysis.

Urinalysis. Increased urine bilirubin is noted. Hemoglobinuria occurs once hemoglobin binding sites in the plasma, such as haptoglobin and hemopexin, are saturated.

G6PD assay. A G6PD assay measures production of NADPH using a spectrophotometer. G6PD assay may be normal immediately after a hemolytic episode, despite G6PD deficiency, since younger red blood cells (reticulocytes) with normal levels of G6PD will have replaced the older, more deficient population. This screening test should be performed at least 2 weeks after a hemolytic episode. Additional screening tests are also available that utilize dye decolorization techniques that quantify G6PD levels as normal or deficient (<30% normal activity). The limitations of these screening tests are that they do not detect heterozygotes and are only helpful for steady-state levels; therefore, they are unreliable during or after active hemolysis.

TREATMENT

Supportive care is the mainstay of treatment. Activated charcoal and cathartics are helpful in acute napthalene ingestions. In addition, patients should avoid milk or fatty meals which would aid the absorption of the lipophilic napthalene. The hemolytic anemia may require blood product transfusion if there is hemodynamic instability. Otherwise, hemoglobin levels will return to normal in 3-6 weeks without intervention. Hemoglobinuria rarely leads to the development of renal failure in children.

SUGGESTED READINGS

1. Cohen AR. Hematologic emergencies. In: Fleisher GR, Luwdig S, eds. *Textbook of Pediatric Emergency Medicine*. 4th ed. Philadelphia: Lippincott Williams & Wilkins; 2000:859-863.
2. Desforges, J. Glucose 6 phosphate dehydrogenase deficiency. *N Engl J Med*. 1991;324:169-194.
3. Luzzato L. Hemolytic anemias. In: Nathan D, Orkin S, eds. *Hematology of Infancy and Childhood*. 5th ed. Philadelphia: WB Saunders; 1988:704-722.
4. Wason S, Siegel E. Mothball toxicity. *Pediatr Clin N Am*. 1986;33:369-374.

CASE 8-3

Nine-Year-Old Boy

JENNIFER L. McGUIRE

HISTORY OF PRESENT ILLNESS

The patient is a previously healthy 9-year-old boy who presented to his pediatrician 3 days prior to admission with complaints of headache and malaise. Crackles were noted in the right lung and he was treated with azithromycin for suspected community-acquired pneumonia. The next day he developed low grade fevers with decreased oral intake, emesis, lethargy, and weakness. His mother described him as "being out of it." His symptoms worsened over the next 2 days and he was admitted to an outside hospital with disorientation, slurred speech, diffuse weakness, drooling, and bradykinesia. A noncontrast cranial computed tomography (CT) was normal, but magnetic resonance imaging (MRI) of the brain revealed bilateral basal ganglia T2-hyperintensities without restricted diffusion. He was transferred to a regional Children's Hospital for further evaluation and management. There was no history of trauma, drug or toxin exposure, ill contacts, or any chronic changes in his behavior or school performance.

MEDICAL HISTORY

The medical history was remarkable for bronchiolitis requiring hospitalization at 3 months of age. He had a history of primary enuresis that had improved over the past 6 months. He was a third grader who did well in school. His older half-brother had attention-deficit and hyperactivity disorder, but there was no other family history of neurologic or developmental disorders. The boy had been placed in foster care at age 5; however, he had returned to live with his mother, stepfather, stepbrother, and stepsister 2 years ago.

PHYSICAL EXAMINATION

T 39°C; HR 60 bpm; RR 28/min; BP 114/64 mmHg; Oxygen saturation 94% in room air

Weight 50th percentile; Height 50th percentile

General examination revealed a pale boy with masked facies who was occasionally tearful sitting up in bed. He was oriented to person and place, but was confused regarding the date and reason for his hospitalization. He had minimal spontaneous movement. Pupils were equally round and reactive to light. There were no Kaiser-Fleischer rings and optic disc margins on undilated fundoscopic examination were sharp. Extraocular movements were full without nystagmus. Facial sensation was full and symmetric bilaterally. Facial strength was full and symmetric, but he had diminished voluntary facial movement throughout. His tongue, uvula, and palate were midline. Motor examination revealed a resting tremor in bilateral hands. He had normal tone but diminished strength throughout. Sensory examination was intact and symmetric in all four extremities to light touch, temperature, and proprioception. He had coordinated but slow movement with finger-nose-finger.

Deep tendon reflexes were normal. Babinski reflexes were downgoing bilaterally. There were no murmurs on cardiac examination. Crackles were appreciated bilaterally with diminished breath sounds at the left lung base.

DIAGNOSTIC STUDIES

Laboratory results from the outside hospital were as follows: A complete blood count (CBC) revealed a WBC count of 4600/mm³ (57% segmented neutrophils, 33% lymphocytes, 8% monocytes, and 2% eosinophils). Serum electrolytes, blood urea nitrogen, creatinine, and calcium were normal. The serum glucose was 124 mg/dL. Liver function tests were significant for an elevated lactic dehydrogenase level 228 U/L. Ammonia level was 19 mcg/dL. Serum ceruloplasmin and lead levels were normal. Carboxyhemoglobin level was normal. Urinalysis and urine tests for heavy metals were negative. Lumbar puncture revealed clear cerebrospinal fluid with a glucose of 65 mg/dL and protein of 40 mg/dL. There were 20 CSF WBC/mm³ and no red blood cells (RBC). Viral and bacterial cultures of blood, urine, and CSF were negative. CSF herpes simplex virus (HSV) and enteroviral polymerase chain reaction (PCR) were also negative. Plasma and cerebrospinal fluid (CSF) amino acids, pyruvate, and lactate were normal. The initial chest radiograph was abnormal (Figures 8-3A and 8-3B).

COURSE OF ILLNESS

The child was hospitalized. His medications on arrival included acyclovir, vancomycin, cefotaxime, and eythromycin. He was started on nasogastric feeds due to the profound weakness of his oropharyngeal muscles and difficulty swallowing. He showed no evidence of respiratory or cardiovascular compromise, although the bradykinesia and tremor worsened during the 48 hours following admission and his ability to communicate verbally deteriorated. A Parkinsonian-like clinical picture prompted initiation of amantadine. A chest CT was also abnormal and suggested a potential cause (Figure 8-3C). The results from a CSF PCR confirmed the diagnosis.

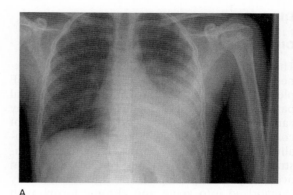

A

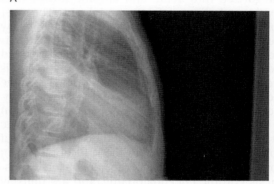

B

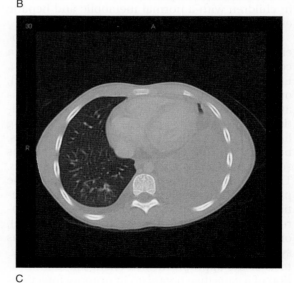

C

FIGURE 8-3. **A.** Chest radiograph, anterior-posterior view. **B.** Chest radiograph, lateral view. **C.** Chest CT.

DISCUSSION CASE 8-3

DIFFERENTIAL DIAGNOSIS

This child presented with encephalopathy, weakness, and bradykinesia, in the context of a CSF pleocytosis and MRI demonstrating focal bilateral basal ganglia T2 hyperintensities. Encephalopathy can be defined as a depressed or altered level of consciousness, lethargy, or a change in personality for more than 24 hours; this child demonstrated progressive lethargy and disorientation over 5 days. Encephalopathy in children is broadly categorized into acute and chronic forms, with toxic, metabolic, or infectious etiologies. The most notorious of the toxins causing encephalopathy are carbon monoxide and lead; however, toxic etiologies do not typically demonstrate a fever and pleocytosis, and ideally an exposure history is present. Multiple metabolic disorders that involve the basal ganglia may cause encephalopathy, including Wilson disease (copper accumulation in the brain, liver, and cornea) and pantothenate kinase-associated neurogeneration (deposition of iron-containing material in the substantia nigra); however, these are rare disorders that usually present as chronic encephalopathy, and are unlikely in children with a normal metabolic and hepatic evaluation.

Encephalitis, or inflammation of the brain associated with clinical neurologic dysfunction, is a common cause of encephalopathy in children. Encephalitis may be related to a primary infection, or may be a postinfectious immunologically mediated phenomenon. Primary infectious encephalitis is most commonly caused by viruses, including herpes simplex virus, enterovirus, or arboviruses, but may also be caused by nonviral pathogens such as *Borrelia burgdorferi* and *Rickettsia species*. The clinical diagnosis of encephalitis rests on the presence of encephalopathy requiring hospitalization, in conjunction with fever, seizures, focal neurologic findings (such as bradykinesia in this case), or other objective measures of central nervous system (CNS) inflammation (such as a CSF pleocytosis or the appropriate MRI changes). Identification of a causative organism in primary infectious cases rests on specific microbial testing in the CSF and periphery using organism-appropriate PCR and serologies. No causative agent is found in up to 65% of clinical encephalitis cases.

Mycoplasma pneumoniae, varicella, and influenza are among the few infectious agents causing pneumonia concurrently with encephalitis. Central nervous system findings in varicella more classically cause a postinfectious cerebellitis.

DIAGNOSIS

The chest radiograph (Figures 8-3A and 8-3B) revealed a moderate-size left pleural effusion and left lower lobe consolidation. The chest CT (Figure 8-3C) confirmed poorly enhancing left lower lobe consolidation with a left pleural effusion with compressive atelectasis of the left upper lobe as well as a small right pleural effusion. The child's pneumonia raised the possibility of a common etiology for both his respiratory disease and CNS disease. *Mycoplasma pneumoniae* PCR assay of the CSF and nasopharyngeal aspirate were positive. **The diagnosis of *Mycoplasma pneumoniae* encephalitis was confirmed.**

INCIDENCE AND EPIDEMIOLOGY

Mycoplasma pneumoniae, the smallest free-living organism, accounts for one-third of all pneumonias in children 5-9 years old and 70% of all pneumonias in children aged 9-15 years. Less than 0.1% of these cases have central nervous system complications. In one Toronto series of 159 children with encephalitis, *M. pneumoniae* was implicated as the etiology in 7% of children. In the California Encephalitis project, 111 (5.6%) of 1988 patients enrolled had evidence of recent or current *M. pneumoniae* infection. The median age of children with *M. pneumoniae*-associated encephalitis is about 11 years old; there does not appear to be a seasonal or gender predominance.

CLINICAL PRESENTATION

Mycoplasma pneumoniae pneumonia most commonly presents as a gradual onset of headache, malaise, fever, and rhinorrhea and progresses to cough, dyspnea, and bronchpneumonia. Extrapulmonary manifestations are commonly reported.

Systemic manifestations of infection include a maculopapular rash, erythema multiforme, and/or Stevens-Johnson syndrome. Central nervous system involvement may be related to direct CNS viral invasion (aseptic meningitis, meningoencephalitis, or encephalitis), vascular occlusion (systemic or focal cerebral vasculitis), and/or immune-mediated injury (Guillain-Barré, transverse myelitis). CNS manifestations are protean and vary according to pathogenesis. In *M. pneumoniae*-related encephalitis, symptoms commonly include encephalopathy, meningeal signs (headache, stiff neck, fever >39°C), and/or seizures. Encephalitis may occur without respiratory symptoms, or may follow onset of respiratory symptoms by up to a week. Immune mediated *M. pneumoniae* white matter injury may follow respiratory symptoms by several weeks.

DIAGNOSTIC APPROACH

Detection of *M. pneumoniae*. Diagnosis of *M. pneumoniae* infection is typically based on one of three possible findings: (1) fourfold change in serum complement fixing IgG antibodies to *M. pneumonia*; (2) positive serum IgM antibodies in combination with a positive respiratory sample PCR; or (3) positive *M. pneumoniae* CSF PCR. However, the subsequent diagnosis of *M. pneumoniae* as the definitive cause of a case of clinical encephalitis is significantly more complicated and fraught with potential difficulties. First, *M. pneumoniae* is widely prevalent in the respiratory tract in healthy patients. Therefore, when serologies are positive or an organism is isolated from the periphery in a clinical case of encephalitis, it is unclear whether that is a definitively causative source of CNS infection, or an incidental finding related to baseline population prevalence. Among the 111 patients in the California Encephalitis Project with evidence of recent or current *M. pneumoniae* infection, 85% were positive by serology alone (*Mycoplasma* IgM-positive), 11% were positive by respiratory PCR alone, and 2% had positive CSF PCR for *M. pneumoniae*. Second, if an older child or adult who has been exposed to *M. pneumoniae* in the past is reinfected, they may not mount a typical IgM response to infection. Therefore, infection may be present in

the absence of IgM antibodies. This problem is one reason why acute and convalescent serologies are helpful. Third, IgM titers may persist for months after a primary infection, therefore an elevated IgM may not indicate a concurrent infection that is causative for the clinical presentation of encephalitis. Finally, the actual pathophysiologic role of *M. pneumoniae* in the CNS is unclear. Hence, some have argued that when the organism is isolated from the CSF it may be a contaminant, and may not be clinically important. Therefore, diagnosis should be made with caution, in the context of a combination of positive tests and exclusion of alternate diagnoses.

Lumbar puncture. Cerebral spinal fluid is normal in 45%-70% of patients with *M. pneumoniae* encephalitis. Abnormalities, when present, include a mild-to-moderate mononuclear CSF pleocytosis (<100 WBCs). The CSF protein may be normal or mildly elevated, and the glucose is normal.

Neuroimaging. Cranial CT is often normal in *M. pneumoniae*-related encephalitis. However, cranial MRI is abnormal in up to 49% of cases, typically demonstrating nonspecific focal, multifocal, or diffuse edema or ischemia, enhancing lesions, or white matter lesions. MRI is most helpful to exclude other causes of encephalopathy and fever.

Electroencephalogram (EEG). EEG findings are abnormal in up to 79% of children with *M. pneumoniae*-related encephalitis. Most cases demonstrate nonspecific diffuse slowing; fewer cases demonstrate focal dysfunction or epileptiform activity.

TREATMENT

There are no clear-cut guidelines to the treatment of *M. pneumoniae* encephalitis. *M. pneumoniae* does not have a cell wall; therefore, it is resistant to penicillins and cephalosporins. Macrolide antibiotics (erythromycin, clarithromycin, azithromycin), tetracyclines, and fluoroquinolones effectively eradicate the organism in vitro, but have limited ability to cross the blood-brain barrier, and have not been demonstrated to clinically alter the course of the neurologic illness. There is anecdotal evidence that corticosteroids and intravenous immunoglobulin may be beneficial in treating CNS infection with *M. pneumoniae,* particularly in cases with prominent white matter disease, when a postinfectious immune-mediated mechanism is suspected.

Mortality rates of 8% and morbidity rates of 23% have been reported in *M. pneumoniae*-related encephalitis. Common long-term neurologic sequelae include cognitive problems, movement disorders, and seizures.

SUGGESTED READINGS

1. Beskind DL, Keim SM. Choreathetotic movement disorder in a boy with *Mycoplasma pneumoniae* encephalitis. *Ann Emer Med J.* 1994;23:1375-1378.
2. Bitnun A, Ford-Jones EL, Petric M, et al. Acute childhood encephalitis and *Mycoplasma pneumoniae. Clin Infect Dis.* 2001;32:1674-1684.
3. Bitnun A, Richardson SE. *Mycoplasma pneumoniae:* innocent bystander or a true cause of central nervous system disease? *Curr Infect Dis Rep.* 2010;12:282-290.
4. Carpenter TC. Corticosteroids in the treatment of severe mycoplasma encephalitis in children. *Crit Care Med.* 2002;30:925-927.
5. Christie LJ, Honarmand S, Talkington DF, et al. Pediatric encephalitis: what is the role of *Mycoplasma pneumoniae? Pediatrics.* 2007;120:305-313.
6. Glaser CA, Honarmand S, Anderson J, et al. Beyond viruses: clinical profiles and etiologies associated with encephalitis. *Clin Infect Dis.* 2006;43:1565-1577.
7. Koskiniemi, M. CNS manifestations associated with Mycoplasma pneumoniae infections: summary of cases at the University of Helsinki and review. *Clin Infect Dis.* 1993;17(1):S52-S57.
8. Lehtokoski-Lehtiniemi E, Koskiniemi MJ. *Mycoplasma pneumoniae* encephalitis: severe entity in children. *Pediatr Infect Dis J.* 1989;8:651-653.
9. Powell DA. Mycoplasmal infections. In: Behrman RE, Kliegman RM, Jenson HB, eds. *Nelson Textbook of Pediatrics.* 16th ed. Philadelphia, PA: WB Saunders; 2000:914-917.
10. Rautonen J, Koskiniemi M, Vaheri A. Prognostic factors in childhood acute encephalitis. *Pediatr Infect Dis J.* 1991;10:441-446.
11. Thomas NH, Collins JE, Robb SA, Robinson RO. *Mycoplasma pneumoniae* infection and neurological disease. *Arch Dis Child.* 1993;69:573-576.

CASE 8-4

Eight-Month-Old Boy

NATHAN TIMM

HISTORY OF PRESENT ILLNESS

A previously well 8-month-old male was brought to the emergency department because of increased sleepiness. The mother reports that her son was well earlier in the day, but during the last few hours she has noticed him to be extremely drowsy. Her son had two episodes of nonbloody nonbilious emesis during this period but no diarrhea. There was no history of fever, cough, or rash. The parents reported, however, that they had been cleaning the house with bleach, and although they did not witness any ingestion, his drowsiness seemed to coincide with the cleaning. There were no prescription medications in the house.

MEDICAL HISTORY

The child was full-term infant delivered via Cesarean section for fetal distress; however, the infant did well and was discharged to home after 48 hours. The pregnancy had been complicated by preecclampsia. The remainder of the past history was unremarkable.

PHYSICAL EXAMINATION

T 36.7°C; HR 133 bpm; RR 55/min; BP 118/57 mmHg; SpO_2 99% in room air

Weight greater than 90 percentile; Height 75-90 percentile

In general, the child was well-developed and appeared lethargic. He had moist mucus membranes with no oral ulcers or burns. His pupils were equally round and reactive to light. His neck was supple. Cardiac and lung examination was unremarkable. The abdomen was nontender with active bowel sounds. There were no masses. Testes were descended bilaterally and there were no hernias. Rectal examination revealed normal tone with brown, hemoccult positive stool. The neurologic examination was significant for a lethargic appearing child who moved all four extremities, had symmetric facies, and responded to painful stimulation.

DIAGNOSTIC STUDIES

The complete blood count revealed a WBC count of 7100 cells/mm³ (70% segmented neutrophils, 1% eosinophils, 23% lymphocytes, 6% monocytes); hemoglobin, 12.0 g/dL; and platelet count, 274 000/mm³. Serum electrolytes, calcium, blood urea nitrogen, and creatinine were normal. The serum glucose was 111 mg/dL.

COURSE OF ILLNESS

An abdominal radiograph suggested a diagnosis (Figure 8-4).

DISCUSSION CASE 8-4

DIFFERENTIAL DIAGNOSIS

The etiology of a depressed mental status as described in this patient is diverse; however, clues from the history and physical can lead to the diagnosis. Ingestion should be high on the list in this particular age group. Parents were concerned about cleaning products. However, household bleach, soaps, and detergents cause mainly gastrointestinal irritation resulting in vomiting and mild diarrhea. Other possible ingestions resulting in a depressed mental status include alcohol, carbon monoxide, iron, clonidine, opiates, and sedative hypnotics. Closed head injury with expanding mass lesion should also be considered in a previously well child who presents with lethargy and

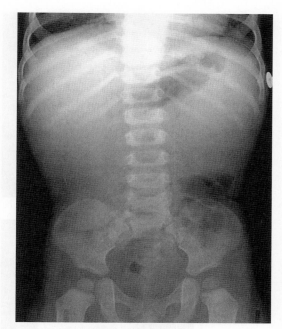

FIGURE 8-4. Abdominal radiograph.

vomiting. Although an infectious cause is unlikely given the absence of fever, early shigellosis is possible given the vomiting, abdominal pain, and hemoccult positive stool. However, shigellosis is an uncommon infection, and there is a much more common diagnosis that occurs in this age group that would explain the vomiting, hemoccult positive stool, and a depressed mental status.

DIAGNOSIS

The history of lethargy and emesis, the finding of hemoccult positive stool, and the presence of tachypnea were worrisome. The radiograph showed a paucity of bowel gas in the right abdomen as well as a soft tissue density protruding into a gas-filled loop of transverse colon. These findings were concerning for intussusception. A barium enema identified an intussusception in the mid-transverse colon that was easily reduced leading to flow of contrast into the nondilated bowel loops (see Figure 8-5). **The diagnosis is ileocolic intussusception.**

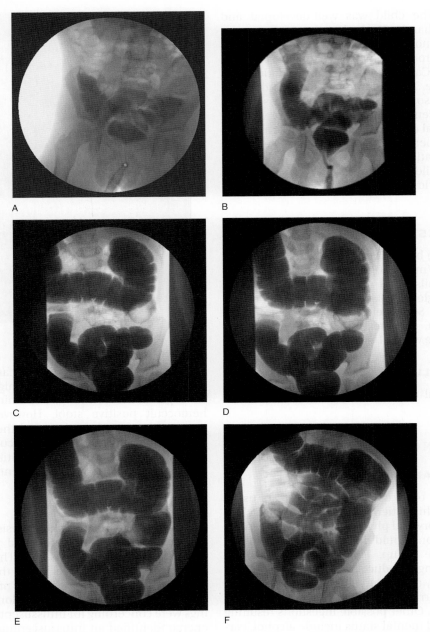

FIGURE 8-5. Barium enema. The patient is prone so the right side of the image is the patient's right side and the left side of the image is the patient's left side. The images show a sequence from contrast injection into the rectum **(A)** with flow through the descending colon **(B)**, past the splenic flexure, across the transverse colon, past the hepatic flexure **(C)** and then you see the intussusceptum **(D)** and its reduction **(E)** followed by very brisk flow to the small bowel as the insussusception is reduced **(F)**.

INCIDENCE AND EPIDEMIOLOGY

Intussusception is the most common cause of intestinal obstruction in children between the ages of 3 months and 2 years. Sixty percent occur in children who are less than 1 year old, and males are four times more likely to be affected than females. Ninety percent of the cases are idiopathic, and the most common type occurs when the distal ileum telescopes into the proximal colon. The other 10% have a lead point such as a Meckel diverticulum, polyp, or lymphoma.

CLINICAL PRESENTATION

The classic presentation of intussusception is a previously well child who develops intermittent episodes of colicky abdominal pain with "currant jelly" stools and an abdominal mass. Nevertheless, nearly 15% of children present without abdominal pain, only 40% have hematochezia, and 25% have a palpable mass. Therefore, nonspecific signs and symptoms such as vomiting, irritability, and decreased oral intake may be only indication that intussusception is present. Lethargy is a well described presenting complaint of intussusception. Although most cases described were also associated with other findings (hematochezia, abdominal mass), a high level of suspicion for intussusception must be maintained for any child presenting with altered mental status. Lethargy may be due to dehydration, shock, or cytokine release by the entrapped bowel wall.

DIAGNOSTIC APPROACH

History and physical examination findings will raise the clinical suspicion of intussusception.

Abdominal radiograph. Plain radiography is a helpful next step. Free air and obstruction can be identified on abdominal films; however, nearly 30% of patients with intussusception will have normal abdominal radiographs.

Abdominal ultrasound. Ultrasound, if available, provides a highly sensitive and specific test to diagnose or exclude intussusception. Additional benefits of ultrasound are patient safety and comfort, the ability to characterize lead points, and

make alternative diagnoses. High-risk features such as absence of blood flow and fluid within the intussusception can be detected with the use of ultrasound.

Air or barium contrast enema. If ultrasound is not available then an air or barium contrast enema should be performed for the diagnosis and treatment of intussusception. Successful reduction rates are 90% or air and 65%-85% for barium or water soluble contrast enemas. Contraindications for the use of barium contrast enema include free air on plain films or clinical peritonitis.

TREATMENT

Barium enema has been the standard diagnostic and therapeutic tool for intussusception for the past 3 decades. Success rates at reduction approach 80%, yet drop off when symptoms have persisted for greater than 48 hours. Water-soluble contrast, air, and ultrasound guided saline enemas have also been described with equal effectiveness at reduction compared with barium, yet have the benefits of cleaner methods, less radiation exposure, and reduced risk of chemical peritonitis if perforation occurs. Surgical correction is necessary if enema reduction fails. Recurrence rate of intussusception is greater in children with definable lead points. Ten percent will recur after enema reduction, while surgical correction has a 2%-5% recurrence rate.

SUGGESTED READINGS

1. Birkhahn R, Fiorini M, Gaeta TJ. Painless intussusception and altered mental status. *Am J Emer Med.* 1999;17:345-347.
2. Del-Pozo G, Albillos JL, Tejedor D, et al. Intussusception in children: current concepts in diagnosis and enema reduction. *Radiographics.* 1999;19:299-319.
3. Harrington L, Connolly B, Hu X, et al. Ultrasonographic and clinical predictors of intussusception. *J Pediatr.* 1998;132:836-839.
4. Kupperman N, O'Dea T, Pinckney L, Hoecker C. Predictors of intussusception in young children. *Arch Pediatr Adol Med.* 2000;15:250-255.
5. Losek JD, Intussusception: don't miss the diagnosis! *Pediatr Emer Care.* 1993;9:46-51.

6. Lui KW. Air enema for diagnosis and reduction of intussusception in children: clinical experience and fluoroscopy time. *J Pediatr Surg*. 2001;36:479-481.

7. Luks FI, Yazbeck S, Perreault G, Desjardins JG. Changes in the presentation of intussusception. *Am J Emer Med*. 1992;10:574-576.

8. McGuigan MA. Bleach, soaps, detergents and other corrosives. In: Haddad LM, Shannon MW, Winchester JF, eds. *Clinical Management of Poisoning and Drug Overdose*. 3rd ed. Philadelphia: WB Saunders; 1998;830-835.

9. Myllyla V. Intussusception in infancy and childhood. *Rontgenblatter*. 1990;43:94-98.

10. Sargent MA. Plain abdominal radiography in suspected intussusception: a reassessment. *Pediatr Radiol*. 1994; 24:17-20.

11. Schnaufer L, Mahboubi S. Abdominal emergencies. In: Fleisher GR, Ludwig S, eds. *Textbook of Pediatric Emergency Care*. 4th ed. Philadelphia: Lippincott Williams & Wilkins; 2000;1519-1521.

12. Wyllie R. Intussusception. In: Behrman RE, Kliegman RM, Jenson HB, eds. *Nelson Textbook of Pediatrics*. 16th ed. Philadelphia: W.B. Saunders Company; 2000: 1072-1074.

CASE 8-5

Fourteen-Year-Old Girl

NATHAN TIMM

HISTORY OF PRESENT ILLNESS

A previously healthy 14-year-old girl is brought to the emergency department after she was found semiconscious on the floor next to an open bottle. Her mother reports that she had been upset lately because her boyfriend was recently diagnosed with HIV. In the ambulance, she was uncooperative en route and refused vital signs. Although combative upon arrival, within a few minutes she became less and less responsive. Supplemental oxygen was administered. Her initial set of vitals included a heart rate of 100 bpm and a blood pressure of 100/70 mmHg. Her serum glucose was 110 mg/dL. Naloxone and flumazenil were administered without impact on her deteriorating mental status. She was now only responsive to painful stimulation. The patient required endotracheal intubation. Nasogastric lavage did not reveal pill fragments. Activated charcoal was administered via nasogastric tube. While awaiting a head CT, the patient's heart rate increased to 180 bpm and she became hypotensive. Electrocardiogram revealed supraventricular tachycardia. Her blood pressure improved after cardioversion with adenosine.

MEDICAL HISTORY

The girl's medical history was unremarkable. She had never attempted suicide. She did not take any prescription medications. Her father had a history of depression.

PHYSICAL EXAMINATION

T 39.0°C; HR 120 bpm; RR 16/min; BP 110/70 mmHg

Physical examination revealed an intubated patient who responded only to painful stimulation. Her head and neck examination revealed no evidence of head injury. There was no hemotympanum. The oropharynx was clear. Pupils were 5 mm and reactive to light. Sharp disc margins were present on fundoscopic examination. She was mildly tachycardiac without murmurs, rubs, or gallops. Lungs were clear bilaterally. Abdomen was soft with absent bowel sounds and no organomegaly. She was incontinent of stool that was hemoccult negative. Her skin examination was significant for linear excoriations on her left wrist. Her neurologic examination was significant for a Glasgow coma scale of 4 with response to deep pain only. A gag reflex was present. Babinski reflexes were downgoing bilaterally.

DIAGNOSTIC STUDIES

Complete blood count revealed a WBC count of 6600/mm^3 (54% segmented neutrophils, 35%

lymphocytes); hemoglobin, 11.4 g/dL; and 180 000 platelets/mm^3. Electrolytes were normal. Calcium, magnesium, and phosphorous were normal. Blood urea nitrogen was 8 mg/dL with a creatinine of 0.6 mg/dL. Prothrombin time, partial thromboplastin time, and liver enzymes were unremarkable. Urinalysis and pregnancy test were both negative. A urine toxicology screen was negative for drugs of abuse including phencyclidine, cocaine, amphetamines, cannabinoid, opiates, and barbiturates. Acetaminophen and aspirin levels were undetectable. Head CT was negative. Electrocardiogram revealed a QTC of 0.42 seconds with a QRS duration of 0.110 seconds.

COURSE OF ILLNESS

The patient remained endotracheally intubated and had two additional episodes of supraventricular tachycardia that responded well to adenosine. Her father arrived soon after her last cardioversion and provided the team with the identity of the bottle's contents.

DISCUSSION CASE 8-5

DIFFERENTIAL DIAGNOSIS

An open bottle next to the young lady is an important clue to the diagnosis; however, additional diagnoses beyond overdose need to be considered. Sepsis, meningitis, or encephalitis should always be considered in someone with fever and rapid mental deterioration. Furthermore, an intracranial bleed either spontaneous or from trauma should be excluded. Nevertheless, the history directs the differential diagnosis toward an ingestion. The presence of an anticholinergic toxidrome (altered mental status, increased temperature, dilated pupils, absent bowel sounds) leads to a number of possible medications: antihistamines, antipsychotics, and muscle relaxants. Ingestion of jimsonweed and certain species of mushrooms produce similar anticholinergic effects. In addition to the specific anticholinergic toxidrome, a prolonged QRS duration was present on the electrocardiogram. Class IA and IC antiarrythmics, cocaine, propranolol, and digoxin can prolong

the QRS duration. However, the father's history of depression provided the final clue to the diagnosis.

DIAGNOSIS

The father reported that his bottle of Doxepin was missing. He was taking the tricyclic antidepressant for his depression. He reported that they were 100 mg tablets and there were approximately 20 pills in the bottle.

INCIDENCE AND EPIDEMIOLOGY

Tricyclic antidepressants (TCAs) are the leading cause of death from a prescription drug overdose in the United States. Despite this propensity for significant mortality following overdose, TCAs continue to be a commonly prescribed medication in the pediatric population for disorders such as enuresis, attention deficit hyperactivity disorder, and depression. Amitriptyline, imipramine, nortriptyline, clomipramine, and doxepin constitute the most commonly prescribed TCAs. Although each is unique in clinical effectiveness, the entire group acts similarly in overdose. Ingestions of 1 g of TCA can result in life-threatening consequences in adults; however, in children only 10-20 mg/kg, or just two 50 mg tablets, can be equally devastating.

CLINICAL PRESENTATION

The clinical picture of TCA toxicity includes the following: hypotension, arrythmias, seizures, altered level of consciousness, and hyperthermia. Alpha-adrenergic blockade results in refractory hypotension—the most common cause of death from TCA overdose. Myocardial depression from sodium channel blockade results in PR, QT, and classically, QRS interval prolongation. Wide-complex tachycardia either supraventricular or ventricular in origin is characteristic of the life-threatening arrhythmia from TCA overdose. However, the most common arrhythmia is sinus tachycardia, a result of the anticholinergic properties of TCAs. Altered levels of consciousness and hyperthermia constitute the other significant components of the anticholinergic effects. Seizures may occur, usually 1-2 hours after ingestion and are usually generalized and brief. Ten to twenty percent of those with seizures will quickly go on to develop cardiovascular deterioration. The clinical picture can change rapidly with TCA overdose requiring prompt diagnosis, therapy, and monitoring.

DIAGNOSTIC APPROACH

Electrocardiogram (ECG). The most helpful diagnostic tool is an electrocardiogram.

Measurement of the QRS interval is a good prognostic aid. QRS intervals greater than 0.1 second reflect significant risk of seizure, while QRS intervals greater than 0.16 second are associated with increased risk of ventricular arrythmias. An additional ECG finding is a large R wave > 3 mm in aVR (Figure 8-6).

Other studies. Laboratory testing should be performed including electrolytes, blood urea nitrogen, creatinine, hemoglobin, prothrombin time, and a screen for additional ingested drugs. Serum

TCA levels are not helpful in the immediate management of a TCA ingestion. TCAs have a large volume of distribution with tissue concentrations exceeding blood concentrations by 10- to 100-fold; therefore, levels do not correlate well with toxicity.

TREATMENT

Patients with suspected TCA toxicity are at great risk for rapid clinical deterioration; therefore, evaluation and treatment should be started without delay, and frequent reassessment is a necessity. Attention to airway, breathing, and circulation are the critical components of the initial assessment. Mechanical ventilation may be required to secure the airway, and careful attention to perfusion and temperature is crucial. Cardiac monitoring is mandatory, and a 12-lead ECG should be performed immediately to assess for any evidence of cardiac toxicity reflected in a prolonged QRS interval, R wave height is greater than 3 mm in aVR or ventricular arrhythmias.

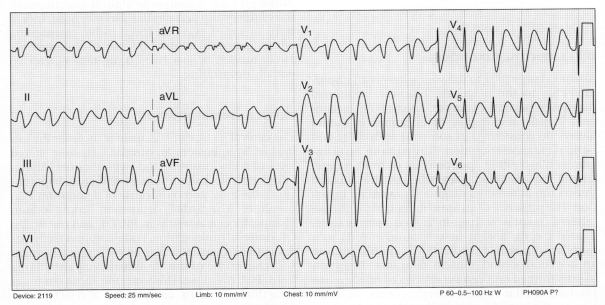

Device: 2119   Speed: 25 mm/sec   Limb: 10 mm/mV   Chest: 10 mm/mV   P 60–0.5–100 Hz W   PH090A P?

FIGURE 8-6. TCA Electrocardiogram. A 12-lead ECG of a patient who ingested a massive quantity of a tricyclic antidepressant, demonstrating QRS widening. (*Reproduced, with permission, from Knoop K, Stack L, Storrow A, Thurman RJ, eds.* Atlas of Emergency Medicine, *New York: McGraw-Hill, 2009*). (*Photo contributors: Thomas Babcock, MD and Clay Smith, MD.*)

If cardiac toxicity is evident as conduction delays, hypotension or wide-complex tachycardia, serum alkalinization with hypertonic sodium bicarbonate is the treatment of choice. Empiric treatment should not be initiated in the absence of cardiac toxicity given the potential arrhythmias, hypocalcemia, and seizures from profound alkalemia. Although the exact mechanism of alkalinization's effectiveness in treating TCA toxicity is unknown, two theories are the correction of acidosis and decreasing the pharmacologically active drug through protein binding. Nevertheless, numerous animal models and anecdotal evidence supports the use of alkalinization in reducing QRS prolongation, increasing blood pressure and reversing ventricular arrhythmias.

The goal for alkalinization is a serum pH of 7.50-7.55. This can be accomplished using 1-2 mEq/kg boluses of sodium bicarbonate (1 mEq/mL) administered over 1-2 minutes followed by an infusion of sodium bicarbonate (150 mEq of $NaHCO_3$ in 1 L of 5% dextrose in water). If arrhythmias are not responding to alkalinization, hypoxia, acidosis, hyperthermia, and hypotension should be corrected and lidocaine may be used as an antiarrhythmic. Hypotension is the most common cause of death from TCA overdose and should be managed with normal saline boluses (up to 30 cc/kg) and alkalinization. However, if the hypotension is refractory to fluid administration norepinephrine and low-dose dopamine may be effective.

Alkalinization should be continued until mental status is back to baseline, hypotension resolved, and electrocardiogram abnormalities improved. Observation for 24 hours after resolution of toxicity is appropriate. However, patients can be safely discharged to psychiatry services if they have received activated charcoal and show no signs of TCA toxicity after 6 hours of observation.

SUGGESTED READINGS

1. Harrigan RA, Brady WJ. ECG abnormalities in tricyclic antidepressant ingestion. *Am J Emer Med.* 1999;17:387-393.
2. Osterhoudt KC, Shannon MD, Henretig FM. Toxicologic emergencies. In: Fleisher GR, Ludwig S, eds. *Textbook of Pediatric Emergency Medicine.* 4th ed. Philadelphia: Lippincott Williams & Wilkins, 2000:925-927.
3. Pentel PR, Keyler DE, Haddad LM. Tricyclic antidepressants and selective serotonin reuptake inhibitors. In: Haddad LM, Shannon MW, Winchester JF, eds. *Clinical Management of Poisoning and Drug Overdoses.* 3rd ed. Philadelphia: WB Saunders; 1998:437-451.
4. Shannon M, Liebelt EL. Toxicology reviews: Targeted management strategies for cardiovascular toxicity from tricyclic antidepressant overdose: the pivotal role for alkalinization and sodium loading. *Pediatr Emer Care.* 1998;14:293-298.

CASE 8-6

Four-Year-Old Boy

NATHAN TIMM

HISTORY OF PRESENT ILLNESS

A 4-year-old African-American male presented to the emergency department with a 2-day history of fever. He awoke the day prior to admission and complained of neck pain and headache in the back of his head. She also noted that he would crawl down the stairs instead of walking and was unable to put food into his mouth. The mother also reported that he appeared confused. She asked him to bring her a hat and he returned with a book. She states that he has no history of medication ingestions, vomiting, diarrhea, head injury, or rashes. There were no ill contacts.

MEDICAL HISTORY

The boy was born at 32 weeks gestation and had a history of unconjugated hyperbilirubinemia. He had been hospitalized in the neonatal intensive care unit for 2 weeks, but did not require endotracheal intubation or antibiotics. He also had a history of plumbism with a peak lead level of 25 mcg/dL; however, a lead level 2 weeks ago was

10 mcg/dL. He did not take any medication and had no allergies.

PHYSICAL EXAMINATION

T 37.5°C; HR 110 bpm; RR 24/min; BP 100/65 mmHg

Height 50th percentile; Weight 50th percentile

In general, he was a well-appearing boy who was sitting quietly in his mother's arms. He was appropriately interactive during the examination. He had no nuchal rigidity, tympanic membranes were clear and had normal fundoscopic examination. Cardiac, pulmonary, and abdominal examinations were normal. The cranial nerves were grossly intact. He had brisk reflexes symmetrically with downgoing toes. Tone and strength were normal and symmetric throughout. The child displayed truncal ataxia while sitting and was unable to walk without assistance due to ataxia. He also had dysmetria with finger-nose-finger. A rash suggested the diagnosis (Figure 8-7).

DIAGNOSTIC STUDIES

The complete blood count revealed a WBC count of 7800 cells/mm³ (34% segmented neutrophils, 51% lymphocytes, 10% monocytes, 5% eosinophils), a hemoglobin of 12.2 g/dL, and a platelet count of 275000/mm³. Electrolytes, urinalysis, PTT, PT, ammonia, and liver function tests were normal. His serum glucose was 84 mg/dL. Head CT was negative. Cerebral spinal fluid revealed 3 WBCs/mm³ and

FIGURE 8-7. Patient's rash.

1 RBC/mm³, with a glucose of 54 mg/dL and protein of 15 mg/dL. There were no bacteria on CSF Gram stain. Lead level was 8 mcg/dL.

COURSE OF ILLNESS

The child was admitted to the hospital and treated empirically with vancomycin, cefotaxime, and acyclovir.

DISCUSSION CASE 8-6

DIFFERENTIAL DIAGNOSIS

The life-threatening causes of ataxia that must be addressed are acute bacterial meningitis, cerebellar abscess, neoplasm, and metabolic disturbances including hypoglycemia, hyponatremia, and hyperammonemia. Toxin ingestions, particularly alcohol, benzodiazepines, and phenytoin, must also be considered. Posterior fossa tumors and metastatic malignancies may present with ataxia. Guillain-Barré may also present as ataxia with lower extremity weakness in an otherwise healthy child. Infectious causes include bacterial meningitis and *Listeria* rhombencephalitis. Measles, mumps, and rubella were common precipitants of cerebellar ataxia prior to widespread vaccination. However, the vast majority of children with ataxia will fall into the postinfectious acute cerebellar ataxia. Common inciting agents are enteroviruses, influenza, Epstein-Barr virus, and varicella.

DIAGNOSIS

The next day the boy developed a puritic vesicular rash on his face and trunk. The rash consisted of clear fluid-filled vesicles with a surrounding irregular margin of erythema resembling "dewdrops on a rose petal." Several stages of the rash were present in the same area, a finding consistent with varicella (Figure 8-7). **The diagnosis is acute cerebellar ataxia secondary to varicella infection.**

INCIDENCE AND EPIDEMIOLOGY

Prior to the availability of the varicella vaccine, approximately 4 million cases of varicella occurred in the United States. Nearly 100000 hospitalizations and 100 deaths occurred each year in the

United States from the infection. Ninety-five percent of the cases occurred in people under the age of 20 years, and nearly half of the deaths occurred in children. However, the vaccine licensed in 1995 has resulted in a marked decrease in severe varicella infection in the United States. The vaccine prevents 70%-85% of mild disease and greater than 95% of severe disease.

CLINICAL PRESENTATION

Varicella is contagious 24-48 hours prior to the eruption of the rash until all of the vesicles have crusted over. The incubation period is 10-21 days and prodromal symptoms include fever, headache, and malaise. The lesions initially occur on the face and trunk and spread to the extremities. They begin as erythematous macules that evolve to form clear, fluid-filled vesicles with irregular surrounding erythema (Figure 8-7). These vesicles are classically described as "dewdrops on a rose petal." New lesions erupt as older lesions are crusting. The lesions are typically pruritic.

Varicella is usually benign and a self-limited infection and complications are rare; however, the two most common complications of varicella are secondary bacterial infections and neurologic disturbances. Group A beta-hemolytic *Streptococcus* and *Staphylococcus aureus* are the notorious causes of bacterial superinfection. Neurologic manifestations include cerebellar ataxia and meningoencephalitis. Cerebella ataxia is characterized by gait disturbance, nystagmus, and slurred speech. Signs of meningoencephalitis include seizures, altered level of consciousness, and nuchal rigidity. The neurologic sequelae usually develop 3-7 days after the eruption of the rash but, as in this case, may also appear during the incubation phase making the diagnosis difficult if there is no history of varicella exposure. The etiology of the neurologic complications is unknown; however, direct invasion by the virus and an autoimmune response are proposed theories.

DIAGNOSTIC APPROACH

A thorough history focused on possible ingestions, trauma, associated symptoms, or viral syndromes is necessary with any child presenting with ataxia. Close attention to vital signs, an altered level of consciousness, or weakness help distinguish between life-threatening and more benign causes of ataxia.

Lumbar puncture. Cerebrospinal fluid examination may be normal or reveal a mild lymphocytic pleocytosis (fewer than 200 WBCs/mm^3) and elevated protein (50-200 mg/dL).

Varicella detection. Varicella may be detected in the cerebrospinal fluid and from lesion scrapings by polymerase chain reaction (PCR). The sensitivity and specificity of PCR for detection of varicella in skin lesions are >98%. If PCR is not available, direct fluorescent-antibody staining of epithelial cells from the base of newly formed vesicles detects viral antigens and is a reasonable alternative (sensitivity, ~85%; specificity, ~90%). This rapid test readily differentiates varicella from herpes simplex virus, which can present with similar lesions. Isolation of varicella from tissue culture provides definitive diagnosis but identification requires 3-7 days. Thus, viral culture serves to confirm a diagnosis already made by clinical examination or PCR or rapid antigen testing. Varicella IgM antibody detection should not be used for clinical diagnosis since the test results in many false-positives and false-negatives.

Neuroimaging. MRI should be considered to exclude posterior fossa tumors. Neuroimaging is necessary if there is a history of trauma, focal neurologic examination, or increased intracranial pressure.

Other studies. Testing of serum and urine for toxic ingestions may help narrow the differential diagnosis. Laboratory studies including glucose and serum electrolytes are also appropriate in the evaluation.

TREATMENT

Acyclovir is the drug of choice for the treatment of varicella in high-risk patients, including neonates and immunocompromised children. Patients with disseminated varicella disease (e.g., pneumonia, encephalitis) also benefit from intravenous acyclovir. However, acyclovir is not recommended in cases of cerebellar ataxia since it does not alter the course of the illness. Otherwise healthy patients may benefit from acyclovir if the drug is initiated within 24 hours after the appearance of the initial skin lesions; however, this practice is not universally recommended.

SUGGESTED READINGS

1. American Academy of Pediatrics, Committee on Infectious Disease. Varicella vaccine update. *Pediatrics*. 2000;105:136-140.
2. Arvin AM. Varicella Zoster virus. In: Behrman RE, Kliegman RM, Jenson HB, eds. *Nelson Textbook of Pediatrics*. 16th ed. Philadelphia: W.B. Saunders; 2000:973-977.
3. Dangond F, Engle E, Yessayan L, Sawyer MH. Pre-eruptive varicella cerebellitis confirmed by PCR. *Pediatr Neurol*. 1993;9:491-493.
4. DeAngelis C. Ataxia. *Pediatr Rev*. 1995;16:114-155.
5. Gieron-Korthals MA, Westberry KR, Emmanuel PJ. Acute childhood ataxia: 10 year experience. *J Child Neurol*. 1994;9:381-384.
6. Haslam RHA. Varicella Virus Infection. In: Behrman RE, Kliegman RM, Jenson HB, eds. *Nelson Textbook of Pediatrics*. 16th ed. Philadelphia: W.B. Saunders; 2000: 1793-1803.
7. Klassen TP, et al. Acyclovir for treating varicella in otherwise healthy children and adolescents: a systemic review of randomized controlled trials. *BMC Pediatrics*. 2002;2: (abstract).
8. Skull SA, Wang EL. Varicella vaccination: a critical review of the evidence. *Arch Dis Child*. 2001;85:83-90.
9. Ziebold C, von Kries R, Lang R, Weigl J, Schmitt HJ. Severe complications of varicella in previously healthy children in Germany: a 1 year survey. *Pediatrics*. 2001;108:E79.
10. Wilson DA, Yen-Lieberman B, Schindler S, Asamoto K, Schold JD, Procop GW. Should varicella-zoster virus culture be eliminated? A comparison of direct immunofluorescence antigen detection, culture, and PCR with a historical review. *J Clin Micro*. 2012;50:4120-4122.

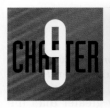

RASH

KARA N. SHAH

DEFINITION OF THE COMPLAINT

Rash is a general term applied to any acute or chronic skin eruption, and is the presenting problem or secondary complaint for 20%-30% of pediatric visits to pediatricians, emergency rooms, and primary care practitioners. Rash is variably used to describe the dermatologic manifestations of a variety of disorders, and as most rashes are benign and many are self-limiting, patients with skin complaints may receive only cursory physical examinations and overly hasty diagnoses. However, the astute clinician should remember that cutaneous findings may indicate an underlying systemic disease, and therefore all patients presenting with a rash should receive a thorough history and physical examination.

MEDICAL HISTORY

The history is vitally important in narrowing the differential diagnosis of a rash. Since cutaneous manifestations can be the primary sign of systemic disease, general questions relating to the child's overall health and review of systems are important. In particular, elicitation of a history of fever, pharyngitis, and joint symptoms can be helpful. Determination of age, gender, and racial or ethnic background may be useful, as some skin disorders are found only in particular age groups or are seen more commonly in specific subsets of the population. It is important to ask about any sick contacts, recent exposure to new medications, in particular antibiotics and antiepileptic medications, and travel and outdoor activities such as camping and hiking that might have served as a source for exposure to arthropod vector-borne infectious disease.

An understanding of the course of the rash is vital in formulating a differential diagnosis. Specific questions that will help narrow down the diagnosis include the following:

- What was the progression of the rash over time and the duration of the rash?
  —Viral exanthems often manifest predictable pattern of progression. For example, measles begins at the scalp and hairline and progresses caudally, whereas scarlet fever begins on the upper trunk. Duration may be variable, but some rashes have relatively defined duration with resolution expected within a specific time.

- What is the configuration of the rash?
  —The configuration or grouping or individual lesions is often very helpful. Linear or geometric configurations may be seen with allergic contact dermatitis. Herpes zoster presents in a dermatomal configuration. Annular configuration of vesicles and bullae are characteristic of linear IgA disease of childhood.

- Where is the rash distributed on the body?
  —If contact dermatitis is being considered, the distribution of the rash must be consistent with the areas in contact with the inciting agent. Scabies rarely involves the face, except in infants. Atopic dermatitis favors the flexural areas of the extremities in older children.

- What is the color of the rash?
  —Pigment changes can include hyperpigmenta-tion and hypopigmentation and usually indicate postinflammatory changes due to increases or decreases in melanin production or deposition. Erythema may indicate an inflammatory process or a vascular reaction.

- What symptoms are present?
  —Elicitation of symptoms, such as pain or pruritis, can be very helpful. Cellulitis is typically painful, while contact dermatitis, which is often misdiagnosed as cellulitis, is usually pruritic.

PHYSICAL EXAMINATION

Although the presenting concern may appear to involve only the skin, it is important to thoroughly examine the hair, nails, and mucous membranes (including the oropharynx and conjunctivae) in all patients. Appropriate lighting is essential, and the patient should be undressed whenever pos-sible to ensure that the entire skin surface area is examined. The skin examination should include not only a visual examination of the skin but palpa-tion as well.

When evaluating a rash, it is important to differ-entiate between primary and secondary lesions. The primary lesion is the most representative lesion and arises from the disease process itself without alteration by patient manipulation, evolu-tion of the underlying process, or by therapeutic intervention. Identification of the primary lesion is the most helpful step in creating a differential diagnosis. Secondary lesions result from changes caused by the patient, by the natural evolution of the pathophysiologic process, or by other influ-ences such as application of topical medications or secondary infection. Therefore, in any given patient, there may be lesions of different morphol-ogies, including that of the primary lesion and one or more distinct secondary lesions.

Use of correct terminology when defining the primary and secondary lesions is critical. A sum-mary of common morphologic terms is provided in Table 9-1. A *macule* is a flat, nonpalpable lesion less than 1 cm in greatest diameter, while a *patch* is a flat lesion greater than 1 cm in diameter. *Pap-ules* are raised lesions less than 0.5 cm in diame-ter. *Nodules* are larger raised lesions greater than

0.5 cm in diameter, while *tumors* are even larger nodules, generally over 2 cm in diameter. *Plaques* are well-circumscribed, raised but flat-topped lesions with a diameter usually greater than the height. *Wheals* are raised, edematous papules and plaques that are transient in nature. *Vesicles* are raised, fluid-filled lesions less than 1 cm in diam-eter, while *bullae* are similar but greater than 1 cm in diameter. *Pustules* are raised well-demarcated lesions containing purulent material. *Cysts* are cir-cumscribed tumors which may be fluid filled or solid. *Erythema* refers to an area of blanchable red-ness. *Telangiectasia* are small, superficial, blanch-able dilated capillaries. *Petechiae* are caused by the leakage of blood into the skin from damaged capil-laries and appear as pinpoint areas of nonblanch-able erythema. *Purpura* is the leakage of blood into the skin such as may occur from damage to larger blood vessels and appears as either nonblanch-able red-to-violaceous patches (nonpalpable) or papules and plaques (palpable). *Burrows* are linear papules caused by the movement of parasites in the superficial layers of the skin. *Annular* lesions present as round patches or plaques with central clearing, whereas *arciform* lesions are arc-like or semicircular; both may be seen in urticaria.

Secondary lesions include *scales*, which repre-sent accumulation of dried layers of squamous cells. Scales can appear greasy, yellow, white, or silvery. *Crusts* are composed of dried exudate, which may be hemorrhagic. *Erosions* represent denuded epidermis, while *ulcers* signify damage of the dermis and/or subcutaneous tissue. *Exco-riations* are usually caused by scratching, and are linear erosions. *Fissures* are linear clefts involving the epidermis and dermis. *Lichenification* refers to an exaggeration of skin markings that result from chronic skin rubbing or scratching. A *scar* results from the development of dermal fibrosis that occurs after injury. *Hyperkeratosis* describes the development of thick and adherent scale. *Atrophy* is the loss or thinning of the epidermis or dermis and often presents as depressed areas of skin with translucency and/or a cigarette paper-like appear-ance. Additionally, there are two terms that define a constellation of findings rather than primary or secondary lesions. *Eczematous* lesions are ery-thematous, inflammatory patches, and plaques that have poorly defined borders and, when acute,

TABLE 9-1. Common morphologic patterns of dermatologic disease.

Morphology	Description	Examples
Primary lesions		
Macule	A flat lesion < 1 cm in diameter	Leukocytoclastic vasculitis
Papule	A raised lesion < 1 cm in diameter	Molluscum contagiosum
Patch	A flat lesion > 1 cm in diameter	Erythema chronicum migrans (Lyme disease)
Plaque	A raised lesion with a flat top > 1 cm in diameter	Verucca vulgaris

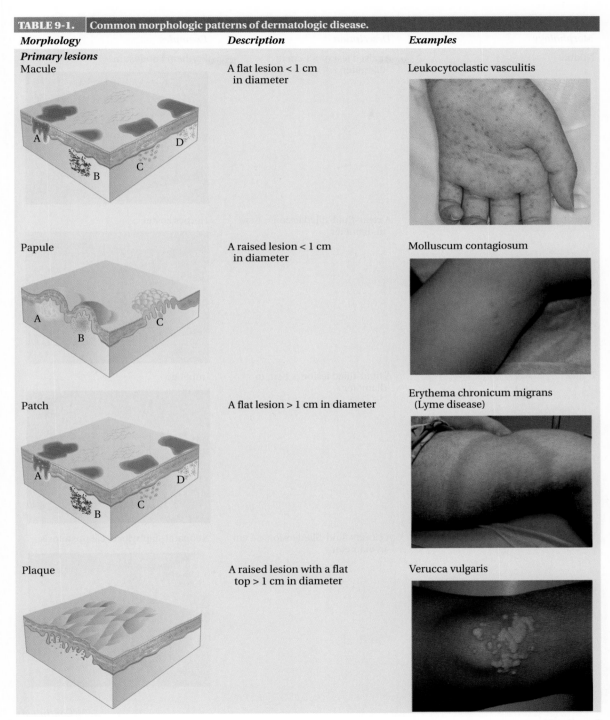

(*Continued*)

TABLE 9-1.	Common morphologic patterns of dermatologic disease. (Continued)	
Morphology	**Description**	**Examples**
Nodule	A raised lesion > 1 cm in diameter	Erythema nodosum
Vesicle	A clear-fluid-filled lesion < 1 cm in diameter	Herpes zoster
Bullae	A fluid-filled lesion > 1 cm in diameter	Impetigo
Pustule	A cloudy fluid-filled lesion < 1 cm in diameter	Neonatal staphylococcal pustulosis

(Continued)

TABLE 9-1.	Common morphologic patterns of dermatologic disease. (Continued)	
Morphology	*Description*	*Examples*
Erosion	A loss of the epidermis (superficial)	Streptococcal intertrigo
Wheal	A transient edematous lesion, often with blanching or pallor centrally with surrounding erythema	Urticaria
Ulcer	A loss of the epidermis and part of the dermis and sometimes the subcutis (deep)	Echthyma gangrenosum
Fissure	A linear cleft or ulcer	Angular chelistis (*Candida albicans*)

(Continued)

TABLE 9-1.	Common morphologic patterns of dermatologic disease. (Continued)	
Morphology	*Description*	*Examples*
Erythroderma 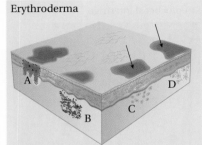	Confluent erythema resulting from vasodilation or capillary leak	Toxic epidermal necrolysis 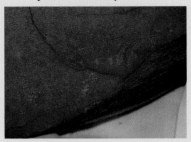
Purpura 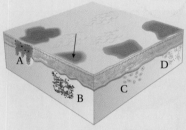	Nonblanchable erythema or violaceous areas	Cutaneous vasculitis 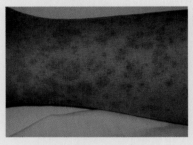
Excoriation 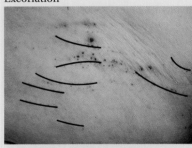	A superficial abrasion, often self-induced from scratching	Scabies 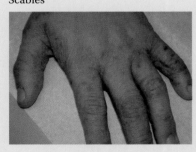
Scale 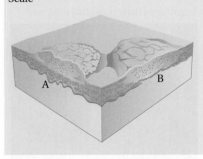	Superficial epidermal desquamation	*Tinea faciei* 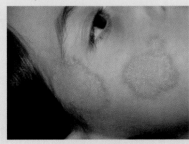

(Continued)

TABLE 9-1. Common morphologic patterns of dermatologic disease. (Continued)

Morphology	Description	Examples
Crust	Dried exudate	Impetigo
Atrophy	Thinning of the skin that may involve the epidermis, dermis, or subcutis; may present with hypopigmentation and a fine, wrinkled appearance to the epidermis	Lichen sclerosis et atrophicus
Lichenification	Accentuation of normal skin markings with epidermal thickening and hyperpigmentation; results from chronic rubbing or scratching	Chronic atopic dermatitis
Shape and configuration		
Individual	Singly dispersed lesions	Ecthyma, *S. aureus*

(Continued)

TABLE 9-1.	Common morphologic patterns of dermatologic disease. (Continued)

Morphology	*Description*	*Examples*
Grouped	Multiple similar lesions present within a localized area	Herpes simplex virus infection
Annular	Ring-shaped	Urticaria
Targetoid	"Bulls-eye" appearance with central dusky zone surrounded by a ring of pallor (edema) and a peripheral rim of erythema	Erythema multiforme
Serpiginous	A wavy, linear grouping of lesions	Cutaneous larva migrans

(Continued)

TABLE 9-1. | Common morphologic patterns of dermatologic disease. (Continued)

Morphology	Description	Examples
Arcuate	Incomplete rings and arcs	Urticaria
Polycyclic	Linked ring-shaped lesions	Urticaria
Dermatomal	Confined to one or more areas of cutaneous sensory nerve innervation	Herpes zoster

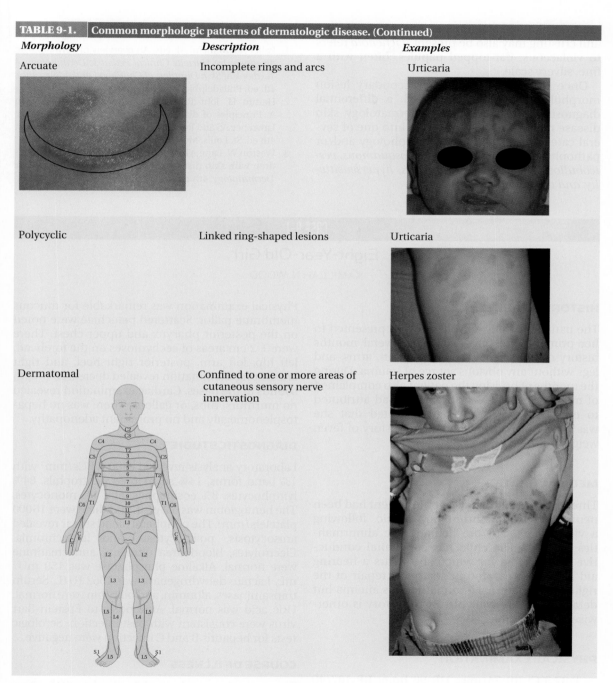

Reprinted with permission from Rash. In: Shah SS, eds. *Pediatric Practice: Infectious Diseases.* New York, NY: McGraw-Hill; 2008:108-119.

may develop vesiculation and exudate. Scaling and crusting may also be present. *Lichenoid* refers to violaceous, flat-topped papules, often with a fine, silvery scale.

Once the primary and any secondary lesion morphology has been identified, a differential diagnosis can be generated. In dermatology, skin disease may be broadly classified into one of several categories as defined by morphology and/or pathophysiology, including *papulosquamous, vesicobullous, exfoliative, eczematous, hypersensitivity, and vascular dermatoses.*

SUGGESTED READINGS

1. Paller AS, Mancini AJ, eds. An overview of dermatologic diagnosis. In: *Hurwitz Clinical Pediatric Dermatology: A Textbook of Skin Disorders of Childhood and Adolescence.* 4th ed. Philadelphia: W. B. Saunders Company; 2011:1-9.
2. Hamm H, Johr R, Ersoy-Evans S, Hernandez-Martin A. Principles of diagnosis in pediatric dermatology. In: Lawrence AS and Ronald CH, eds. *Pediatric Dermatology.* 4th ed. St. Louis: Mosby Elsevier; 2011:69-114.
3. Weston W, Lane AT, Morelli JG, eds. Evaluation of children with skin disease. In: *Color Textbook of Pediatric Dermatology.* 4th ed. St. Louis: Mosby; 2007:11-24.

CASE 9-1

Eight-Year-Old Girl

KAMILLAH N. WOOD

HISTORY OF PRESENT ILLNESS

The patient is an 8-year-old girl who presented to her primary care physician with several months history of bruising of the chest, groin, arms, and legs without any obvious source of trauma. During the months of bruising the patient also complained of mild leg pain, which the family had attributed to excessive exercise. A relative noted that she was increasingly pale. She had no history of fever, weight loss, or night sweats.

MEDICAL HISTORY

Three years prior to this visit the patient had been neutropenic and thrombocytopenic following a viral illness, but the hematologic abnormalities resolved. The child has congenital conductive hearing loss for which she wears a hearing aid in the left ear and had surgical repair of the right ear. A maternal grandfather has anemia but details were not available. Birth history is otherwise unremarkable.

PHYSICAL EXAMINATION

T 37.3°C; RR 24/min; HR 96 bpm; BP 107/46 mmHg

Height 5-10th percentile; Weight 5-10th percentile

Physical examination was remarkable for mucous membrane pallor. Scattered petechiae were noted on the posterior pharynx and upper chest. There were 1-2 cm areas of ecchymoses on the forehead, left hip, left arm, posterior right heel, and right knee. Lung examination revealed decreased breath sounds at the bases. Cardiac examination revealed no murmurs, rubs, or gallops. There was no hepatosplenomegaly and no prominent adenopathy.

DIAGNOSTIC STUDIES

Laboratory analysis revealed 2300 WBCs/mm³ with 1% band forms, 14% segmented neutrophils, 84% lymphocytes, 8% eosinophils, and 1% monocytes. The hemoglobin was 6.2 g/dL and there were 16000 platelets/mm³. The peripheral blood smear revealed anisocytosis, poikilocytosis, and hypochromia. Electrolytes, blood urea nitrogen, and creatinine were normal. Alkaline phosphatase was 159 mU/mL. Lactate dehydrogenase was 1062 IU/L. Serum transaminases, albumin, and bilirubin were normal. Uric acid was normal. Antibodies to Epstein-Barr virus were consistent with past infection. Serologic tests for hepatitis B and C infection were negative.

COURSE OF ILLNESS

The patient was admitted to the hospital where bone marrow biopsy (Figure 9-1) and a hematologic test were diagnostic for the patient's condition.

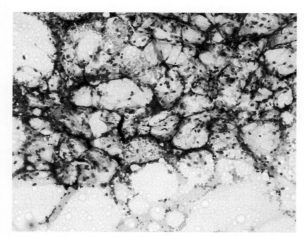

FIGURE 9-1. Bone marrow biopsy. *(Photo courtesy of Marybeth Helfrich, MT, ASCP.)*

DISCUSSION CASE 9-1

DIFFERENTIAL DIAGNOSIS

Bruising and petechiae are types of vascular rashes. Because of the location of the lesions in areas where accidental trauma was unlikely, first on the differential in this age child would be coagulation disorders such as leukemia or immune thrombocytopenic purpura (ITP). Leukemia is possible given the bone complaints and pancytopenia. ITP is an acute and self-limited illness presenting with bruising and petechiae 2-4 weeks after a minor illness. The timing of this patient's symptoms and the effect on all three cell lines rather than on the platelets alone makes ITP unlikely. Because of the slow evolution of her illness and the lack of other systemic symptoms, acute illness causing vasculitis would also be less likely. It is the fact that all three cell lines were affected which caused clinicians to suspect a congenital or acquired aplastic anemia.

DIAGNOSIS

Bone marrow biopsy revealed a markedly hypocellular marrow with only rare hematopoietic cells (Figure 9-1). There was also stromal edema and focal hemosiderosis. Peripheral blood lymphocytes were cultured in the presence of diepoxybutane (DEB),

an alkylating agent. The DEB test was considered positive by the presence of consistent chromosomal abnormalities. This indicated the diagnosis of **Fanconi anemia, or congenital aplastic anemia**.

INCIDENCE AND EPIDEMIOLOGY OF FANCONI ANEMIA

Fanconi anemia is transmitted in an autosomal recessive inheritance pattern. More than 600 cases have been reported in many ethnic groups since the disorder was first described by Professor Fanconi in Switzerland in 1927, but is seen in higher frequency among Ashkenazi Jews. Scientists have identified 15 Fanconi anemia or Fanconi anemia-like genes. Although usually transmitted as an autosomal recessive fashion, there is one gene that is X-linked. It is estimated that approximately 1000 persons worldwide are living with Fanconi anemia, and genetic counseling and testing is recommended for families that may be carriers.

CLINICAL PRESENTATION OF FANCONI ANEMIA

There are three features of Fanconi anemia: chromosome breakage, pancytopenia, and congenital anomalies (Table 9-2). Although chromosomal breakage and pancytopenia are universal features of the disease, congenital anomalies and resultant dysmorphic features are not. Over one-half

TABLE 9-2.	Congenital abnormalities of Fanconi anemia.
Developmental delay	
Microcephaly	
Microphthalmia	
Ear malformations, hearing loss	
Cardiac murmur	
Skin hyperpigmentation	
Renal malformations	
Hypospodias, cryptorchidism	
Scoliosis, thumb abnormalities (supernumery thumb, absent thumb), absent radius, congenital hip dislocation, short stature	

of patients with Fanconi anemia have skeletal abnormalities including thumb abnormalities or absence of the radii, and one-third have renal abnormalities. Other findings in some include short stature and hyperpigmentation. In this case, the absence of obvious congenital anomalies led to delays and difficulties in the diagnosis.

Although genetically determined, pancytopenia does not usually present until after 5 years of age. The onset of progressive bone marrow failure is initially manifested by petechiae and ecchymosis secondary to thrombocytopenia between ages 2 and 22 (mean age 7 years). Anemia and neutropenia develop later. In addition to the cytopenias, recent studies have also identified specific immune dysfunctions with patients with Fanconi anemia, including deficits in natural killer cell function.

DIAGNOSTIC APPROACH

Complete blood count. Disordered erythropoesis is demonstrated by macrocytosis and elevated levels of fetal hemoglobin before marrow failure. Thrombocytopenia is usually noted at presentation with pancytopenia ultimately developing.

Bone marrow biopsy. Serial bone marrow aspirates show progressive hypocellularity and finally frank aplasia.

Chromosomal breakage test. The laboratory diagnosis is made by finding an increased incidence of chromosome breakage induced by alkylating agents, such as nitrogen mustards, mitomycin C, and diepoxybutane (DEB), as in this case. Fanconi anemia cells are characteristically hypersensitive to these DNA cross-linking agents, with new testing developments allowing for testing on fetal blood, chorionic villus, and amniotic cells, offering prenatal diagnosis. An increased incidence of spontaneous chromosome breakage is seen in these patients.

TREATMENT

Supportive therapy including transfusions of erythrocytes and platelets are only of temporary benefit. In the past, 75% of these patients died within 2 years of diagnosis. Therapy administered with pharmacologic doses of androgenic hormones give hematologic benefit in more than two-thirds of the patients and may be maintained for several years. However, complications of androgenic therapy are common and most patients eventually become refractory to therapy. Bone marrow transplantation has been successful and curative in patients who find a successful donor match.

SUGGESTED READINGS

1. De Kerviler E, Guermazi A, Zagdanski AM, Gluckman E, Frija J. The clinical and radiological features of Fanconi's anaemia. *Clin Radiol.* 2000;55:340-345.
2. Giampietro PF, Davis JG, Auerbach AD. Fanconi's anemia. *N Engl J Med.* 1994;330:720-721.
3. Joenje H, Patel KJ. The emerging genetic and molecular basis of Fanconi's anaemia. *Nature Rev Genetics.* 2001;2:446-457.
4. Martin PL, Pearson HA. Hypoplastic and aplastic anemias. In: McMillan JA, DeAngelis CD, Feigin RD, Warshaw JB, eds. *Oski's Pediatrics: Principles and Practice.* 3rd ed. Philadelphia: Lippincott Williams & Wilkins; 1999:1459-1460.
5. Woods CG. DNA repair disorders. *Arch Dis Child.* 1998;78:178-184.
6. Su X, Huang J. The Fanconi anemia pathway and DNA interstrand cross-link repair. *Protein Cell.* 2011;704-711.
7. Kiato H, Takata M. Fanconi anemia: a disorder defective in the DNA damage response. *Int J Hematol.* 2011; 93(4):417-424.
8. Myers KC, Bleesing JJ, Davies SM, et al. Impaired immune function in children with Fanconi anemia. *Br J Haematol.* 2011;154(2):234-240.
9. Glanz A, Fraser FC. Spectrum of anomalies in Fanconi anaemia. *J Med Genetics.* 1982;19:412-416.

CASE 9-2

Eleven-Week-Old Girl

JOANNE N. WOOD

HISTORY OF PRESENT ILLNESS

The patient, an 11-week-old Caucasian girl, presented for evaluation of unexplained bruising. Her mother reported that she had noticed several small purple bruises on her right arm and a linear bruise across her left cheek at 3 weeks of age. Her mother noted linear and circular bruises along her buttocks and legs at 5 weeks of age. Her mother denied any history of trauma that may have caused the bruises. Laboratory evaluation at that time included a complete blood count, prothrombin time (PT), activated partial thromboplastin time (aPTT), international normalized ratio (INR), thrombin time (TT), von Willebrand factor activity, von Willebrand factor antigen, and factor VIII. All test results were in the normal range.

At 11 weeks of life the patient was brought to the emergency department after her mother again noted her to have purple, red lesions on her face and back. Her mother reported that she noticed the marks that evening after she returned home from work and bathed the infant. Her father reported that she had been unusually fussy during the day and cried whenever she was picked up. She also had decreased oral intake during the day. There was no recent history of fever, vomiting, or diarrhea, and no history of trauma. Immunizations had been given 2 days prior.

MEDICAL HISTORY

The child was the full term, 3500 g product of an uncomplicated pregnancy. She was delivered vaginally without complication. She did not have a history of prolonged bleeding from her umbilical stump. She had been evaluated for the bruising at her pediatrician's office at 3 and 5 weeks of age. Her pediatrician had performed a full physical examination at that time and noted no other abnormalities or signs of injuries. Her pediatrician had referred her to a hematologist who had performed the laboratory evaluation detailed above. Family history is significant for an uncle with frequent nosebleeds and a first cousin who was born with a "platelet problem" requiring platelet transfusion at birth. Social history reveals that she lives at home with her mother, father, and a pet cat. Her father cares for her while her mother is at work.

PHYSICAL EXAMINATION

T 37.0°C; RR 43/min; HR 180 bpm; BP 113/53 mmHg

Height 50th percentile; Weight 50th percentile

Physical examination revealed an alert infant who was calm while lying still in the crib but cried when picked up. Her anterior fontanel was flat and soft. Pupils were equal and reactive to light. Cardiac examination revealed tachycardia but no murmurs, rubs, or gallops. Lung examination was clear. Her abdomen was soft and nontender without hepatosplenomegaly. No prominent adenopathy. Her skin examination was remarkable for a hemangioma of the left occiput, a hematoma of the tip of the tongue and two ecchymotic areas on the right mandible, each about 1 cm in diameter. She had three 3-4 cm ecchymotic areas on the left back. Neurologically she was moving all extremities and had normal tone. No tenderness or deformity was noted with palpation of her extremities. Palpation of her left chest caused her to cry and elicited crepitus which felt like rough surfaces grinding. The rest of her examination was normal.

DIAGNOSTIC STUDIES

Laboratory analysis revealed 18 800 WBCs/mm^3 with 39% segmented neutrophils, 49% lymphocytes, and 11% monocytes. The hemoglobin was 11.4 g/dL and there were 406 000 platelets/mm^3. Prothrombin and partial thromboplastin times were normal. Electrolytes, blood urea nitrogen, and creatinine were normal. Alkaline phosphatase was 270 mU/mL. Other liver function studies were ALT, 100 IU/L; AST, 220 IU/L; and GGT, 46 IU/L.

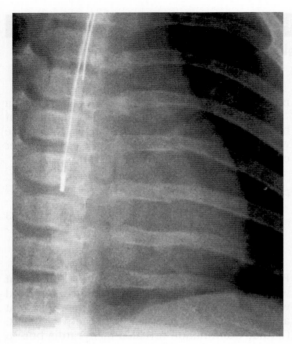

FIGURE 9-2. Chest radiograph.

COURSE OF ILLNESS

Examination of the chest radiograph (Figure 9-2), in conjunction with the clinical examination, suggested a diagnosis. Patient was admitted to the intensive care unit for further evaluation and management.

DISCUSSION CASE 9-2

DIFFERENTIAL DIAGNOSIS

The differential diagnosis of "bruises" in a young infant includes dermatologic conditions, hematologic, and oncologic diseases, connective tissue disorders, vasculitis, folk remedies, and trauma (Table 9-3).

Dermatologic conditions that may be mistaken for bruises include dermal melanosis or Mongolian spots which are characterized by blue-gray macules. Lesions typically have less distinct borders than bruises and do not appear inflamed. Unlike bruises, dermal melanosis lesions will remain unchanged in color and size over days to weeks. The red-purple color of a superficial hemangioma may also be mistaken for a bruise but can be distinguished by its typical pattern of rapid growth for the first 6 months of life, then a slowing of growth until 12-18 months, followed by involution. Other dermatologic conditions that may be mistaken for bruises are phototoxic reactions to psoralens (a chemical in citrus fruits) and other plants and photoallergic reactions to bergamot which may be found in perfumes. The locations of these lesions, the child's age, and the lack of contact with psoralens or bergamots made such a diagnosis unlikely.

Hematologic disorders both inherited and acquired can lead to bruising in infants following minor trauma or even in the absence of trauma and were considered in this case. The type and pattern of bruising and bleeding may suggest a particular hematologic disorder. A history of easy bruising, epistaxis, gingival bleeds, and menorrhagia may suggest Von Willebrand disease, the most common inherited bleeding disorder. Male children with hemophilia (Factor VIII and IX deficiency) may have a history of excessive bleeding following circumcision, present with bleeding into the muscles and joints and have a prolonged PTT. Infants who did not receive appropriate vitamin K supplementation following birth are at increased risk for developing vitamin K deficiency bleeding (VKDB) and will have a prolonged PT and possibly prolonged PTT. Idiopathic thrombocytopenic purpura (ITP), an acute and usually self-limited illness that presents with bruising and petechiae, could be considered in the differential but is excluded in this case due to the normal platelet count. Disseminated intravascular coagulation (DIC) is unlikely in this case given the several week time frame over which the bruises occurred, well appearance of the infant, lack of signs of associated illness and normal coagulation studies, and platelet count. Several other less common hematologic disorders including platelet function defects, factor deficiencies (VII, X, XI, and XIII), $\alpha2$-antiplasmin deficiency and fibrinogen deficiencies may cause easy bruising. Many, but not all, of these hematologic disorders will cause abnormalities in the screening coagulation studies this infant underwent. Oncologic diseases including leukemia can present with

TABLE 9-3.	Differential diagnosis of bruises in infants and young children.
Disease	*Key Features*
Bleeding Disorders: Inherited and Acquired	
Hemophilia	• Factor VIII and IX deficiency • Male children with excessive bleeding after circumcision • Bleeding into the muscles and joints • Prolonged PTT
Idiopathic Thrombocytopenic Purpura	• Acute, usually self-limited illness with bruising and petechiae • Low platelet count
Disseminated Intravascular Coagulation (DIC)	• Secondary to other illness • Prolonged coagulation studies, decreased platelet count, reduced fibrinogen, and elevated d-dimers
Vitamin K Deficiency Bleeding (VKDB)	• Lack of appropriate vitamin K supplementation after birth • Prolonged PT +/- prolonged PTT • Early onset presents within 24 hours after birth. Related to in utero medication exposures • Classic onset VKDB presents at 1-7 days of life • Late-onset VKDB presents between 2 weeks-6 months with bruising, gastrointestinal bleeding, and intracranial hemorrhage • May occur in patients with liver dysfunction, or cystic fibrosis or after ingestion of warfarin
Von Willebrand Disease	• Most common inherited bleeding disorder. Can vary in severity • Family history: easy bruising, epistaxis, gingival bleeds, menorrhagia
Other Less Common Disorders	• Platelet function defects, factor deficiencies (VII, X, XI, and XIII), α2-antiplasmin deficiency and fibrinogen deficiencies • Not all cause abnormalities in screening coagulation studies
Dermatologic Conditions	
Dermal Melanosis (Mongolian spots)	• Blue-gray macules often located on the buttocks • Most common in black, Latino, Asian, and Native American infants • Less distinct borders than bruises and do not appear inflamed • Remain unchanged in color and size over days to weeks • May fade during childhood
Phototoxicity: Psoralens	• Chemical in citrus fruits and other plants • Erythematous or purple marks, erosions, blisters, and hyperpigmented regions may occur after exposure to sunlight
Photoallergy: Bergamot	• Chemical which may be found in perfume • Blisters and hyperpigmented lesions occur after exposure to sunlight
Hemangioma	• Benign congenital vascular neoplasm • Superficial hemangiomas composed of purple/red telangiectatic macules and papules • Deep hemanigiomas may appear as poorly defined bluish nodules • Rapid growth for the first 6 months of life, then slowing of growth until 12-18 months, followed by involution
Connective Tissue	
Elhers-Danlos Syndrome	• Congenital defect in collagen synthesis • Skin hyperextensibility, joint hypermobility, and skin fragility • Bruising and lacerations can occur after minor trauma

(Continued)

TABLE 9-3.	Differential diagnosis of bruises in infants and young children. (Continued)
Disease	**Key Features**
Folk Remedies	
Cao Gio (coin rolling)	• Used in Southeast Asia • Back or chest is coated with ointment and rubbed with an object • Linear petechiae and purpura
Cupping	• Alcohol-soaked cotton ball is ignited in a cup to form a vacuum and then the cup is applied to the skin • Circular areas of erythema, petechiae, and occasionally burns
Moxibustion	• A rolled moxa herb is ignited, placed on the skin, and allowed to burn • Areas of redness and possibly burns
Oncologic Disorders	
Leukemia, Neuroblastoma, etc.	• May have easy bruising • Bilateral periorbital bruising can occur with neuroblastoma • Systemic symptoms • Abnormal CBC
Trauma	
Accidental	• Common in ambulatory children • Typically over bony prominences • Accompanied by a history of trauma
Child Abuse	• Bruises in nonambulatory infants without verifiable history of trauma • Bruises to torso, neck, ears, and over soft tissue areas • Patterned bruises
Self-harm	• Child with history of self-injurious behavior • Injuries on areas of body accessible to child
Vasculitis	
Henoch-Schönlein Purpura (HSP)	• Most commonly occurs in children 2-7 years old • Palpable purpura on buttocks and extensor surfaces of extremities • Arthritis and abdominal pain • May have elevated ESR and platelets, hematuria, and proteinuria

bruising but are less likely in this case based on the normal complete blood count and lack of other symptoms.

Elhers-Danlos syndrome is a congenital defect in collagen synthesis characterized by skin hyperextensibility, joint hypermobility, and skin fragility which may lead to cutaneous injury including bruising and lacerations following minor trauma. Henoch-Schönlein purpura (HSP), a vasculitis that most commonly occurs in children 2-7 years old, causes palpable purpura that may be confused with bruises.

Although there is a broad differential for the causes of bruises, trauma and nonaccidental trauma must be considered in a young nonambulatory child presenting with bruises.

DIAGNOSIS

Chest radiograph revealed fractures of the left 6th and 7th posterior ribs (Figure 9-2). A complete skeletal survey was performed which revealed metaphyseal fractures of the left distal femur, left proximal tibia, and right distal radius. A computed tomography (CT) of the head demonstrated bilateral chronic and acute subdural hemorrhages. Ophthalmologic examination showed multiple intraretinal hemorrhages in both eyes. **The diagnosis was child abuse.** The parents denied any knowledge of trauma to the child and reported they were the sole caretakers. A report was made to child protective services (CPS), prompting an investigation.

INCIDENCE AND EPIDEMIOLOGY OF CHILD ABUSE AND BRUISES FROM ABUSE

Each year more than 120 000 children are substantiated as victims of physical abuse in the United States, but the true incidence is likely higher. Infants under the age of 1 year are at the highest risk of experiencing and dying from child abuse and neglect.

CLINICAL PRESENTATION OF CHILD PHYSICAL ABUSE

Victims of child physical abuse may present for medical care in several ways. A caregiver who is unaware that the child has been injured may bring the child for care as a result of symptoms he or she observed. Alternatively, perpetrators of the abusive injury sometimes bring the children for care but may provide a misleading history. In other cases, children are brought for care after someone witnesses an abusive event or notes a suspicious injury and makes a report. Lastly, injuries from physical abuse may be noted during the course of medical evaluations performed for unrelated concerns.

Cutaneous injuries such as bruising are the most common manifestation of physical abuse and have been reported in up to 92% of children hospitalized due to suspected abuse. Although bruises are common in active children, they are unusual in young, nonambulatory infants and should raise suspicion for abuse or underlying disorder. In a prospective study of 973 infants and toddlers seen for well-child care visits, only 0.6% of infants less than 6 months of age and 1.7% of infants less than 9 months of age had any bruises. Only 2.2% of nonambulatory children had bruises, but 17.8% of children who were walking with support and 51.9% of children walking without support had bruises. Bruises in certain locations should also raise the possibility of abuse. The majority of accidental bruises are located over bony prominences such as anterior tibia, knees, elbows, and forehead. Bruises on the torso, neck, and ear are uncommon accidental bruises and in the absence of a clear confirmatory history of accidental trauma should prompt a consideration of possible inflicted trauma. Patterned bruises should also prompt suspicion for inflicted trauma.

Other injuries that child victims of physical abuse may present, which include but are not limited to, are fractures, traumatic brain injury, burns, bites, and abdominal injuries. Traumatic brain injury is the most common cause of morbidity and mortality from physical abuse.

DIAGNOSTIC APPROACH

Although the majority of injuries in children are accidental and not abusive, it is important to maintain a high index of suspicion for abuse when evaluating young injured children. Retrospective studies have demonstrated that medical professionals frequently fail to recognize and evaluate abuse resulting in children suffering from medical complications related to untreated injuries and further abusive injuries, including fatal injuries.

A thorough and detailed history including mechanism of injury should be performed in all cases of suspected physical abuse. A list of potential red flags on history for physical abuse is included in Table 9-4. Family history of diseases that may increase the severity of injury following minimal trauma should be obtained. A social history including a prior history of maltreatment should be performed. Physical examination should include an evaluation of growth to identify failure to thrive or malnutrition. A thorough skin examination for bruises, burns, and bite marks should be performed as well as an oral examination

TABLE 9-4.	Findings on history that may suggest inflicted trauma.
• Lack of history to explain injury	
• History that changes with time	
• Histories provided by different caregivers are conflicting	
• History that is inconsistent with the developmental level of the child	
• History that is inconsistent with the injury	
• Unexplained delay in bringing child for care	
• History of home resuscitative efforts causing the injuries	
• History of siblings causing the injuries	

The findings outlined above have been identified as potential red flags for child abuse.

for soft tissue injury, tooth fractures, and dental neglect. An abdominal examination should be performed to identify any tenderness or other signs of abdominal injuries. The extremities, ribs, and head should be carefully palpated to identify signs of acute or healing fractures.

Radiologic studies may be needed to evaluate for occult injuries. Fractures, the most common type of occult injury, are identified on skeletal surveys in approximately one-third of physical abuse victims less than 2 years old. Occult head injuries including skull fractures and intracranial hemorrhage are also common in young victims of physical abuse. Thus, physicians should have a low threshold for performing head imaging in young children with injuries from suspected abuse. Although less common than occult fractures and occult head injury, occult intra-abdominal injuries can occur and thus screening for occult abdominal trauma should be considered. Finally, an ophthalmologic examination to evaluate for retinal hemorrhages should be conducted if there is any traumatic brain injury. A summary of recommendations for occult injury screening in suspected victims of abuse is provided below.

Diagnostic studies to consider include the following:

Skeletal survey. A skeletal survey should be performed in all suspected victims of child physical abuse under age 2 years. Follow-up skeletal surveys performed 2 weeks after the initial skeletal survey should be considered as they can help to clarify tentative findings on the initial radiographs and show healing injuries that were not visible in the acute stage on initial radiographs.

Head imaging. Head imaging with CT or MRI should be performed in all cases in which intracranial injury is suspected based on history or physical examination findings. Head imaging should also be strongly considered to evaluate for occult head injuries in children under the age of 2 years with injuries suggestive of a shaken or impact mechanism.

Abdominal laboratory studies. Consider obtaining the following laboratory tests in cases of suspected physical abuse, even in the absence of signs or symptoms of abdominal injuries: serum amylase, serum lipase, liver function tests, urinalysis for erythrocytes.

Abdominal imaging. An abdominal CT should be performed in suspected victims of child physical abuse with symptoms, signs, or laboratory values suggestive of abdominal injury.

Laboratory evaluation for other causes of injuries. Additional laboratory studies to evaluate for alternate diagnoses should be performed if indicated based on history and physical. In the case of infant with bruising (with or without intracranial hemorrhage), an evaluation for hematologic disorders is indicated especially if there are not additional injuries to support a diagnosis of abuse. There is not, however, consensus regarding the extent of the evaluation. To screen for common, severe coagulopathies, a CBC, PT, PTT, and thrombin time should be performed. If screening test results are normal and a bleeding disorder is suspected based on clinical presentation or family history, consultation with a hematologist and further testing for other hematologic disorders may be indicated.

Fundoscopic examination for retinal hemorrhages. Consider in any infant or young child with injuries from suspected abuse.

TREATMENT

The injuries suffered by the child should be managed as medically indicated. A report to CPS must be made in any case in which there is a reasonable suspicion of child abuse. In all states and in the District of Columbia, physicians and nurses are included as mandatory reporters, and in many states medical providers may face penalties for failure to report suspected child physical abuse. Medical providers should be familiar with the child abuse reporting laws of their state. In this case, a report was made to CPS. Under the direction of CPS, when medically ready the child was discharged in the care of her grandparents. At follow-up in 3 months her grandparents reported that she had not had any further bruising.

SUGGESTED READINGS

1. Makoroff KL, McGraw ML. Skin conditions confused with child abuse. In: Jenny C, ed. *Child Abuse and Neglect: Diagnosis, Treatment, and Evidence.* 1st ed. Philadelphia: Elsevier; 2011:252-259.

2. Mudd S, Findlay J. The cutaneous manifestations and common mimickers of physical child abuse. *J Pediatr Health Care.* 2004;18(3):123-129.

3. Smolinski KN, Yan AC. Hemangiomas of infancy: clinical and biological characteristics. *Clin Pediatr (Phila).* Nov-Dec 2005;44(9):747-766.

4. Paller AS, Mancini AJ, eds. Photosensitivity and photoreactions. In: *Hurwitz's Clinical Pediatric Dermatology: A Textbook of Skin Disorders of Childhood and Adolescence.* Philadelphia: Elsevier; 2011:436-443.

5. Sarnaik A, Kamat D, Kannikeswaran N. Diagnosis and management of bleeding disorder in a child. *Clin Pediatr (Phila).* May 2010;49(5):422-431.

6. Brousseau TJ, Kissoon N, McIntosh B. Vitamin K deficiency mimicking child abuse. *J Emerg Med.* 2005;29(3):283-288.

7. Chalmers EA. Neonatal coagulation problems. *Arch Dis Child Fetal Neonatal Ed.* Nov 2004;89(6):F475-F478.

8. Liesner R, Hann I, Khair K. Non-accidental injury and the haematologist: the causes and investigation of easy bruising. *Blood Coagul Fibrinolysis.* May 2004;15 Suppl 1:S41-S48.

9. Sedlak A, Mettenburg J, Basena M, et al. *Fourth national incidence study of child abuse and neglect (NIS–4): report to congress.* Washington, D.C.: U.S. Department of Health and Human Services; 2010.

10. U.S. Department of Health and Human Services, Administration on Children, Youth, and, Families. Child maltreatment 2010. Washington, DC: U.S. Government Printing Office; 2011.

11. Kellogg ND, American Academy of Pediatrics Committee on Child Abuse and Neglect. Evaluation of suspected child physical abuse. *Pediatrics.* Jun 2007;119(6):1232-1241.

12. McMahon P, Grossman W, Gaffney M, Stanitski C. Soft-tissue injury as an indication of child abuse. *J Bone Joint Surg.* 1995;77(8):1179-1183.

13. Harris TL, Flaherty EG. Bruises and skin lesions. In: Jenny C, ed. *Child Abuse and Neglect: Diagnosis, Treatment, and Evidence.* 1st ed. Philadelphia: Elsevier; 2011:239-250.

14. Maguire S, Mann MK, Sibert J, Kemp A. Are there patterns of bruising in childhood which are diagnostic or suggestive of abuse? A systematic review. *Arch Dis Child.* Feb 2005;90(2):182-186.

15. Sugar NF, Taylor JA, Feldman KW. Bruises in infants and toddlers: those who don't cruise rarely bruise. Puget Sound Pediatric Research Network. *Arch Pediatr Adolesc Med.* Apr 1999;153(4):399-403.

16. Pierce MC, Kaczor K, Aldridge S, O'Flynn J, Lorenz DJ. Bruising characteristics discriminating physical child abuse from accidental trauma. *Pediatrics.* Jan 2010;125(1):67-74.

17. Rubin DM, Christian CW, Bilaniuk LT, Zazyczny KA, Durbin DR. Occult head injury in high-risk abused children. *Pediatrics.* 2003;111(6):1382-1386.

18. Jenny C, Hymel KP, Ritzen A, Reinert SE, Hay TC. Analysis of missed cases of abusive head trauma. *JAMA.* Feb 1999;281(7):621-626.

19. Oral R, Blum KL, Johnson C. Fractures in young children: are physicians in the emergency department and orthopedic clinics adequately screening for possible abuse? *Pediatr Emerg Care.* Jun 2003;19(3):148-153.

20. Oral R, Yagmur F, Nashelsky M, Turkmen M, Kirby P. Fatal abusive head trauma cases: consequence of medical staff missing milder forms of physical abuse. *Pediatr Emerg Care.* 2008;24(12):816-821.

21. Ravichandiran N, Schuh S, Bejuk M, et al. Delayed identification of pediatric abuse-related fractures. *Pediatrics.* 2010;125(1):60-66.

22. Kellogg N. Oral and dental aspects of child abuse and neglect. *Pediatrics.* Dec 2005;116(6):1565-1568.

23. Day F, Clegg S, McPhillips M, Mok J. A retrospective case series of skeletal surveys in children with suspected non-accidental injury. *J. Clin Forensic Med.* 2006;13(2):55-59.

24. Belfer RA, Klein BL, Orr L. Use of the skeletal survey in the evaluation of child maltreatment. *Am J Emerg Med.* Mar 2001;19(2):122-124.

25. Hicks RA, Stolfi A. Skeletal surveys in children with burns caused by child abuse. *Pediatr Emerg Care.* 2007;23(5):308-313.

26. Rubin DM, Christian CW, Bilaniuk LT, Zazyczny KA, Durbin DR. Occult head injury in high-risk abused children. *Pediatrics.* 2003;111(6):1382-1386.

27. Laskey AL, Holsti M, Runyan DK, Socolar RR. Occult head trauma in young suspected victims of physical abuse. *J Pediatr.* Jun 2004;144(6):719-722.

28. American Academy of Pediatrics. Diagnostic imaging of child abuse. *Pediatrics.* May 2009;123(5):1430-1435.

29. Kleinman PK, Nimkin K, Spevak MR, et al. Follow-up skeletal surveys in suspected child abuse. *AJR Am J Roentgenol.* Oct 1996;167(4):893-896.

30. Zimmerman S, Makoroff K, Care M, Thomas A, Shapiro R. Utility of follow-up skeletal surveys in suspected child physical abuse evaluations. *Child Abuse Negl.* Oct 2005;29(10):1075-1083.

31. Feldman KW. The bruised premobile infant: should you evaluate further? *Pediatr Emerg Care.* Jan 2009;25(1):37-39.

32. Child Welfare Information Gateway. Mandatory Reporters of Child Abuse and Neglect: Summary of State Laws. 2008. http://www.childwelfare.gov/systemwide/laws_policies/statutes/manda.cfm#fn1. Accessed 8/1/2012.

33. Hettler J, Greenes DS. Can the initial history predict whether a child with a head injury has been abused? *Pediatrics.* 2003;11(3):602-607.

34. Sirotnak A, Grigsby T, Krugman R. Physical abuse of children. *Pediatr Rev.* 2004;25(8):264-277.

CASE 9-3

Four-Year-Old Girl

CHRISTINE T. LAUREN

HISTORY OF PRESENT ILLNESS

A 4-year-old Caucasian girl presented for evaluation of an eruption on her lower extremities. Four days prior to admission, she presented to her primary physician for evaluation of left knee pain. At that time she had mild swelling and tenderness of the joint without erythema. She was started on ibuprofen with some relief. One day later she developed abdominal pain, and was evaluated at a nearby hospital. Physical examination and abdominal radiograph with obstructive series were normal. Rectal examination was normal with negative stool guaiac. The patient was sent home, but the severe, intermittent abdominal pain persisted. On the day of admission the child's mother noted the development of "small red bumps" all over both legs while giving the child a bath. The lesions became larger and continued to spread on her lower extremities throughout the day. There was no history of fever, vomiting, or diarrhea. The patient ate well between episodes of abdominal pain. She had some nasal congestion and rhinorrhea 1 week prior to the onset of her symptoms. There was no history of tick bites or ingestions.

MEDICAL HISTORY

The child was a full-term infant with an uncomplicated birth history. There was no significant family history, travel, or exposures.

PHYSICAL EXAMINATION

T 37.7°C; RR 22/min; HR 124 bpm; BP 98/65 mmHg

Height 50th percentile; Weight 50th percentile

Physical examination was remarkable for 2-10 mm nonblanching, erythematous papules on the lower extremities from the dorsum of her feet to waist bilaterally. A horizontal 4-cm wide purpuric plaque on the left leg at the sock line was also noted (Figure 9-3). Lung examination was normal. Cardiac examination revealed no murmurs, rubs, or gallops. There were active bowel sounds, a soft nondistended abdomen, and no hepatosplenomegaly. Rectal examination was normal with soft heme-negative stool in the vault. There was no prominent adenopathy. Joint and neurologic examinations were normal.

DIAGNOSTIC STUDIES

Laboratory analysis revealed 10 700 WBCs/mm^3 with 50% segmented neutrophils, 40% lymphocytes, 4% eosinophils, and 6% monocytes. The hemoglobin was 10.9 g/dL and there were 436 000 platelets/mm^3. Electrolytes, blood urea nitrogen, and creatinine were normal. Erythrocyte sedimentation rate was 22 mm/h. Urinalysis demonstrated a specific gravity of 1.010, with no protein, white blood cells, or red blood cells. Blood cultures were obtained.

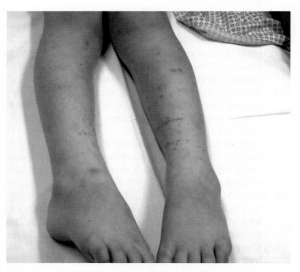

FIGURE 9-3. Rash on the lower extremities.

COURSE OF ILLNESS

The patient was admitted to the hospital where she received medication to manage her abdominal pain. The distribution and character of the rash suggested the diagnosis (Figure 9-3).

DISCUSSION CASE 9-3

DIFFERENTIAL DIAGNOSIS

The differential diagnosis of a nonblanching eruption includes both endogenous and exogenous causes (Table 9-5). When isolated to the

TABLE 9-5.	Select causes of acute petechiae/purpura in children.

Infectious
  Meningococcemia
  Rickettsial disease
  Parvovirus

Hematologic
  Thrombocytopenia
    Idiopathic thrombocytopenic purpura (ITP)
    Hemolytic uremic syndrome (HUS)
    Thrombotic thrombocytopenic purpura (TTP)
    Leukemia
  Coagulopathy
    Vitamin K deficiency
    Hepatic dysfunction
    Disseminated intravascular coagulation
  Prothrombotic state
    Protein C, S deficiency

Drugs
  Anticoagulants
  Corticosteroids

Vasculitis
  Rheumatologic
    Lupus
    ANCA associated vasculitis
  Infectious
    Viral (e.g., Hepatitis, HIV)
  Idiopathic
    Henoch-Schölein Purpura (HSP)
    Acute hemorrhagic edema of infancy (AHEI)

Idiopathic
  Pigmented purpuric dermatoses

Exogenous
  Traumatic purpura
  Nonaccidental trauma
  Self-inflicted trauma/factitial disorder

lower extremities, ecchymoses due to trauma in a healthy child must be considered. However, extent and bilaterally symmetric nature of the lesions, as well as the timing of the eruption in relation to her symptoms makes this less likely. Purpura can be seen in a variety of coagulopathies and in association with joint and gastrointestinal pain may reflect underlying hematologic malignancy (leukemia), idiopathic thrombocytopenic purpura, hemolytic uremic syndrome, or septicemia. Purpura due to meningococcemia or rickettsial disease should also be considered. Screening studies including normal complete blood count, blood urea nitrogen, and creatinine mitigate these diagnoses. Vasculitis in association with infection or underlying inflammatory or rheumatologic disease, such as lupus, must be considered. Although joint complaints can be seen in setting of juvenile idiopathic arthritis, the morphology of her skin lesions was not the evanescent pink lesions seen in this condition.

DIAGNOSIS

The characteristic palpable purpuric lesions on the lower extremities, especially along the sock line of the left leg (Figure 9-3) along with the constellation of symptoms in this patient led to the clinical diagnosis of **Henoch-Schönlein purpura (HSP), also known as anaphylactoid purpura**. One of the most common vasculitic syndromes affecting children, HSP is characterized by purpuric papules and plaques on the buttocks and lower extremities, polyarthritis, colicky abdominal pain, nephritis, or any combination of these symptoms. It is an IgA mediated leukocytoclastic vasculitis that involves inflammation of the precapillary, capillary, and postcapillary vessels in the skin, joints, gastrointestinal tract, and kidneys.

INCIDENCE AND EPIDEMIOLOGY

HSP can occur at any age, with peak incidence at 4-5 years; it is less common before age 1 or after age 10. Variable sex and ethnicity predominance has been reported. The incidence increases in the fall suggesting an infectious trigger and variable viral and bacterial infections have been described as inciting events.

CLINICAL PRESENTATION

The clinical picture of HSP is similar to this case: a previously healthy child acutely develops a distinctive eruption often preceded by arthritis or arthralgias, and/or abdominal pain. The rash is seen in all patients, and half the patients initially present with the skin rash. The eruption often occurs on the buttocks, lower extremities, and other areas of dependency. In severe cases it may include the face, trunk, and arms. The classic lesions are nonblanching erythematous macules and papules that last days with recurrences for up to 1-2 months. Nonpitting edema may be found in dependent areas. Arcuate purpura with a facial predominance may be a manifestation of acute hemorrhagic edema of infancy, a primarily cutaneous vasculitis that mimics HSP in younger children.

Arthralgia or arthritis are seen in 65%-85% of patients and may precede the eruption in 25% of the patients. The large joints are most commonly affected. These symptoms usually resolve within a few days.

Gastrointestinal manifestations can be seen in as many as three-fourths of patients. Abdominal pain is usually colicky in nature. Pain may be severe, mimicking appendicitis. Vomiting is common. Abdominal symptoms occasionally precede other manifestations by up to several weeks. While stools often contain occult blood, massive gastrointestinal bleeding occurs rarely. Other gastrointestinal complications include intussusception, bowel infarction, perforation, pancreatitis, and hydrops of the gallbladder. Intussusception, which occurs in 3% of cases, is usually ileo-ileal (rather than ileo-colic) and is seen in older children.

Renal manifestations range from transient hematuria or proteinuria to nephritis, nephrotic syndrome, and end-stage renal disease. While microscopic hematuria is a constant feature, up to 40% of patients have gross hematuria. Proteinuria occurs in conjunction with hematuria in two-thirds of patients, but proteinuria alone is rarely, if ever, a manifestation of HSP nephritis. Nephritis develops in 20%-50% of children with HSP. It usually appears days or weeks after the initial symptoms of HSP. Though it usually resolves, 2% may progress to renal failure. The histopathology of HSP renal disease demonstrates an IgA nephropathy. Those children who present with renal disease with nephritic and nephrotic features are at the highest risk to develop end stage renal disease.

Neurologic findings, including headaches and behavioral changes are seen in about one-third of the cases. Seizures, focal neurologic deficits, and peripheral neuropathies are rare. These symptoms may be seen in 2%-8% of those with the disease. Most neurologic findings are transient.

Orchitis develops in up to 10% of boys. Symptoms may mimic testicular torsion. Recurrences occur in a minority of patients and are manifested by appearance of symptoms after a period of resolution of 2 weeks or greater. Gastrointestinal and skin symptoms are most common.

DIAGNOSTIC APPROACH

The diagnosis is made clinically, as there are no specific laboratory tests to diagnose HSP. Laboratory studies may reveal suggestive features or complications of HSP but are more important to help differentiate HSP from other potential causes.

Complete blood count. Leukocytosis is seen in two-thirds of the children. Eosinophilia is occasionally present. Anemia is more commonly seen with Crohn disease and ulcerative colitis than HSP.

Serum IgA level. Serum IgA is elevated during the acute illness in approximately 50% of patients.

Complement levels. C3 and C4 levels are normal in HSP nephritis but may be low in lupus nephritis and poststreptococcal glomerulonephritis.

Urinalysis. Urinalysis should be performed on all the patients to look for findings suggestive of nephritis or nephrotic syndrome, including hematuria and proteinuria. Urinalysis should be repeated every 7 days while the disease is still active to monitor for the development of nephritis and renal function should be monitored for 3-6 months after disease onset given cases of late onset disease.

Radiologic studies. When gastrointestinal signs are present, contrast radiologic studies of the gastrointestinal tract demonstrate small bowel involvement with thickened folds, hypomotility and "thumb-printing," characteristic of submucosal hemorrhage. Ultrasound may help diagnose intussusception, as intussusception proximal to the ileo-colic location may be missed by air or liquid contrast enemas.

Other studies. The erythrocyte sedimentation rate (ESR) may be elevated but is rarely helpful in diagnosing HSP. The ESR is always elevated with Crohn disease and ulcerative colitis. The prothrombin time and partial thromboplastin time are normal in children with HSP but are frequently elevated in children with meningococcemia, sepsis, and other coagulation disorders presenting with purpura. Blood cultures should be performed in ill-appearing children when HSP cannot be readily distinguished from meningococcemia or sepsis. Renal biopsy should be considered in children with nephritis complicated by nephrotic syndrome, hypertension, or substantial renal insufficiency to predict prognosis more precisely. Skin biopsy for routine histology and immunofluorescence in severe or atypical cases is warranted: unlike other small vessel vasculitic processes, HSP classically manifests with cutaneous IgA and C3 deposition on immunofluorescence.

TREATMENT

Specific treatment is not usually required and most children can be managed in the outpatient setting. Hospital admission should be considered in children who develop gastrointestinal hemorrhage, colicky abdominal pain suggestive of intussusception, significant renal disease, or changes in mental status. The duration of illness is typically 3-4 weeks. Relapses are uncommon but have occurred in up to 15% of children in some studies.

The use of prednisone (1-2 mg/kg/day) has been suggested to hasten improvement of abdominal pain as well as improve outcomes in hospitalized patients with HSP. This may also reduce the risk of intussusception. Some reports suggest that corticosteroids alone or combined with other immunosuppressive agents, such as azathioprine or cyclophosphamide, reduce the risk of renal failure in children with HSP nephritis, although prospective trials are still needed.

The prognosis for children who develop HSP is generally good. Approximately 95% of children have complete recovery. However, of those children who required renal biopsy to evaluate persistent renal disease, 18% ultimately developed chronic renal failure. The risk factors for renal failure include age at onset greater than 7 years, severe abdominal symptoms, and persistent purpura.

SUGGESTED READINGS

1. Al-Sheyyab M, El-Shanti H, Ajlouni S, Sawalha D, Daoud AS. The clinical spectrum of Henoch-Schönlein purpura in infants and young children. *Eur J Pediatr.* 1995;154:969-972.
2. Hyams JS. Corticosteroids in the treatment of gastrointestinal disease. *Curr Opinion Pediatr.* 2000;12:451-455.
3. Lanzkowsky S, Lanzkowsky L, Lanzkowsky P. Henoch-Schönlein purpura. *Pediatr Rev.* 1992;13:130-137.
4. Saulsbury FT. Henoch-Schönlein purpura in children: report of 100 patients and review of the literature. *Medicine.* 1999;78:395-409.
5. Walker WA, Higuchi L. Henoch-Schönlein syndrome. In: McMillan JA, DeAngelis CD, Feigin RD, Warshaw JB, eds. *Oski's Pediatrics: Principles and Practice.* 3rd ed. Philadelphia: Lippincott Williams & Wilkins; 1999:2176-2179.
6. Sano H, Izumida M, Shimizo H, et al. Risk factors of renal involvement and significant proteinuria in Henoch-Schönlein purpura. *Eur J Pediatr.* 2002;161:196-201.
7. Shah D, Goraya JS, Poddar B, et al. Acute infantile hemorrhagic edema and Henoch-Schönlein purpura overlap in a child. *Pediatr Dermatol.* 2002;19:92-93.
8. Praid D, Amir J, Nussinovitch M. Recurrent Henoch-Schonlein purpura in children. *J Clin Rheumatol.* 2007;13:25-28.
9. Mills JA, Michel BA, Bloch DA, et al. The American College of Rheumatology 1990 criteria for the classification of Henoch-Schönlein purpura. *Arthritis Rheum.* 1990;33:1114-1121.
10. Weiss PF, Klink AJ, Localio R, et al. Corticosteroids may improve clinical outcomes during hospitalization for Henoch-Schönlein purpura. *Pediatrics.* 2010 Oct;126(4):674-81. Epub 2010 Sep 20.

CASE 9-4

Fourteen-Year-Old Boy

KARA N. SHAH

HISTORY OF PRESENT ILLNESS

A 14-year-old boy presented to the emergency department complaining of a facial rash. Seven days prior to admission he had developed low-grade fevers, sore throat, myalgias, and malaise. He was evaluated by his primary pediatrician, who diagnosed him with influenza. His symptoms gradually improved until the day of admission when he developed fever to 39.0°C, a rapidly worsening cough, and rash on his face. In the emergency department he had an episode of hemoptysis (approximately 250 mL) and subsequently became hypotensive, requiring treatment with multiple normal saline boluses and a packed red blood cell transfusion. He did not have a history of abdominal or chest pain. The patient recalled striking his head in the shower while coughing, a fact that he had not mentioned to his parents.

MEDICAL HISTORY

The patient had a history of recurrent rectal prolapse at 4 years of age that resolved without sequelae. His mother noted that he had a tendency to bruise easily and often had gingival bleeding after brushing his teeth. He had not undergone any surgical procedures. He had no allergies and his immunizations were up-to-date. He was adopted at the age of 4 weeks. His biologic mother died after delivery due to complications of uterine rupture. Additional details of the family history were not known.

PHYSICAL EXAMINATION

T 38.5°C; RR 50/min; HR 130 bpm; BP 100/55 mmHg

Height 50th percentile; Weight 25th percentile

Physical examination revealed an ill-appearing but alert boy. He had a very thin and narrow face. His sclerae were mildly injected. There was no blood in the nares and no hemotympanum. His neck was supple. He had mild suprasternal retractions with dullness to percussion approximately half way up the back on the right. There were rales in the region of the right lower and middle lobes. Cardiac examination was notable for thread femoral pulses that improved after fluid resuscitation; no murmur was appreciated. He had mild tenderness to palpation at the right costal margin but the remainder of the abdominal examination was normal. Examination of the skin was remarkable for a large ecchymoses on the patient's forehead (3 cm) that was tender to palpation. There were numerous thin, atrophic scars on his extremities, especially overlying the joints.

DIAGNOSTIC STUDIES

Arterial blood gas demonstrated the following: pH, 7.35; PCO_2, 26 mmHg; and PO_2, 60 mmHg in room air. The WBC count was 1600/mm^3 (26% band forms; 26% segmented neutrophils; 44% lymphocytes); hemoglobin, 9.8 g/dL; and platelets, 270 000/mm^3. Erythrocyte sedimentation rate was 35 mm/h. The prothrombin and partial thromboplastin times were 13.1 seconds and 35.7 seconds, respectively. The fibrinogen was 749 mg/dL and fibrin split products were 20 mcg/mL. The creatinine kinase was 120 U/L. Serum electrolytes were as follows: sodium, 136 mmol/L; potassium, 3.6 mmol/L; chloride, 104 mmol/L; bicarbonate, 18 mmol/L; blood urea nitrogen, 16 mg/dL; creatinine, 1.0 mg/dL; and glucose, 169 mg/dL. Serum aminotransferases and total bilirubin were normal. Urinalysis was normal. A blood culture was obtained. The chest radiograph revealed areas of consolidation in the right lower and right middle lobes with a moderate right-sided pleural effusion.

COURSE OF ILLNESS

The patient received empiric vancomycin and gentamicin for presumed bacterial sepsis. Computed tomography of the chest revealed extensive consolidation involving the entire right lower lobe and part of the left lower lobe with moderate pleural effusions. A chest tube was placed, draining approximately 500 mL of pleural fluid. The pleural fluid contained 7350 WBCs/mm^3 and 650 RBCs/mm^3. His chest tube was removed on the third day of hospitalization. Initial blood cultures grew *Staphylococcus aureus*, while cultures of the pleural fluid were negative. Antibiotic coverage was changed to oxacillin and he recovered uneventfully, completing a 4-week course of antibiotics. The patient was diagnosed with influenza complicated by *S. aureus* pneumonia and bacteremia. A detailed cutaneous examination suggested an underlying diagnosis that predisposed the patient to bruising, hemoptysis, and poor wound healing. The diagnosis was confirmed by skin biopsy.

DISCUSSION CASE 9-4

DIFFERENTIAL DIAGNOSIS

In this case, the bruising, atrophic scars, and bleeding indicated increased vascular permeability or weakness. The use of corticosteroids or Cushing syndrome could result in the development of atrophic scars as well as easy bruising and bleeding, but there was no history of corticosteroid use nor did the patient demonstrate Cushingoid features. Scurvy, secondary to a dietary lack of vitamin C, may present with bruising, bleeding, and poor wound healing, but is unlikely in a patient in the United States with a normal diet and no history of malnutrition.

Thrombocytopenia, especially due to immune thrombocytopenic purpura or sepsis, may occur in patients with a history of recent illness and fever, but can be excluded based on the normal platelet count. Von Willebrand disease is a relatively common disorder involving a deficiency of a circulating plasma protein related to factor VIII. This results in decreased platelet aggregation and a prolonged bleeding time. There is usually a history of mild to moderate bleeding involving the mucous membranes, including epistaxis and prolonged bleeding after dental procedures. This patient had a history of gingival bleeding with routine dental care, nosebleeds, and easy bruising, but von Willebrand disease does not explain the presence of atrophic scars.

Osteogenesis imperfecta (OI) is a congenital abnormality of quality or quantity of Type I collagen synthesis. Of the four subtypes of OI, Type I is associated with easy bruising. However, this child did not display the other signs of OI, which include frequent fractures, blue sclera, hearing impairment, osteopenia, bony deformities, or excessive laxity of his joints. Ehlers-Danlos syndrome (EDS) is also a congenital defect in collagen synthesis. There are multiple forms of EDS, identified by clinical features (major and minor criteria) and biochemical and molecular findings (Table 9-6). Most of the forms of EDS are associated with skin hyperextensibility and joint hypermobility.

DIAGNOSIS

Close examination of the patient's skin revealed dramatic hyperextensibility. Numerous atrophic, cigarette paper-like (papyraceous) scars most prominently overlying the large joints of the extremities were also present. Additional history revealed that the patient had a history of wound dehiscence after suture placement for a skin laceration. These findings together with the history of easy bruising, history of rectal prolapse, and mother's death from uterine rupture suggest a diagnosis of Ehlers-Danlos syndrome. The diagnosis was confirmed by skin biopsy with fibroblast culture, which revealed decreased secretion of Type III procollagen consistent with the diagnosis of Ehlers-Danlos, vascular type (previously classified as EDS Type IV).

INCIDENCE AND EPIDEMIOLOGY OF EHLERS-DANLOS SYNDROME

Ehlers-Danlos syndrome, vascular type is the most severe form of the Ehlers-Danlos syndromes. It occurs as a result of mutations on the COL3A1 gene which encodes Type III collagen. Type III collagen is found in highly vascular structures such as liver and blood vessels. EDS, vascular type is inherited as an autosomal dominant condition. This is a very rare condition with a prevalence of less than 1 per 100 000. Possibly as a result of its rarity, the diagnosis is often made only after catastrophic or fatal complication.

TABLE 9-6.	The Ehlers-Danlos syndromes: clinical subtypes and associated defects.		
Villefranche Type/(OMIM)	*Clinical Features*	*Inheritance*	*Protein/(Gene Defect)*
Classical/(130000 and 130010)	Hyperextensible skin; easy bruising; wide, atrophic scars; hypermobile joints	AD	Collagen Type V/(*COL5A1*, *COL5A2*)
Hypermobility/(130020)	Smooth, velvety skin; joint hypermobility	AD/AR	Unclear for most; collagen Type III; tenascin XB/ (*COL3A1*; *TNXB*)[a]
Vascular/(130050)	Thin, translucent skin with easy bruising; arterial and visceral rupture; typical facies	AD	Collagen Type III/(*COL3A1*)
Kyphoscoliosis/(225400 and 229200)	Atrophic scars, easy bruising; neonatal hypotonia; scoliosis; ocular rupture; marfanoid habitus	AR	Lysyl hydroxylase/(*PLOD1*)
Arthrochalasia/(130060)	Hyperextensible and fragile skin; severe joint hypermobility; congenital hip dislocation	AD	Collagen Type I/(*COL1A1*; *COL1A2*)
Dermatosparaxis/(225410)	Severely fragile, sagging, redundant skin; hernias and premature rupture of fetal membranes	AR	Procollagen I N-peptidase/ (*ADAMTS2*)
Other types[a]			
Progeroid variant/(130070)	Wrinkled, loose facial skin, curly fine hair, scanty eyebrows and eyelashes	AR	Due to mutations in galactosyltransferase

AD,autosomal dominant; AR,autosomal recessive; OMIM, Online Mendelian Inheritance in Man

[a]Few reported cases, including X-linked EDS, periodontitis type, and progeroid EDS

Reprinted with permission from *Fitzpatrick's Dermatology in General Medicine*, 6th edition, Table 139-1.

CLINICAL PRESENTATION OF EHLERS-DANLOS SYNDROME

The clinical diagnosis of EDS, vascular type is made on the basis having at least two of four major clinical criteria: easy bruising, thin skin with visible veins, characteristic facial features (thin faces, pinched nose, large eyes), and fragility or rupture of arteries, uterus, or intestines (Table 9-6). Minor features include acrogeria, hypermobility of small joints, tendon or muscle rupture, congenital clubfoot, early onset varicose veins, and pneumothorax (Figure 9-4). Because EDS, vascular type is a heterogeneous genetic disorder, various clinical presentations may be seen. Diagnosis is often delayed until the second or third decade of life in the absence of a known family history, as vascular complications typically present during the third decade of life. The median age of survival is 48 years, with death most commonly occurring as a result of an arterial dissection or rupture;

spontaneous bowel perforation and organ rupture (heart, uterus, spleen, or liver) are the other leading cause of catastrophic death. Although present in this patient, the hypermobility of the large joints and hyperextensibility of the skin, characteristic of the more common forms of EDS, are only occasionally seen in the vascular type.

DIAGNOSTIC APPROACH

In addition to the clinical criteria noted above, diagnosis may be confirmed by the demonstration of abnormal Type III procollagen molecules in cultured fibroblasts or by the identification of a mutation in the gene for Type III procollagen (COL3A1).

TREATMENT

Unfortunately, the prognosis in patients with EDS, vascular type is poor. In a study of 220 patients with vascular EDS, more than 80% of affected

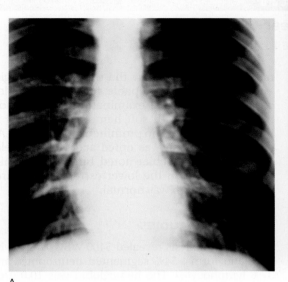

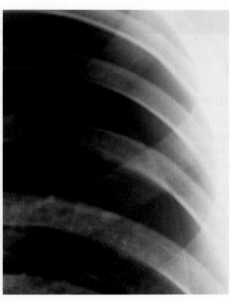

A   B

FIGURE 9-4. Chest radiograph showing pneumothorax in the anterior-posterior projection with images of the **A.** Entire chest radiograph. **B.** A close-up image.

patients suffered a complication (arterial dissection or rupture, spontaneous bowel perforation, or organ rupture) by age 40 years, and 12% died after the first event. Women have a significant risk of death with each pregnancy due to uterine or vascular rupture, with a reported 11.5% mortality rate.

Genetic evaluation and counseling is crucial for patients diagnosed with this disorder. It is transmitted in an autosomal dominant pattern; thus patients and families need to be informed of the 50% risk of transmission to an affected individual's offspring. Although management is limited to symptomatic treatment and precautionary measures, use of celiprolol, a beta(1)-adrenoceptor antagonist/beta(2)-adrenoceptor agonist has been associated with a reduction in arterial events in adults (rupture or dissection). Knowledge of the diagnostic features of vascular EDS is critical in the recognition and management of emergency, surgical, and obstetrical issues.

SUGGESTED READINGS

1. Beighton P, De Paepe A, Steinmenn B, Tsipouras P, Wenstrup RJ. Ehlers-Danlos syndromes: revised nosology, Villefranche, 1997. *Am J Med Genet.* 1998;77:31-37.
2. Drera B, Zoppi N, Riteli M, et al. Diagnosis of vascular Ehlers-Danlos syndrome in Italy: clinical findings and novel COL3A1 mutations. *J Dermatol Sci.* 2011; 64:237-248.
3. Fernandes NF, Schwartz RA. A "hyperextensive" review of Ehlers-Danlos syndrome. *Cutis.* 2008;82:242-248.
4. Germain DP, Herrera-Guzman Y. Vascular Ehlers-Danlos syndrome. *Ann Genet.* 2004;47:1-9.
5. Ong KT, Perdu J, De Backer J, et al. Effect of celiprolol on prevention of cardiovascular events in vascular Ehlers-Danlos syndrome: a prospective randomized, open, blinded-endpoints trial. *Lancet.* 2010;376: 1476-1484.
6. Pepin M, Schwarze U, Superti-Furga A, Byers P. Clinical and genetic features of Ehlers-Danlos syndrome type IV, the vascular type. *N Engl J Med.* 2000;342: 673-680.

Sixteen-Year-Old Girl

CHRISTINE T. LAUREN

HISTORY OF PRESENT ILLNESS

A 16-year-old Caucasian girl presented to the emergency department with acute onset of epistaxis lasting 3-4 hours. Her parents estimated her blood loss to be several cups with no slowing of bleeding noted with compression. She reported a history of intermittent epistaxis since she was 8 years of age. She noted at least one nosebleed per year lasting 20-30 minutes each time. Her most recent episode was 1 year prior lasting approximately 4 hours. Her review of symptoms was notable for "easy bruising" without prolonged bleeding at sites of prior lacerations/abrasions. She reported an 18-month history of lower extremity pain, primarily in the ankles and knees. This pain would usually last for minutes and occurred twice weekly. She had no history of fractures. She endorsed worsening fatigue over recent months. Her menstrual periods were monthly with heavy flow during the first 2 days of her cycle. She denied fever, weight loss, or night sweats.

MEDICAL HISTORY

She was born at term and pregnancy was uncomplicated. There was no significant travel or exposures. Family history was remarkable for a brother with deletion of the short arm of chromosome 7, also with a history of epistaxis. Systemic lupus erythematosus was present in maternal aunt.

PHYSICAL EXAMINATION

T 37.4°C; RR 36/min; HR 110 bpm; BP 151/83 mmHg

Height 50th percentile; Weight 50th percentile

Physical examination was remarkable for nonicteric sclera, a small amount of bleeding from the left nostril and dried blood in the oropharynx. Lung examination was normal. Cardiac exam revealed no murmurs, rubs, or gallops. Abdomen was soft and nondistended; however, the liver was noted to be 4 cm below the right costal margin, and the spleen was palpable 4 cm below the left costal margin. Rectal examination revealed normal rectal tone with soft heme-positive stool in the vault. There was no prominent adenopathy. An erythematous rash was noted across her cheeks. There were no petechiae noted, but there was mild bruising found on the lower extremities. Neurologic examination was normal.

DIAGNOSTIC STUDIES

Laboratory analysis revealed 5400 WBCs/mm³ with 4% band forms, 54% segmented neutrophils, and 37% lymphocytes. The hemoglobin was 10.0 g/dL and there were 46000 platelets/mm³. Reticulocyte count was 2.7%. Prothrombin and partial prothrombin times were 12.6 seconds and 34.7 seconds, respectively. Serum electrolytes, blood urea nitrogen, and creatinine were normal. Lactate dehydrogenase was normal and uric acid was 6.3 mg/dL. The erythrocyte sedimentation rate was 35 mm/h. Antinuclear antibodies, antidouble stranded DNA, rapid plasma reagin test, and monospot were negative.

COURSE OF ILLNESS

Hemostasis was achieved without immediate intervention other than pressure applied to her nares. The patient was admitted to the hospital where she underwent further evaluation for the bleeding and associated symptoms. Bone marrow biopsy (Figure 9-5) suggested a diagnosis that was confirmed by a blood test.

DISCUSSION CASE 9-5

DIFFERENTIAL DIAGNOSIS

Bruising and easy bleeding in this older child suggests a hematologic condition. The differential includes malignancy such as leukemia, lymphoma, or immune thrombocytopenia purpura.

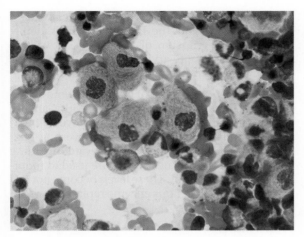

FIGURE 9-5. Bone marrow biopsy. *(Photo courtesy of Marybeth Helfrich, MT, ASCP.)*

Idiopathic thrombocytopenia purpura (ITP) would be unlikely due to the prolonged duration of the symptoms, as ITP is an acute, often self-limited condition. Chronic forms of ITP can occur; however, it would be atypical for the acute phase of the illness to have resolved undetected. The enlargement of the liver and spleen caused consideration of an oncologic, autoimmune, or metabolic conditions. The differential diagnosis was somewhat narrowed due to the relatively low sedimentation rate and negative autoimmune serologies. Infectious causes of thrombocytopenia and enlarged liver and spleen including Epstein-Barr virus or cytomegalovirus-associated infectious mononucleosis were considered less likely in setting of laboratory results.

DIAGNOSIS

The bone marrow biopsy revealed macrophages with the characteristic "wrinkled tissue paper" appearance of Gaucher cells (Figure 9-5). The leukocyte glucocerebrosidase activity was 0.85 nmol/h/mg/protein (<10% of normal values), consistent with the diagnosis of Gaucher disease. Radiographs of the right femur revealed undertabulation of the distal femoral metaphysis with marked cortical thinning and sclerosis. Additionally, an elevated tartrate-resistant acid phosphatase

level of 6.1 U/L (reference range, 2.0-4.2 U/L) was noted. MRI revealed diffuse infiltration of her liver, spleen, and bone marrow. **All of these findings were consistent with Gaucher disease, Type I.**

INCIDENCE AND EPIDEMIOLOGY OF GAUCHER DISEASE

Gaucher disease, the most common lysosomal storage disease, is an autosomal recessive disorder associated with deficient activity of the catabolic enzyme beta-glucocerebrosidase with resultant accumulation of glucocerebroside. In Gaucher disease, macrophages, the major site of catabolism of glycolipids, accumulate glucocerebroside. There are three forms of the disorder, with varying severity. This child had Type I Gaucher disease, the most common sphingolipid storage disorder. The highest incidence is found in people of Eastern European Jewish ancestry.

CLINICAL PRESENTATION OF GAUCHER DISEASE

Macrophages are most numerous in the liver, spleen, bone, and lung and, therefore, it is not surprising that manifestations of Gaucher disease are often related to these organs. Patients with Gaucher disease Type I can present at any age, though more severely affected present during childhood with splenomegaly and pancytopenia. Patients may complain of easy bruising and chronic fatigue. They may also have hepatomegaly and mild elevation of hepatic transaminases. Cirrhosis and liver failure may develop. As seen in this case, infiltration of the bone marrow interferes with bone mineralization and growth and compounds the pancytopenia. Skeletal complications include osteopenia, osteonecrosis, and recurrent bone pain. Pulmonary glycolipid accumulation may lead to respiratory dysfunction.

In general, the disease is slowly progressive with many individuals living well into adulthood. The disease may achieve a steady state between lipid accumulation and lipid degradation or loss. Individuals with the mildest disease may be identified incidentally as adults during routine evaluation. The central nervous system is spared in Type I Gaucher disease, and affected children have normal intelligence. Neurologic symptoms develop early in life for infants with Type II disease with death occurring by 2 years of age. In Type III disease, children develop visceromegaly early in life and late-onset neurologic complications.

DIAGNOSTIC APPROACH

The diagnosis of Gaucher disease can now be made by measurement of enzyme levels or by gene mutation analysis. In some states, Gaucher disease will be screened for as part of routine newborn testing programs.

Glucocerebrosidase levels. Since the glucocerebrosidase gene has been mapped to chromosome 1q21, identification of the underlying enzymatic defect in Gaucher disease is possible from peripheral blood. Decreased level of glucocerebrosidase activity in peripheral blood leukocytes (usually 10%-30% of normal levels) is diagnostic of Gaucher disease.

Gene analysis. DNA-based diagnosis can be used if findings from enzymatic testing are equivocal, as is occasionally the case in heterozygotes. The detection of mutations is, however, limited to the previously defined mutations. DNA analysis will detect most mutations (95%) in Ashkenazi Jews but only a few mutations in other populations who have a greater diversity of mutations.

Bone marrow biopsy. Once considered the diagnostic method of choice, bone marrow biopsy has fallen out of favor as a diagnostic tool in Gaucher disease since less invasive and more reliable diagnostic modalities have become available. Bone marrow biopsy findings include the detection of large, lipid-laden, fusiform macrophages with dense eccentric nuclei that resemble wrinkled tissue paper or crumpled silk (Gaucher cells). These cells are not pathognomonic of Gaucher disease, since the same type of cell can be found in various leukemias and some infectious disorders. This test is often performed to exclude malignancy in the child presenting with pancytopenia.

Complete blood count. Patients with untreated disease may have anemia, thrombocytopenia, and leukopenia.

Radiologic imaging. Radiographs, CT, or MRI of the femur will show the Erlenmeyer-flask deformity, due to expansion of the cortex, as well as cyst-like changes of varying sizes. MRI of various bones will show infiltration of bone marrow.

Other studies. A number of plasma enzyme activities are greatly increased in patients with Gaucher disease. Serum acid phosphatase levels, beta-hexosaminidase, and angiotensin-converting enzyme have all been found to be elevated in these patients. Acid phosphatase levels are used to monitor response to therapy. These levels become normal with adequate exogenous enzyme replacement.

TREATMENT

Management includes symptomatic treatment, exogenous administration of the missing enzyme, and allogeneic bone marrow transplantation. Gene transfer is being explored for future therapy.

Symptomatic measures are used to improve quality of life. Surgical splenectomy can correct the thrombocytopenia, and complete or partial splenectomy is used when the splenomegaly has become symptomatic. Patients are advised to avoid activities that put stress on the skeleton that can result in fractures. In some cases joint replacement may be necessary.

Type I Gaucher disease is particularly responsive to exogenous replacement of the defective enzyme because the central nervous system is not involved. This enzyme is a macrophage-targeted modified glucocerebrosidase. Patients require enzyme replacement (alglucerase) every 2 weeks. Enzyme replacement therapy has been effective in regression of the visceral and hematologic manifestations, and to a lesser extent the skeletal manifestations of Gaucher disease. Recently, the enzyme inhibitor Miglustat has also become available for the treatment of Type 1 disease.

Bone marrow stem cell transplantation may be considered in some patients. Since macrophages are derived from the hematopoietic stem cells, the stem cell transplantation can be expected to cure Gaucher disease. Indeed, allogeneic bone marrow transplantation has led to the correction of the clinical manifestations of the disease. However, marrow transplantation carries substantial risks, and is currently reserved for a small subset of patients.

SUGGESTED READINGS

1. Balicki D, Beutler E. Gaucher disease. *Medicine.* 1995;74:305-323.
2. Beutler E, Grabowski GA. Gaucher disease. In: Scriver CR, Beaudet AL, Sly WS, Valle D, eds. *The Metabolic and Molecular Basis of Inherited Disease.* 8th ed. New York: McGraw Hill; 2001:3635-3668.
3. Charrow J, Esplin JA, Gribble TJ, et al. Gaucher disease: recommendations on diagnosis, evaluation, and monitoring. *Arch Intern Med.* 1998;158:1754-1760.
4. Rosenthal DI, Doppelt SH, Mankin HJ, et al. Enzyme replacement therapy for Gaucher disease: skeletal responses to macrophage-targeted glucocerebrosidase. *Pediatrics.* 1995;96:629-637.
5. Chen M, Wang J. Gaucher disease: review of the literature. *Arch Pathol Lab Med.* 2008 May;132(5):851-853.
6. Hughes DA, Pastores GM. Haematological manifestations and complications of Gaucher disease. *Curr Opin Hematol.* 2012 Oct 25. [Epub ahead of print]
7. Somaraju UR, Tadepalli K. Hematopoietic stem cell transplantation for Gaucher disease. *Cochrane Database Syst Rev.* 2012 Jul 11;7:CD006974.
8. Venier RE, Igdoura SA. Miglustat as a therapeutic agent: prospects and caveats. *J Med Genet.* 2012 Sep;49(9):591-597. doi: 10.1136/jmedgenet-2012-101070. Epub 2012 Aug 14.

CASE 9-6

Eighteen-Month-Old Girl

KARA N. SHAH

HISTORY OF PRESENT ILLNESS

An 18-month-old girl was brought to the office by her mother for evaluation of a rash and low-grade fevers. The mother reported that the child was a bit fussy and not eating quite as well as usual. There was no history of irritability, vomiting, or loose stools. The infant did attend daycare but there were no known sick contacts.

MEDICAL HISTORY

There was no significant medical history. Immunizations were up-to-date.

PHYSICAL EXAMINATION

T 39.5°C; RR 24/min; HR 120 bpm; BP 95/50 mmHg

Height 50th percentile; Weight 50th percentile

Physical examination revealed a well-appearing, playful toddler. Numerous 2-3 mm nontender erythematous papules and oval vesicles on an erythematous base were diffusely scattered on the torso and extremities with increased concentration on the hands, knees, and buttocks (Figure 9-6). The mucous membranes were normal. Of note, the mother was noted to have a few discrete inflammatory vesicles on her hands (Figure 9-7).

DIAGNOSTIC STUDIES

No laboratory testing was performed.

COURSE OF ILLNESS

The rash and fever resolved without treatment over the course of 7 days.

DISCUSSION CASE 9-6

DIFFERENTIAL DIAGNOSIS

The differential diagnosis of a diffuse papulovesicular exanthem in a young child includes viral exanthems such as primary varicella, herpes simplex virus, and enterovirus infection, most commonly hand, foot, and mouth disease; scabies; and an id hypersensitivity reaction. Unusual causes include Gianotti-Crosti syndrome, also called papular acrodermatitis of childhood, and acropustulosis of infancy.

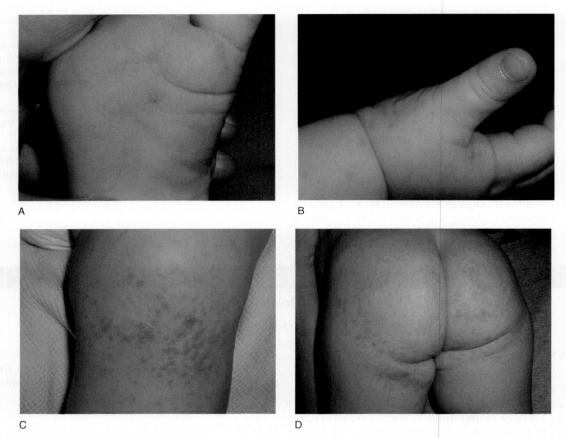

A

B

C

D

FIGURE 9-6. Typical cutaneous manifestations of hand, foot, and mouth disease on a toddler. **A.** Inflammatory vesicles on the hand. **B.** Inflammatory vesicle on the foot; **C, D.** Numerous small erythematous papules and vesicles on the knees and buttocks.

Primary varicella typically presents with low-grade fever, malaise, cough, coryza, and sore throat. The classic dewdrop on a rose petal exanthem presents first on the face and trunk, then spreads centripetally and appears as crops of red macules that progress to papules, vesicles, and pustules before crusting and resolving over 2-3 weeks. An enanthem with shallow oral ulcers may occur. The hallmark of the disease is the simultaneous presence of different clinical stages of the exanthem. With the initiation of routine immunization to the varicella-zoster virus in children, primary varicella is uncommon in immunocompetent children. Transmission occurs via respiratory droplets.

In children under age 5 years, the most common clinical presentation of primary herpes simplex virus

(HSV) infection is acute herpetic gingivostomatitis, which usually presents with fever, irritability, gingival inflammation, and painful grey vesicles and shallow ulcers on the tongue, buccal mucosa, and palate which may extend to the lips and face. Drooling and decreased oral intake are common, and tender submandibular or cervical adenopathy may be seen. Symptoms usually resolve over 10-14 days. Infection is usually caused by HSV-1. Reactivation usually presents as more localized, grouped vesicles on an erythematous base localizing on the vermillion border of the lips or less frequently on the face and associated with pain, pruritus, burning, or tingling. Primary and recurrent cutaneous HSV infection without mucosal involvement may also occur, typically with involvement localized to a single area

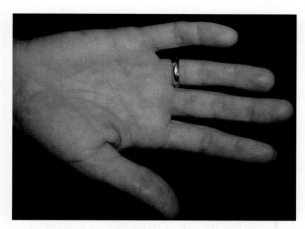

FIGURE 9-7. Typical small inflammatory vesicles on the hand of an adult.

and manifest as grouped vesicles on an inflammatory base that quickly rupture, leaving shallow ulcerations. In children, transmission of herpes simplex virus typically occurs via oral contact from adult caregivers such as may occur from kissing or sharing of cups; caregivers may have obvious colds sores or may be asymptomatically shedding the virus. Disseminated HSV infection is usually seen only in neonates or immunocompromised individuals. Affected patients are generally ill-appearing and multiorgan involvement is common.

Gianotti-Crosti syndrome, also known as papular acrodermatitis of childhood, is an exanthem seen most commonly in association with EBV infection, although association with other viruses and with some bacteria, including influenza, coxsackievirus A16, enteroviruses, and group A Streptococcus has been reported and the entity was first described in association with acute hepatitis B virus infection. Gianotti-Crosti presents with an asymptomatic, acute, cutaneous eruption that develops over several days and appears as monomorphous pale, pink-to-flesh-colored or erythematous 1- to 10-mm papules or papulovesicles localized symmetrically and acrally over the extensor surfaces of the extremities, the buttocks, and the face. The number of lesions ranges from few to many. The trunk, knees, elbows, palms, and soles are rarely involved, and, in general, extensive involvement of the trunk is not consistent with a diagnosis of Gianotti-Crosti syndrome. Complete resolution

typically takes more than 2 months, and the condition is self-limited. Fever and other signs and symptoms related to the primary infection may be seen, but in general children are well appearing.

Enteroviruses may cause a number of cutaneous manifestations, including a morbilliform exanthem, petechiae, and vesicular exanthems, which classically present as herpangina and hand, foot, and mouth disease. Herpangina manifests as shallow oral aphthae on the buccal mucosa and palate, lacks the gingival involvement of primary herpetic gingivostomatitis, and is milder in severity. Enteroviruses are transmitted by oral-oral and fecal-oral transmission; presumably, enterovirus infection may also be transmitted through direct contact with fluid from these cutaneous and mucosal lesions. Of the many enteroviral subtypes, coxsackieviruses, echoviruses, and enterovirus-71 are the subtypes which have been associated with cutaneous manifestations. Coxsackie A4 and echovirus 11 have been associated with a diffuse vesicular exanthem; echoviruses 2 and 9 with a rubelliform eruption; echoviruses 6, 9, 11, and 25 with a morbilliform eruption; echoviruses 11 and 19 with a petechiae exanthema, and echovirus 19 with a macular eruption.

Scabies is not an uncommon infestation caused by the *Sarcoptes scabei* mite. Transmission occurs via contact, and infestation of several household or other close contacts is not uncommon. Scabies classically presents as diffusely distributed, intensely pruritic inflammatory papules, vesicles, and burrows, which are often excoriated. The palms, soles, axillae, and scalp are often involved preferentially in infants, whereas in older children and adults, areas of involvement typically include the web spaces between the fingers and of the wrists, axillae, and waist.

Id hypersensitivity reactions (autoeczematization) occur as an immunologic reaction to a primary cutaneous infection or inflammatory disease. Id reactions present as a symmetric eruption of small erythematous, pruritic papules, and vesicles which may favor an acral distribution or may involve the head, torso, and extremities more diffusely. In children, id reactions typically are seen in association with dermatophyte skin infections, such as tinea capitis, or in association with a contact dermatitis, other eczematous dermatitis, or bacterial skin infection such as cellulitis.

Acropustulosis of infancy, also known as infantile acropustulosis, is a recurrent, pruritic vesicopustular dermatitis that typically involves the hands and feet, although milder involvement of the torso, face, arms, or legs is occasionally seen. It classically presents in infants and toddlers, with each episode lasting 1-2 weeks and recurring every 3-4 weeks, and generally resolves by age 3 years. Although the etiology is unknown, some cases appear to begin after scabies infestation, suggesting that acropustulosis may represent a hypersensitivity reaction to scabies.

DIAGNOSIS

On the basis of the clinical presentation, a diagnosis of hand, foot, and mouth disease (HFMD) was carried out.

INCIDENCE AND EPIDEMIOLOGY

HFMD is a common and mild, self-limited disease usually seen in children under 10 years of age. The most common cause of HFMD is Coxsackievirus A type 16, although HFMD has also been associated with coxsackievirus A5, A7, A9, A10, B2, and B5 infection. In Japan and other Pacific countries, enterovirus 71 infection has been associated with HFMD and neurologic complications, including a polio-like syndrome, aseptic meningitis, encephalitis, encephalomyelitis, and acute cerebellar ataxia. HFMD most commonly occurs in epidemics during the summer and fall, although low levels of endemic cases occur throughout the year. Coxsackievirus is a subgroup of the enteroviruses and is a member of the Picornaviridae family consisting of small, nonenveloped, single-stranded RNA viruses. The virus is transmitted via the fecal-oral route or via contact with skin lesions and oral secretions. Viremia develops, followed by invasion of the skin and mucous membranes.

CLINICAL PRESENTATION

The cutaneous manifestations of HFMD present as anywhere from several to over 100 erythematous macules and papules that evolve into oral, gray vesicles on an erythematous base. As suggested by the name, involvement of the hands and feet is characteristic, and lesions favor the lateral aspects on the fingers and toes as well as periungual. Mucosal involvement characteristically involves the hard palate, tongue, buccal mucosa, and gums and presents as erythematous macules, papules, and fragile vesicles that rupture easily, resulting in shallow painful ulcers surrounded by an erythematous halo; associated pain may interfere with oral intake, and irritability is common. Both the cutaneous and oral lesions typically resolve over 7-10 days without intervention and without sequelae, although aseptic meningitis may also be seen with enteroviral infection.

DIAGNOSTIC APPROACH

HFMD is usually diagnosed clinically, although the virus can be detected from appropriate samples, including blood, stool, and skin lesions. Identification methods include culture, immunoassay, polymerase chain reaction (PCR), and microarray technology. PCR may also be performed on urine and will remain positive for longer than PCF of blood specimens.

TREATMENT

Management of HFMD is symptomatic. Affected children should be encouraged to drink cool, soothing liquids to maintain hydration and to avoid hot and spicy foods and drinks. Appropriate pain control medications, such as oral acetaminophen or ibuprofen, and use of topical analgesics should be provided as necessary. Topical analgesic preparations include "Magic Mouthwash," which is typically composed of equal volume of liquid diphenhydramine and Maalox®; 2% viscous lidocaine may be added if the child is old enough to swish and spit the medication but is best avoided in infants and younger children to avoid swallowing of medication and risk of lidocaine toxicity. Topical benzocaine gel is also helpful.

SUGGESTED READINGS

1. Cherry JD, Krogstad P. Enteroviruses and parechoviruses. In: Feigin RD, Cherry JD, Demmler-Harrison GJ, Kaplan SL, eds. *Feigin and Cherry's Textbook of Pediatric Infectious Diseases*. 6th ed. Philadelphia, PA: Saunders Elsevier; 2009:2110-2169.
2. Modlin JF. Enteroviruses: coxsackieviruses, echoviruses, and newer enteroviruses. In: Long SS, Pickering LK, Prober CG, eds. *Principles and Practice of Pediatric Infectious Diseases*. 3rd ed. Philadelphia, PA: Churchill Livingstone Elsevier; 2008:1149-1157.

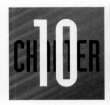

10 PALLOR

STEPHEN LUDWIG

BRANDON C. KU

DEFINITION

The complaint of pallor indicates a perceived decrease in rubor in the skin and mucous membranes of a child, which is associated with decreased oxyhemoglobin delivery to the skin or mucous membranes. Potential causes include decreased blood flow, which may be regional (e.g., thrombosis) or systemic (e.g., shock), and normal blood flow with decreased oxygen-carrying capacity (e.g., anemia).

In most cases, the finding of pallor demands that anemia first be considered as this is the most common cause. Exceptions include children who have a constitutional cause of pallor due to their fair complexion and lack of exposure to sunlight. However, most children with pallor should be considered to have low hemoglobin, which should be measured. Ordinarily, a complete blood count with differential count, red blood cell (RBC) indices, and reticulocyte count guide the clinician in differentiating the many causes of anemia and in determining unusual situations in which pallor is not related to anemia. In addition, a peripheral smear with examination of RBC morphology may further guide the clinician in determining the etiology of anemia.

CAUSE AND FREQUENCY

Pallor may be divided into causes involving normal hemoglobin (Table 10-1) and those involving a low hemoglobin level. The etiology of anemia may be separated into causes due to decreased RBC production, increased RBC destruction, or acute blood loss. Causes due to decreased RBC production are generally associated with low reticulocyte count while causes due to increased RBC destruction or acute blood loss are generally associated with increased reticulocyte count. Anemia may also be considered in relation to mechanism, such as trauma, toxin, metabolic tumor, congenital, or mixed etiology (Table 10-2), or in relation to RBC morphology (Table 10-3).

QUESTIONS TO ASK AND WHY

- Is there hemodynamic instability or need for emergent intervention?
  —The most important question to ask is whether a child's pallor is secondary to severe anemia with hemodynamic compromise that requires emergent intervention and stabilization with fluid resuscitation until transfusion of packed RBCs. This question also helps to determine whether severe anemia is secondary to acute external hemorrhage that may require immediate surgical intervention. One can also elucidate if a child's pallor is secondary to decreased blood flow from acute thrombosis or systemic shock further guiding therapy.

- What are the child's dietary habits?
  —Because the most common cause of pallor is iron deficiency anemia, important clarifying questions pertain to diet. Diets containing large quantities of cow's milk may raise concern for iron deficiency due to lack of iron intake and loss of appetite for iron-rich foods.

TABLE 10-1. | **Pallor with anemia.**

Decreased erythrocyte or hemoglobin production

Nutritional deficiencies
  Iron deficiency
  Folic acid and vitamin B_{12} deficiency or associated
    metabolic abnormalities

Aplastic or hypoplastic anemias
  Diamond-Blackfan anemia
  Fanconi anemia
  Aplastic anemia[a]
  Transient erythroblastopenia of childhood
  Malignancy: leukemia, lymphoma, neuroblastoma[a]

Anemia of chronic disease

Abnormal heme and hemoglobin synthesis
  Lead poisoning[a]
  Sideroblastic anemias
  Thalassemias

Increased Erythrocyte Destruction

Erythrocyte membrane defects: hereditary spherocytosis,
  elliptocytosis, stomatocytosis, pyknocytosis, paroxysmal
  nocturnal hemoglobinuria

Erythrocyte enzyme defects
  Defects of hexose monophosphate shunt: G6PD
    deficiency most common
  Defects of Embden-Meyerhof pathway: pyruvate
    kinase deficiency most common

Hemoglobinopathies
  Sickle cell syndrome[a]
  Unstable hemoglobins

Immune hemolytic anemia

Autoimmune hemolytic anemia (e.g., Evans syndrome)

Isoimmune hemolytic anemia

Infection
  Viral: mononucleosis, influenza, coxsackie, measles,
    varicella, cytomegalovirus
  Bacterial: *Escherichia coli*, Pneumococcus,
    Streptococcus, thyphoid fever, Mycoplasma

Drugs: antibiotics, methyldopa

Inflammatory and collagen vascular disease

Malignancy[a]

Microangiopathic anemias
  Disseminated intravascular coagulation[a]
  Hemolytic uremic syndrome[a]
  Thrombotic thrombocytopenic purpura
  Cavernous hemangioma

Blood Loss

Severe trauma[a]

Anatomic lesions
  Meckel diverticulum
  Peptic ulcer
  Idiopathic pulmonary hemosiderosis[a]

[a]Can present as life-threatening emergencies

TABLE 10-2. | **Etiology of anemia by mechanism (common causes of pallor).**

Mechanism	Examples
Trauma	Blood loss
Infection	Sepsis Viral suppression of bone marrow production
Toxin	Lead poisoning Aplastic anemia
Metabolic-inherited or Acquired	Iron deficiency Thalassemia Sideroblastic anemia Sickle cell disease Diamond-Blackfan anemia Hereditary spherocytosis and elliptocytosis G6PD deficiency Pyruvate kinase deficiency Allergic-immunologic Immune hemolytic anemia Goodpasture syndrome Hemolytic uremic syndrome Systemic lupus erythematosus
Tumor	Leukemia Lymphoma Neuroblastoma Myelodysplastic syndrome Marrow infiltration

• Is there a family history of anemia, splenectomy, or gallbladder surgery?
—Many RBC membrane disorders are inherited. Some disorders, such as hereditary spherocytosis and elliptocytosis, frequently necessitate splenectomy due to RBC sequestration. Inherited diseases causing hemolysis, such as sickle cell disease, may be recognized in some families by a history of gallbladder surgery for gallstones.

• Are there signs of systemic illness, fatigue, growth failure, weight loss, or lymphadenopathy?
—The presence of these signs or symptoms should raise concern for malignancy.

• Was there exposure to certain medications or toxins?
—Questions regarding exposure to toxins or medications should be asked as these may cause anemia by hemolysis (e.g., sulfonamide or nitrofurantoin exposure in a patient with glucose-6-phosphate dehydrogenase [G6PD deficiency]) or

by suppressing bone marrow production of RBCs (e.g., trimethoprim/sulfamethoxazole).

- Did pallor develop quickly or gradually?
  — Information about the progression of anemia provides clues about the cause. Gradual onset suggests iron deficiency while acute onset with jaundice suggests hemolysis. In cases of gradual development of pallor, additional questions should focus on sources of iron loss or blood loss, such as history of heavy menstruation, blood in stool or melena, or multiple blood draws for diagnostic testing.

SUGGESTED READINGS

1. Poncz, M. Pallor. In: Schwartz MW, ed. *Pediatric Primary Care: A Problem-Oriented Approach.* 2nd ed. Chicago, London, Boca Raton, Littleton, MA: Year Book Medical Publishers; 1987.
2. Segel GB, Hirsh MG, Feig SA. Managing anemia in pediatric office practice: Part I. *Pediatr Rev.* 2002;23:75-84.
3. Shah S. Pallor. In: Fleisher GR, Ludwig S, eds. *Textbook of Pediatric Emergency Medicine.* 6th ed. Philadelphia: Lippincott Williams & Wilkins; 2010.
4. Bizzaro M, Colson E, Ehrenkranz R. Differential diagnosis and management of anemia in the newborn. *Pediatr Clin North Am.* 2004;51:1087-1107.

CASE 10-1

Three-Week-Old Boy

MAYA A. JONES

HISTORY OF PRESENT ILLNESS

The patient was a 3-week-old Caucasian male, born at 38 weeks gestation, who presented to an outpatient clinic for evaluation of anemia. Shortly after birth, he was noted to be pale in the newborn nursery. At that time, his hemoglobin was 12.3 g/dL with a mean corpuscular volume (MCV) of 120 fL. The hemoglobin was repeated at 2 weeks of age and was 8.1 g/dL with a reticulocyte count of 1.2%. He had initial problems with weight gain that improved after his mother started pumping and giving him breast milk via bottle in addition to breastfeeding. His parents thought he was often "sleepy" and were specifically concerned that he frequently fell asleep during feeds. He had no vomiting, diarrhea, fever, or cough. He had normal gold-colored bowel movements. There had been no change in urine color and he had no rash.

MEDICAL HISTORY

The infant was a twin born via vaginal delivery at 38 weeks gestational age following in vitro fertilization. He had transverse lie and was delivered vertex after external manipulation. The mother had anemia during pregnancy and her only medication was prenatal vitamins. Her blood type was

O positive. The birth weight was 2470 g; the infant's twin sibling weighed 2900 g at birth. On his first day of life, the infant was noted to have a swollen right upper leg with significant bruising. The initial radiograph was normal but a subsequent film showed evidence of a healing fracture that was presumably related to birth trauma. There was no history of jaundice in the newborn nursery.

The infant received multivitamin with iron. He did not have any known allergies. He received a diet of breast milk with occasional formula supplementation.

The family history was remarkable for the mother's anemia, which did not require treatment. The maternal grandmother also had a history of anemia. Both the maternal grandmother and aunt required cholecystectomy for gallstones.

PHYSICAL EXAMINATION

T 36.7°C; HR 166-230 bpm; RR 46-66/min; BP 70/37 mmHg

Weight 3.1 kg (25th percentile); Height 50 cm (50th percentile); Head circumference 36 cm (~75th percentile)

On examination, the infant was remarkably pale appearing, awakened easily, and cried. The anterior

TABLE 10-3.	Etiology of anemia by red blood cell morphology.

Microcytic Anemia

Iron deficiency

Lead poisoning

Thalassemias

Hemoglobinopathies

Sideroblastic anemia

Normocytic Anemia

Low reticulocyte count
  Anemia of chronic disease
  Transient erythoblastopenia of childhood
  Diamond-Blackfan anemia
  Infection
  Myelosuppression from medication side effect
  Renal disease
  Leukemia
  Marrow infiltration
  Aplastic anemia

Elevated reticulocyte count
  Blood loss
  Pulmonary hemosiderosis
  Goodpasture syndrome
  Immune hemolytic anemia
  Hemoglobinopathies
  Hereditary spherocytosis and elliptocytosis
  G6PD deficiency
  Pyruvate kinase deficiency
  Hemolytic-uremic syndrome
  Thrombotic thrombocytopenic purpura
  Kasabach-Merritt syndrome (hemangioma thrombocytopenia syndrome)

Macrocytic Anemia

Low reticulocyte count
  Folate or vitamin B_{12} deficiency
  Aplastic anemia
  Diamond-Blackfan anemia
  Transient erythroblastopenia of childhood

Elevated reticulocyte count
  Hemolytic anemia and high reticulocyte count
  Autoimmune hemolytic anemia

Secondary folate deficiency in hemolytic anemia

fontanel was open and flat. The conjunctivae were pale and the sclerae were anicteric. Mucous membranes were moist. The clavicles were intact. The infant was tachypneic but the lungs were clear to auscultation. On cardiac examination, the patient had a normal S1 and S2 and there was a 3/6 systolic murmur best appreciated at the left upper sternal border but not heard along the back. There were no gallops or rubs. The liver edge was palpable but the spleen was not. On musculoskeletal examination, the site of known extremity fracture had minimal edema but no tenderness and the right distal femur appeared larger than the left. The remainder of the examination was normal.

DIAGNOSTIC STUDIES

Complete blood count revealed the following: hemoglobin, 3.9 g/dL; 11 300 WBCs/mm³ (1% metamyelocytes, 43% segmented neutrophils, 34% lymphocytes, and 19% monocytes); 430 000 platelets/mm³; MCV, 117 fL; red cell distribution width, 17; and reticulocyte count, 0.3%. The peripheral blood smear revealed a few small spherocytes but no schistocytes, burr cells, or target cells.

COURSE OF ILLNESS

The infant was admitted for supportive care and a diagnostic evaluation begun. What are the likely cause for his anemia?

DISCUSSION CASE 10-1

DIFFERENTIAL DIAGNOSIS

Table 10-4 lists the differential diagnosis of anemia in an infant. This patient presented with pallor during infancy and no history of jaundice, which lessened the likelihood of hemolysis. There was no concern of a dietary etiology because of the baby's young age, there was no chronic illness apparent, and no history of blood loss; therefore, the focus shifted to a congenital defect in red cell production. There was a remarkable drop in the hemoglobin along with a very poor bone marrow response as far as production of reticulocyte. The white cells and platelets were normal and the anemia was macrocytic. The sum of these findings indicated a defect of red cell production. There was also the physical examination finding of a possible skeletal anomaly in the distal right femur.

Red cell aplasia may be congenital or acquired. Most of the acquired forms occur during adulthood or adolescence. In childhood the major causes of red cell aplasia are Diamond-Blackfan anemia,

TABLE 10-4.	Causes of anemia during infancy.	
Decreased Production	**Increased Destruction**	**Blood Loss**
Diamond-Blackfan anemia	Rh disease	Intracranial bleed
Transient erythroblastopenia of childhood	ABO incompatibility	Fetal-maternal transfusion
Aplastic crisis	G6PD	Twin-twin transfusion
Fanconi anemia	Hereditary spherocytosis	Placental abruption
Sickle cell disease	Elliptocytosis	Delayed cord clamping
Aplastic anemia	Thalassemia	
Iron deficiency	Unstable hemoglobinopathies	
TORCH infections	Sepsis	
Congenital leukemia	Metabolic disorders	
Nutritional deficiencies	Vitamin E deficiency	
Physiologic nadir		

transient erythroblastopenia of childhood, and acquired aplasia of red cells associated with chronic hemolysis (as seen in sickle cell disease).

In this case, there was no evidence of acute or chronic hemolysis and the patient was too young to be considered for transient erythroblastopenia of childhood. Another possible etiology to be considered was Fanconi anemia. Fanconi anemia is an autosomal recessive disorder associated with aplastic anemia, short stature, skeletal defects, pigmentation changes, and other abnormalities. Some cases of Fanconi anemia are diagnosed in the first year of life. The anemia involves all cell lines and the diagnosis is established via bone marrow analysis and genetic studies. However, the patient had anemia without abnormalities in the white blood cell or platelet count, thus Diamond-Blackfan was the most plausible diagnosis.

DIAGNOSIS

The infant was admitted with the diagnosis of anemia secondary to a hypoproductive state. The infant was felt to have symptomatic anemia (difficulty feeding); therefore, he was transfused with a total of 15 mL/kg of packed red blood cells administered in three separate aliquots. He underwent bone marrow aspiration, which revealed absence of red cell precursors with normal granulocyte

precursors, a finding consistent with Diamond-Blackfan anemia. Following the packed red cell transfusion, the infant's hemoglobin was 8.7 g/dL. He was more active and was no longer in respiratory distress. The baby received corticosteroids at 2 mg/kg/day, and was given an additional 5 mL/kg of packed red blood cells prior to discharge. **The final diagnosis in this case was Diamond-Blackfan anemia.**

INCIDENCE AND EPIDEMIOLOGY OF DIAMOND-BLACKFAN ANEMIA

The precise incidence is unknown; however, it is estimated that there are 300-1000 new cases of red cell aplasia annually in the United States. Diamond-Blackfan occurs primarily in infancy. Studies show that 10% of patients are anemic at birth, 25% by 1 month, 50% by 3 months, and 70% by 1 year. It is seen in all ethnic groups but primarily in Caucasians. There is no gender predominance.

CLINICAL PRESENTATION OF DIAMOND-BLACKFAN ANEMIA

Pallor caused by anemia in the early months of life characterizes this form of anemia. About one-third of patients have at least one associated finding, including characteristic facies, thumb anomalies, short stature, eye abnormalities including glau-coma, renal anomalies, hypogonads, skeletal anom-alies, congenital heart disease, and mental retarda-tion. There is a wide range of involvement. Some patients progress to full aplastic anemia and about 5% may develop leukemia or myelodysplasia.

DIAGNOSTIC APPROACHES

Complete blood count and peripheral blood smear. The mean hemoglobin level for all patients with Diamond-Blackfan anemia is 7 g/dL at diag-nosis. Infants diagnosed in the first 4 months of life typically have hemoglobin levels of 4 g/dL at presentation. The reticulocyte count is decreased or zero. The peripheral blood smear reveals mac-rocytes, anisocytosis, and teardrops. The WBC counts are normal in most patients; though in 20%, WBC counts are less than 5000/mm^3.

Bone marrow aspirate. Bone marrow aspirates and biopsies show normal cellularity, myeloid cells, and megakaryocytes. Approximately 90% of patients have erythroid hypoplasia or aplasia. The remaining 10% of patients have either normal erythroblast number and maturation or erythroid hyperplasia with maturation arrest. Despite the variable marrow findings, all patients have reticu-locytopenia, indicating some form of ineffective erythropoiesis and delayed precursor maturation.

Other studies. Serum iron, ferritin, folate, vitamin B$_{12}$, and erythropoietin are all elevated. In most cases, there is an increase in erythrocyte adenos-ine deaminase (eADA). Among patients with bone marrow failure syndromes, eADA had a sensitivity of 84%, specificity of 95%, and positive and nega-tive predictive values of 91% for the diagnosis of Diamond-Blackfan anemia. Genetic studies have shown one site on chromosome 19 and other gene defects have also been associated.

TREATMENT

The treatment includes use of corticosteroids. The current recommended dose is 2 mg/kg/day of prednisone, administered in 3-4 divided doses. Reticulocytes appear within 1-2 weeks but the rise

in hemoglobin is delayed for several more weeks. Once the hemoglobin level reaches 10 g/dL, the steroid dose is gradually tapered until the patient receives a single daily dose that adequately main-tains appropriate hemoglobin levels. Response followed by steroid dependence is seen in 60% of patients. Approximately one-fifth of the steroid-responsive patients may ultimately be maintained without steroids.

Approximately 30%-40% of patients have poor or no response to steroids and require chronic trans-fusion therapy to maintain normal hemoglobin. These children require leukocyte-depleted packed red blood cell transfusions every 3-6 weeks with the goal of keeping the hemoglobin level greater than 6 g/dL. Concurrent chelation of iron with subcutane-ously administered desferrioxamine may decrease some chronic transfusion-related complications. Complications of chronic transfusion therapy are similar to other conditions that employ this modal-ity (e.g., thalassemia). Bone marrow transplanta-tion has been successful for some patients.

Median survival is 43 years of age but approxi-mately 13% of patients die within the first six years of life. Deaths occur from complications of iron overload, pneumonia, sepsis, and occasionally from transplant-related complications, leukemia, and pulmonary emboli.

SUGGESTED READINGS

1. Alter BP. Inherited bone marrow failure syndromes. In: Nathan DG, Orkin SH, Ginsburg D, Look AT, eds. *Nathan and Oski's Hematology of Infancy and Child-hood*. 6th ed. Philadelphia: Saunders; 2003:280-365.
2. Ball SE, McGuckin CP, Jenkins G, et al. Diamond-Blackfan anaemia in the UK: analysis of 80 cases from a 20 year birth cohort. *Br J Haematol.* 1996;94:645-653.
3. Willing TN, Draptchinskaia N, Dianzani I, et al. Muta-tions in ribosomal protein S19 gene and Diamond Blackfan anaemia: wide variations in phenotypic expression. *Blood.* 1999;94:4294-4306.
4. Willing TN, Gazda H, Sieff CA. Diamond Blackfan anaemia. *Curr Opin Haematol.* 2000;7:85-94.
5. Fargo JH, Kratz CP, Giri N, et al. Erythrocyte adenosine deaminase: diagnostic value for Diamond-Blackfan anemia. *Br J Haematol.* 2012 [Epub ahead of print, PMID 23252420].

Twelve-Month-Old Girl

MAYA A. JONES

HISTORY OF PRESENT ILLNESS

A 12-month-old Caucasian girl presented to the emergency department with pallor. On the day of arrival, the grandparents had arrived from Florida and were alarmed at her appearance (Figure 10-1) prompting a visit to the emergency department. The child had last been seen by her grandparents a few months prior and at that time she appeared well. The parents conceded that she did appear more pale than usual. There was no fever, rash, vomiting, or diarrhea and her activity level was normal. She had no jaundice and had not traveled recently, although the parents had visited Puerto Rico 2 weeks ago.

MEDICAL HISTORY

The birth history was unremarkable. She had a febrile illness at 6 months of age but did not require hospitalization. Evaluation at that time included

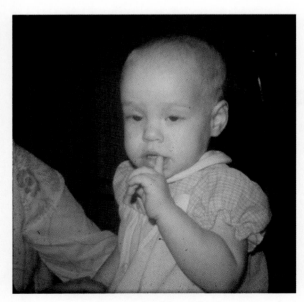

FIGURE 10-1. Photograph of the child showing marked pallor.

a complete blood count (see Diagnostic Studies) and a blood culture positive for *Staphylococcus epidermidis,* which was felt to be a contaminant. Her immunizations were up-to-date. She was breast fed until 6 months of age after which she began drinking whole milk. She was a finicky eater but had been growing well. There were no pets in the home and her development was normal.

PHYSICAL EXAMINATION

T 36.1°C; HR 145 bpm; RR 38/min; BP 97/53 mmHg; SpO$_2$ 99% in room air

The girl was pale but alert and playful. The conjunctivae were also pale but without injection or discharge. There was no lymphadenopathy and her neck was supple. A 2/6 systolic murmur was heard at the left upper sternal border without radiation. The lungs were clear to auscultation. On abdomen examination, there was no splenomegaly or hepatomegaly and there were no rash or petechiae on skin.

DIAGNOSTIC STUDIES

At 6 months of age, the complete blood count revealed the following: WBCs, 15 200/mm^3 (71% segmented neutrophils, 25% lymphocytes, and 4% monocytes); hemoglobin, 11.2 g/dL; 365 000 platelets/mm^3, with an MCV of 78 fL and an RDW was 17.3.

Her current studies revealed the following: WBCs, 8300/mm^3 (58% segmented neutrophils, 31% lymphocytes, and 11% monocytes); hemoglobin, 3.4 g/dL; and 410 000 platelets/mm^3 with an MCV 59 fL and an RDW of 15.1. The reticulocyte count was 1.4%. Stool was hemoccult negative.

COURSE OF ILLNESS

The history, examination (Figure 10-1), and laboratory findings suggested a diagnosis that was subsequently confirmed.

DISCUSSION CASE 10-2

DIFFERENTIAL DIAGNOSIS

Table 10-5 lists the differential diagnosis of microcytic anemia in children. Causes of iron deficiency include poor bioavailability, decreased iron absorption, blood loss, insufficient intake, and disruption of enteric mucosa or loss of functional bowel. Alkaline gastric pH reduces the solubility of inorganic iron, impeding absorption. Chronic use of acid pump blockers, vagotomy (for severe gastroesophageal reflux), and impaired gastric parietal cell function in pernicious anemia may compromise iron absorption. Iron absorption may also be disrupted after surgical bowel resection often following volvulus or intussusception. Iron deficiency in such cases develops slowly and may not become evident for several years. Blood loss is a leading cause of iron deficiency. Common causes of gastrointestinal blood loss in children include Meckel diverticulum, cow milk protein allergy, and parasitic infestation; however, blood loss from hematuria or pulmonary hemorrhage can also occur. In this case, the dietary history suggested a likely cause.

DIAGNOSIS

On examination the child was extremely pale (Figure 10-1). **The combination of a hypochromic microcytic anemia and paucity of dietary iron implicated iron deficiency as a cause of this child's pallor.** Subsequent tests, including iron level, ferritin, and total iron-binding capacity, supported this diagnosis. The child received a packed red blood cell transfusion followed by daily iron supplements. Studies performed 1 month later revealed a hemoglobin level of 9.7 g/dL. This case illustrates the importance of the red cell distribution width as a marker of iron deficiency that precedes anemia.

INCIDENCE AND EPIDEMIOLOGY

In developed countries, routine iron fortification of formulas and cereals led to a significant decrease in early childhood anemia. However, iron deficiency remains a leading cause of anemia. Currently, the prevalence of iron deficiency is approximately 7% and one-third of these children develop anemia. Children living below the poverty level are at greatest risk. Anemia is only one manifestation of iron deficiency. Even in the absence of anemia, children with iron deficiency may have neurocognitive and behavioral problems. Only some of these problems are reversible with iron supplementation, highlighting the importance of prevention.

CLINICAL PRESENTATION

The clinical examination in children with mild iron deficiency is usually normal. With moderate

TABLE 10-5.	Evaluation of microcytic anemia.			
	Iron Deficiency	*Lead*	*Thalassemia Trait*	*Chronic Disease*
Hemoglobin	↓	Normal or ↓	↓	↓
MCV	Normal or ↓	Normal or ↓	↓	Normal or ↓
RDW	Normal or ↑	Normal or ↑	Normal	Normal
RBC No.	↓	↓	Normal or ↓	↓
FEP	↑	↑	Normal	↑
Serum iron	↓	Normal	Normal	↓
TIBC	↑	Normal	Normal	Normal or ↓
% Transferrin saturation	↓	Normal	Normal or ↑	↓
Ferritin	↓	Normal	Normal	Normal or ↑

Abbreviations: MCV, mean corpuscular volume; RDW, red cell distribution width; RBC No., red blood cell number; FEP, free erythrocyte protoporphyrin; TIBC, total iron-binding capacity

or severe iron deficiency the findings may be similar to other causes of anemia including fatigue and pallor. If the anemia develops gradually, as in the child presented here, immediate family members may not notice changes in pigmentation. Other findings may include pica, the compulsive consumption of nonnutritive substances such as soil or ice. Longstanding iron deficiency may lead to angular stomatitis, glossitis, and softening of the fingernails leading to concave deformities descriptively termed "spooning (koilonychia)."

DIAGNOSTIC APPROACH

Complete blood count. In children, an elevated red cell distribution width is usually the earliest hematologic finding in iron deficiency. As the deficiency progresses, other hematologic parameters are affected (Table 10-5).

Peripheral blood smear. Peripheral blood smear in early disease may reveal anisocytosis. Red blood cells become microcytic and hypochromic as the iron deficiency progresses. With severe iron deficiency, red blood cells may be deformed and misshapen and demonstrate poikilocytosis.

Other studies. In the absence of a concurrent inflammatory disease state, the ferritin level decreases, reflecting diminished total tissue iron stores. With continued iron deficiency, reticuloendothelial macrophage iron stores become depleted and serum iron levels decrease. At this point, the total iron-binding capacity increases without a change in hemoglobin levels. When the transferrin saturation decreases to approximately 10%, the availability of iron becomes the rate-limiting step for hemoglobin synthesis. This leads to the accumulation of heme precursors called free erythrocyte protoporphyrins. Ultimately, the red blood cells become smaller as their hemoglobin content decreases.

TREATMENT

Treatment of iron deficiency depends on its etiology. For children with suspected dietary deficiency, treatment is supplemental iron. In children with anemia, an initial therapeutic trial often eliminates the need for expensive laboratory testing in determining the diagnosis. The reticulocyte count usually increases within several days and the hemoglobin increases within 3 weeks. Patients should be treated until the hemoglobin reaches the normal range and then continued for at least one additional month to replete the iron stores. Failure of the hemoglobin level to rise within 1 month indicates either poor compliance with iron therapy or incorrect diagnosis. The use of iron-fortified foods can reduce the likelihood of iron deficiency anemia.

SUGGESTED READINGS

1. Oski FA. Iron deficiency in infancy and childhood. *N Engl J Med*. 1993;329:190-193.
2. Segel GB, Hirsh MG, Feig SA. Managing anemia in pediatric office practice: part I. *Pediatr Rev*. 2002;23:75-83.
3. Andrews NC. Disorders of iron metabolism and sideroblastic anemia. In: Nathan DG, Orkin SH, Ginsburg D, Look AT, eds. *Nathan and Oski's Hematology of Infancy and Childhood*. 6th ed. Philadelphia: Saunders; 2003:456-497.
4. Lozoff B, Jimenez E, Wolf AW. Long-term developmental outcome of infants with iron deficiency. *N Engl J Med*. 1991;325:687-694.
5. Aslan D, Altay C. Incidence of high erythrocyte count in infants and young children with iron deficiency anemia: re-evaluation of an old parameter. *J Pediatr Hematol Oncol*. 2003;25:303-306.
6. Centers for Disease Control and Prevention. Iron deficiency-United States, 1999-2000. *MMWR*. 2002;51: 897-899.
7. Athe R, Vardhana Rao MV, Nair KM. Impact of iron-fortified foods on Hb concentration in children (<10 years): a systematic review and meta-analysis of randomized controlled trials. *Public Health Nutr*. 2013 [Epub ahead of print, PMID 23388159].

CASE 10-3

Five-Month-Old Boy

STEPHEN LUDWIG

BRANDON C. KU

HISTORY OF PRESENT ILLNESS

A 5-month-old African-American boy presented with pallor, difficulty breathing, and lethargy. He was in his usual state of good health until 4 days prior to admission when he developed a fever to 102-103°F with rhinorrhea. There was no coughing, vomiting, or diarrhea. The patient otherwise seemed well at the time. During the next few days, he developed increased work of breathing with decreased appetite. One day prior to admission, the mother noted that he seemed lethargic and irritable. Oral intake was significantly decreased; the infant was taking in only 8 ounces rather than his typical 48 ounces over the day. The patient was brought to the emergency department. In retrospect, the father noted that his abdomen seemed to be increasing in size and firmness over the last month with some tenderness.

MEDICAL HISTORY

The infant was born at term after an uncomplicated pregnancy. He was taken home on the second day of life. He had no known allergies. He did not receive any medications. Immunizations appropriate for age had been promptly administered, including two doses of the pneumococcal conjugate vaccine. The family history was notable for sickle cell disease in a paternal cousin and reactive airway disease, cervical cancer, and ovarian cancer in several maternal relatives. A great uncle died of "jaundice" at 3 years of age and a cousin at 10 years of age.

PHYSICAL EXAMINATION

  T 38.4°C; HR 160 bpm; RR 58/min; BP 83/38 mmHg; Weight 5.7 kg

In general, the child was lethargic and responsive only to painful stimuli. He also had severe respiratory distress. The anterior fontanel was sunken. The pupils were equal, round, and reactive to light. The conjunctivae and oral mucosa were pale. The lips were dry and cracked. There were white patches on the buccal mucosa that were easily removed with scraping. There was shotty anterior and posterior cervical adenopathy. The lungs were clear to auscultation but the child had mild grunting and flaring. There was a 2/6 systolic ejection murmur at the left lower sternal border. The abdomen was firm with a liver edge palpable 5 cm below the right costal margin. The spleen was palpable at the level of the umbilicus. Bowel sounds were present. The extremities were cool with delayed capillary refill (5 seconds). On neurologic examination, the child localized pain but had decreased tone and diminished spontaneous activity.

In the emergency department, the patient had an oxygen saturation of 94% in room air. He received several normal saline boluses as well as sodium bicarbonate and intravenous dextrose. Blood and urine cultures were obtained. The patient received intravenous cefotaxime for presumed sepsis.

DIAGNOSTIC STUDIES

White blood 14 300 cells/mm^3 (2% band forms; 52% segmented neutrophils, 42% lymphocytes, 2% eosinophils, 2% atypical lymphocytes). Hemoglobin, 2.6 g/dL; platelets, 184 000/mm^3; MCV, 88 fL; red sell distribution width, 17.4; total bilirubin, 4.6 mg/dL with an unconjugated level of 3.8 mg/dL; hepatic transaminases were normal; lactate dehydrogenase level was 2984 IU/L (normal range, 934-2150). Chest radiograph was normal. There was no cardiomegaly, infiltrates, or mediastinal masses.

COURSE OF ILLNESS

The peripheral blood smear (Figure 10-2), in conjunction with other laboratory findings, suggested the diagnosis.

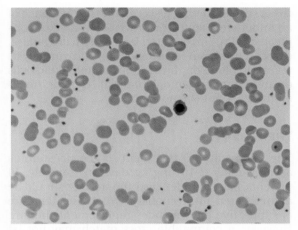

FIGURE 10-2. Peripheral blood smear.

DISCUSSION CASE 10-3

DIFFERENTIAL DIAGNOSIS

This child came to the hospital with significant severe pallor of acute onset. The child has had no medications or unusual exposures. It was clear that the child was critically ill. Despite the severe illness, white blood cell and platelet counts were normal. The most significant finding was the severe anemia. The increased unconjugated bilirubin and lactate dehydrogenase levels suggested a hemolytic process. Other causes of hemolytic anemia were considered in this case, including drug associated hemolytic anemia, disorders of red cell membrane and cytostructure (e.g., hereditary spherocytosis), abnormalities of red blood cell metabolism (e.g., glucose-6-phosphate-dehydrogenase deficiency), as well as sepsis with disseminated intravascular coagulation. The patient was given antibiotics to cover this later possibility. Parvovirus B19 infection may cause severe anemia but usually due to bone marrow suppression rather than hemolysis.

Patients with a microangiopathic hemolytic anemia such as hemolytic uremic syndrome and thrombotic thrombocytopenic purpura usually have schistocytes rather than spehrocytes on peripheral blood smear. Both of these conditions usually present with severe thrombocytopenia. A child of this age should be closely examined for physical abnormalities seen with Diamond-Blackfan syndrome and Fanconi anemia. Laboratory studies allowed differentiation of the diagnostic possibilities.

DIAGNOSIS

The peripheral blood smear revealed a nucleated red cell (erythroid progenitor cell) prematurely released from the bone marrow into the peripheral circulation (Figure 10-2). There were also many small spherocytes. Polychromasia was also noted because the bone marrow releases large numbers of reticulocytes and nucleated red blood cells to compensate for accelerated red cell destruction. A direct antiglobulin test (DAT or Coombs) was positive, confirming the presence of antibodies to circulating red blood cells. Specifically, this test was positive for IgG and negative for C3, consistent with the diagnosis of warm agglutinin autoimmune hemolytic anemia. **The patient had autoimmune hemolytic anemia of the warm agglutinin type.**

INCIDENCE AND EPIDEMIOLOGY OF AUTOIMMUNE HEMOLYTIC ANEMIA (AHA)

Autoimmune hemolytic anemia (AHA) occurs as a result of antibody, antibody and complement complex, or complement binding to the red blood cell. The resulting immunologic reaction destroys red cells and causes anemia. Infectious agents, drugs, and other agents may stimulate the process. Some autoimmune disease such as systemic lupus erythematosus may also generate anti-red cell antibodies and red cell destruction. The true incidence of AHA is unknown but is estimated at 1-3 cases per 100000 population per year. Acute AHA usually presents in the first 4 years of life.

CLINICAL MANIFESTATION OF AUTOIMMUNE HEMOLYTIC ANEMIA

Children usually present with signs and symptoms of severe anemia. In younger children, parents or other family members may note pallor or weakness. Older children may complain of exercise intolerance or dizziness. Jaundice and scleral icterus result from the recycling of unconjugated bilirubin released from hemolyzed red blood cells.

Dark urine suggests hemoglobinuria. On examination there is usually mild or moderate splenic enlargement. Some patients present with congestive heart failure related to the rapid development of anemia.

DIAGNOSTIC APPROACH

Complete blood count. The anemia of acute onset AHA is usually significant. Most children have a hemoglobin level of 4-7 g/dL. The MCV may be relatively normal, reflecting the weighted average of small microspherocytes and large reticulocytes. Erythrocyte agglutination within the sample tube may artifactually raise the MCV on an automated counter. An elevated red cell distribution width may be a clue that several different red cell populations are present such as microspherocytes forming after partial splenic ingestion and large reticulocytes. There is an increase in reticulocytes once the bone marrow has a chance to respond. The white blood cell and platelet counts are typically normal. Concurrent thrombocytopenia indicates Evan syndrome, aplastic anemia, hemolytic uremic syndrome, or other conditions rather than isolated autoimmune hemolytic anemia.

Direct antiglobulin (Coombs) test. A positive Coombs test confirms the suspected diagnosis. To establish a diagnosis there must be antibody and evidence of hemolysis. The red cell antibodies that react at 37°C (warm antibodies) are usually IgG and do not cause spontaneous agglutination of cells unless Coombs antiserum is added. Cold antibodies are usually IgM and react at 4°C. These are considered complete antibodies because no antiserum needs to be added to cause the red blood cell destructive process. There are also cases of mixed-type autoimmune responses.

Other studies. Other tests can provide evidence of an underlying hemolytic process: elevated unconjugated bilirubin, elevated lactate dehydrogenase, decreased serum haptoglobin, and urinalysis revealing blood on dipstick but no red blood cells on microscopy (hemoglobinuria). Hepatic transaminases should be normal.

TREATMENT

The mainstay of treatment is corticosteroids administered 2-10 mg/kg/day. In severely ill patients, like our index case, the steroids should be administered intravenously. Otherwise, the care is supportive and includes replacement therapy. However, a compatible cross match may not be possible. But if the patient is in extremis blood type group O, RH-negative blood should be used in aliquots that are given slowly and in amounts sufficient to stabilize the cardiovascular system. The patient should be adequately hydrated to avoid renal involvement. At times, splenectomy may be necessary for those who fail steroid therapy.

SUGGESTED READINGS

1. Gehrs BC, Friedberg RC. Autoimmune hemolytic anemia. *Amer J Hematol.* 2002;69:258-271.
2. Flores G, Cunningham-Rundles C, Newland AC, et al. Efficacy of intravenous immunoglobulin in the treatment of autoimmune hemolytic anemia: results in 73 patients. *Am J Hematol.* 1993;44:237-242.
3. Ware RE. Autoimmune hemolytic anemia. In: Nathan DG, Orkin SH, Ginsburg D, Look AT, eds. *Nathan and Oski's Hematology of Infancy and Childhood.* 6th ed. Philadelphia: Saunders, 2003;521-559.
4. Naithani R, Agarwal N, Mahapatra M, et al. Autoimmune hemolytic anemia in children. *Pediatr Hematol and Oncolog.* 2007;24:309-315.

Six-Year-Old Girl

STEPHEN LUDWIG

BRANDON C. KU

HISTORY OF PRESENT ILLNESS

A 6-year-old Caucasian girl developed fever, abdominal pain, and pallor 3 days prior to admission. She had one episode of nonbilious emesis. Two days before admission, the family thought she was pale and then "yellow." On the day of admission, she had a rash on her buttocks and extremities. She complained of feeling dizzy in the morning. She had decreased oral intake and her urine appeared slightly dark. She also had several loose stools.

MEDICAL HISTORY

Six years prior, the patient had been admitted for dehydration and was noted to have anemia at that time. Past surgical history was notable for three surgeries for cleft palate and cleft lip repair. There were no known allergies and she did not require any medications. Her immunizations were up to date. She had also received the hepatitis A vaccination series prior to her vacation in Mexico 1 year ago. There had been no recent travel. She lived with her parents. There were no pets. The mother had her spleen removed after blunt abdominal trauma suffered in a car accident. The mother also required supplemental iron therapy for treatment of anemia. A maternal aunt required removal of her gallbladder at 19 years of age. Multiple family members suffered from diabetes mellitus.

PHYSICAL EXAMINATION

T 38.5°C; HR 142 bpm; RR 24/min; BP 100/50 mmHg; Weight 25 kg (50th percentile)

On general examination, the patient was very pale but alert and oriented. The scelera were mildly icteric. The oropharynx had mild erythema but no exudates or vesicles. The lungs were clear to auscultation. A gallop was appreciated on cardiac examination. The abdomen was soft. A tender spleen was palpated 4 cm below the left costal margin. There was no tenderness in the right upper quadrant. The capillary refill was brisk. The remainder of the examination was normal.

DIAGNOSTIC STUDIES

White blood 6300 cells/mm^3 (64% segmented neutrophils, 30% lymphocytes, and 6% monocytes). Hemoglobin, 4.5 g/dL; platelets, 179 000/mm^3; red cell distribution width was elevated at 16.9; mean corpuscular volume, 78 fL; mean corpuscular hemoglobin concentration, 37 mg/dL; reticulocyte count, 8.4%; total bilirubin, 3.3 mg/dL; unconjugated bilirubin, 2.4 mg/dL; uric acid, 2.3; lactate dehydrogenase, 1136; serum albumin, transaminases, and electrolytes were normal.

COURSE OF ILLNESS

This child was admitted for fever and abdominal pain. Significant anemia was noted on complete blood count. The presence of a gallop with severe anemia prompted a gradual packed red blood cell transfusion. She received empiric ceftriaxone after a blood culture was obtained. The peripheral blood smear suggested a diagnosis (Figure 10-3).

DISCUSSION CASE 10-4

DIFFERENTIAL DIAGNOSIS

The history of gallbladder surgery in a young aunt certainly raises the possibility of an inherited hemolytic disorder. The mother's history of splenectomy may be related to splenic laceration due to trauma; however, the history of anemia is intriguing. The differential diagnosis is that of other hemolytic anemias both congenital and acquired. There are other disorders of the red cell membrane and cytoskeleton including spherocytosis, elliptocytosis, and stomatocytosis. Also under consideration are disorders of red cell enzymes (e.g., glucose-6-phosphate

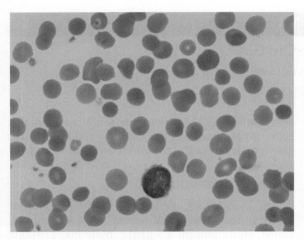

FIGURE 10-3. Peripheral blood smear.

dehydrogenase deficiency), drug associated, and autoimmune hemolytic anemia. The differential diagnostic possibilities are broad but spherocytosis is the most common of the congenital causes. Basic laboratory testing allows for the establishment of the correct diagnosis.

DIAGNOSIS

The peripheral blood smear revealed numerous small spherocytes (note the lack of central pallor seen in normal red blood cells), wide variation in red blood cell size (anisocytosis), and a paucity of normal red blood cells (Figure 10-3). Causes of spherocytosis include conditions that lead to red cell membrane damage such as immunohemolytic anemias (e.g., autoimmune hemolytic anemia), clostridial toxin, severe burns, Wilson disease, and hereditary spherocytosis. **This child had hereditary spherocytosis (HS),** a congenital hemolytic anemia caused by defects in proteins comprising the red blood cell skeleton. Subsequent evaluation of other family members revealed mild hereditary spherocytosis in the mother and maternal aunt. The grandparents declined testing.

INCIDENCE AND EPIDEMIOLOGY OF HEREDITARY SPHEROCYTOSIS

Spherocytosis incidence in the United States is 1 in 5000 live births. It is most common in individuals of Northern European descent but does occur in other ethnic groups. Inheritance is usually autosomal dominant but in up to a quarter of the cases family history is negative. In some cases, family members have only minor manifestations. A family history of gallbladder surgery or splenectomy should raise suspicion for underlying hemolytic diseases, including hereditary spherocytosis. In other situations there may be a new mutation or a recessive pattern of inheritance. The defects for this condition are found on chromosomes 1, 8, 14, 15, and 17.

CLINICAL PRESENTATION OF HEREDITARY SPHEROCYTOSIS

Presentation depends to some extent on severity of the spherocytosis. Fatigue due to anemia or episodic jaundice are common complaints. Jaundice may be noted more frequently during viral infections. Most children have splenomegaly (50% of infants and 75%-90% of older children). During the newborn period some cases are detected by severe or prolonged hyperbilirubinemia. Some patients present with gallstones.

DIAGNOSTIC APPROACH

Complete blood count. Patients with hereditary spherocytosis have varying degrees of anemia, reticulocytosis, elevated mean corpuscular hemoglobin, and hyperbilirubinemia. In mild forms, the hemoglobin may be normal (compensated hemolysis). Those with moderate or moderately severe spherocytosis have a hemoglobin level that ranges from 6 to 10 g/dL and a reticulocyte count of 8% or greater. Those with severe spherocytosis typically have hemoglobin levels less than 6 g/dL and reticulocyte counts greater than 10%. The MCHC exceeds the normal value in about one-third of affected patients. The finding of an MCHC greater than 35 g/dL has a sensitivity of 70% and a specificity of 86% in diagnosing hereditary spherocytosis. The MCV is usually normal but the red cell distribution width is elevated due to the mixed population of small spherocytes and large reticulocytes.

Peripheral blood smear. The finding of spherocytes on peripheral blood smear is characteristic. Spherocytes are round, dense, hyperchromic red cells that lack the typical central pallor and biconcavity of normal red blood cells. They are present in 25%-35% of patients with mild spherocytosis but on almost all patients with moderate or severe disease. In contrast to some other causes of hemolytic disease, spherocytes and microspherocytes are the only abnormal cells visualized on the peripheral blood smear in patients with hereditary spherocytosis. In severe hereditary spherocytosis, the spherocytes may appear dense, contracted, or budding. Nucleated red blood cells are not usually seen. Howell-Jolly bodies are seen in only 4% of patients prior to splenectomy.

Osmotic fragility test. Normal red blood cells have a high surface-to-volume ratio (more membrane than they need). When normal red blood cells are suspended in a hypotonic saline solution they expand due to the influx of fluid. The extra membrane present allows the cells to expand and gradually take the shape of a sphere, a conformation that efficiently minimizes the surface area relative to volume. As the solution becomes progressively hypotonic, the normal red cells become more spherical and ultimately burst, releasing hemoglobin into the solution. In spherocytes, the red cell surface area is already decreased relative to volume at the start. Cells that start with a low surface-to-volume ratio (e.g., spherocytes) reach the spherical limit at a higher saline (less hypotonic) concentration than normal cells. The fragility is calculated by measuring the percent lysis at specific saline concentrations.

Other studies. The glycerol lysis test measures the rate rather than extent of hemolysis. The hypertonic cryohemolysis test is based on the fact that spherocytes are particularly sensitive to cooling in hypertonic solutions. In contrast to the other tests, this test is independent of the surface-to-volume ratio. Other findings in children with hereditary spherocytosis such as unconjugated hyperbilirubinemia and increased fecal urobiloinogen reflect chronic hemolysis.

TREATMENT

Patients with hereditary spherocytosis require folic acid supplementation to keep up with their chronic hemolysis (usually 0.5-1 mg/day orally). Patients with spherocytosis may require transfusion in the acute phase. Splenectomy can reduce or eliminate the need for transfusion. Most often splenectomy is delayed until the patient reaches 5 or 6 years of age, a time when the risk of pneumococcal sepsis has decreased considerably. Children evaluated for splenectomy should receive vaccination with both the heptavalent pneumococcal conjugate and the pneumococcal 23-valent polysaccharide vaccines. Postsplenectomy, penicillin prophylaxis is generally recommended.

Complications related to hereditary spherocytosis include gallstones, hemolytic crises, and aplastic crises. Bilirubinate gallstones can be asymptomatic or can cause cholecystitis or biliary obstruction. Ultrasonography detects these pigmented stones and some specialists recommend routine abdominal ultrasounds every 5 years. Hemolytic crises occur commonly in children with hereditary spherocytosis, usually in association with viral syndromes. Transient jaundice, emesis, and abdominal pain characterize the hemolytic crisis. Most children do not require specific treatment but the development of severe anemia may lead to hospitalization and packed red blood cell transfusion. Aplastic crises occur less frequently than hemolytic crises but severe anemia may precipitate congestive heart failure. Aplastic crises frequently occur following parvovirus B19 infection.

SUGGESTED READINGS

1. Michaels LA, Cohen AR, Zhao HMA, et al. Screening for hereditary spherocytosis by use of automated erythrocyte indexes. *J Pediatr.* 1997;130:957-960.
2. Evans TC, Jehle D. The red cell distribution width. *J Emerg Med.* 1991;9:72-74.
3. Gallagher PG, Lux SE. Disorders of the erythrocyte membrane. In: Nathan DG, Orkin SH, Ginsburg D, Look AT, eds. *Nathan and Oski's Hematology of Infancy and Childhood.* 6th ed. Philadelphia: Saunders; 2003:560-684.
4. Tse WT, Lux SE. Red blood cell membrane disorders. *Br J Haematol.* 1999;104:2-13.
5. Delhommeau F, Cynober T, Schischmanoff PO, et al. Natural history of hereditary spherocytosis during the first year of life. *Blood.* 2000;95:393-397.
6. Bolton-Maggs PH, Langer JC, Iolascon A, et al. Guidelines for the diagnosis and management of hereditary spherocytosis – 2011 update. *Br J Haematol.* 2012;156:37-49.
7. Casale M, Perrotta S. Splenectomy for hereditary spherocytosis: complete, partial or not at all. *Expert Rev Hematol.* 2011;4:627-635.

CASE 10-5

Five-Year-Old Girl

STEPHEN LUDWIG

BRANDON C. KU

HISTORY OF PRESENT ILLNESS

A 5-year-old African-American girl was brought to the emergency department for complaints of pallor and fatigue. For the past 3-4 days she seemed tired. She had not been eating or drinking as usual and had been relatively inactive. There have been no fevers. She denied nausea, vomiting, and diarrhea. Her urinary pattern has not changed. She has no specific sites of pain or discomfort. The mother stated that her eyes are always somewhat yellow and the color had not changed.

MEDICAL HISTORY

The girl was full-term product of a spontaneous vaginal delivery. At 2 years of age she developed painful swelling of her hands. Her 5-year-old sibling had witnessed a "bee sting." She was treated with diphenhydramine and corticosteriods for a possible allergic reaction. The swelling resolved over the course of several days. She required emergency department evaluation at 4 years of age for persistent left knee and back pain after falling. Radiographs of her spine, hips, and left femur, tibia, and fibula were normal. She was treated with a combination of ibuprofen and oxycodone. She has not received any medications recently. She was born in Jamaica and moved to the United States at 2 years of age. Her immunizations were reportedly up-to-date although written confirmation was not available.

PHYSICAL EXAMINATION

T 37.3°C; HR 140 bpm; RR 30/min; BP 100/60 mmHg; SpO$_2$ 95% in room air; Weight 5th percentile

Physical examination revealed a thin child with obvious scleral icterus. She was in mild respiratory distress. The neck was supple. There were several small cervical lymph nodes palpable. The lungs were clear. There was a 1/6 systolic ejection murmur at the lower left sternal border. The abdomen was soft. The liver edge was palpable 1-2 cm below the right costal margin. The spleen was massively enlarged and could be felt at the pelvic brim. The remainder of the examination was normal.

DIAGNOSTIC STUDIES

A WBC count of 8200/mm^3 (2% band forms, 23% segmented neutrophils, 61% lymphocytes, 12% monocytes, and 2% eosinophils) Hemoglobin, 4.6 g/dL; platelets, 156000/mm^3; reticulocyte count, 16%; total bilirubin, 2.4 mg/dL; hepatic function panel was normal; chest radiograph was normal.

COURSE OF ILLNESS

The peripheral blood smear revealed the diagnosis (Figure 10-4).

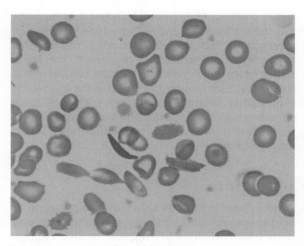

FIGURE 10-4. Peripheral blood smear.

DISCUSSION CASE 10-5

DIFFERENTIAL DIAGNOSIS

The findings on peripheral blood smear were suggestive of sickle cell disease (see below). In patients known to have sickle cell disease who present with the signs of pallor and fatigue, the differential diagnosis consists of four elements—infection, acute red cell aplasia (aplastic crisis), acute hemolytic crisis, or sequestration. Infections until recently were the major cause of mortality in children. Infection is usually heralded by fever. Any fever in a patient with sickle cell disease or one of the variants must be taken seriously and treated aggressively. Acute red cell aplasia occurs when red cell production fails to keep up with the need produced by a shortened red cell survival. Often parvovirus B19 is the cause of this type of acute drop in hemoglobin. Acute hemolysis may also occur and cause a worsening of anemia. Often parents will detect an increase in jaundice or a darkening of the child's urine. Sequestration can be diagnosed by clinical examination and tends to occur in young children whose spleens have not yet auto-infarcted. Table 10-6 shows the comparison of findings in the different manifestations of sickle cell disease.

DIAGNOSIS

The peripheral blood smear revealed numerous blunted and boxy sickled cells more typically seen with SC type sickle cell disease (Figure 10-4).

This diagnosis was confirmed by hemoglobin electrophoresis. **The clinical picture in light of the peripheral blood smear suggested the diagnosis of sickle cell disease (SC type) with associated splenic sequestration.** In retrospect, the episode of hand swelling at 2 years of age may have been dactylitis, a complication of sickle cell disease in young children. The episode of pain requiring narcotics may have been a vasoocclusive episode causing pain. Obviously, this would be difficult to prove in retrospect. She promptly received penicillin prophylaxis.

INCIDENCE AND EPIDEMIOLOGY OF SICKLE CELL DISEASE WITH SEQUESTRATION

The cultural incidence of sequestration is not known. Sickle cell disease affects one in every 400-500 African-Americans. It also occurs in people of Mediterranean, Arabic, and Indian origins. There are three major forms of sickle cell disease in the United States population: Hgb SS Disease (60%), Hgb SC Disease (30%), and Sickle B+ Thalassemia (10%). In patients with Hgb SS type, sequestration usually occurs early in life since the spleen ultimately undergoes auto infarction. Children with milder forms of disease, typically SC type, may develop sequestration as late as 10 or 11 years of age.

CLINICAL PRESENTATION OF SICKLE CELL DISEASE WITH SEQUESTRATION

The manifestations of sequestrations are varied. The patient may have a mild form of sequestration with only a minor drop in hemoglobin or may

TABLE 10-6.	Comparison of findings in sequestration, aplastic, and hemolytic crises in sickle cell disease.		
	Sequestration Crisis	*Aplastic Crisis*	*Hemolytic Crisis*
Onset	Sudden	Gradual	Sudden
Pallor	Present	Present	Present
Jaundice	Normal	Normal	Increased
Abdominal pain	Present	Absent	Absent
Hemoglobin level	Very low	Low or very low	Low
Reticulocytes	Unchanged or increased	Decreased	Increased
Marrow erythroid activity	Unchanged or increased	Decreased	Increased

Source: Cohen A, Hematologic emergencies. In: Fleisher G, Ludwig S, eds. *Textbook of Pediatric Emergency Medicine*. 4th ed. Philadelphia: Lippincott Williams & Wilkins; 2000.

present in full cardiovascular collapse. In all cases, there is splenic enlargement and evidence of a decrease in circulating blood volume. There may be a fatal outcome if therapeutic response is not adequate. Splenic sequestration may recur.

DIAGNOSTIC APPROACH

The diagnosis is established by having a high index of suspicion and a careful physical examination. Laboratory studies will rule out other conditions in the differential diagnosis but there is no single laboratory test to confirm sequestration. Part of the high index of suspicion comes in having a well-educated patient and patient population that is capable of recognizing and reporting every sign and symptom.

Hemoglobin electrophoresis. Hemoglobin electrophoresis establishes the diagnosis of sickle cell disease. In a patient with homozygous sickle cell disease, electrophoresis reveals more than 80% HbSS, less than 20% HbF (fetal hemoglobin), and less than 4% HbA2. Patients with hemoglobin SC disease, as in this case, will have equal proportions of HbS and HbC. In contrast, carriers will have approximately 35% HbSS and more than 60% HbA.

Complete blood count. The hemoglobin concentration in children with homozygous sickle cell disease (HbSS) is low, typically less than 9 g/dL. In contrast, the hemoglobin concentration of children with hemoglobin SC disease is higher, typically 10-12 g/dL.

Peripheral blood smear. The peripheral blood smear reveals characteristic sickle cells. Other findings include target cells (excess red cell membrane relative to the amount of hemoglobin) and, as a result of hemolysis, schisocytes.

Reticulocyte count. The reticulocyte count is elevated, but the value depends on the extent of hemolysis.

Other studies. Laboratory findings that indicate hemolysis include increased lactate dehydrogenase, increased unconjugated bilirubin, reduced serum haptoglobin, and hemoglobinuria.

TREATMENT

In mild cases with hemodynamic stability, hydration and careful watching in an inpatient setting may be all that is required. In severe cases, prompt transfusion therapy is required. Some patients are placed on a routine transfusion program. In frequently recurring episodes, splenectomy may be indicated. Splenic infarct occurs over time and the splenic function is usually already compromised.

SUGGESTED READINGS

1. Ohene-Frempong K. Abnormalities of hemoglobin structure and function. In: Rudolph A, ed. *Rudolph's Pediatrics*. 21st ed. New York: McGraw-Hill; 2003.
2. Kinney TR, Ware RE, Schultz WH, et al. Long-term management of splenic sequestration in children with sickle cell disease. *J Pediatr*. 1990;117:194-199.
3. Piccone CM. Sickle cell disease. In: Florin TA, Ludwig S, eds. *Netter's Pediatrics*. Philadelphia: Elsevier; 2011.
4. Brousse V, Elie C, Benkerrou M, et al. Acute splenic sequestration crisis in sickle cell disease: cohort study of 190 paediatric patients. *Br J Haematol*. 2012;156:643-648.
5. Rezende PV, Viana MB, Murao M, et al. Acute splenic sequestration in a cohort of children with sickle cell anemia. *J Pediatr*. 2009;85:163-169.

CASE 10-6

Two-Year-Old Boy

STEPHEN LUDWIG

BRANDON C. KU

HISTORY OF PRESENT ILLNESS

The patient was a 2-year-old boy who was in his usual state of good health until the day of admission when he visited his grandmother who felt his "color was off." She had not seen him for 4 weeks. The mother took his temperature, which was normal. He did not have fever, vomiting, or diarrhea and his activity level had not changed. At the grandmother's insistence, he was taken to the hospital for evaluation. He had not received any medications recently. He had an upper respiratory infection approximately 6 weeks ago, which resolved without intervention.

MEDICAL HISTORY

The infant was born at term by spontaneous vaginal delivery after an uncomplicated pregnancy. The birth weight was 3400 g. He had not required any hospitalizations or undergone any surgical procedures. He reportedly had a "rash" with amoxicillin approximately 1 year ago during treatment of an otitis media. He had received the appropriate immunizations for his age. He had traveled to Lake George in New York State 2 months ago. His developmental history was normal. There were no siblings. The family history was unremarkable.

PHYSICAL EXAMINATION

T 38.0°C; HR 120 bpm; RR 25/min; BP 113/54 mmHg; SpO_2 98% in room air

In general, the child was alert and in no acute distress. However, he was extremely pale. The conjunctivae were anicteric. The tympanic membranes were normal in appearance. The lungs were clear to auscultation. There were no murmurs on cardiac examination. Distal pulses were strong. The abdomen was soft without hepatomegaly or splenomegaly. The palmar creases were remarkable for the loss of pigmentation.

DIAGNOSTIC STUDIES

The complete blood count revealed the following: WBCs 8400/mm³; hemoglobin, 7.2 g/dL; platelets, 326000/mm³; MCV, 81 fL; Red cell distribution width, 12.4; Reticulocyte count was 0.2%. Serum electrolytes, blood urea nitrogen, glucose, transaminases, albumin, and lactate dehydrogenase were all normal. Direct Coombs test was negative. Parvovirus IgM and IgG were also negative.

COURSE OF ILLNESS

The child was noted to be pale by his grandmother when he went to see her for a visit. This history speaks of the insidious onset of this child's pallor. His mother who lived with him day by day did not notice the change. The child had been well except for a mild viral illness. He had no other symptoms. There was no family history of anemia and no previous complete blood counts that suggested any problem. His examination was normal except for the pallor and when laboratory studies were obtained he had a normocytic normochromic anemia and a reticulocyte count of virtually zero. None of the other cell lines was abnormal. The findings indicated a need for a bone marrow aspirate and analysis that confirmed the diagnosis (Figure 10-5).

DISCUSSION CASE 10-6

DIFFERENTIAL DIAGNOSIS

The differential diagnosis of acquired red cell aplasia includes transient erythroblastopenia of childhood (TEC), anemia associated with parvovirus B19, drug and chemical involved, and idiopathic. The condition may also be confused with congenital red cell aplasia (Diamond-Blackfan) but the age of onset of TEC is usually older and there are no associated anomalies. Also, TEC is a normocytic

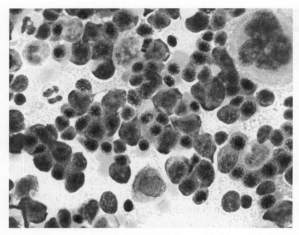

FIGURE 10-5. Bone marrow aspirate.

anemia while Diamond-Blackfan anemia is usually macrocytic.

DIAGNOSIS

The bone marrow aspirate revealed numerous young (nucleated) red blood cells all in the same stage of maturation (Figure 10-5). **This finding combined with the normal MCV and low reticulocyte count suggested the diagnosis of transient erythroblastopenia of childhood on the verge of recovery.** It is one of the most common acquired red cell aplasias.

INCIDENCE AND EPIDEMIOLOGY OF TRANSIENT ERYTHROBLASTOPENIA (TEC)

Transient erythroblastopenia (TEC) is a condition that occurs in previously well children. The age of diagnosis is usually around 2 years with a typical range of 1- 3 years. There is often a history of a preceding upper respiratory tract infection or other viral illness but no single agent has been identified. Parvovirus infection is usually not an etiologic agent in this diagnosis.

CLINICAL MANIFESTATION OF TRANSIENT ERYTHROBLASTOPENIA

The presenting signs and symptoms are usually pallor and fatigue. Sometimes tachycardia and

feelings of palpitations prompts a visit to the physician's office and subsequent detection. There are no other common significant manifestations but there have been sporadic cases of TEC associated with neurologic conditions including papilledema and transient hemiplegia. One recent report links TEC and breath holding.

DIAGNOSTIC APPROACHES

The suspicion for TEC comes with a patient of the appropriate age who has insidious onset of anemia and no reticulocyte response.

Complete blood count. The median hemoglobin value at presentation is 5-6 g/dL but varies significantly depending on whether the diagnosis occurs early or late in the course of disease. Reticulocyte counts are less than 1% except for those children on the cusp of recovery. White blood cell and platelet counts are typically normal, though exceptions are possible. The MCV in TEC is usually normal while the MCV in Diamond-Blackfan anemia is usually elevated. Other features also help distinguish between TEC and Diamond-Blackfan anemia (Table 10-7).

Bone marrow aspirate. During the illness, the bone marrow reveals significant erythroblastopenia with

TABLE 10-7.	Features of transient erythroblastopenia of childhood and Diamond-Blackfan anemia.	
Feature	TEC	DBA
Age >1 year at diagnosis	80%	10%
Physical anomalies	0%	30%
Adenosine deaminase	Normal	Elevated
Elevated mean corpuscular volume at diagnosis	5%	80%
Elevated fetal hemoglobin (HbF) at diagnosis	20%	100%
Elevated i antigen at diagnosis	20%	100%

Abbreviations: TEC, transient erythroblastopenia of childhood; DBA, Diamond-Blackfan anemia

Adapted from Alter BP. Inherited bone marrow failure syndromes. In: Nathan DG, Orkin SH, Ginsburg D, Look AT, eds. *Nathan and Oski's Hematology of Infancy and Childhood.* 6th ed. Philadelphia: Saunders; 2003:280-365.

maturation arrest. During the recovery phase, patients with TEC produce a cohort of "fetal-like" erythrocytes that evolve into normal red blood cells. All marrow red blood cells are at the same stage of maturation.

Other studies. Interpretation of MCV, fetal hemoglobin, and i antigen depends on stage of illness. During the recovery phase the MCV, fetal hemoglobin, and i antigen may all be elevated. Ultimately, the distinction is often made when the patient with TEC begins recovery.

TREATMENT

Treatment is supportive. A blood transfusion may be needed for hemodynamic instability. Resolution typically occurs within 1-3 months after diagnosis. Approximately 5%-10% of children have

begun to recover by the time medical care is sought. There are no other associated hematologic problems. The prognosis is excellent.

SUGGESTED READINGS

1. Skeppner G, Kreuger A, Elinder G. Transient erythroblastopenia of childhood: prospective study of 10 patients with special reference to viral infections. *J Pediatr Hem/Onc.* 2002;24:294-298.
2. Chan GC, Kanwar VS, Williams J. Transient erythroblastopenia of childhood associated with transient neurologic deficit: report of a case and review of the literature. *J Paediatr Child Health.* 1998;34:299-301.
3. Tam DA, Rash FC. Breath-holding spells in a patient with transient erythroblastopenia of childhood. *J Pediatr.* 1997;130:651-653.
4. Shaw J, Meeder R. Transient erythroblastopenia of childhood in siblings: a case report and review of the literature. *J Pediatr Hematol Oncol.* 2007;29:659-660.

CHAPTER 11

FEVER

SAMIR S. SHAH

DEFINITION OF THE COMPLAINT

The complaint of fever accounts for a large portion of ambulatory pediatric visits. While classically defined as a temperature greater than 38.0°C for neonates and greater than 38.5°C for older children, the term "fever" is subject to significant interpretation. An isolated temperature measurement of 38.0°C in a toddler may not be meaningful; however recurrent daily temperatures of 38.0°C during a period of several weeks may indicate an underlying pathology.

Practitioners must also remember that body temperature normally fluctuates throughout the day. Body temperature tends to be lower in the early morning and peaks in the evening. Certain conditions or activities, such as exercise, warm baths, or hot drinks, also affect the measured temperature. Additionally, temperature values of axillary measurements may be 0.5°C-1.0°C lower than oral, rectal, or tympanic measurements. To compensate for such discrepancies, parents are sometimes instructed to add 0.5°C or 1.0°C to axillary measurements to approximate the "real" temperature. Such "corrections" may further cloud evaluation of the febrile child.

COMPLAINT BY CAUSE AND FREQUENCY

Fever may develop in response to injury, infection, autoimmune disease, or malignancy. The release of endogenous pyrogens triggers a cascade of reactions that ultimately raise the hypothalamic set-point. Fever may also be caused when the body's heat production or environmental heat overwhelms heat loss mechanisms or when heat loss mechanisms are deficient. Viruses are the most common cause of fever in children. Specific common causes of fever are too numerous to list here but less common causes of fever are listed in Table 11-1.

CLARIFYING QUESTIONS

The clarifying questions listed below may help provide clues to the diagnosis.

• What temperature value is the parent using to define a fever?
  —While 98.6°F is commonly considered the normal body temperature, normal body temperature exhibits significant daily variation with a nadir in the early morning and a peak in the early evening.

• Are there symptoms of specific illness?
  —The presence of certain complaints such as bloody diarrhea, cough, and stiff neck suggests specific diagnostic categories.

• Is there exposure to animals?
  —Animal exposure refers not only to pets within the home but also to contact with animals owned by the school or by friends and acquaintances. Inquire about contact with rodents and farm animals as well as consumption of unpasteurized dairy products and raw or undercooked meats. For example, exposure to house mice may suggest lymphocytic choriomeningitis virus, while exposure to farm animals suggests brucellosis as a potential cause. The animal-exposure history should also elicit participation in recreational

TABLE 11-1.	Less common causes of fever.
Diagnostic Category	*Examples*
Infection	Endemic fungi (histoplasmosis, blastomycosis) Enteric diseases (*Salmonella* spp., *Shigella* spp.) Human immunodeficiency virus Infectious mononucleosis (Epstein-Barr virus, cytomegalovirus) Protozoa (malaria, toxoplasma) Tickborne diseases (Lyme, Rocky Mountain spotted fever) Tuberculosis Zoonoses (cat-scratch, tularemia, brucellosis)
Collagen Vascular Disease	Systemic juvenile rheumatoid arthritis Systemic lupus erythematosus Dermatomyositis Scleroderma Sarcoidosis Vasculitis (e.g., Kawasaki, Behçet, Wegener granulomatosis)
Malignancy	Leukemia Lymphoma
Inflammatory Bowel Disease	Crohn disease Ulcerative colitis
Drug Fever	Penicillins Cephalosporins Sulfonamides Phenytoin Methylphenidate Cimetidine Acetaminophen
Factitious Fever	Pseudofever Munchausen syndrome by proxy
Recurrent Fever Syndromes	Familial Mediterranean fever Hyper-IgD syndrome PFAPA syndrome Tumor necrosis factor receptor-associated periodic fever
Centrally Mediated Fever	

activities such as hunting or triathlons that include a fresh-water swimming component. An outbreak of leptospirosis, a cause of prolonged fever, occurred in athletes and community residents following a triathlon; 11% of triathletes and 6% of community residents contracted leptospirosis.

Household contacts with occupational exposure to potentially infectious animals should also be sought.

- Were there recent tick bites?
  —Tularemia, ehrlichiosis, anaplasmosis, Rocky Mountain spotted fever, babesiosis, and Lyme disease may be acquired in this manner.

- Was there any recent travel?
  —Travel to regions where certain diseases are endemic may shift the differential diagnosis. For example, travel to the Indian subcontinent raises the suspicion for typhoid fever, and malaria. Coccidioidomycosis would be included in the differential diagnosis of a child with atypical pneumonia who has traveled to the Southwestern United States.

- What medications is the child receiving?
  —Medications may cause fever. Some of the most common mechanisms include altered thermoregulatory regulation (e.g., cimetidine, anticholinergic agents) and idiosyncratic reactions. Medications commonly implicated as a cause of fever include penicillins, cephalosporins, acetaminophen, anticonvulsants, and methylphenidate. Medication-related fever may occur any time after initiation of therapy but typically occurs within 1-2 weeks of medication initiation. Children with medication-related fever typically appear well rather than ill.

- What is the pattern of fever?
  —The evaluation of acute, prolonged, and recurrent fevers differs dramatically. When distinguishing between prolonged and recurrent fevers is difficult, documenting the fevers in a "fever diary" may help clarify the pattern. It is also important to clarify the method used ("felt warm" vs. actual measurement), duration of thermometer insertion, location (tympanic membrane, oral, axillary, or rectal), time of day, and whether the elevated temperature—in cases of prolonged fever or fever of unknown origin—was confirmed by more than one person.

- What is the patient's ethnicity?
  —Some causes of recurrent fever occur more commonly among certain ethnic groups: familial Mediterranean fever (Armenian, Arab, Turkish, Sephardic Jews), Hyper-IgD (Dutch, French), and

tumor necrosis factor receptor-associated peri-odic fever syndrome (TRAPS) (Irish, Scottish).

SUGGESTED READINGS

1. Calello DP, Shah SS. The child with fever of unknown origin. *Pediatr Case Rev.* 2002;2:226-239.
2. Nizet V, Vinci RJ, Lovejoy FH Jr. Fever in children. *Pediatr Rev.* 1994;15:127-135.
3. Saper BC, Breder CD. The neurologic basis of fever. *N Engl J Med.* 1994;330:1880-1886.
4. Tunnessen WW Jr. Fever. In: Tunnessen WW Jr., ed. *Signs and Symptoms in Pediatrics.* 3rd ed. Philadelphia: Lippincott Williams & Wilkins; 1999:3-7.
5. Morgan J, Bornstein SL, Karpati AM, et al. Outbreak of leptospirosis among triathlon participants and community residents in Springfield, Illinois, 1998. *Clin Infect Dis.* 2002;34:1593-1599.

CASE 11-1

Eighteen-Month-Old Girl

REBECCA TENNEY-SOEIRO

HISTORY OF PRESENT ILLNESS

An 18-month-old girl presented with a 1-day history of fever to 38.0°C and cough. While in the examination room, she had tonic flexion of her upper extremities and her "eyes rolled back." This episode lasted 10 minutes and resolved spontaneously. Mild perioral cyanosis developed just before the end of the seizure. Afterward, the child was tired and irritable. There was no history of rash, eye pain, neck pain, or emesis. There were no alterations in gait or balance. There was no antecedent witnessed trauma. The only pet was a recently acquired goldfish. Several children at her daycare had symptoms of upper respiratory infection. The remainder of the review of systems was unremarkable.

MEDICAL HISTORY

The girl was born at term after an uncomplicated pregnancy. She had not previously required hospitalization. Her immunizations were up-to-date and included the pneumococcal conjugate vaccine. The child received supplemental iron starting at 12 months of age for treatment of "anemia." The maternal grandmother had type 2 diabetes treated with glyburide, a sulfonylurea oral hypoglycemic agent. There was no family history of febrile seizures but one relative supposedly had a seizure and drowned while swimming. The family was not able to provide further details.

PHYSICAL EXAMINATION

T 39.1°C; HR 132 bpm; RR 26/min; BP 97/53 mmHg; SpO$_2$ 98% in room air

Weight 25th percentile

The child was crying and seemed mildly disoriented. There were no bruises or abrasions on her face or scalp. Her tympanic membranes were mildly erythematous but mobile. There was copious purulent nasal discharge. The neck was difficult to assess due to the child's lack of cooperation. While yelling and screaming, she was able to arch her back and neck without apparent limitation. There was no cervical lymphadenopathy. The heart and lung sounds were normal. The abdomen was soft without organomegaly. There were no focal neurologic deficits but the child appeared groggy and irritable and was slow to respond to her mother's voice. Several hyperpigmented macules were noted on her skin as her clothes were removed for the lumbar puncture (Figure 11-1).

DIAGNOSTIC STUDIES

Complete blood count revealed the following: 15 500 WBCs/mm^3 (61% segmented neutrophils, 22% lymphocytes, 15% monocytes, and 2% eosinophils); hemoglobin, 12.1 g/dL; and 282 000 platelets/mm^3. Serum electrolytes, calcium, and

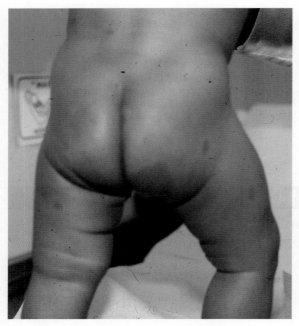

FIGURE 11-1. Photo of patient's skin findings.

glucose were normal. Urinalysis revealed no white blood cells or nitrites. Lumbar puncture revealed 2 WBCs/mm^3 and 19 RBCs/mm^3. No bacteria were visualized on Gram stain. The CSF protein and glucose were normal. Blood and CSF cultures were subsequently negative.

COURSE OF ILLNESS

The skin findings (Figure 11-1) suggested a diagnosis that was subsequently confirmed with further evaluation.

DISCUSSION CASE 11-1

DIFFERENTIAL DIAGNOSIS

This child presented with fever and seizures. Given the age and difficult examination, a lumbar puncture was performed to exclude meningitis as a cause of seizures. The reassuring CSF findings led to other diagnostic considerations. The maternal grandmother used an oral hypoglycemic agent making an ingestion-induced hypoglycemic seizure

possible. However, the child's serum glucose was normal. The history of a relative drowning during a reported seizure raised the specter of cardiac conditions, such as prolonged QT syndrome, Wolf-Parkinson White syndrome, and hypertrophic cardiomyopathy, as possible causes of hypoxic seizures. The EKG, performed in light of this history, was normal.

In an 18-month-old girl presenting with a brief (<10 minute) seizure in the context of fever, simple febrile seizure is the most likely diagnosis. However, it is possible that the fever lowered the seizure threshold in a child with an underlying seizure disorder. Potentially important clues in this case were the hyperpigmented macules on the child's skin. Café-au-lait spots, while characteristic for neurofibromatosis type 1, may also be noted in unaffected children and in other disorders. The critical factor in this case is the number of spots seen; fewer than 0.1% of normal individuals have more than six café-au-lait spots. Inherited disorders associated with café-au-lait spots are summarized in Table 11-2.

DIAGNOSIS

Examination of the skin revealed approximately 15 hyperpigmented macules substantially greater than 5 mm in diameter (Figure 11-1). Axillary freckling was also noted on physical examination. An ophthalmology examination revealed findings suspicious for an optic glioma. These findings confirmed the diagnosis of neurofibromatosis type 1 (NF1). Given her age, it is likely that this child had a febrile seizure; however, the possibility of NF1 was considered by the treating physicians on the basis of the child's skin findings. This child did not have structural brain lesions to suggest a specific cause of seizures attributable to NF.

EPIDEMIOLOGY AND INCIDENCE

NF1 and NF2 are genetic disorders in which affected patients develop both benign and malignant tumors at increased frequency. NF1 is associated with cutaneous lesions, vision loss, and skeletal problems, while cataract formation and hearing loss are more typically associated with NF2. NF1, also known as von Recklinghausen NF or peripheral NF, is an autosomal dominant condition. One-half of cases occur

TABLE 11-2.	Inherited multisystem diseases associated with café-au-lait spots.
Disease	*Key Features*
Ataxia telangiectasia	Bulbar telangiectasia, progressive ataxia, oculomotor apraxia, recurrent sinopulmonary infection
Bannayan-Riley-Ruvalcaba syndrome (formerly Riley-Smith, Ruvalcaba-Myhre, and Bannayan syndromes)	Macrocephaly, subcutaneous lipomas, pigmentary changes of penis, polyposis of colon, hypotonia, joint hyperextensibility, seizures
Bloom syndrome	Short stature, malar hypoplasia, facial telangiectatic erythema, propensity to develop malignancy
Fanconi syndrome	Pancytopenia, mental retardation, hypoplastic radii and thumbs, microcephaly, microphthalmia, genitourinary tract anomalies, generalized hyperpigmentation
McCune-Albright syndrome	Polyostotic fibrous dysplasia, precocious puberty, nevi with irregular ("coast of Maine") borders
Multiple lentigines syndrome (LEOPARD syndrome)	*L*entigenes, *E*KG abnormalities, *O*cular hypertelorism, *P*ulmonic stenosis, *A*bnormal genitalia, *R*etardation of growth, *D*eafness
Multiple endocrine neoplasia type 2b	Medullary thyroid carcinoma, pheochromocytoma, parathyroid adenoma, marfanoid habitus, mucosal neuromas
Neurofibromatosis type 1	See text
Russell-Silver syndrome	Intrauterine growth retardation, congenital hemihypertrophy, precocious puberty, small/triangular face
Tuberous sclerosis	Abnormal hair pigmentation, adenoma sebaceum, shagreen patches, seizures

in patients with a family history of NF1 and the other half occur as spontaneous mutations. The incidence is approximately 1 in 3000. The clinical manifestations of NF1 result from alterations of the NF1 gene located on chromosome 17. The gene product, termed neurofibromin, is thought to function as a negative growth regulator.

CLINICAL PRESENTATION

Despite advances in our understanding of the molecular basis for NF1, the diagnosis remains one largely based on clinical criteria. Clinical diagnosis of NF1 requires the presence of at least two of the seven National Institutes of Health consensus criteria (Table 11-3). Children with sporadic rather than inherited cases may not meet the NIH diagnostic criteria until later in life. At 1 year of age, approximately 50% of sporadic cases lack two or more of the cardinal clinical features permitting diagnosis but by age 8 years 95% meet NIH criteria.

The most visible features of NF1 are flat, evenly pigmented macules known as café-au-lait spots. These macules, often present at birth, increase in both number and size over the first few years of life. One or two café-au-lait macules are present in up to 25% of the normal population but the presence of six or more macules should raise suspicion for NF1. These macules are easier to visualize using a Wood lamp. Skinfold freckling, another pigmentary change associated with NF1, usually occurs in the axillae, inguinal region, nape of the neck, or above the eyelids. By 6 years of age, approximately 80% of children with NF1 demonstrate axillary or inguinal freckling.

Lisch nodules are benign pigmented hamartomas of the iris occurring in patients with NF1. These nodules do not interfere with vision. Lisch nodules may not be apparent in young children but are present in more than 95% of adolescent and adult patients. Detection of Lisch nodules on bedside examination is challenging and diagnosis frequently requires a slit-lamp examination by an experienced ophthalmologist. In contrast to Lisch nodules, optic nerve tumors, such as optic nerve gliomas, primarily occur in younger children. They are often associated with asymmetric noncorrectable visual loss, diminished peripheral vision and color discrimination, and proptosis.

TABLE 11-3.	Diagnostic criteria for neurofibromatosis type 1.

Diagnostic Criteria*

1) Six or more café-au-lait spots
   –Greater than 1.5 cm in postpubertal children
   –Greater than 0.5 cm in prepubertal children
2) Greater than 2 neurofibromas or any type of greater than1 plexiform neurofibroma
3) Freckling in the axillary or inguinal regions (Crowe sign)
4) Optic glioma
5) Two or more Lisch nodules
   –Benign iris hamartomas
6) Distinctive bony lesions
   –Dysplasia of sphenoid bone or long bone cortex
7) First-degree relative with neurofibromatosis type 1
   –Includes parent, sibling, or offspring

*Diagnostic for neurofibromatosis type 1 if two or more criteria present

Subcutaneous or cutaneous (dermal) neurofibromas are rarely seen in young children but appear during or just before adolescence. Neurofibromas are present in 48% of 10-year-old patients and 84% of 20-year-old patients. Cutaneous lesions frequently begin as small papules on the face, scalp, trunk, and extremities. Deep lesions may be detected only through palpation. These lesions represent a major cosmetic problem but do not transform into malignant tumors. In contrast, plexiform neurofibromas surround soft tissue and bone causing aberrant growth. Plexiform neurofibromas, present in 30% of patients, are locally invasive and may transform into malignant peripheral nerve sheath tumors. They may be accompanied by overlying hyperpigmentation or hypertrichosis. Fluorodeoxyglucose positron emission tomography (FDG-PET) imaging is proving to be useful to differentiate benign plexiform neurofibromas from MPNSTs. Other tumors that occur with higher frequency in patients with NF1 include pheochromocytomas, juvenile chronic myeloid leukemia, and rhabdomyosarcomas.

Seizures occur in approximately 5% of patients with NF1. Seizures may be generalized or partial. In a study by Korf et al., 22 of 359 NF1 patients developed seizures. The seizures were most often characterized as complex-partial (9 patients), febrile (6 patients), or generalized epilepsy (3 patients).

Cardiovascular manifestations include hypertension, congenital heart disease, and vasculopathy. The arterial system is most affected by vasculopathy and renal artery stenosis is the most common manifestation. Other manifestations of NF1 include learning disabilities, behavioral abnormalities, pain, scoliosis, tibial dysplasia, headaches, stroke, and bowel or bladder complications (secondary to pelvic plexiform neurofibromas).

DIAGNOSTIC APPROACH

NF1 is diagnosed by the presence of clinical features mentioned previously. Evaluation should focus on symptoms associated with NF1, such as neurocognitive deficits, visual complaints, progressive neurologic deficits, altered bowel or bladder function, weakness, seizures, and headaches. Other medical complications associated with NF1 include hypertension, short stature, and precocious puberty. Once the diagnosis is made, the following management strategies should be considered.

Orthopedic referral. Tibial dysplasia appears at birth with anterolateral bowing of the lower leg. The presence of tibial bowing should prompt referral to an orthopedic surgeon familiar with the management of orthopedic problems in children with NF1. Patients should also be referred if scoliosis is noted.

Ophthalmologic referral. Symptomatic optic gliomas are diagnosed in the first year of life in 1% of NF1 patients though they typically develop between 4 and 6 years of age. They are ultimately present in 15% of patients with NF1 and cause symptoms in 2%-5% of cases. An annual vision evaluation by an experienced ophthalmologist is part of the routine follow-up for children with NF1.

Head MRI. Routine presymptomatic screening for CNS tumors is *not* necessary. However, any evidence of optic nerve dysfunction, seizures, or neurologic abnormalities warrants neuroimaging with special attention to the orbits.

Other radiology studies. Plain radiographs may detect a variety of bony abnormalities. They should be ordered when clinical findings suggest bony erosion secondary to an adjacent plexiform neurofibroma, scoliosis, or bone pain.

Genetic evaluation. Families who have a child with NF1 may benefit from genetic counseling. Genetic testing can be difficult due to the large number of possible mutations. Linkage analysis is offered but is not helpful in sporadically affected individuals. The use of complementary techniques permits detection of approximately 95% of mutations in those who fulfill diagnostic criteria.

Other studies. Children with NF1 should be monitored for blood pressure elevations associated with renal artery stenosis or pheochromocytomas. Approximately 6% of NF1 patients develop hypertension and a secondary cause (e.g., renal artery stenosis) is identified in one-third of cases. Learning disabilities are seen in 40%-60% of children with NF1. Children should undergo evaluation for cognitive and motor function with prompt referral or intervention as required. Plexiform neurofibromas grow in early childhood, are difficult to remove, and tend to regrow. A multidisciplinary team that includes the primary pediatrician as well as surgeons, radiologists, and oncologists should manage these neurofibromas.

TREATMENT

No specific therapy is currently available. In the future, targeted therapies for NF1-associated tumors may be designed to inhibit growth-promoting pathways activated in the absence of neurofibromin. Other potential therapies focus on blockade of angiogenic factors that could potentially decrease tumor growth.

Routine office visits should focus on detection and management of complications as discussed earlier. Annual ophthalmologic examinations are important to detect optic nerve lesions. Interval history should focus on subtle sensory or motor symptoms, such as paresthesia or muscle atrophy. Pediatricians should also inquire about incontinence given the risk of spinal cord neurofibromas. Consultation with specific surgical specialists is warranted based on the location of neurofibromas. Laser treatment has not yet been proven to be successful in permanently removing café-au-lait spots.

SUGGESTED READINGS

1. Williams V, Lucas J, Babcock M, et al. Neurofibromatosis type 1 revisited. *Pediatrics.* 2009;123:124-133
2. DeLucia T, Yohay K, Widmann R. Orthopaedic aspects of neurofibromatosis: update. *Curr Opin Pediatr.* 2011;23:46-52.
3. Brenner W, Friedrich RE, Gawad KA, et al. Prognostic relevance of FDG PET in patients with neurofibromatosis type 1 and malignant peripheral nerve sheath tumours. *Eur J Nucl Med Mol Imaging.* 2006;33:428-432.
4. DeBella K, Szudek J, Friedman JM. Use of the National Institutes of Health criteria for diagnosis of neurofibromatosis 1 in children. *Pediatrics.* 2000;105:608-614.
5. Lynch TM, Gutmann DH. Neurofibromatosis 1. *Neurologic Clin.* 2002;20:841-865.
6. Riccardi VM, Eichner JE. Neurofibromatosis: past, present, and future. *N Engl J Med.* 1991;324:1283-1285.
7. Tekin M, Bodurtha JN, Riccardi VM. Café au lait spots: the pediatrician's perspective. *Pediatr Rev.* 2001;22:82-90.

CASE 11-2

Ten-Year-Old Boy

MATTHEW TEST

SAMIR S. SHAH

HISTORY OF PRESENT ILLNESS

A 10-year-old boy presented with a 4-day history of worsening cough with occasional episodes of hemoptysis. Three days before presentation, he developed chills and fever to 38.9°C. Two days prior to presentation he had increasingly frequent posttussive emesis. He complained of abdominal pain with coughing. He also complained of "not having any energy." There was no weight loss or night sweats. There were no known contacts with a chronic cough or history of tuberculosis. No family members lived or worked in nursing homes. He had not traveled outside of the state of Pennsylvania. Prior to this illness, he was actively participating in soccer at school. He had also assisted with household chores that included washing dishes, mowing the lawn, and sweeping the chimney.

MEDICAL HISTORY

The boy's birth history was unremarkable. He required hospitalization at 1 year of age for *Salmonella* gastroenteritis leading to dehydration. Epidemiologic investigation attributed a local *Salmonella* outbreak occurring during that time to a pet store engaging in improper import of reptiles. The family turtle, purchased from that store, was held culpable for this child's illness and removed from the home at the family's request. The only other pet was a healthy cat acquired 2 years ago. The patient did not require any medication. He received appropriate childhood immunizations. A paternal uncle suffered from adult-onset diabetes.

PHYSICAL EXAMINATION

   T 38.3°C; HR 108 bpm; RR 24-28/min; BP 111/72 mmHg; SpO$_2$ 97% in room air

   Weight 95th percentile

On examination, the patient was observed to be alert and cooperative. His oropharynx was clear. There was no cervical lymphadenopathy. There were no crackles or wheezing on lung examination. Heart sounds were normal. There was no hepatomegaly or splenomegaly. There were two mildly tender erythematous nodules on the anterior aspect of his left tibia. There were no other rashes.

DIAGNOSTIC STUDIES

A complete blood count revealed the following: 20 400 WBCs/mm^3 (83% neutrophils, 5% eosinophils, and 11% lymphocytes); hemoglobin, 12.2 g/dL; and 372 000 platelets/mm^3.

COURSE OF ILLNESS

Chest radiograph revealed ill-defined pulmonary nodules. A chest computed tomography was

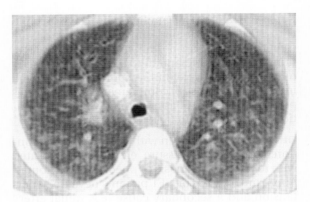

FIGURE 11-2. Chest computed tomogram.

performed to better delineate the radiographic findings (Figure 11-2). Tuberculous skin testing was negative.

DISCUSSION CASE 11-2

DIFFERENTIAL DIAGNOSIS

The differential diagnosis of reticulonodular infiltrates on chest radiograph or chest CT includes tuberculosis as well as pulmonary disease caused by endemic fungi, such as blastomycosis, coccidioidomycosis, and histoplasmosis. Tuberculosis is possible, particularly given the hemoptysis, but is less likely with a negative tuberculin skin test. Knowledge of this patient's travel history virtually excludes blastomycosis and coccidioidomycosis. In an adolescent, *Mycoplasma pneumoniae* may cause hilar adenopathy as well as diffuse lung infiltrates.

Hypersensitivity pneumonitis, sarcoid, and vasculitis (particularly Wegener granulomatosis) may cause similar findings. Sarcoidosis, a multisystem granulomatous disease, usually presents with generalized lymphadenopathy and prominent cervical involvement. Associated findings include erythema nodosum and uveitis. Granuloma formation occurs in the eyes, skin, liver, spleen, and parotid glands. Blacks are more commonly affected than whites. Wegener granulomatosis is relatively uncommon in children.

DIAGNOSIS

The chest CT revealed bilateral hilar lymphadenopathy (Figure 11-2). The largest hilar lymph node on the right measured 1.7 × 2.2 cm. The CT also revealed numerous pulmonary nodules ranging in size from a few millimeters to 1 cm. No acid-fast bacilli were detected in serial sputum samples. *Mycoplasma pneumoniae* polymerase chain reaction (PCR) of a nasopharyngeal aspirate was negative. Antigens to influenza A and B, parainfluenza types 1, 2, and 3, adenovirus, and respiratory syncytial virus were not detected by immunofluorescence of nasopharyngeal washings. **The diagnosis of pulmonary histoplasmosis was confirmed by detection of *Histoplasma capsulatum* antigen in the urine and a fourfold increase in *H. capsulatum* antibody between acute and convalescent serum samples.** The chimney cleaning likely contributed to the development of pulmonary histoplasmosis. He improved clinically during the next 3 days without specific treatment. A repeat chest radiograph was normal 2 weeks later.

EPIDEMIOLOGY AND INCIDENCE

Histoplasma capsulatum is a dimorphic fungus that grows as a yeast-like organism at temperatures greater than 37°C and as a spore-forming mold at lower temperatures. It is endemic in certain areas of the United States and Latin America. Between 1958 and 1965, a total of 275 558 military recruits raised in different areas of the United States underwent *Histoplasma* skin testing. Recruits from states of the Ohio and Mississippi River valleys along with Maryland and Virginia had the highest rates of reaction. Histoplasma was also prevalent in parts of Pennsylvania and Texas. This study by Edwards et al. remains the largest study of histoplasmosis endemicity in the United States.

Histoplasma capsulatum resides in the soil in endemic areas. Excretions of birds and bats facilitate growth of the organism. As a consequence, *H. capsulatum* infections are associated with aerosolization of debris from sites where birds or bats roost, as may occur by cutting firewood, sweeping chimneys, or playing in hollow trees, barns, or caves. Infection occurs after inhalation of spores that transform to the yeast phase in the lung. Hematogenous dissemination may occur after primary pulmonary infection. Rarely, the skin or intestinal mucosa serves as the portal of entry.

CLINICAL PRESENTATION

Severity of illness depends on the intensity of exposure and host's immune status. Low-intensity exposure usually results in asymptomatic infection in immunocompetent hosts. Higher intensity exposures lead to pulmonary infection, manifested as fever, cough, malaise, and poor appetite. Some patients experience pleuritic chest pain. Rales and wheezing may also occur. Erythema nodosum and other hypersensitivity reactions to infection occasionally develop. Symptoms are self-limited and last 2 or 3 days. In a small number of children, symptoms persist for more than 2 weeks. Symptoms persisting longer than 3 weeks after acute histoplasmosis suggest progressive disease or dissemination. In the immunocompetent host, extrapulmonary dissemination is rare. Infants younger than 2 years of age are at higher risk of disseminated disease than older children. Features of disseminated histoplasmosis include prolonged fever, failure-to-thrive, and hepatosplenomegaly. Pericardial and pleural effusions occur rarely.

In the immunocompromised host, the illness begins with fever and cough, followed by worsening respiratory distress. Disseminated histoplasmosis is more likely to occur in immunocompromised patients. These patients usually have diarrhea, weight loss, hepatomegaly, splenomegaly, and skin lesions. Less commonly, dissemination leads to bone marrow involvement, meningitis, pericarditis, or chorioretinitis.

DIAGNOSTIC APPROACH

Histoplasma capsulatum does not comprise the normal flora of humans, so its isolation from mucous membranes, skin lesions, deep organs, or body fluids usually indicates infection.

Chest radiograph. In those with respiratory symptoms, chest radiograph abnormalities include hilar adenopathy and localized or diffuse reticulonodular lung infiltrates. In patients with previous pulmonary infection (symptomatic or subclinical), single or multiple calcified nodules may be detected in the lungs, hilar lymph nodes, spleen, or liver. Cavitary lesions resembling tuberculosis may be seen in those with chronic pulmonary histoplasmosis (rare in children). Among immunocompromised children with disseminated disease, 40%-50% have normal chest radiographs.

Culture. Culture of the organism on standard mycologic media, including brain-heart infusion agar or broth, requires a 2- to 6-week incubation period, making culture methods less useful in the acute setting (but important for confirmation of the organism in certain cases). Specimens appropriate for culture depend on the site of infection (pulmonary, cutaneous, or disseminated) and include sputum (for pulmonary disease), skin lesion biopsy specimens, blood, bone marrow, and organ biopsy specimens. Culture is most sensitive in patients with disseminated infection, being positive in greater than 75% of cases.

Histoplasmin skin test. The histoplasmin skin test has several limitations that limit its usefulness as a diagnostic tool. First, in endemic areas, the prevalence of skin test positivity because of previous asymptomatic infection approaches 60% among young adults. Second, the skin test is unable to reliably distinguish asymptomatic past infection from symptomatic current infection. Third, administration of the skin test has been associated with falsely elevated antibody titers in 15%-25% of patients, meaning that use of the skin test may complicate the interpretation of other diagnostic methods. Its use is now limited to epidemiologic investigations.

Serum *H. capsulatum* antibody. This test is recommended for routine detection of infection in otherwise healthy children. Antibodies are detectable 2-4 weeks after infection. Antibody titers greater than 1:8 or a fourfold increase between acute and convalescent titers suggests acute infection. Titers revert to negative 12-18 months after infection. Serologic tests are positive in 90% of patients with symptomatic disease; however, their utility is limited in immunocompromised patients. Cross-reaction from *Blastomyces* or *Coccidioides* antibodies can occur, but the travel history usually differentiates these from *H. capsulatum*.

Histoplasma capsulatum urinary antigen detection. This test is most useful in diagnosing

disseminated disease in young children or infection at any site in immunocompromised patients, in whom antibody titers can be falsely negative. It is also positive in 80% of patients with acute pulmonary infection. Sensitivity is increased when combined with serum antigen testing. In a study by Fojtasek et al., *H. capsulatum* antigenuria was detected in all 22 children with disseminated histoplasmosis. Declining antigenuria levels correlate with clinical improvement. Like antibody titers, false positive antigen tests have been reported in patients with *Blastomyces* and *Coccidiodes*.

Histologic examination of tissue. Severely immunocompromised patients with disseminated histoplasmosis commonly have negative antibody titers and normal chest radiographs. They occasionally have negative urine antigen tests as well. In the severely ill, immunocompromised patients with negative *H. capsulatum* testing but continued suspicion of infection, a bone marrow biopsy should be considered for early detection and management of this life-threatening illness. In these patients, ovoid yeast forms are frequently visible on microscopic examination of bone marrow and biopsy specimens. Grocott-Gomori methenamine-silver nitrate and periodic acid-Schiff (PAS) stains are most useful for identifying *H. capsulatum* infection.

Other studies. Any child with hilar adenopathy requires evaluation, including tuberculin skin testing, to exclude tuberculosis. Findings in disseminated infection may include pancytopenia, anemia, coagulopathy, elevated liver enzymes, and increased serum ferritin.

TREATMENT

Antifungal treatment clearly benefits those with progressive forms of histoplasmosis (e.g., disseminated infection). Other manifestations for which antifungal therapy should be considered include pulmonary infection with protracted symptoms (4 weeks), severe acute pulmonary infection (e.g., hypoxia), and granulomatous adenitis obstructing critical structures such as blood vessels and bronchi. Antifungal therapy is generally not recommended in children with mild-to-moderate acute pulmonary disease.

Options for treatment include ketoconazole, itraconazole, and amphotericin B (deoxycholate or lipid preparations). Fluconazole is less effective than either itraconazole or amphotericin B. Ketoconazole, although effective, is poorly tolerated compared with the other antifungal agents and is associated with a higher rate of hepatoxicity. Voriconazole and posaconazole, newer triazole antifungal agents, demonstrate comparable or better in vitro activity than either itraconazole or amphotericin against *H. capsulatum*. These agents have also shown success in a small number of patients but require additional clinical evaluation. Amphotericin B deoxycholate is generally well tolerated in children and is preferred over lipid preparation. In general, patients with severe acute pulmonary histoplasmosis should receive a short course of amphotericin B, followed by a prolonged course of itraconazole while those with disseminated disease should receive a prolonged course of amphotericin B.

Duration of therapy depends on the type of histoplasmosis and the underlying host immunocompetence. Those with acute pulmonary disease who require treatment generally receive 1-2 weeks of amphotericin B, followed by 12 weeks of itraconazole. Disseminated infection requires 4-6 weeks of amphotericin B in otherwise healthy patients, but those with acquired immunodeficiency syndrome (AIDS) require lifelong suppressive therapy with itraconazole. Prolonged therapy may be necessary for those with serious *H. capsulatum* infections, immunosuppression, or primary immunodeficiency syndromes. For these patients, duration of therapy is usually determined in conjunction with an infectious diseases specialist.

Antigen levels should be monitored during therapy to evaluate the response to treatment and for 12 months following completion of therapy to monitor for relapse.

SUGGESTED READINGS

1. Edwards LB, Acquaviva FA, Livesay VT. An atlas of sensitivity to tuberculin, PPD-B, and histoplasmin in the United States. *Am Rev Respir Dis.* 99;1:1969.
2. Fischer GB, Mocelin H, Severo CB, Oliveira FM, Xavier MO, Severo LC. Histoplasmosis in children. *Pediatr Resp Rev.* 2009;10:172-177.
3. Flynn PM, Hughes WT. Histoplasmosis. In: Chernick V, Boat TF, eds. *Kendig's Disorders of the Respiratory Tract in Children.* 6th ed. Philadelphia: W.B. Saunders Company; 1998:946-953.
4. Fojtasek MF, Kleiman MB, Connolly-Stringfield P, Blair R, Wheat LJ. The *Histoplasma capsulatum* antigen assay in disseminated histoplasmosis in children. *Pediatr Infect Dis J.* 1994;13:801-805.
5. Kleiman MB. Histoplasma capsulatum (Histoplasmosis). In: Long SS, Pickering LK, Prober CG, eds. *Principles and Practice of Pediatric Infectious Diseases.* 2nd ed. New York: Churchill Livingstone; 2003:1233-1238.
6. Leggiardo RJ, Barrett RD, Hughes WT. Disseminated histoplasmosis of infancy. *Pediatr Infect Dis J.* 1986;7:799-805.
7. Wheat J, Freifeld AG, Kleiman MB, et al. Practice guidelines for the management of patients with histoplasmosis. *Clin Infect Dis.* 2007;45:807-825.

CASE 11-3

Fourteen-Year-Old Boy

MATTHEW TEST

SAMIR S. SHAH

HISTORY OF PRESENT ILLNESS

A 14-year-old boy was brought to the emergency department for evaluation of prolonged fever and new seizures. Eight days prior to admission, he developed fever to 38.3°C. Two days prior to admission, he complained of headache and continued fevers. On the day before admission he was standing in the kitchen talking to his aunt when he fell to the floor and had tonic flexion of his arms associated with eye deviation. This event lasted approximately 2 minutes. He was evaluated at a nearby hospital. His temperature was 38.6°C, but the physical examination was normal. He was discharged after a normal noncontrast head CT was obtained. On the day of admission, he was taken to his pediatrician's office for evaluation of continued fever. Shortly after arriving at the office, he had a similar event with arm flexion and eye deviation. It did not resolve spontaneously, and the boy was rushed to the hospital by ambulance. He received several doses of lorazepam without termination of apparent seizure activity. He required endotracheal intubation due to respiratory failure. Seizures were ultimately controlled with the combination of fosphenytoin and valproic acid.

The boy's aunt, the primary caretaker, related that during the past month he had several episodes of fecal soiling. Additionally, he had a documented 8-pound weight loss. The most striking information, however, was the marked deterioration in handwriting that occurred during the same time period. Furthermore, in the past month he had frequently neglected his household chores, a change from his baseline demeanor that was attributed to "teenage hormones." Aside from the two recent events, she did not recall any seizure activity. There were no rashes, emesis, or diarrhea. He performed well in school except during the past month, during which he failed several tests. This change in school performance was attributed to poor vision, and an ophthalmology appointment had been scheduled for later in the month.

MEDICAL HISTORY

The boy had not previously required hospitalization. He was adopted by his aunt in infancy while his biological mother struggled with drug addiction. She had died recently, but the aunt did not know the cause of death. The patient lived in an urban area and had no pets.

PHYSICAL EXAMINATION

T 38.4°C; HR 93 bpm; RR 18/min; BP 193/98 mmHg

Prior to endotracheal intubation his Glasgow Coma Score was 8. After stabilization, corneal reflexes were present. The gag reflex was intact. The tongue was midline. However, there was no spontaneous eye opening. Although he did not respond to voice or blink with direct visual confrontation, he localized painful stimuli. His tone was increased in the lower extremities. Babinski sign was negative bilaterally. His neck was supple. Heart and lung sounds were normal. The liver was palpable 3 cm below the right costal margin, with a total span of 11 cm.

DIAGNOSTIC STUDIES

Serum electrolytes were normal. Serum glucose was 119 mg/dL. Serum ammonia level was normal. Complete blood count revealed the following: 11 500 WBCs/mm^3 (73% segmented neutrophils and 22% lymphocytes); hemoglobin, 11.7 g/dL; and 785 000 platelets/mm^3. Prothrombin and partial thromboplastin times, fibrinogen, and fibrin split products were normal. Noncontrast head CT, obtained before lumbar puncture, revealed normal-sized ventricles and no masses. CSF analysis revealed 1 WBC/mm^3 and 630 RBCs/mm^3. The protein and glucose concentrations were 53 mg/dL and 52 mg/dL, respectively.

COURSE OF ILLNESS

Gram stain of the cerebrospinal fluid revealed some yeast forms. Magnetic resonance imaging of the head was significantly abnormal (Figure 11-3). What is the most likely diagnosis?

DISCUSSION CASE 11-3

DIFFERENTIAL DIAGNOSIS

The boy's initial complaint of prolonged fever precipitated medical evaluation. However, the history of behavioral changes, worsening school performance, and seizures was even more alarming. The development of status epilepticus at the pediatrician's office ultimately prompted a more thorough investigation of his symptoms. It was not clear at this point whether the patient has an encephalitis or encephalopathy. Although bacterial meningitis causes fever and seizures, the absence of CSF pleocytosis and the chronicity of symptoms made typical bacterial meningitis unlikely. Bacterial causes of encephalitis include

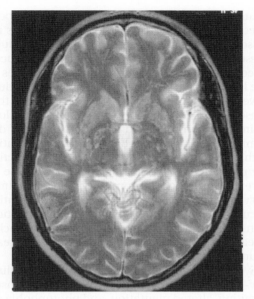

FIGURE 11-3. Magnetic resonance image of the head.

Borrelia burgdorferi, *Bartonella henselae* (cat-scratch disease), *Rickettsia rickettsia*, and *Anaplasma phagocytophilum*. Residence in an urban area made *B. burgdorferi*, the causative agent of Lyme disease, unlikely. Patients critically ill with *R. rickettsia* (Rocky Mountain spotted fever) infection typically have hyponatremia, hypoalbuminemia, anemia, and mild thrombocytopenia, findings not present in this case. Most, but not all, patients with cat-scratch disease have a clear history of contact with a cat or, more likely, a kitten. Again, the chronic symptoms, if related to the fever and seizures, are not typically seen with any of the above illnesses.

Viral causes of encephalitis include enteroviruses, arthropod-borne viruses (e.g., West Nile virus, St. Louis encephalitis virus, Eastern equine encephalitis virus), herpes simplex virus, Epstein-Barr virus, adenovirus, influenza, and human immunodeficiency virus (HIV). In adolescents, herpes simplex virus usually causes focal seizures and radiologic changes localized to the temporal lobe. There were no clear risk factors for HIV based on the initial history. The other viruses do not usually cause the progressive neurologic symptoms seen in this child.

Although this child's history did not have worrying indications for immunodeficiency, several infectious conditions can present with subacute symptoms in immunocompromised patients. Patients with humoral deficiencies may develop a chronic enteroviral meningoencephalitis. Those with cell-mediated immune deficiencies are at risk for subacute herpes simplex virus encephalitis, varicella-zoster virus encephalitis, and progressive multifocal leukoencephalopathy. Patients with AIDS can develop central nervous system infection with *Toxoplasma gondii* and *Cryptococcus neoformans*, an encapsulated yeast. These patients can also develop HIV-related encephalopathy.

The finding of yeast forms upon CSF Gram stain is helpful. Occasionally, degenerating WBCs are mistaken for yeast forms but additional investigation of this finding is clearly warranted. Meningitis due to *Candida* species typically occurs in patients with indwelling venous catheters, sustained neutropenia, and hyperglycemia due to diabetes, glucocorticoids, or hyperalimentation; none of which was present in this patient. In this case, the finding of yeast forms upon Gram stain of the CSF strongly suggested the diagnosis of cryptococcal meningitis.

Noninfectious causes include acute drug or medication ingestions as well as lead intoxication. Central nervous system vasculitis caused by either systemic lupus erythematous or polyarteritis nodosa should be strongly considered in the differential diagnosis.

DIAGNOSIS

Head MRI revealed dilatation of the Virchow-Robin spaces in the white matter, especially in the basal ganglion and thalamus, a finding seen with cryptococcal meningitis (Figure 11-3). The MRI also revealed dilatation of the lateral and third ventricles and sulci seen with HIV encephalitis. There was also abnormally increased signal in the periventricular white matter bilaterally, a finding consistent with HIV-related encephalitis. *Cryptococcus neoformans*, the yeast identified on Gram stain of the CSF, was isolated from cultures of the blood and CSF. Serum cryptococcal antigen was positive at 1:1024. The CSF cryptococcal antigen was also elevated at 1:512. HIV antibody testing was positive. Additional data, gathering by the family revealed the patient's birth mother had died from HIV-related complications. The family did not previously know the birth mother's HIV status, and as a consequence the patient had never undergone HIV testing. **The diagnosis was perinatally acquired HIV infection manifesting as cryptococcal meningitis and HIV encephalitis.** The patient died on the third day of hospitalization.

EPIDEMIOLOGY AND INCIDENCE

Cryptococcus neoformans, a ubiquitous encapsulated yeast, causes diseases ranging from asymptomatic pulmonary colonization to life-threatening meningitis. Cryptococcal infection may occur in healthy persons, but most infected patients have some immunocompromising factor such as immune suppression related to organ transplantation or HIV infection. Other predisposing conditions of childhood include primary immunodeficiency (e.g., hyper-immunoglobulin M syndrome) and certain malignancies (e.g., acute lymphoblastic leukemia). Primary infection occurs through the inhalation of aerosolized soil particles containing *C. neoformans*. Central nervous system involvement results from hematogenous dissemination.

Cryptococcal infection has been documented in up to 2.8% of organ transplant recipients, most often in those receiving renal transplants (80% of infections), but occasionally after liver (10% of infections) or heart (5% of infections) transplantation. Cryptococcal infection occurs in up to 15% of HIV-infected adults, typically when CD4+ T-lymphocyte count declines to less than 50 cells/mm^3. In contrast, this infection occurs in fewer than 2% of HIV-infected children, probably reflecting their lower exposure to sources of *C. neoformans* in the environment. *Cryptococcus neoformans* antibodies are detectable in only 4% of school-age children but in two-thirds of adults. Sources of *Cryptococcus* include pigeon droppings and soil.

Neonatal cryptococcal infection has been rarely reported. Transplacental vertical transmission has been implicated as the cause in these cases.

CLINICAL PRESENTATION

Cryptococcal infection may present with acute or chronic symptoms. In children, findings in acute primary pulmonary infection have not been adequately characterized, because most cases are disseminated at the time of diagnosis. In adults, presentation of primary pulmonary cryptococcal infection ranges from asymptomatic nodules in the lungs to severe pneumonia. One half of adults develop cough and chest pain. Less often, they present with fever, hemoptysis, and weight loss. In immunocompromised patients, the risk of dissemination is high enough that patients presenting with findings of pulmonary cryptococcal infection are presumed to have extrapulmonary disease. In severely immunocompromised patients, pulmonary involvement may be minimal if dissemination occurs shortly after exposure. On examination, signs of respiratory involvement include tachypnea, accessory muscle use, and decreased breath sounds.

Symptoms of cryptococcal meningitis include low-grade fever, malaise, and headache. Nausea, vomiting, altered mentation, and photophobia are less common. Stiff neck, focal neurologic deficits, and seizures are rare. Physical examination findings of cryptococcal meningitis are not sufficiently characteristic to distinguish it from other causes of meningitis. Findings may include nuchal rigidity and photophobia; however, these are typically not observed, particularly in immunocompromised patients.

Although the lungs and CNS are the most common sites of infection, dissemination occasionally affects other organs, including the skin, liver, spleen, adrenal glands, kidneys, bone, and joints. Cutaneous manifestations of cryptococcal infection include erythematous or verrucous papules, nodules, or pustules. Occasionally acneiform lesions or granulomas are noted. The lesions are usually located on the face and neck but may occur anywhere on the body.

DIAGNOSTIC APPROACH

Sputum culture. The sputum fungal culture can be used to diagnose cryptococcal pneumonia. Although isolation from the sputum may be helpful, it is important to note that asymptomatic colonization of the respiratory tract does occur.

Blood culture. *Cryptococcus neoformans* may grow in 3 days but occasionally takes up to 3 weeks.

Cryptococcal polysaccharide antigen by latex agglutination. The cryptococcal antigen test can be performed on serum and CSF specimens. This test should be performed on the serum of any HIV-infected patient who develops pneumonia and has a CD4+ count less than 200/mm³. This test should also be performed in any patient with suspected cryptococcal pneumonia. A positive serum test indicates disseminated infection. The serum antigen test is positive in 85%-90% of patients with central nervous system involvement. False negative results can occur at both very low and very high antigen concentrations. At high antigen concentration, this is known as the prozone phenomenon, and it is thought to occur as a result of interference with appropriate antigen-antibody interaction necessary for a positive test result. This phenomenon can be overcome through serial dilution of the sample.

Lumbar puncture. CSF should be examined in all immunocompromised patients with suspected cryptococcal infection, even if signs and symptoms of meningitis are absent. CSF specimens should be sent for cell count, protein, glucose, cultures for bacterial, fungal, and viral pathogens, and cryptococcal polysaccharide antigen by latex agglutination. Lumbar puncture classically reveals an increased opening pressure. There are typically less than 100 WBCs/mm³ (mostly lymphocytes and monocytes), although some patients may not demonstrate a pleocytosis. The glucose is less than 50 mg/dL in 65% of patients, and there may be a mild elevation of the CSF protein. Positive CSF culture on Sabouraund agar remains the gold standard in the diagnosis of cryptococcal meningitis. Cultures are positive in 90% of patients with central nervous system disease. CSF cryptococcal antigen titers of 1:4 or higher also confirm the diagnosis. CSF antigen testing is positive in nearly all patients with cryptococcal meningitis. Budding yeasts are visualized by India ink stain in 50% of cases, but this test is not required if cryptococcal antigen testing is performed. Real-time polymerase chain reaction assays have been developed for the identification of *C. neoformans*. These assays have sensitivities similar to that of cryptococcal antigen testing.

Serum electrolytes. Hyponatremia complicates cryptococcal meningitis, and its development portends a poor prognosis.

Radiologic studies. Chest radiography may reveal parenchymal infiltrates with air bronchograms, diffuse nodular infiltrates and, occasionally, small bilateral pleural effusions. However, in many cases, chest radiography is unremarkable. CT or MRI of the head may demonstrate granulomatous lesions (cryptococcomas), white matter changes, and increased intracranial pressure.

HIV testing. All patients diagnosed with cryptococcal meningitis or disseminated cryptococcal infection should undergo evaluation for immune deficiency, particularly HIV infection.

Cryptococcal antigen dipstick. A point-of-care dipstick for the detection of cryptococcal antigen has been developed for use on whole blood, serum, or urine. Identification of antigen with the dipstick was strongly correlated with ELISA-identification of cryptococcal antigen. Although not yet widely used, this test has the potential to improve cryptococcal diagnosis, particularly in resource-limited settings, due to its low cost, ease of use, and noninvasiveness.

TREATMENT

Clinical management varies depending on the extent of disease and immune status of the host. An asymptomatic normal host with isolated pulmonary nodules does not require treatment if the serum cryptococcal antigen test is negative. Patients with mild-to-moderate pulmonary disease require treatment with fluconazole for 6-12 months. Immunocompromised and immunocompetent patients with either severe pulmonary disease or cryptococcemia are treated in the same manner as patients with central nervous system disease. After primary therapy is complete, there is no consensus on how long HIV-negative immunocompromised patients require fluconazole prophylaxis. Most experts suggest providing prophylaxis for 1 year after the completion of acute antifungal treatment and then reassess its ongoing need based on the level of immunosuppression at that time. Treatment may be discontinued when the immune function returns to normal (e.g., after completion of chemotherapy).

HIV-positive patients and organ transplant patients with meningitis are treated with intravenous amphotericin plus flucytosine for at least

2 weeks; if the CSF culture is negative on repeat lumbar puncture, they may receive fluconazole for an additional 8 weeks. Non-HIV infected, nontransplant hosts should receive intravenous amphotericin plus flucytosine for 4 weeks, followed by 8 weeks of fluconazole. The strength of the recommendations for non-HIV infected, nontransplant hosts is impacted by the limited number of studies in this population. Additionally, the available studies are further limited by heterogeneous patient populations, ranging from normal hosts to those with malignancy and liver disease, and the administration of lower doses of antifungal therapy than are currently recommended.

Regardless of immune status, extended therapy with amphotericin and flucytosine may be considered for any patient with neurologic complications, prolonged coma, clinical deterioration or lack of improvement, and/or persistence of CSF infection.

HIV-infected patients with pulmonary or disseminated cryptococcal infection require treatment with fluconazole that continues indefinitely. The rate of relapse in HIV-infected patients is 100% without maintenance of antifungal therapy. The relapse rate decreases from 18% to 25% with itraconazole prophylaxis and 2% to 3% with fluconazole prophylaxis. Due to advances in antiretroviral therapy, some authors propose discontinuation of secondary prophylaxis for cryptococcal meningitis in HIV-infected patients if the CD4 cell count has increased above $100/mm^3$ and HIV viral load has been low or undetectable for longer than 3 months. If maintenance therapy is discontinued, monitoring for relapse of infection and regular monitoring of cryptococcal antigen and CD4+ cell count are recommended.

Untreated cryptococcal infection in HIV-infected patients is uniformly fatal. Survival rates are high with early diagnosis and treatment, but relapse rates are high without lifelong antifungal prophylaxis.

Factors associated with poor prognosis include low weight, hyponatremia, high CSF antigen titre, low CSF WBC count, and alteration in mental status at the time of diagnosis.

SUGGESTED READINGS

1. Buchanan KL, Murphy JW. What makes *Cryptococcus neoformans* a pathogen? *Emerg Infect Dis.* 1998;4:71-83.
2. Chuck SL, Sande MA. Infections with *Cryptococcus neoformans* in the acquired immunodeficiency syndrome. *N Engl J Med.* 1989;321:794-799.
3. Gonzalez CE, Shetty D, Lewis LL, Mueller BU, Pizzo PA, Walsh TJ. Cryptococcis in human immunodeficiency virus-infected children. *Pediatr Infect Dis J.* 1996;15:796-800.
4. Husain S, Wagener MM, Singh N. *Cryptococcus neoformans* infection in organ transplant recipients: variables influencing clinical characteristics and outcome. *Emerg Infect Dis.* 2001;7:375-381.
5. Jackson A, van der Horst C. New insights in the prevention, diagnosis, and treatment of Cryptococcal meningitis. *Curr HIV/AIDS Rep.* 2012;9:267-277.
6. Mirza SA, Phelan M, Rimland D, et al. The changing epidemiology of cryptococcosis: an update from population-based active surveillance in 2 large metropolitan areas, 1992-2000. *Clin Infect Dis.* 2003;36:789-794.
7. Pappas PG, Perfect JR, Cloud GA, et al. Cryptococcosis in human immunodeficiency virus-negative patients in the era of effective azole therapy. *Clin Infect Dis.* 2001;33:690-699.
8. Powderly WG. Current approach to the acute management of cryptococcal infections. *J Infect Dis.* 2000; 41:18-22.
9. Perfect JR, Dismukes WE, Dromer F, et al. Practice guidelines for the management of cryptococcal disease. *Clin Infect Dis.* 2010;50:291-322.
10. Saag MS, Powderly WG, Cloud GA, et al. Comparison of amphotericin B with fluconazole in the treatment of acute AIDS-associated cryptococcal meningitis. *N Engl J Med.* 1992;326:83-89.
11. Severo CB, Xavier MO, Gazzoni AF, Severo LC. Cryptococcosis in children. *Ped Resp Rev.* 2009;10:166-171.

CASE 11-4

Seven-Month-Old Girl

REBECCA TENNEY-SOEIRO

HISTORY OF PRESENT ILLNESS

A 7-month-old Japanese girl developed fever to 102°F associated with cough, rhinorrhea, and loose stools. During the next few days, the respiratory symptoms and diarrhea resolved; however, her fever persisted. Six days prior to admission, she was evaluated by her primary pediatrician and diagnosed with cellulitis involving the labia majora. She was treated with cephalexin, an oral first-generation cephalosporin. She presented to the emergency department due to continued fevers and worsening cellulitis and was admitted for intravenous antibiotic therapy and additional evaluation.

MEDICAL HISTORY

The girl's birth history was remarkable for unconjugated hyperbilirubinemia. Her bilirubin level peaked at 16 mg/dL and returned to normal without phototherapy. Two months ago, she developed otitis media that resolved after treatment with a 10-day course of amoxicillin. Cephalexin was her only medication at the time of admission. She had received all of the appropriate immunizations, including three doses of the heptavalent pneumococcal conjugate vaccine. The family history was remarkable for hepatitis A in the maternal grandmother approximately 2 months ago.

PHYSICAL EXAMINATION

T 40.3°C; HR 160 bpm; RR 50/min; BP 104/60 mmHg; SpO$_2$ 98% in room air

Weight, 75th percentile

Examination revealed an ill but nontoxic appearing infant. The anterior fontanelle was open and flat. Tympanic membranes were mildly erythematous but had normal mobility bilaterally. There were no oropharyngeal lesions. Capillary refill was brisk. The heart and lung sounds were normal.

The spleen was palpable just below the left costal margin. Examination of the genitalia revealed significant erythema and induration of the left labia majora with mild fluctuance. There was no crepitus. There were no other skin lesions.

DIAGNOSTIC STUDIES

The WBC count was 3100/mm^3 with 2% segmented neutrophils, 28% monocytes, and 70% lymphocytes. The absolute neutrophil count (ANC) was 62 cells/mm^3. Hemoglobin and platelets were 12.3 mg/dL and 337000/mm^3, respectively. A repeat complete blood count revealed similar results. Lactate dehydrogenase and uric acid were normal. Urinalysis did not reveal pyuria or hematuria. Blood and urine cultures were obtained.

COURSE OF ILLNESS

Gram-stain after percutaneous drainage of the labial abscess demonstrated many Gram-negative rods. She received vancomycin and piperacillin-tazobactam to provide adequate coverage for *Staphylococcus aureus* (including methicillin-resistant *S. aureus* isolates) and Gram-negative organisms, including *Pseudomonas aeruginosa*. A bone marrow aspirate suggested the underlying diagnosis (Figure 11-4).

DISCUSSION CASE 11-4

DIFFERENTIAL DIAGNOSIS

Neutropenia, defined as an absolute decrease in the number of circulating neutrophils in the blood, can be due to decreased production, increased peripheral utilization, or increased destruction. The absolute neutrophil count (ANC) is calculated by multiplying the total white blood cell (WBC) count by the percentage of band forms and segmented neutrophils [ANC = total WBC × (percent

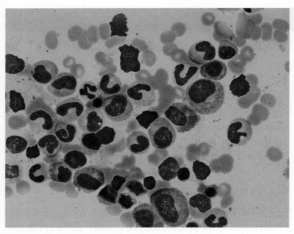

FIGURE 11-4. Bone marrow aspirate.

TABLE 11-4.	Differential diagnosis of neutropenia in infancy.
Category	*Examples*
Congenital	Kostmann syndrome Cyclic neutropenia Fanconi syndrome
Metabolic	Shwachman-Diamond-Oski syndrome Propionic academia Glycogen storage disease type Ib Methylmalonic acidemia
Immune-mediated	Alloimmune neonatal neutropenia Autoimmune neutropenia in infancy Secondary autoimmune neutropenia Felty syndrome Systemic lupus erythematosus
Nutritional	Vitamin B_{12} deficiency Folate deficiency Copper deficiency
Primary Immunodeficiency	X-linked agammaglobulinemia Hyper-IgM syndrome Common variable immune deficiency Reticular dysgenesis Cartilage-hair hypoplasia
Hematologic	Aplastic anemia Myelodysplastic syndromes
Drug-induced	Antibiotics (sulfonamides, penicillin) Barbiturates Propylthiouracil Penicillamine Others
Infection	Epstein-Barr virus Rickettsiae Human immunodeficiency virus Malaria Others

bands + percent segmented neutrophils)]. In general, patients may be characterized as having mild (1000-1500 cells/mm³), moderate (500-1000 cells/mm³), or severe (<500 cells/mm³) neutropenia. Blacks tend to have lower neutrophil counts, and therefore, in some patients an ANC equal to 900 cells/mm³ may be considered normal.

The differential diagnosis of neutropenia in infancy includes a wide range of conditions (Table 11-4). In a child who was previously healthy, the most likely causes include alloimmune neonatal neutropenia, cyclic neutropenia, autoimmune neutropenia in infancy, and Kostmann syndrome. Alloimmune neutropenia, a condition occurring in neonates, is analogous to Rh hemolytic disease. Maternal sensitization to fetal neutrophils results in maternal IgG antibodies crossing the placenta and causing an immune-mediated destruction of fetal neutrophils. Neutropenia lasts several weeks but rarely persists beyond 6 months of age, making it an unlikely diagnosis in this 7-month-old infant. Cyclic neutropenia can be diagnosed by following serial white blood cell counts.

Less likely cause includes neutropenia related to infection. Neutropenia associated with increased peripheral utilization is possible in the context of a serious cellulitis. Infections such as Epstein-Barr virus and parvovirus B19 infection can also cause neutropenia but the normal hemoglobin and platelet count make these infections less likely.

The mother does not have autoimmune neutropenia, a finding that sometimes leads to transient secondary neutropenia in newborn infants.

DIAGNOSIS

Bone marrow aspirate revealed a hypercellular marrow (Figure 11-4). There was an increased number of granulocytes with maturation to the band stage but there were no mature neutrophils. Quantitative serum immunoglobulins (IgA, IgE, IgG, IgM) were normal. **These findings combined with the neutropenia suggest the diagnosis of autoimmune neutropenia of infancy.** Antibodies to the neutrophil-specific cell surface antigen NA1 were detected confirming the diagnosis of autoimmune neutropenia of childhood. Culture of the labial cellulitis revealed *P. aeruginosa*. The patient's infection resolved with a 10-day course of piperacillin-tazobactam. Serial absolute neutrophil counts during the next 6 weeks revealed persistent neutropenia, effectively excluding the diagnosis of cyclic neutropenia. She experienced no additional infections. Her neutropenia resolved by 20 months of age. The episode of otitis media did not appear to be related to her neutropenia.

EPIDEMIOLOGY AND INCIDENCE

Autoimmune neutropenia (AIN) can occur as an isolated phenomenon (primary AIN) or in association with a known precipitating factor (secondary AIN), such as other autoimmune disorders, infections, medications, and malignancies. In infants and young children, the term primary AIN usually refers to autoimmune neutropenia in infancy (formerly chronic benign neutropenia). The average age at diagnosis of AIN in infancy is 8 months (range, 1-38 months). Two-thirds of patients are diagnosed between 5 and 15 months of age. The estimated frequency is 1 per 100000 children, making it more common than the severe chronic neutropenias, such as cyclic neutropenia.

CLINICAL PRESENTATION

Most patients with AIN in infancy suffer from mild infections, such as otitis media, gastroenteritis, lymphadenitis, superficial skin infections, or upper respiratory tract infections. In one series, 6 (23%) of the 26 girls developed cellulitis of the labia majora; 3 of these 6 infections were caused by *P. aeruginosa*. Approximately, 10%-15% suffer from serious infections including pneumonia, sepsis, or meningitis. In approximately 10% of children, the diagnosis will be suspected only after a routine complete blood count reveals neutropenia.

DIAGNOSTIC APPROACH

Complete blood count. The complete blood count reveals neutropenia (absolute neutrophil count <1000/mm³). Eosinophilia occasionally occurs. Patients with other causes of neutropenia may have anemia or thrombocytopenia (as occurs with Evan syndrome).

Neutrophil-specific antibodies. Anti-neutrophil antibodies are not consistently identified during the period of neutropenia. Therefore, such testing is not necessary in children with a normal hemoglobin and platelet count or with a bone marrow aspirate result consistent with the diagnosis of autoimmune neutropenia of infancy.

Coombs test. A Coombs test should be considered to evaluate for the presence of a concomitant red blood cell autoantibody.

Bone marrow aspirate. This test is not routinely required, particularly if the patient appears well and has a normal hemoglobin level and platelet count. When performed, the bone marrow aspirate is usually normocellular to hypercellular. The marrow contains a reduced number of mature neutrophils and occasionally there is maturation arrest at earlier stages. Bone marrow examination is normal in 30% of cases and hypocellular in 3% of cases.

Other studies. Serum immunoglobulins (IgA, IgG, IgE, IgM) should be sent if an underlying primary immunodeficiency associated with neutropenia is suspected. Examples include X-linked agammaglobulinemia, hyper-IgM syndrome, and common variable immunodeficiency. Serum vitamin B_{12} and red blood cell folate levels are indicated in patients with suspected nutritional deficiency. Other tests to consider in the patient with neutropenia include antinuclear antibody (ANA; collagen vascular disease), serum copper level, and evaluation for metabolic diseases (e.g., glycogen storage disease type Ib, Shwachman-Diamond-Oski syndrome).

TREATMENT

Most patients only require antibiotics to treat bacterial infections as they occur. Prophylactic antibiotics are not routinely used because the efficacy is not definite. Some patients benefit from antibacterial mouthwashes for occasional mouth sores and gingivitis. G-CSF, corticosteroids, and intravenous gamma globulin administration are not routinely required but they have been used to increase neutrophil counts in patients with *serious* or *recurrent* infections (15% of patients with AIN in infancy). In such cases, approximately 50% of children respond to corticosteroids and 75% respond to gamma globulin. G-CSF is effective in almost all patients. The neutropenia resolves spontaneously in 95% of patients, usually in 7-24 months. Disappearance of autoantibodies precedes spontaneous normalization of the neutrophil count.

SUGGESTED READINGS

1. Bux J, Behrens G, Jaeger G, Welte K. Diagnosis and clinical course of autoimmune neutropenia in infancy: analysis of 240 cases. *Blood.* 1998;91:181-186.

2. Taniuchi S, Masuda M, Hasui M, et al. Differential diagnosis and clinical course of autoimmune neutropenia: comparison with congenital neutropenia. *Acta Paediatr.* 2002;91:1179-1182.

3. Bruin M, Dassen A, Buddelmeyer L, et al. Primary autoimmune neutropenia in children: a study of neutrophil antibodies and clinical course. *Vox sanguinis.* 2005;88:52-59.

4. Boxer LA. Neutrophil abnormalities. *Pediatr Rev.* 2003; 24:52-61.

5. Jonsson OG, Buchanan GR. Chronic neutropenia during childhood: a 13-year experience in a single institution. *AJDC.* 1991;145:232-235.

6. Alario AJ, O'Shea JS. Risk of infectious complications in well-appearing children with transient neutropenia. *AJDC.* 1989;143:973-976.

CASE 11-5

Six-Year-Old Boy

MATTHEW TEST

SAMIR S. SHAH

HISTORY OF PRESENT ILLNESS

A 6-year-old boy presented with a 2-week history of low-grade fevers. One week prior to admission, he had an episode of nonbilious emesis and subsequently began complaining of neck pain. There was no cough, diarrhea, rash, or abdominal or joint pain. Although he never complained that light bothered his eyes, he did not play outside with his friends during the day. His mother initially attributed this to the summer heat. He received several doses of ibuprofen for complaints of headache. He was brought for evaluation after the mother learned of a meningococcal meningitis outbreak at local school from the evening news broadcast. She became concerned about the possibility of meningitis and, after speaking with her pediatrician, rushed the child to the emergency department. There were no ill contacts. Neither the child nor his two siblings attended the school where several children had developed meningitis.

MEDICAL HISTORY

The child had an unremarkable birth history. At the age of 8 months he required hospitalization for management of rotavirus gastroenteritis-induced dehydration. Two months before admission, he was bitten on the hand while feeding deer during a hiking trip in the Pocono Mountains in Pennsylvania. Three weeks before admission, he developed a severe contact dermatitis on his arms and face that was attributed to poison ivy. He recovered uneventfully after treatment with oral antihistamines and cool compresses. The family history was unremarkable. The child lived with his parents and two brothers in Southern New Jersey.

PHYSICAL EXAMINATION

T 38.1°C; HR 100 bpm; RR 28/min; BP 101/53; mmHg; SpO$_2$ 100% in room air

Weight 50th percentile for age

In general, the child was a lean but healthy-appearing boy. He had mild photophobia. There was no Kernig or Brudzinski sign, but there was difficulty with terminal neck flexion. There was no cervical lymphadenopathy. The heart and lung sounds were normal. There was no hepatomegaly or splenomegaly. The cranial nerve examination was normal. The skin examination revealed a rash that had appeared recently. The rash suggested the diagnosis (Figure 11-5).

DIAGNOSTIC STUDIES

Complete blood count revealed the following: 8600 WBCs/mm^3 (71% segmented neutrophils, 22% lymphocytes, and 7% monocytes); hemoglobin, 11.1 g/dL; and 461000 platelets/mm^3. Serum glucose was 96 mg/dL. Lumbar puncture revealed 21 WBCs (3% segmented neutrophils, 77% lymphocytes, and 20% monocytes) and 1 RBC/mm^3. The CSF protein and glucose were 23 mg/dL and

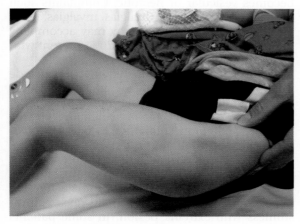

FIGURE 11-5. Photograph of patient's rash.

63 mg/dL, respectively. No bacteria were noted on the CSF Gram stain. The CSF and blood cultures were subsequently negative.

COURSE OF ILLNESS

The diagnosis suggested by the rash was confirmed by additional testing.

DISCUSSION CASE 11-5

DIFFERENTIAL DIAGNOSIS

Aseptic meningitis refers to a syndrome of meningeal inflammation without evidence of pathogens by traditional bacterial culture methods. A specific cause is identified in fewer than 60% of cases. Enteroviruses, including echoviruses, coxsackie viruses, and numbered enteroviruses, are the most common cause of aseptic meningitis. They account for up to 95% of cases when a specific pathogen is implicated. In the summer, other infectious causes of aseptic meningitis include Lyme disease (*Borrelia burgdorferi*), Rocky Mountain spotted fever (*Rickettsia rickettsii*), anaplasmosis, and arboviruses such as West Nile virus, St. Louis encephalitis virus, and Eastern and Western equine encephalitis viruses. Some parainfluenza viruses occur throughout the year, including summer. Other viruses include herpes simplex virus, varicella zoster virus, Epstein-Barr virus, and human herpesvirus 6. Less common causes of aseptic meningitis include tuberculosis, syphilis, various fungi (e.g., *Cryptococcus neoformans*), and parasites. Noninfectious causes include Kawasaki disease, systemic lupus erythematosus, and polyarteritis nodosum.

This relatively well-appearing child presented with subacute symptoms and a CSF pleocytosis. The CSF WBC count does not point to a particular etiology. Although tuberculous meningitis is important to consider in any patient with aseptic meningitis, it usually manifests with characteristic CSF findings including a dramatically elevated protein and a low glucose concentration—findings not present in this case. Although a rash is associated with several of the above-mentioned conditions, children with Rocky Mountain spotted fever, anaplasmosis, herpes simplex virus, varicella, or syphilis are often quite ill. Additionally, children with Rocky Mountain spotted fever and anaplasmosis typically have leukopenia and thrombocytopenia. The rash of herpes simplex virus and varicella, when present, is characteristic and does not resemble the rash on this patient. The CSF WBC differential with a mononuclear cell predominance (i.e., predominance of lymphocytes and monocytes rather than neutrophils) argues against a bacterial process. The rash shown in Figure 11-5 was characteristic of early disseminated Lyme disease.

DIAGNOSIS

Examination of the skin revealed multiple annular lesions on the chest, back, and legs, ranging from 5 to 15 cm in diameter (Figure 11-5). These macular erythematous lesions with partial to complete central clearing were characteristic of erythema migrans (EM). **This finding of multiple EM lesions combined with headache, photophobia, and mononuclear CSF pleocytosis suggested the diagnosis of Lyme meningitis.** Serum antibodies revealed an IgM titer of 27.3 (reference, 0-0.8) and an IgG titer of 0.4 (reference, 0-0.8). This positive IgM test was also confirmed by Western blotting. CSF enterovirus PCR and bacterial culture were negative. An electrocardiogram did not reveal evidence of heart block, a feature associated with early disseminated Lyme disease. The child was treated with intravenous ceftriaxone for 3 weeks and recovered completely.

EPIDEMIOLOGY AND INCIDENCE

Lyme disease, caused by the tick-borne spirochete, *B. burgdorfei,* was initially identified during investigation of a cluster of children with arthritis in Lyme, Connecticut. Features of the disease had been previously described in Europe under various names including erythema chronicum migrans, acrodermatitis chronica atrophicans, and Bannwarth syndrome. Lyme disease is now endemic in more than 15 states. The infection is also common in middle Europe, Scandinavia, and parts of Russia, China, and Japan. Several closely related ticks that are part of the *Ixodes ricinus* complex (*Ixodes scapularis, Ixodes pacificus, Ixodes ricinus,* and *Ixodes persulcatus*) comprise the

vectors of Lyme disease. They vary in their geographic distribution. In the United States, *I. scapularis* is the vector in the northeast and midwest, while *I. pacificus* predominates on the west coast. New England, the mid-Atlantic States, Minnesota, and Wisconsin have the highest prevalence of infected ticks. Lyme disease has a bimodal age distribution, with the greater number of cases occurring between the ages of 5 and 9 years and between the ages of 45 and 59 years.

Most infections occur between May and July. After injection of *B. burgdorferi* by the *Ixodes* tick into the skin, the spirochete multiplies locally at the site of the bite and within days to weeks may disseminate to other sites. The risk of Lyme disease after a tick bite will be discussed later.

CLINICAL PRESENTATION

Lyme disease typically manifests in three stages: localized infection, early (disseminated) infection, and late infection. Localized infection generally occurs 7-14 days (range, 3-32 days) after the tick bite. Early infection occurs 2-6 weeks after the tick bite, and late infection occurs 6-12 weeks (range, up to 12 months) after the tick bite. Localized infection refers to development of EM lesions at the site of the tick bite. It usually begins as an erythematous macule or papule and expands to a median diameter of 15 cm, with intensely erythematous macular borders and central clearing or induration. Occasionally, the central area becomes vesicular or necrotic. Complaints such as malaise, headache, arthralgias, myalgias, fever, and regional lymphadenopathy may accompany the lesion. Most children (60%-70%) present with the localized form of Lyme disease.

Features of early disseminated infection include multiple EM lesions (23% of all Lyme disease cases), carditis (0.5%), cranial nerve palsy (3%), meningitis (2%), and acute radiculopathy (<0.5%). The most common cranial nerve palsy involves the seventh (facial) nerve but palsy of cranial nerves III, IV, or VI may develop. Most children with Lyme meningitis have symptoms for 2-3 weeks before the diagnosis. They initially develop low-grade fevers, followed by mild neck pain or stiffness with extreme flexion. In some patients with Lyme meningitis, EM rash or concomitant cranial nerve palsy, rather than neck pain, brings the child to medical attention, and the findings of EM, cranial nerve palsy, or papilledema are helpful in distinguishing Lyme meningitis from viral meningitis. Cardiac manifestations include fluctuating degrees of atrioventricular block (first degree, Wenckebach, or complete) and, less commonly, myocarditis, pericarditis, or cardiomegaly. Earlier reports suggested that carditis may occur in 5% of untreated patients with Lyme disease, but more recent studies have found a much lower incidence.

Arthritis is the most common late manifestation of Lyme disease, occurring in up to 10% of untreated patients. Children are more likely than adults to develop Lyme arthritis and are also more likely to have arthritis as their presenting complaint. It involves the knee in 90% of cases. The spirochete occasionally affects the hip, ankle, wrist, elbow, or temporomandibular joint. The joint is swollen and warm but, in contrast to bacterial septic arthritis, only mildly tender. If left untreated, Lyme arthritis is often intermittent, with episodes of inflammation lasting weeks to months. Signs and symptoms of systemic illness are rare.

DIAGNOSTIC APPROACH

The diagnosis is usually suspected on characteristic clinical findings, history of exposure in an endemic area, and antibody testing. Diagnosis of Lyme meningitis requires a high level of suspicion, careful history and examination, serum antibody studies, and lumbar puncture. Diagnosis of other manifestations of Lyme disease is discussed later.

Serologic diagnosis. For serologic testing, the U.S. Centers for Disease Control and Prevention recommends a two-tiered approach to testing. An enzyme-linked immunoassay (EIA) is performed initially. The EIA test is very sensitive but false-positive results occur due to cross-reactive antibodies in patients with other spirochetal infections or certain viral infections or autoimmune diseases. Those with equivocal or positive results by EIA should undergo confirmatory testing by Western blot of the initial sample. An IgM determination is considered positive if two of three specific bands (23, 39, or 41 kd) are detected by Western blotting. An IgG Western blot is considered positive if at least 5 of 10 specific bands are present.

Only 40% of children with localized EM have detectable antibodies. On repeat testing 4 weeks after detection of the EM lesion, 70% will have detectable antibodies, thereby suggesting that early antibiotic treatment of the EM lesion may blunt antibody response. In children with early disseminated infection such as Lyme meningitis, IgM antibodies are present in more than 95% of cases and IgG antibodies are present in 70%. Children with late infection should have detectable IgG and may have detectable IgM.

Peripheral blood smear. As *Ixodes* is a vector for multiple infective agents, patients with Lyme disease frequently are coinfected with another tick-borne pathogen. In a study by Krause et al., 22% of patients with Lyme disease were coinfected with basbesiosis, and 4% were coinfected with human granulocytic anaplasmosis. The diagnosis of babesiosis depends on microscopic identification of intraerythrocytic parasites in Giemsa- or Wright-stained thick and thin blood smears. In approximately 50% of patients with anaplasmosis, morulae are detected in peripheral blood neutrophils. Peripheral blood smears should be examined in any patient with Lyme disease who has continued symptoms despite appropriate therapy. These coinfecting pathogens should also be considered in any patient with a more severe presentation than is typically observed with Lyme disease alone or a patient presenting with accompanying leukopenia, thrombocytopenia, anemia, hemolysis, or jaundice—findings that are more typical of other tickborne diseases rather than Lyme disease.

Lumbar puncture. In children with Lyme meningitis, CSF analysis reveals a mild mononuclear (lymphocytes and moncoytes) pleocytosis (mean, 100 WBCs/mm^3; range, 10-500/mm^3). In a study by Turnquist et al., 23 of 24 children with Lyme meningitis had less than 10% segmented neutrophils in the CSF. The CSF glucose is normal and the protein may be normal or mildly elevated. CSF antibody studies may provide supporting evidence of Lyme meningitis. CSF Lyme PCR is generally not useful in diagnosing Lyme meningitis due to low bacterial counts in the CSF and subsequent poor sensitivity. There have been recent improvements in PCR methods for identification of *B. burgdorferi* DNA but many laboratories are not capable of accurately performing the test, and its clinical utility remains limited.

Joint aspiration. In cases of Lyme arthritis, joint aspiration typically reveals between 30 000 and 50 000 WBCs/mm³, often with neutrophil predominance. Results of Lyme PCR testing of joint fluid are positive in approximately 85% of patients with suspected Lyme arthritis. False-positive PCR results from joint fluid are uncommon.

Electrocardiogram. An electrocardiogram should be performed in patients with signs and symptoms of cardiac disease, and should be considered in patients with concern for Lyme arthritis. Approximately one-third of children with Lyme meningitis will have ECG abnormalities; heart block and prolongation of the corrected QT interval are most common. ECG abnormalities occur in 50% of children with Lyme meningitis who have fever for 5 or more days and those who are 13 years of age or older at the time of diagnosis; the probability of ECG abnormalities was 83% (95% confidence interval: 50%-96%) in children with both of these findings. As most ECG abnormalities will resolve without consequence, the relevance of detecting these abnormalities is uncertain.

Other studies. There is *no* role for Lyme PCR testing of urine or blood samples. Because clinically it may be difficult to distinguish Lyme meningitis from other causes of aseptic meningitis, studies to detect other causes (e.g., enteroviral CSF PCR, serum antibodies, and CSF PCR for arboviruses) should be considered. Results of additional studies such as peripheral WBC count and erythrocyte sedimentation rate are relatively nonspecific for Lyme disease, but certain findings (e.g., leukopenia) can suggest an alternate or concomitant infection. If coinfection with *Babesia* or anaplasmosis is suspected, serologic testing may be indicated, as antibody detection is more sensitive than blood smear in the identification of these conditions.

TREATMENT

Treatment of Lyme disease depends on the clinical manifestation (Table 11-5). Localized disease may be treated with amoxicillin or cefuroxime for 14-21 days, or if the patient is 8 years of age or older, doxycycline for 10-21 days. For patients intolerant

to these agents, macrolides should be considered, although they have been shown to be less effective. Some controversy exists as to the appropriate management of children with facial nerve palsy. Although some experts recommend CSF evaluation on all patients with a Lyme-associated cranial palsy, others reserve lumbar puncture for those with clinical evidence of CNS infection (e.g., headache, neck stiffness, or photophobia). An oral regimen, as discussed, is reasonable to treat isolated cranial nerve palsy due to Lyme disease.

Children with carditis may be treated either orally or parenterally depending on the severity of cardiac involvement. Children with first-degree atrioventricular heart block may be treated with oral antibiotics. Hospitalization and parenteral antibiotic therapy is recommended for children with second- or third-degree atrioventricular heart block, for those with first-degree heart block in whom the PR interval is prolonged to 30 milliseconds or longer, and for those with symptoms (e.g., syncope, dyspnea, chest pain). A 14-day course (range, 10-28 days) of ceftriaxone is the preferred parenteral regimen, but administration of cefotaxime and penicillin G are reasonable alternatives. These children are often transitioned to oral antibiotics for completion of their treatment course. This decision is frequently made in conjunction with an infectious diseases specialist.

Children with evidence of Lyme meningitis or radiculopathy should receive parenteral therapy for 14 days (range, 10-28 days), as described previously. Children with Lyme arthritis often respond well to 28 days of oral therapy. For those with poor initial response to oral therapy, parenteral ceftriaxone should be considered. Children with Lyme arthritis may have recurrence of arthritis. Recurrences of arthritis after successful initial treatment can be management with nonsteroidal antiinflammatory agents.

Although early studies of the efficacy of prophylaxis after tick bites failed to show a protective effect, a more recent study of adults showed that a single 200-mg dose of doxycycline administered within 72 hours after a recognized *I. scapularis* bite had an efficacy of 87% in preventing EM when compared to placebo. However, adverse events, including nausea and vomiting, occurred in approximately 30% who received doxycycline.

TABLE 11-5. Manifestations of Lyme disease.

Stage of Disease	Onset After Exposure	Clinical Manifestations	Treatment[a]
Early Localized	3-32 days	Erythem migrans, often accompanied by fever, myalgia, headache, and fatigue	14-21 days oral therapy
Early Disseminated	2-6 weeks	Multiple erythema migrans lesions	14-21 days oral therapy
		Neuroborreliosis (facial nerve palsy or meningitis)	14-21 days oral therapy for facial nerve palsy and 14-28 days parenteral therapy for meningitis
		Carditis, most commonly atrioventricular conduction block	14-21 days oral therapy for first-degree block and 14 days parenteral therapy for second- or third-degree block
Late Disseminated	6 weeks to 12 months	Arthritis, most commonly monoarticular arthritis of the knee	28 days oral therapy

[a]The preferred oral agents are amoxicillin and cefuroxime axetil and the preferred parenteral agent is ceftriaxone

Given these findings, routine administration of antimicrobial prophylaxis or serologic testing following a tick bite is not recommended. However, a single dose of doxycycline may be offered to patients 8 years of age or older if each of the following criteria is met: the attached tick can be reliability identified as an *I. scapularis*, it is estimated to have been attached for 36 hours or longer, based on exposure history and the degree of tick engorgement, prophylactic therapy can be initiated within 72 hours of tick removal, ecologic information suggests that the local *B. burgdorferi* infection rate is 20% or greater among these ticks, and the patient has no contraindications to doxycycline. In those who cannot receive doxycycline, no prophylactic therapy is recommended, as the benefit of other antibiotics is not known.

SUGGESTED READINGS

1. Esposito S, Bosis S, Sabatini C, Tagliaferri L, Principi N. *Borrelia burgdorferi* infection and Lyme disease in children. *Int J Infect Dis.* 2013;17:e153-e158.
2. Feder HM. Lyme disease in children. *Infect Dis Clin N Am.* 2008;22:315-326.
3. Gerber MA, Zemel LS, Shapiro ED. Lyme arthritis in children: clinical epidemiology and long-term outcomes. *Pediatr.* 1998;102:905-908.
4. Gerber MA, Shapiro ED, Burke GS, et al. Lyme disease in children in Southeastern Connecticut. *N Engl J Med.* 1996;335:1270-1274.
5. Hayes EB, Piesman J. How can we prevent Lyme disease? *N Engl J Med.* 2003;348:2424-2430.
6. Krause PJ, McKay K, Thompson CA, et al. Disease-specific diagnosis of coinfecting tickborne zoonoses: babesiosis, human granulocytic ehrlichiosis, and Lyme disease. *Clin Infect Dis.* 2002;34:1184-1191.
7. Nadelman RB, Nowakowski J, Fish D, et al. Prophylaxis with single-dose doxycycline for the prevention of Lyme disease after an *Ixodes scapularis* tick bite. *N Engl J Med.* 2001;345:79-84.
8. Newland JG, Zaoutis TE, Shah SS. The child with aseptic meningitis. *Pediatr Case Rev.* 2003;3(4):218-221.
9. Stanek G, Wormser GP, Gray J, Strle F. Lyme borreliosis. *Lancet.* 2012;379(9814):461-473.
10. Steere AC. Lyme disease. *N Engl J Med.* 2001;345:115-125.
11. Turnquist JL, Shah SS, Zaoutis TE, Hodinka RL, Coffin SE. Clinical and laboratory features allowing early differentiation of Lyme and enteroviral meningitis in children. *Pediatr Res.* 2003;53:106A.
12. Welsh EJ, Cohn KA, Nigrovic LE, et al. Electrocardiograph abnormalities in children with Lyme meningitis. *J Pediatr Infect Dis Soc.* 2012;1:293-298.
13. Wormser GP, Dattwyler RJ, Shapiro ED, et al. The clinical assessment, treatment, and prevention of Lyme disease, human granulocytic anaplasmosis, and babesiosis. *Clin Infect Dis.* 2006;43:1089-1134.

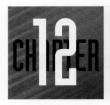

CONSTIPATION

HEIDI C. WERNER

DEFINITION OF THE COMPLAINT

Constipation, a common problem in childhood, accounts for 10%-25% of all referrals to pediatric gastroenterologists. Although constipation is usually characterized by the painful passage of hard stool, the term refers to both the consistency and frequency of stools. A precise definition of constipation is difficult since the normal stooling pattern differs among individuals and varies by age. The frequency of stools in most children decreases from a mean of four per day in the first week of life to two per day by 16 weeks of age, and one stool per day at 4 years of age.

All cases of constipation involve a failure to evacuate the lower colon completely with a bowel movement. Thus, a child who has two small stools per day may not have evacuated the colon, whereas the child who has two large stools weekly may not be constipated. The child who has experienced pain while defecating may aggressively contract the external sphincter to prevent expulsion of stool when the urge to defecate arises. This leads to the collection of increased amounts of stool in the rectum and during a period of weeks to months the rectum gradually dilates, becoming less capable of peristaltic activity.

COMPLAINT BY CAUSE AND FREQUENCY

While functional fecal retention is the most common cause of childhood constipation, several other causes must be considered in the differential diagnosis (Table 12-1).

CLARIFYING QUESTIONS

A diagnosis of constipation can readily be made by the history and physical examination. The following questions may provide clues to the diagnosis:

- What is the stool consistency, caliber, and volume?
  —Small, pellet-like stools indicate incomplete evacuation. Intermittent, massive stools are characteristic of functional fecal retention.

- Did the child have a bowel movement in the first 24 hours of life?
  —A normal bowel movement in the first 24 hours of life can help lower the suspicion of Hirschsprung disease.

- Were there any neonatal complications or surgery?
  —Neonatal gastrointestinal complications such as necrotizing enterocolitis or prior surgery can lead to strictures or adhesions and predispose a child to constipation and small bowel obstruction.

- Is the child going through any transitions such as from breast- to bottle-feeding, diapers to toilet training, or home to childcare or school?
  —Developmental and social transition periods are the most common time for the beginning of functional constipation. Asking about transitions such as a move into childcare can help identify a possible cause of constipation and also provide parents insight into the diagnosis.

TABLE 12-1.	Differential diagnosis of constipation.		
Functional	Fecal retention Protracted vomiting Lack of bulk in diet Toilet phobia/toilet training Depression	**Decreased Sensation/ Motility**	
		Drug induced	Laxative abuse Tricyclic antidepressants Narcotics Vincristine Iron overload Lead poisoning
Mechanical Obstruction	Hirschsprung Pelvic mass Rectal stenosis Anal atresia Meconium ileus Rectal/sigmoid stricture (postoperative)	Neuromuscular disease	Hypotonia syndrome Myelomeningocele Cerebral palsy Tethered cord
Pain on Defecation	Anal fissure Foreign body Sexual abuse Rectal prolapse Perianal streptococcal Infection	Metabolic	Hypothyroidism Hyperparathyroidism Hypercalcemia Diabetes insipidus Renal tubular acidosis Hypokalemia
		Infant botulism	
		Spinal cord tumor	

- Is there a history of sexual abuse?
  —The emotional trauma of sexual abuse can predispose a child to constipation.

- Is the child on any medication?
  —Several medications can cause constipation (Table 12-1).

- Are there any other symptoms (e.g., fever, blood in stool)?
  —Symptoms associated with constipation point to an organic cause.

- Has the family kept a journal of stooling patterns and diet?
  —A 5-7 day journal of stooling patterns and diet can help both the clinician and family objectively assess the true extent of constipation. Diet history can also help identify a cause of constipation and also help as a starting point for therapy for functional constipation.

CASE 12-1

Eleven-Month-Old Girl

HEIDI C. WERNER

HISTORY OF PRESENT ILLNESS

The patient, an 11-month-old girl with a history of chronic constipation, presented to the emergency department with her last bowel movement having been 3 weeks ago. Her regular bowel pattern has been two stools per month, which were accompanied by significant straining. No blood or mucous was noted with any of these stools. Two days prior to this visit she had fever with decreased oral intake and decreased urine output. She also seemed to be having increased abdominal distention. These symptoms did not improve with several phosphate enemas at home. Prior to this episode she had normal weight gain without vomiting or diarrhea.

MEDICAL HISTORY

The patient was delivered at term gestation and there were no complications during the pregnancy. She was evaluated at 4 days of life because she had not passed meconium. Over the next few months there were several interventions for constipation including prune juice, increased water intake, and changes in formula. Each intervention seemed to initially produce more frequent bowel movements, and then the pattern would worsen again. Bowel movements tended to be loose, watery, and small in volume. Otherwise, her review of systems was negative. The patient has been on docusate since 9 months of age. She has had two episodes of otitis media. Thyroid function tests, including thyroid stimulating hormone, were normal.

PHYSICAL EXAMINATION

T 38.2°C; RR 36/min; HR 140 bpm; BP 90/60 mmHg

Weight 8.7 kg (25th-50th percentile); Height 74.5 cm (50th percentile); Head Circumference 45.5 cm (75th percentile)

Initial examination revealed a quiet but uncomfortable infant. Physical examination was remarkable for mild erythema of the posterior oropharynx, and erythematous tympanic membranes with decreased mobility. The abdomen was distended with distant bowel sounds. The abdominal examination also revealed palpable stool in the left quadrant. On the rectal examination, there were no fissures, the anus was patent, and there was no stool in the ampulla.

DIAGNOSTIC STUDIES

Serum chemistries revealed the following: sodium, 130 mEq/L; potassium, 5.0 mEq/L; chloride, 107 mEq/L; bicarbonate, 14 mEq/L; blood urea nitrogen, 66 mg/dL; and creatinine, 0.3 mg/dL. An abdominal obstruction series showed increased stool with dilated loops of bowel but no air-fluid levels (Figure 12-1).

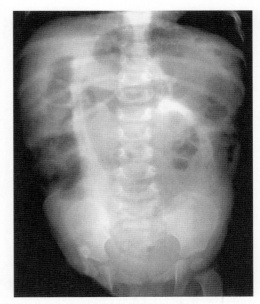

FIGURE 12-1. Abdominal radiograph.

COURSE OF ILLNESS

In the emergency department she was treated for dehydration with intravenous normal saline fluid boluses. She was treated with amoxicillin for otitis media. She also received two pediatric phosphate enemas that produced small amounts of liquid stool. She subsequently had three episodes of bile-tinged emesis. Later, on the first day of admission, she became more irritable with an increasing abdominal girth. Cultures of the blood and urine were negative.

Serial abdominal obstruction series did not show any change during the first 2 days of admission. However, with continuing enemas the patient's abdominal girth decreased (from 48 to 41 cm) as her stool-output increased. On the third day of hospitalization, radiographic barium enema was performed (Figure 12-2) that suggested the diagnosis.

DISCUSSION CASE 12-1

DIFFERENTIAL DIAGNOSIS

Based on the history, the patient has been constipated for her entire life. She also failed to pass

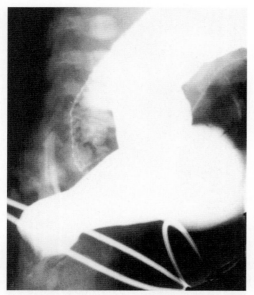

FIGURE 12-2. Radiographic enema from a patient with a similar diagnosis.

TABLE 12-2.	Diagnoses to consider in the patient with delayed passage of meconium.
Condition	**Comments**
Hirschsprung Disease	Abdominal distention and vomiting common, rectal vault may be empty, transition zone on contrast enema
Meconium Ileus	Most patients have cystic fibrosis
Intestinal Obstruction	Consider anterior ectopic anus, anal ring stenosis, volvulus
Functional Ileus	Prematurity, respiratory distress, sepsis, electrolyte disturbances
Small Left Colon	Increased incidence in infants of diabetic mothers
Hypothyroidism	Infants may also have jaundice, lethargy, low body temperature
Drugs Administered to Mother Prior to Delivery	Opiates, magnesium

meconium in the first 48 hours of life. Hirschsprung disease should, therefore, be at the top of a differential list. However, there are several other diagnoses to consider in the infant or child with delayed passage of meconium (Table 12-2).

DIAGNOSIS

The barium enema (Figure 12-2) revealed a funnel-shaped transition zone that suggested the diagnosis of Hirschsprung disease. The transition zone probably would have been more obvious had the patient not received several phosphate enemas prior to the study. Endoscopic rectal suction biopsy was inconclusive. **A full-thickness surgical biopsy showed no ganglion cells in 100 sections and was diagnostic of Hirschsprung disease.** The patient underwent a successful Duhamel pull-through procedure.

INCIDENCE AND HISTORY

Hirschsprung disease, or aganglionosis of the bowel, is the most common cause of lower intestinal obstruction in neonates. It is characterized by abnormal innervation of the distal bowel, beginning at the anus and extending proximally for a variable distance. The defect results from a failure of neural crest cell caudal migration. The primary histologic finding is the absence of meissner and Auerbach plexuses, hypertrophied nerve bundles between the circular and longitudinal muscles and in the submucosa. This abnormal innervation leads to abnormal tone and motility of the bowel, and predisposes to obstruction.

Hirschsprung disease occurs in 1 per 5000 live births. The overall male to female ratio is 3:1. In 80% of patients, the aganglionic segment does not extend above the sigmoid, while the entire colon and some small bowel may be involved in 3%. Recurrent abdominal distention, emesis, failure to thrive, and acute enterocolitis allow diagnosis of 60% of patients by 3 months of age. More than 50% of affected children are diagnosed within the first year of life, and nearly all are diagnosed by within the first 2 years of life; a minority of children with Hirschsprung disease is not diagnosed until adolescence. Hirschsprung disease is associated with Down syndrome, which occurs in 9%-11% of Hirschsprung disease cases, and cardiac anomalies, which occur in 6%-8% of cases. Conditions less commonly associated with Hirschsprung disease include neuroblastoma, deafness, and central hypoventilation syndrome. Additionally, Hirschsprung disease, multiple endocrine neoplasia type 2 (MEN2A), and familial medullary thyroid cancer are all associated with germ line mutations of the RET-protooncogen; up to 5% of patients with Hirschsprung disease carry the MEN2A RET-mutations and consequently have an increased risk of developing medullary thyroid carcinoma.

CLINICAL PRESENTATION

Most (95%) full-term infants with Hirschsprung disease fail to pass meconium during the first 24 hours of life. Normal full-term infants pass meconium within 24 hours (90%) to 48 hours (99%) of life. Therefore, any neonate who fails to pass meconium within 48 hours should be suspected of having Hirschsprung disease. These infants may also develop vomiting and abdominal distention during the first week of life. Enterocolitis, a consequence of delayed diagnosis in a neonate with significant bowel involvement, is characterized by fever, abdominal distention, and explosive, foul-smelling, bloody diarrheal stools. Hirschsprung enterocolitis may be complicated by intestinal necrosis or perforation and sepsis.

Findings in the older child include a history of severe constipation from birth, failure to thrive, and abdominal distention. Older children may come to attention by presenting with either complete intestinal obstruction or enterocolitis. The rectal ampulla is usually empty on digital rectal examination.

DIAGNOSTIC APPROACH

Abdominal radiographs. In children with Hirschsprung disease, a plain-film of the abdomen may show distended loops of colon; air is usually present in the small bowel proximal to the obstruction.

Barium enema. Barium enema is suggestive in approximately 80% of cases. A barium enema should be performed without bowel preparation so that the large rectum dilated with stool can be appreciated. The characteristic appearance of the barium enema occurs because aganglionosis of the distal colon results in hypertonic contraction of the affected bowel. The normal proximal bowel becomes dilated. Between the two segments, a transition zone of bowel develops. This transition zone lacks innervation but partially distends under the influence of the peristaltic activity of the normal bowel pushing the bowel contents into the contracted distal segment. This transition zone is generally funnel-shaped. Variations of this appearance include an abrupt transition from dilated to narrowed bowel and, in some cases, funneling of the bowel incrementally over a long segment of bowel, making the change barely perceptible. Dilation of the rectum to the anal verge is diagnostic of functional constipation and rules out Hirschsprung disease.

Anal manometry. In older children, anal manometry may facilitate the diagnosis of Hirschsprung disease, with a reported sensitivity of 95%. Failure of the internal sphincter to relax in response to inflation of a rectal balloon suggests Hirschsprung disease.

Rectal biopsy. The absence of ganglion cells in the myenteric (Auerbach) and submucous (Meissner) plexus by rectal suction biopsy is diagnostic for Hirschsprung disease. Staining for the presence of acetylcholinesterase may be more reliable than recognizing the absence of ganglion cells. If the suction biopsy is not conclusive, a full-thickness biopsy is mandatory. Complications of mucosal suction biopsy are rare. In a review of 1340 mucosal biopsies, there were three cases of hemorrhage requiring packed red blood cell transfusion and three clinical perforations.

Other studies. In children with enterocolitis, the complete blood count frequently reveals anemia and leukocytosis.

TREATMENT

Emergency management of intestinal obstruction or enterocolitis includes gastric decompression (e.g., nasogastric tube), initiation of parenteral nutrition, avoidance of oral intake, and, for enterocolitis, empiric antibiotic therapy to cover biliary and intestinal pathogens. Empiric antibiotics may include beta-lactam/beta-lactamase inhibitors (e.g., ampicillin-sulbactam, piperacillin-tazobactam) or third-generation cephalosporins in combination with metronidazole.

Operative intervention is necessary to treat Hirschsprung disease. The original operation (Swenson procedure) consisted of removing the defective distal colon and performing end-to-end anastomosis 2 cm above the anal canal. With this procedure, the defective aganglionic tissue is completely resected and the proximal ganglionated colon and anal canal are left in the normal anatomic position.

For total colonic aganglionosis, some surgeons prefer initially performing a defunctionalizing colostomy or an ileostomy to avoid the hazards of enterocolitis. Definitive surgery is usually performed 6 months to 1 year after the initial colostomy. The endorectal pull-through procedure is widely practiced. This procedure involves stripping the aganglionic rectum of its mucosa and then bringing the normally innervated colon through the rectal muscular cuff, bypassing the abnormal bowel from within. The advantage to this procedure is the preservation of rectal function with minimal risk of injury to the pelvis. The other commonly used procedure is the retrorectal transanal pull-through (Duhamel procedure). In the Duhamel procedure, the normally innervated bowel is brought behind the abnormally innervated rectum approximately 1-2 cm above the pectinate line and an end-to-side anastomosis is performed. A neorectum is created with the anterior half having normal sensory receptors and a posterior half with normal propulsion. The advantages to the Duhamel procedure are that it reduces pelvic dissection to a minimum and retains the sensory pathway of rectal reflexes.

The overall mortality rate for surgical repair is low (approximately 1%). The most common immediate postoperative complications include stricture or leakage at the anastomosis site. Some patients experience recurrent enterocolitis. The widely held view that long-term outcomes of bowel function in Hirschsprung disease are generally favorable have been challenged by recent high-quality studies. Controlled studies in which patient follow-up occurred through adolescence demonstrate a high prevalence of impaired bowel function. Long-term sequelae including fecal soiling or incontinence, constipation, and bowel obstruction occur in up to half of children with Hirschsprung disease following repair. Repeat operations are required in up to one-fourth of cases. Contrast enema findings in children with a poor functional outcome (e.g., soiling, bowel obstruction) include a distal narrowed segment due to stricture or aganglionic/transitional zone segment, dilated or hypomotile distal segment, and thickened presacral space due to compressing Soave cuff.

SUGGESTED READINGS

1. Baillie CT, Kenny SE, Rintala RJ, Booth JM, Lloyd DA. Long-term outcome and colonic motility after the Duhamel procedure for Hirschsprung's disease. *J Pediatr Surg.* 1999;34:325-329.
2. Bees BI, Azmy A, Nigam M, Lake BD. Complications of rectal suction biopsy. *J Pediatr Surg.* 1983;18:273-275.
3. Fortuna RS, Weber TR, Tracy TF Jr., Silen ML, Cradock TV. Critical analysis of the operative treatment of Hirschsprung's disease. *Arch Surg.* 1996;131:520-525.
4. Huang EY, Tolley EA, Blakely ML, Langham MR. Changes in hospital utilization and management of Hirschsprung disease: analysis using the KIDS' inpatient database. *Ann Surg.* 2013: [Epub ahead of print, PMID 23263193].
5. Rintala RJ, Pakarinen MP. Long-term outcomes of Hirschsprung's disease. *Semin Pediatr Surg.* 2012;21:336-343.
6. Rescorla FJ, Morrison AM, Engles D, West KW, Grosfeld JL. Hirschsprung's disease: evaluation of mortality and long-term function in 260 cases. *Arch Surg.* 1992;127:934-941.
7. Garrett KM, Levitt MA, Pena A, Kraus SJ. Contrast enema findings in patients presenting with poor functional outcome after primary repair Hirschsprung disease. *Pediatr Radiol.* 2012;42:1099-1106.
8. Swenson O. Hirschsprung's disease: a review. *Pediatrics.* 2002;109:914-918.

Three-Year-Old Boy

HEIDI C. WERNER

HISTORY OF PRESENT ILLNESS

The patient, a 3-year-old boy, was well until approximately 9 months prior to admission. At this time he developed discomfort and difficulty with passage of large stools, which led to further stool withholding; all during the time he was starting to toilet-train. The patient had bowel movements in his pull-ups, but would refuse to sit on the toilet. When stools were passed they were of normal texture, but he would complain of pain. The patient received several enemas followed by mineral oil orally and since then has had passage of stool on a daily basis. However, 1.5 months ago the patient developed perianal irritation. This started as a small pustule around the anus and evolved to a larger lesion. The patient was admitted to an outlying hospital 1 month prior to this admission at which time the anus was described as having 3-4 cm raised, red excoriating lesion concentrically around the anus. The patient was diagnosed with perianal cellulitis and he was treated for cellulitis with intravenous clindamycin followed by an oral first-generation cephalosporin. After a medical and social evaluation, sexual abuse was excluded. The patient continued to have constipation. He subsequently began to complain of neck pain.

MEDICAL HISTORY

The patient's birth history was unremarkable. The patient has had no other hospitalizations or significant illnesses other than those mentioned previously.

PHYSICAL EXAMINATION

T 37.0°C; RR 22/min; HR 122 bpm; BP 94/61 mmHg

Weight 16.2 kg (50th percentile); Height 98 cm (25%)

The patient was alert and in no acute distress. The examination was remarkable for mild neck stiffness with neck pain with extension. There was no neck pain or resistance to flexion or lateral motion. There was a 2 cm circumferential lesion around the anus. The lesion was erythematous and there was purulent exudate soiling in the underpants. A digital rectal examination could not be performed due to the lack of patient cooperation with the examination.

DIAGNOSTIC STUDIES

Laboratory studies showed a WBC count of 9000 cells/mm^3 (45% segmented neutrophils, 49% lymphocytes, and 6% monocytes); hemoglobin, 11.0 g/dL; and platelets, 400 000/mm^3. The mean corpuscular volume was 73 fL and the red cell distribution width was elevated at 19.1. The erythrocyte sedimentation rate was 55 mm/h. Electrolytes, blood urea nitrogen, creatinine, and liver function tests were all normal. The cholesterol was 265 mg/dL.

COURSE OF ILLNESS

The patient underwent an endoscopy and colonoscopy for suspected Crohn disease. On colonoscopy, a verrucous mass was visualized, which was circumferential to the anus up to the anal verge. Multiple biopsies were taken. The descending colon, sigmoid, and rectum appeared normal. The esophagus, stomach, and duodenum were also normal.

During the week following the biopsy the patient developed a rash on his back that, in the clinical context, suggested a diagnosis (Figure 12-3). He was also noted to have increased "swelling" around the eye. On examination, he had left eye proptosis with mild ptosis. Red reflexes were noted, but a full fundoscopic examination could not be obtained. The lateral neck radiograph and CT showed erosion of the third cervical vertebral body (Figure 12-4). The biopsy results became available that same day confirming the diagnosis suggested by the rash and radiologic imaging.

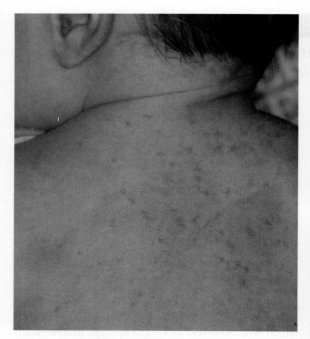

FIGURE 12-3. Photo of a rash.

DISCUSSION CASE 12-2

DIFFERENTIAL DIAGNOSIS

In any 3-year-old boy presenting with difficulty stooling, functional constipation will be first on a differential diagnosis. However, this patient had complicating factors that forced a provider to widen the differential. The perianal lesion should lead us to consider sexual abuse. Inflammatory bowel disease can also present with perianal lesions, but there were no other symptoms such as diarrhea or bloody stools to support that diagnosis. A child with inflammatory bowel disease would also most likely present with other symptoms such as fevers or poor weight gain. Obviously, the symptoms of proptosis and ptosis are worrisome and require additional evaluation. The differential diagnosis of an orbital mass includes leukemia, neuroblastoma, and orbital abscess.

While vertebral osteomyelitis is a diagnostic consideration, this diagnosis would not explain the rash or other findings. Furthermore, lytic destruction of the vertebral body in osteomyelitis

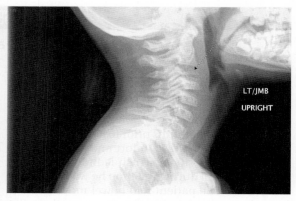

A

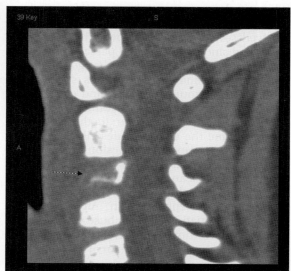

B

FIGURE 12-4. Neck **A.** Radiograph. **B.** CT demonstrating lytic destruction of the third cervical vertebral body with preservation of the posterior elements and transverse foramina. The adjacent disk spaces are preserved. There is also mild bulging of the prevertebral soft tissues in this region.

would typically include encroachment on the disc spaces rather than their preservation.

DIAGNOSIS

The rash consisted of infiltrated, crusted papules and petechiae (Figure 12-3). **The biopsy results** revealed cells consistent with **Langerhans cell histiocytosis (LCH).** Magnetic resonance imaging of the head demonstrated multiple lytic lesions around the skull in the frontal and parietal areas with a left retro-orbital sphenoid mass. The findings of exophthalmos and multiple lytic bone lesions were also characteristic of LCH.

INCIDENCE AND EPIDEMIOLOGY

Langerhans cell histiocytosis (LCH) includes clinical entities such as *eosinophilic granuloma, Hand-Schuller-Christian Disease,* and *Letterer-Siwe disease.* Normally, the Langerhans cell is an antigen-presenting cell of the skin. The hallmark of LCH is the presence of a clonal proliferation of cells of the monocyte lineage containing the characteristic electron microscopic findings of Langerhans cells. LCH is not a malignancy, but rather a manifestation of complex immune dysregulation. The proliferation of these "normal" cells causes destruction or impairment of other organ systems.

LCH affects approximately 4 per million persons with a male to female ratio of 2 to 1. Only 2% of cases are known to be familial but many researchers suspect a genetic basis for the disease. Features that implicate a genetic cause include (1) a greater than expected incidence of malignant disease preceding the onset of LCH, (2) a younger age at onset for identical twins with LCH than for other family pairs, and (3) the finding of monoclonality of the pathologic Langerhans cell in LCH. There is no seasonal or geographic distribution.

CLINICAL MANIFESTATIONS

LCH has an extremely variable presentation depending on sites and extent of involvement (Table 12-3). Approximately 55% of patients have single site disease while the remainder present with multisystem disease. The skeleton may often be the only affected site. Lytic bone lesions may be singular or numerous and are seen most commonly in the skull. These lesions may be asymptomatic or associated with pain and local swelling. Lesions can involve weight-bearing long bones and may result in fractures. Exophthalmos, when present, is often bilateral and caused by retro-orbital accumulation of granulomatous disease. Hypertrophic gingivitis and loose teeth signify underlying mandibular LCH.

TABLE 12-3.	Common sites of presentation of Langerhans cell histiocytosis.
Site	*Frequency*
Bone	77%
Skin	39%
Lymph Nodes	19%
Liver	16%
Spleen	13%
Lung	10%
Central Nervous System	6%

Skin involvement usually presents as a seborrheic dermatitis of the scalp or diaper region, which can spread to involve the back, palms, and soles. The rash frequently consists of infiltrated, crusted papules with areas of hemorrhage. Lymphadenopathy may be part of disseminated disease or associated with local disease affecting adjacent skin or bone. Various degrees of hepatic malfunction can also occur, including jaundice and ascites. In severe cases, liver fibrosis and failure occur. Lung involvement is common in multisystem disease. Children with uncontrolled LCH can develop pulmonary cysts, pneumothorax, and chronic respiratory failure. Central nervous system involvement may also occur. Approximately 15% of children develop diabetes insipidus as a consequence of hypothalamic and pituitary histiocytic involvement. Subtle neurologic defects such as hyporeflexia, ataxia, vertigo, nystagmus, and tremor may develop later during the course of illness. Early treatment may prevent the development of some of these features.

The most severely affected patients may have systemic manifestations such as fever, weight loss, malaise, irritability, and failure to thrive. Bone marrow involvement causes anemia and thrombocytopenia. Mortality is highest in patients presenting with disseminated LCH and organ dysfunction within the first 2 years of life.

DIAGNOSIS

Plain radiography. Plain radiography remains the first-line approach for detecting bone lesions.

Chest radiography may reveal nodular or interstitial infiltrates with relative sparing of the costophrenic angles. Skeletal radiograph may reveal irregularly marginated lytic lesions, usually with adjacent soft tissue swelling. Common sites of bone involvement in multifocal LCH include the skull, mandible, vertebrae, and humerus.

Other radiologic studies. Fluorodeoxyglucose positron emission tomography (FDG PET) may be useful in identifying multiple sites of activity as well as measuring response to treatment. There is high FDG uptake in bone lesions with high concentrations of histiocytes, and thus FDG PET delineates metabolically active LCH. Technetium bone scanning may show lesions before plain radiography but has limited sensitivity in identifying bone lesions compared with FDG PET and MRI. MRI or CT of the head and spine will identify skull and vertebral lesions.

Bone marrow biopsy. Bone marrow infiltration occurs in 18% of patients with multisystem disease and in 33% of patients with hematologic system involvement.

Tissue biopsy. Diagnostic tissue biopsy is easiest to perform on skin or bone lesions.

Other studies. Once the diagnosis has been made, a thorough clinical and laboratory evaluation should be undertaken. This should include a series of laboratory tests (complete blood count, liver function tests, coagulation studies, chest X-ray, urine osmolality, and skeletal survey) and a detailed evaluation of any affected organ system as suspected by history, physical examination, or the above studies.

TREATMENT AND PROGNOSIS

Single-system disease carries a high chance of spontaneous remission, and is generally benign. Therefore, treatment should be minimal and focus on arresting the progression of a lesion that could result in permanent damage. Local radiation therapy is the treatment of choice for single-system disease.

For multisystem or systemic disease, chemotherapy is the treatment of choice. The intensity of the regimen is modified after risk stratification. Children with no organ dysfunction have a better prognosis than those with one or more involved organs. The initial response rate of children without pulmonary, hepatosplenic, or hematopoietic involvement is 90% with a survival rate of 100%. In those with an unfavorable prognosis, the mortality rate ranges from 20%-50%. The mortality rate is more than 90% in children with multisystem LCH who had a poor response to initial therapy with prednisolone, vincristine, and etoposide. Other chemotherapeutic agents with activity against LCH include glucocorticoids, vinblastine, and methotrexate.

SUGGESTED READINGS

1. Arceci RJ, Brenner MK, Pritchard J. Controversies and new approaches to treatment of Langerhans cell histiocytosis. *Hematol Oncol Clin North Am.* 1998;12:339-357.
2. Arico M, Egeler RM. Clinical aspects of Langerhans cell histiocytosis. *Hematol Oncol Clin N Am.* 1998;12:247-258.
3. Gadner H, Heitger A, Grois N, Gatterer-Menz I, Ladisch S. A treatment strategy for disseminated Langerhans cell histiocytosis. *Med Pediatr Oncol.* 1994;23:72-80.
4. Grois N, Tsunematsu Y, Barkovich AJ, Favara BE. Central nervous system disease in langerhans cell histiocytosis. *Br J Cancer.* 1994;70:s24-s28.
5. Grois N, et al. Risk factors for diabetes insipidus in Langerhans cell histiocytosis. *Pediatr Blood Cancer.* 2006;46(2):228.
6. Ladisch S, Jaffe ES. The histiocytoses. In: Pizzo PA, Poplack DG, eds. *Principles and Practice of Pediatric Oncology.* 3rd ed. Philadelphia: Lippincott-Raven, 1997:615-631.
7. Minkov M, Grois N, Heitger A, et al. Response to initial treatment of multisystem Langerhans cell histiocytosis: a prognostic indicator. *Med Pediatr Oncol.* 2002;39:581-585.
8. Willman CL, Busque L, Griffith BB, et al. Langerhans cell histiocytosis (histiocytosis X): a clonal proliferative disease. *N Engl J Med.* 1994;331:154-160.

Three-Month-Old Boy

SAMIR S. SHAH

HISTORY OF PRESENT ILLNESS

A 3-month-old boy was referred from his pediatrician to the emergency department for evaluation. The parents state that 5 days ago they noticed a change in his stooling pattern. Instead of the usual 4 stools per day, he began passing only one stool per day and now he has not stooled in 2 days. He was taken to the pediatrician for evaluation of his constipation. They note that his feeding intake had decreased from vigorous breastfeeding every 3 hours to relatively poor feeding attempts, often requiring to be wakened for feeds. On the day of admission, they commented that he was not holding onto his pacifier well and that he has been drooling more over the past week. He was also not holding his head up as well as he did 2 weeks ago. He has had no fevers and otherwise his review of systems was negative.

MEDICAL HISTORY

There were no complications during the mother's pregnancy or the infant's birth. His birth weight was 4100 g. Nasolacrimal duct obstruction that was noted shortly after birth resolved by 2 months of age. His development had been progressing normally.

PHYSICAL EXAMINATION

T 36.5°C; RR 47/min; HR 175 bpm; BP 87/39 mmHg; SpO$_2$ 96% on room air; Weight 6.3 kg

The initial examination revealed an infant in no acute distress. He was awake and alert, but not making any vigorous movements. He had a weak cry, moderately weak gag. His heart sounds were normal. Femoral pulses were strong and capillary refill was brisk. His abdomen was soft without organomegaly. He had poor truncal tone. The remainder of the physical examination was normal.

DIAGNOSTIC STUDIES

Electrolytes, blood urea nitrogen, creatinine, and glucose were normal except for a bicarbonate level of 16 mEq/L. Serum aminotransferases and bilirubin were normal. The WBC count was 11 400/mm^3 (71% segmented neutrophils, 25% lymphocytes, 3% monocytes); hemoglobin, 9.5 g/dL; and platelets, 425 000/mm^3. Examination of the cerebrospinal fluid (CSF) revealed 3 WBCs/mm^3 and 10 RBCs/mm^3. CSF protein was 24 mg/dL and glucose was 67 mg/dL. There were no organisms on CSF Gram stain. Blood, CSF, and urine cultures were obtained.

COURSE OF ILLNESS

The infant was treated with intravenous cefotaxime for presumed bacterial infection while awaiting culture results. On the third day of hospitalization, his respiratory effort worsened, he had difficulty handling oral secretions, and his gag reflex was diminished requiring endotracheal intubation. What is the most likely diagnosis?

DISCUSSION CASE 12-3

DIFFERENTIAL DIAGNOSIS

Infectious diseases such as meningitis and encephalitis must be considered in any child presenting with lethargy. Dehydration can cause lethargy and altered stooling patterns. Children with viral or bacterial gastroenteritis usually have vomiting or diarrhea though constipation may be present in the severely dehydrated child. Neonatal myasthenia gravis may cause with neurologic abnormalities including lethargy and ptosis but does not usually cause constipation or changes in stooling pattern. Additionally, myasthenia gravis typically presents with a waxing and waning course. Several inborn errors of metabolism may present with lethargy but usually cause other symptoms such as vomiting or irritability. Congenital myopathies (e.g., myotubular myopathy, central core disease, nemaline rod disease) can cause muscular weakness and hypotonia. Focusing on the change in stooling pattern in this patient, hypothyroidism must also be considered as a cause. Tick paralysis is rare in infants but manifests as symmetrical ascending flaccidity; gait abnormalities are the initial manifestation in older children. Guillain-Barré syndrome, though rare in children, should also be considered. Guillain-Barré syndrome manifests as an ascending paralysis resulting from an acute inflammatory polyradiculoneuropathy; a key clinical finding is cytoalbuminemic dissociation (elevated CSF protein without elevation of CSF white blood cells). The Miller-Fisher variant of Guillain-Barré syndrome presents with the triad of ataxia, areflexia, and ophthalmoplegia. Other possible diagnoses include poliomyelitis, anticholinergic poisoning, intracranial hemorrhage from accidental or nonaccidental trauma, cerebrovascular accident, and intussusception. However, the constellation of neurologic changes associated with the change in stooling pattern most strongly suggest infant botulism.

DIAGNOSIS

On examination, the infant had marked hypotonia. Due to the rather rapid progression of symptoms, infant botulism was suspected. EMG revealed a modest decremental response, consistent with infant botulism. **A stool sample was positive for** *Clostridium botulinum* **toxin, confirming the diagnosis of infant botulism.** He received botulism immune globulin on the fourth day of hospitalization. He was extubated on the tenth day of hospitalization and required nasogastric feeds for a total of 3 weeks.

INCIDENCE AND EPIDEMIOLOGY

Botulism results from exposure to *Clostridium botulinum* spores (e.g., infant botulism, wound botulism) or toxin (i.e., foodborne botulism, following injection of botulinum toxin for treatment of hyperhidrosis, muscle spasticity, cervical dystonia, and blepharospasm). Infant botulism occurs

due to an intestinal infection by *C. botulinum*, an anaerobic, Gram-positive, spore-forming bacillus. *Clostridium botulinum* spores are ubiquitous in the environment and can be cultured from soil and many agricultural products. Honey is one dietary source linked to infant botulism by laboratory testing and epidemiologic studies. Corn syrup does not appear to be a risk factor for infant botulism. In the 1980s, a Food and Drug Administration study found botulism spores in commercially prepared corn syrup. Following changes in corn syrup production, spores have not been identified in corn syrup.

Clostridium botulinum spores from various sources are ingested by infants. These spores colonize the colon and release the organism. The organism produces a toxin that causes the disease. In contrast, the adult form occurs after ingestion of the preformed toxin. Botulism toxin is divided into types A-G, with types A, B, E, and F producing human disease. Cases occur in infants less than 1 year old, with 95% occurring during the first 6 months of life. The age-related vulnerability may be due to the lack of competitive flora and possibly to pH and motility. Affected infants are most commonly breastfed, Caucasian, and reside in rural or suburban areas. The intestinal microflora of breast fed infants as compared with bottle fed infants may make them more susceptible to colonization with *C. botulinum*. The organism produces a neurotoxin that is taken up by nerve endings and irreversibly blocks acetylcholine release in peripheral cholinergic synapses. Cranial nerves are usually affected first, leading to difficulty swallowing and loss of protective airway reflexes. The recovery phase begins when terminal motor neurons regenerate and new motor endplates develop.

CLINICAL MANIFESTATIONS AND COMPLICATIONS

Clinical signs and symptoms usually develop between 2 weeks and 6 months of age. Patients are afebrile. The typical evolution is a symmetric descending paralysis, progressing from muscles innervated by the cranial nerves to the upper and lower extremities proximally and then to the trunk and distal extremities.

Constipation is the classic initial complaint. Additional presenting complaints include poor feeding, weak suck, weak cry, and hypotonia. Although often described as lethargic, the infant is typically alert but unable to move or smile. Within a week of the initial presentation, additional neurologic symptoms are seen including ptosis, facial diplegia, dysconjugate gaze, weak suck, impaired swallowing or gag reflex, and worsening hypotonia. Paralysis develops in a descending manner; all cranial nerves are eventually involved. A normal initial response of the pupillary light reflex will fatigue with repeated stimulation over 1-2 minutes. This can be helpful in distinguishing infant botulism from congenital myasthenia syndromes. Deep tendon reflexes are initially normal despite profound hypotonia; hyporeflexia develops later in the course. Autonomic dysfunction is common. Decreased tearing and salivation gradually develop. Blood pressure and heart rate may fluctuate dramatically.

There are several complications that lead to the morbidity and mortality associated with infant botulism. Most infants have progressive weakness over a 1-2 week period culminating in respiratory failure. Inability to swallow or protect the airway from oral secretions leads to nasogastric tube feeding and endotracheal intubation. The symptoms remain at a nadir for 1-2 weeks before improving. Most infants require hospitalization for 4-5 weeks. The syndrome of inappropriate secretion of antidiuretic hormone (SIADH) occurs due to venous pooling, diminished left atrial filling, and subsequent stimulus for antidiuretic hormone production. SIADH complicates approximately 17% of cases. Secondary infections such as urinary tract infection and aspiration pneumonia also occur.

DIAGNOSIS

The clinical presentation usually suggests infant botulism but the definitive diagnosis is made by testing stool samples.

Detection of organism. A small enema with non-bacteriostatic water (not saline) may be used judiciously to obtain stool for diagnostic testing. The most reliable confirmatory test is detection of *C. botulinum* toxin in the infant's stool using the mouse inoculation toxin neutralization assay. Specimens for toxin assay are transported at 4°C to either the state health department or the Centers for Disease Control and Prevention laboratories for testing. *C. botulinum* can be cultured from stool after anaerobic incubation on selective egg yolk agar; however, this is rarely required given the reliability of the toxin assay. Serum testing reveals the diagnosis in fewer than 10% of cases.

Electromyography (EMG). EMG, though not typically necessary, will reveal the following: (1) motor unit action potentials of brief duration, small amplitude, and abundant motor-unit potentials (BSAP); (2) incremental response in the muscle action potential produced by high frequency stimulation; (3) normal nerve conduction velocity; and (4) no significant response to injection of edrophonium chloride or neostigmine (to distinguish this condition from myasthenia gravis).

Other studies. Lumbar puncture, often performed because of concern for meningitis, reveals normal CSF cell count, protein, and glucose. Once the diagnosis is made, serum electrolytes should be checked periodically to detect SIADH.

TREATMENT

Keys to successful management include early recognition, prompt treatment with Botulinum immune globulin, and attention to supportive care strategies to minimize disease-associated and iatrogenic complications (Table 12-4). Attention

TABLE 12-4.	Important preventable complications of infant botulism.
Aspiration pneumonia	
Urinary tract infection	
Bacteremia/sepsis	
Syndrome of inappropriate antidiuretic hormone secretion	
Seizures (hyponatremia)	
Anemia	
Fractures	
Clostridium difficile-associated colitis	

should be directed at protecting the airway, providing adequate ventilation and nutrition, and preventing complications.

Endotracheal intubation, required by approximately 70% of children with infant botulism, should be performed when impairment of the infant's ability to cough, gag, or swallow occurs. In the past, tracheostomies were performed in up to 50% of patients in anticipation of prolonged requirement for mechanical ventilation. Prior to the use of antitoxin, the mean duration of mechanical ventilation was 21 days. Currently, the duration of mechanical ventilation is shorter (median, 6 days; interquartile range, 2-11 days) and late sequelae of airway trauma induced by prolonged endotracheal intubation (e.g., subglottic stenosis) are rare. Prophylactic tracheostomy is not routinely required.

Nasogastric tube feedings are usually required during the course of illness to prevent aspiration of formula. Small volumes of continuous enteral feeding stimulates gut motility and obviates the need for central venous catheterization. Oral feeding can be resumed when the gag, swallow, and suck reflexes have returned. Intake, output, weight, and serum electrolytes must be carefully monitored during this period due to the risk of SIADH.

Antibiotic therapy is often started empirically while the meningoencephalitis and sepsis are excluded. Specific antibiotic therapy is not required for treatment of infant botulism but may be required to treat hospital-acquired infections. Aminoglycoside antibiotics may precipitate rapid deterioration of infants with infant botulism. They contribute to neuromuscular blockade and should be avoided in children in whom the diagnosis of infant botulism is suspected.

Botulism immune globulin intravenous (BIG-IV) has improved outcomes of patients with infant botulism. BIG-IV, derived from pooled plasma of adult volunteers, neutralizes free toxin. BIG-IV was licensed by the U.S. Food and Drug Administration in 2003 for sale by the California Department of Health Services as BabyBIG®. It has a half-life of approximately 28 days in vivo and a large capacity to neutralize botulinum toxin. A single infusion will neutralize for at least 6 months all botulinum toxin that may be absorbed from the colon of an infant. Treatment should not be delayed for confirmatory testing. While the cost per dose is approximately $50 000, treatment is the most cost-effective strategy.

In a double-blind, placebo-controlled randomized trial of 122 infants, BIG-IV or placebo was administered to infants with infant botulism within 3 days of their initial hospital admission. BIG-IV decreased the mean duration of hospitalization from 5.7 to 2.6 weeks, the duration of mechanical ventilation from 4.4 to 1.8 weeks, the duration of intensive care unit stay from 5.0 to 1.8 weeks, and the duration of nasogastric or intravenous feeding from 10.0 to 3.6 weeks. BabyBIG® is available only through the California Department of Health Services Infant Botulism Treatment and Prevention Program (www.infantbotulism.org or 510-231-7600). It is express-shipped to be given as a single dose. While administration within 3 days of hospitalization is most effective, administration within 4-7 days of hospitalization remains far more effective than no treatment. An open-label study of infants who received BIG-IV found that the mean length of stay was 2.0 weeks for the 287 infants treated within 3 days of hospital admission and 2.9 weeks for the 79 infants treated between 4 and 7 days of hospital admission. The illness usually lasts from 1 to 2 months and the prognosis is excellent. Case fatality rates are less than 1%.

Patients with infant botulism excrete *C. botulinum* toxin and organisms in their stools. These organisms may be excreted in stool for up to 3 months and, rarely, longer. Therefore, infected infants should not have close contact with other infants (e.g., sharing cribs, toys).

Most live virus vaccines (e.g., measles, mumps, rubella, varicella) should be delayed until 5 months after BabyBIG treatment as the antibodies in BabyBIG may interfere with the effectiveness of live vaccines. Most infants will not require delayed vaccine administration because most affected infants are younger than 6 months of age and the live virus vaccines are typically administered after 12 months of age.

SUGGESTED READINGS

1. Long SS. Infant botulism and treatment with BIG-IV (BabyBIG). *Pediatr Infect Dis J.* 2007;26:261-262.
2. Graf WD, Hays RM, Astley SJ, et al. Electrodiagnosis reliability in diagnosis of infant botulism. *J Pediatr.* 1992;120:747-749.

3. Hatheway CL, McCroskey LM. Examination of feces and serum for diagnosis of infant botulism in 336 patients. *J Clin Microbiol.* 1987;25:2334-2338.

4. Long SS. *Clostridium botulinum* (botulism). In: Long SS, Pickering LK, Prober CG, eds. *Principles and Practice of Pediatric Infectious Diseases.* 4th ed. New York: Elsevier Saunders; 2012:970-977.

5. Long SS. Epidemiologic study of infant botulism in Pennsylvania: report of the infant botulism study group. *Pediatrics.* 1985;75:928-934.

6. Olsen SJ, Swerdlow DL. Risk of infant botulism from corn syrup. *Pediatr Infect Dis J.* 2000;19:584-585.

7. Schreiner MS, Field E, Ruddy R. Infant botulism: a review of 12 years' experience at The Children's Hospital of Philadelphia. *Pediatrics.* 1991;87:159-165.

8. Thompson JA, Filloux FM, Van Orman CB, et al. Infant botulism in the age of botulism immune globulin. *Neurology.* 2005;64:2029-2032.

9. Underwood K, Rubin S, Deakers T, Newth C. Infant botulism: a 30-year experience spanning the introduction of botulism immune globulin intravenous in the intensive care unit at Children's Hospital Los Angeles. *Pediatrics.* 207;120:e1380-e1385.

10. Arnon SS, Schechter R, Maslanka SE, Jewell MP, Hatheway CL. Human botulism immune globulin for the treatment of infant botulism. *N Engl J Med.* 2006;354:462-471.

CASE 12-4

Twelve-Month-Old Girl

REBECCA TENNEY-SOEIRO

HISTORY OF PRESENT ILLNESS

The patient, a 12-month-old girl, was brought to her pediatrician for evaluation of constipation. She usually stooled once per day, but recently she was stooling only once per week. There had been no apparent change in her appetite or activity level. She had no fevers or emesis, and her review of systems was otherwise negative. She has had normal growth and development.

MEDICAL HISTORY

The patient had a normal birth history. Her birth weight was 3600 g. She passed meconium in the first 24 hours of life. She has not required previous hospitalization. She does not receive any medications.

PHYSICAL EXAMINATION

T 36.2°C; HR 90 bpm; RR 17/min; BP 90/50 mmHg

Height 25th percentile; Weight 50th percentile

On examination, the patient is a well-appearing girl. Her HEENT examination was significant for a 1 × 1 cm fleshy mass at the base of her tongue that did not appear to cause her any discomfort. The heart and lung sounds were normal. Her abdomen had an easily reducible umbilical hernia with a 1 cm fascial defect. There was a 2 × 2 cm macular area of hypopigmentation on her lower abdomen. Her tone was slightly decreased symmetrically but she was able to sit without support. The neurologic examination was otherwise normal.

DIAGNOSTIC STUDIES

A nuclear medicine test confirmed the diagnosis (Figure 12-5).

DISCUSSION CASE 12-4

DIFFERENTIAL DIAGNOSIS

As with any child who goes from a normal to a constipated stooling pattern, major causes of constipation can be divided into functional versus organic. As in this case, findings on physical examination, that is, the mass at the base of the tongue, umbilical hernia, and hypotonia, may lead to the diagnosis. However, in a 1-year-old with constipation, other causes should be considered.

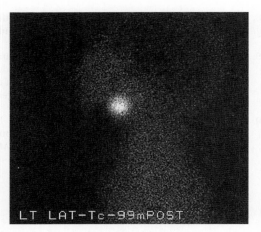

FIGURE 12-5. Radionuclide scan. *(Photo courtesy of Dr. Martin Charron.)*

types of thyroid dysgenesis include aplasia, hypoplasia, and ectopia (ectopic thyroid). The thyroid gland can be totally absent or, as in this case, ectopic. Furthermore, in some cases the deficiency of thyroid hormone can be severe and symptoms will develop in the first weeks of life. As in this case, lesser degrees of deficiency can occur and manifestations are delayed for months. In North America, the incidence of congenital hypothyroidism is 1 in 2000-3000 live births with a 2:1 female to male ratio. One study found a threefold higher incidence of congenital hypothyroidism in multiple (10.1 per 10 000 live births) compared with single (3.2 per 10 000 live births) deliveries. The reason for this finding is unclear, however, the low concordance rate in twins (4.3%) suggests that environmental factors may act as a trigger among those with a susceptible genetic background.

The patient was on no medication, had no evidence of spinal trauma or abnormalities, and no history of lead ingestion or exposure to botulinum.

DIAGNOSIS

Laboratory studies revealed: thyroid-stimulating hormone (TSH) 24.0 U/mL (normal range, 0.6-6.2); free thyroxine (T4) 5.4 mcg/dL (normal range, 6.8-13.5); T4 6.2 mcg/dL (normal range, 5.3-10.8); resin triiodothyronine (T3) uptake 36.9% (normal range, 28.0-47.0%); resin T3 uptake ratio 0.92 (normal range, 0.70-1.18). The patient has an ectopic thyroid gland leading to hypothyroidism. **Thyroid scintigraphy (Figure 12-4) revealed increased uptake at the base of the tongue, confirming the diagnosis of hypothyroidism due to an ectopic thyroid gland.**

PATHOLOGY AND EPIDEMIOLOGY

Causes of congenital hypothyroidism include dyshormonogenesis (deficiency of an enzyme involved in the formation of thyroid hormones), transient congenital hypothyroidism, disorders of thyroxine synthesis, thyroid hormone resistance, and thyroid dysgenesis. Iodide transport defects and iodine organification defects are included among the 15 known disorders of thyroxine synthesis. Thyroid dysgenesis is the most frequent cause of hypothyroidism in infancy. Common

HISTORY AND PHYSICAL EXAMINATION

Most infants with congenital hypothyroidism are asymptomatic at birth, even if there is complete agenesis of the thyroid gland. This is attributed to the transplacental passage of moderate amounts of maternal T4, which accounts for 33% of the infant's T4 levels at birth.

Soon after birth, children with congenital hypothyroidism often develop poor feeding, prolonged hyperbilirubinemia (>7 days), hypotonia, large posterior fontanelle (>1 cm), and macroglossia. Within the first 2 months of life, children who are hypothyroid usually develop constipation and are seen as sedate or placid infants. They also have abdominal distention and an umbilical hernia. There are several other common clinical manifestations: subnormal temperature, edema of the genitals and extremities, slow pulse, cardiac murmurs, cardiomegaly, and goiter. By 3-6 months these symptoms often progress. Development will be delayed as children who are hypothyroid often appear lethargic and are late in learning to sit or stand. Growth retardation is one of the main manifestations in childhood. This growth retardation is accompanied by delayed skeletal maturation.

Children with an ectopic thyroid gland usually have some viable thyroid tissue and symptoms of hypothyroidism are mitigated. These children represent a spectrum of severity of thyroid deficiency.

DIAGNOSTIC TESTS

While neonatal screening programs vary from state to state, most in North America measure levels of T4 and run TSH levels on the lowest 10th percentile for a given day. The false negative rate is 5%-10%. Abnormal tests on a state screen should prompt immediate evaluation of T4 and TSH levels to confirm the diagnosis of hypothyroidism.

Thyroid function tests. Initial evaluation includes TSH and T4. T3 may be performed if ectopic thyroid is suspected initially. A normal or near-normal circulating level of T3 in the presence of a low T4 suggests the presence of residual thyroid tissue.

Thyroid scintigraphy. All children with proven congenital hypothyroidism should undergo radionuclide scanning if possible. The thyroid gland is the only organ in the body that stores iodine to any significant extent, making radioactive isotopes of iodine (e.g., sodium iodide 123, ^{123}I) and ions of similar charge and radius to iodine (e.g., technetium pertechnetate, ^{99m}Tc) useful for thyroid imaging. No uptake of ^{123}I or ^{99m}Tc occurs when the thyroid gland is absent. Ectopic thyroid glands are usually characterized by areas of increased uptake at the base of the tongue but other potential locations include the larynx, mediastinum, and lateral neck. Therefore, images must be obtained from the oropharynx to the upper mediastinum to exclude an ectopic gland. Ectopic thyroid glands are usually hypofunctioning and hence ^{123}I, which produces less background activity than ^{99m}Tc, is the preferred isotope. The demonstration of ectopic thyroid is diagnostic for thyroid dysgenesis and establishes the need for evaluation and treatment of hypothyroidism. A normally placed thyroid with a normal or active uptake of radioisotope in the context of hypothyroidism suggests a defect in thyroid hormone biosynthesis.

THERAPY AND PROGNOSIS

The treatment of choice for children with hypothyroidism is L-thyroxine administered orally. The goal of therapy is to normalize T4 levels as quickly as possible. Levels of T3 and T4 rapidly return to normal in treated infants. TSH levels may not come into the normal range for several weeks even with good T4 values. Treatment is lifelong. If a child was even mildly symptomatic at the time of diagnosis, parents may notice an increase in activity, improvement in feeding, and increased urination and bowel movements soon after treatment begins. If bone maturation was delayed at the time of diagnosis, it will normalize within approximately 1 year. Early diagnosis and treatment usually results in normal IQ and motor development. Delayed diagnosis may result in variable deficits in intelligence that amount to several IQ points for every week of delayed treatment.

To guarantee adequate hormone replacement, T4 levels should be maintained in the upper half of the normal range during therapy. Low T4, high TSH, and poor growth suggest poor compliance or undertreatment. Excessive L-thyroxine over a prolonged period of time (3-6 months) may cause osteoporosis, premature synostosis of cranial sutures, and advancement of bone age. Prognosis is excellent if treatment is begun in the first 4 weeks of life.

SUGGESTED READINGS

1. Bongers-Schokking JJ, Koot HM, Wiersma D, et al. Influence of timing and dose of thyroid hormone replacement on development in infants with congenital hypothyroidism. *J Pediatr.* 2000;136:292-297.
2. Germak JA, Foley TP. Longitudinal assessment of L-thyroxine therapy for congenital hypothyroidism. *J Pediatr.* 1990;117:211-219.
3. Grant DB, Smith I, Fuggle PW, et al. Congenital hypothryoidism detected by neonatal screening: relationship between biochemical severity and early clinical features. *Arch Dis Child.* 1992;67:87-90.
4. Gruters A. Congenital hypothyroidism. *Pediatr Ann.* 1992;21(1):15-28.
5. Eugene D, Djemli A, Van Vliet G. Sexual dimorphism of thyroid function in newborns with congenital hypothyroidism. *J Clin Endocrinol Metab.* 205;90:2696-2700.
6. Harris KB, Pass KA. Increase in congenital hypothyroidism in New York State and in the United States. *Mol Genet Metab.* 2007;91:268-277.
7. Olivieri A, Medda E, De Angelis S, et al. High risk of congenital hypothyroidism in multiple pregnancies. *J Clin Endocrinol Metab.* 2007;92:3141-3147.
8. Pollock AN, Towbin RB, Charron M, Meza MP. Imaging in pediatric endocrine disorders. In: Sperling MA, ed. *Pediatric Endocrinology.* 2nd ed. Philadelphia: Saunders; 2002:725-756.

Nine-Year-Old Girl

PRATICHI K. GOENKA

HISTORY OF PRESENT ILLNESS

A 9-year-old girl who was previously healthy presented with a complaint of constipation. She had developed lower back pain approximately 3 months ago and at that time complained of some difficulty stooling. She tried various therapies including mineral oil, senna, and phosphate supplemented enemas with an improvement in stooling pattern. However, her back pain did not remit. Initially, the pain was intermittent and controlled to some extent with ibuprofen. It began in the lower back and flank and then radiated down the buttocks to both lower legs. It was worse with standing and walking. During the past 2 weeks the pain increased in intensity and was more constant. It now interfered with her daily activities. The mother initially felt that the child was about to start menstruating.

She was evaluated in the emergency department of a nearby hospital about 2 weeks prior to admission where she was diagnosed with pyelonephritis and treated with ciprofloxacin without improvement. One week prior to admission she was reevaluated and computed tomography of the abdomen was normal, specifically there were no renal stones. She now presented in with severe low back pain and had not stooled in 4 days. There had been no recent dysuria, urgency, or frequency. There was no headache, fatigue, weight loss, night sweats, or abdominal pain. Menarche has not occurred. She denies recent trauma or infection.

MEDICAL HISTORY

The girl had problems with constipation as an infant and received mineral oil periodically until 3 years of age. She has not previously required hospitalization. She takes no medications. There is no family history of thyroid disorders or autoimmune diseases.

PHYSICAL EXAMINATION

T 37.4°C; HR 90 bpm; RR 16/min; BP 110/65 mmHg

Weight 25th percentile for age

On examination, she was alert, cooperative, but in obvious distress. She was lying on the examination table moaning and holding her back. Her conjunctivae were pink and anicteric. Her neck was supple. There were no murmurs on cardiac examination. Her abdomen was soft without hepatosplenomegaly. The back was tender along the lumbar spine and flanks bilaterally with significant muscle spasm. The range of motion was limited due to pain. Straight leg raise produced pain in the posterior thighs at approximately 45 bilaterally. The sensation in the lower extremities was intact at all levels. Motor tone was normal. Deep tendon reflexes at the patellar tendon and ankles were normal bilaterally.

LABORATORY STUDIES

Laboratory evaluation included a WBC count, 4100/mm^3 (35% segmented neutrophils, 55% lymphocytes, 8% monocytes, and 2% eosinophils); hemoglobin, 12.0 g/dL; and platelets, 204000/mm^3. Mean corpuscular volume was 87 fL and red cell distribution width was normal at 12.4. Serum chemistries included sodium, 141 mmol/L; potassium, 3.9 mmol/L; chloride, 105 mmol/L; bicarbonate, 25 mmol/L; blood urea nitrogen, 11 mg/dL; creatinine, 0.5 mg/dL; and glucose, 97 mg/dL. The total bilirubin was 0.2 mg/dL and serum albumin, alkaline phosphatse, and transaminases were normal. Urinalysis revealed a specific gravity of 1.011, pH 6.5, and no white blood cells, red blood cells, or protein. Fibrinogen was 411 mg/dL. Prothrombin and partial thromboplastin times were 13.7 seconds and 31.5 seconds, respectively.

HOSPITAL COURSE

Radiographs of the lumbar spine showed no fracture, dislocation, or degenerative changes of the vertebral bodies. MRI of the spine revealed an intradural, intramedullary lesion measuring 5.2 cm × 2.0 cm at the level of T12-L1. There was displacement of the nerve roots and the distal tip of the cauda equina ventrally.

DISCUSSION CASE 12-5

DIFFERENTIAL DIAGNOSIS

While this patient's most consistent symptom is back pain, functional constipation must be considered. Constipation can also lead to difficulty urinating, however this patient has not complained of urinary symptoms despite her earlier diagnosis of pyelonephritis.

Back pain and tenderness along the spine are abnormal and potentially serious findings in a child. Once this history and examination have been elicited, spinal cord processes must be considered. There are several disease processes that can affect the spinal cord and cause the symptoms described. Trauma must be considered in any child with severe back pain. Trauma can lead to hematomas, vertebral fractures, and dislocations in the spine. Bacterial infections can cause epidural abscesses, while viral infections can cause transverse myelitis. Intervertebral disc herniation and spinal tumors also cause back pain in children. Guillain-Barré is occasionally considered in the evaluation of back pain. Table 12-5 includes the differential diagnosis of back pain in the pediatric population. In this child's presentation there was neither a history of trauma nor signs of infection. Imaging studies and biopsy were warranted to make the final diagnosis.

DIAGNOSIS

Diagnosis by frozen section was intramedullary spinal ependymoma.

BACKGROUND

Tumors of the spinal cord can be extramedullary or intramedullary. Extramedullary tumors erode the bony vertebral column and compress sensory and motor tracts located laterally within the spinal cord. Extramedullary lesions are usually due to metastases from primary tumors such as neuroblastoma, sarcoma, and lymphoma. Dysembryoblastic extramedullary tumors are associated with

TABLE 12-5.	Differential diagnosis of back pain in the pediatric population.
Infectious	Discitis
	Epidural abscess
	Osteomyelitis
	Pelvic inflammatory disease
	Pneumonia
	Pyelonephritis
	Pyomyositis
	Retroperitoneal infection
	Septic sacroiliitis
Neoplastic	Bone tumors
	Leukemia
	Lymphoma
	Spinal cord tumors
Musculoskeletal	Herniated disk
	Muscle strain
	Scheuermann kyphosis
	Scoliosis
	Slipped apophysis
	Spondylolisthesis
	Spondylolysis
	Vertebral fracture
Miscellaneous	Chronic recurrent multifocal osteomyelitis
	Nephrolithiasis
	Pancreatitis
	Sickle cell disease
	Syringomyelia

teeth, bones, or calcification and may be associated with a sinus tract leading from the surface and extending intraspinally. Intramedullary tumors are usually either astrocytomas or ependymomas, though oligodendrogliomas also occur.

Ependymomas are CNS intramedullary tumors that arise within or adjacent to the ependymal lining of the ventricular system or the central canal of the spinal cord. They account for 5%-10% of primary childhood CNS tumors. Most ependymomas are located in the posterior fossa but approximately 10% of ependymomas occur in the spinal cord. Ependymomas vary from well-differentiated tumors with no anaplasia and little polymorphism to highly cellular lesions with significant mitotic activity and necrosis.

CLINICAL MANIFESTATIONS

Signs and symptoms of spinal cord tumors can be insidious and misleading. Complaints may be vague and few specific signs occur early in the disease. Most children with a spinal cord tumor ultimately present with a combination of extremity weakness, gait disturbance, scoliosis, and back pain, depending on the location of the tumor. Incontinence as a presenting sign may be overlooked in very young children who may not be fully toilet trained. A clue to the presence of neurogenic bladder is incontinence of urine associated with crying or straining at stool.

Changes in posture, nonspecific complaints of back pain, or even unexplained abdominal pain can be associated with disease of the spinal cord. The child may have difficulty sleeping because of pain. Any pain exacerbated by either valsalva maneuvers, such as straining at stool, or coughing should be evaluated. Tumor attached to nerve roots may cause segmental pain, paresthesias, and weakness. The presence of hyperreflexia, clonus, and up-going toes suggests corticospinal tract disease. Defects in proprioception, vibration sense, or sensory level should also raise suspicion for an intraspinal process.

DIAGNOSTIC APPROACH

Spine radiographs. Obtain anterior-posterior, lateral, and for the cervical spine, oblique projections. Destructive bone lesions are associated with metastatic disease. Increased interpedicular distance suggests a long-standing intramedullary process. Slow-growing spinal tumors may cause scoliosis.

Spine MRI with gadolinium. MRI allows for differentiation of intramedullary from extramedullary masses.

Cystourethrogram. This study can evaluate bladder function and can confirm the diagnosis of neurogenic bladder.

Ophthalmologic examination. Spinal cord tumors are occasionally associated with increased intracranial pressure and papilledema, probably related to decreased CSF absorption due to hemorrhage within the tumor or dramatically elevated CSF protein.

TREATMENT

After confirmation by neurodiagnostic procedures, surgical laminectomy and exploration with removal of the tumor should be considered. Ependymomas expand symmetrically in a rostral caudal fashion. A tissue plane can be readily identified, facilitating surgical excision. Radiation is recommended for most spinal cord tumors but adjuvant chemotherapy is not generally effective. Five-year survival rates for spinal cord ependymomas range from 95% to 100%.

Children with spinal cord tumors often face long-term deficits ranging from partial paralysis of one limb to quadriplegia. Physical therapy, serial casting, and tone-reducing medication may be required for moderate spasticity. Neurogenic bladder problems also require appropriate prophylactic antibiotics, intermittent catheterization, and cystometric evaluation. Multidisciplinary postoperative care includes input from pediatrics, oncology, orthopedics, urology, neurosurgery, and physical therapy.

SUGGESTED READINGS

1. Cohen ME, Duffner PK. Tumors of the brain and spinal cord including leukemic involvement. In: Swaiman KF, Ashwal S, eds. *Pediatric Neurology: Principles and Practice.* 3rd ed. St. Louis: Mosby; 1999:1049-1098.
2. McCormick PC, Torres R, Post KD, et al. Intramedullary ependymoma of the spinal cord. *J Neurosurg.* 1990;72:523-532.
3. Chesney RW. Brain tumors in children. In: Behrman RE, Kliegman RM, Jenson HB, eds. *Nelson Textbook of Pediatrics.* 16th ed. Philadelphia: W.B Saunders Co.; 2000:1858-1862.
4. Garces-Ambrossi GL, McGirt MJ, Mehta VA, et al. Factors associated with progression-free survival and long-term neurological outcome after resection of intramedullary spinal cord tumors: analysis of 101 consecutive cases. *J Neurosurg Spin.* 2009;11:591-599.

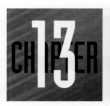

NECK SWELLING

STEPHEN LUDWIG

BRANDON C. KU

DEFINITION

Neck swelling in children is a finding that elicits immediate parental concern and often prompts a visit to the physician. The finding of a neck mass invokes a response because it can be associated with malignancy. Malignancy, though part of the differential diagnosis, is a relatively uncommon cause of neck swelling by far. More common causes include inflammatory conditions, such as reactive lymphadenopathy from viral upper respiratory tract infections, bacterial adenitis, and congenital anomalies with or without bacterial superinfection. Because children often have palpable normal lymph nodes, a significant neck mass is typically defined as swelling that exceeds 2 cm in diameter. In rare cases, smaller nodes may have characteristics that prompt evaluation. Congenital anomalies, although present at birth, may not become clinically apparent until the child is school age or older.

Hospitalization is required if neck masses are present in conjunction with systemic symptoms such as fever, fatigue, or pallor; if the neck masses are large enough to comprise the airway; or if the neck masses have not responded to outpatient therapy.

CAUSE AND FREQUENCY

A differential diagnosis list for neck masses is presented in Table 13-1. Neck masses that require immediate evaluation include those that follow trauma and those that cause airway compromise (Table 13-2). The most common causes of neck swelling include benign reactive lymphadenopathy, bacterial lymphadenitis (including that caused by *Bartonella henselae*), hematoma, congenital causes (e.g., thyroglossal duct cyst, branchial cleft cyst, cystic hygroma), and benign tumors (e.g., lipoma, keloid). Table 13-3 indicates the type of mass by location.

QUESTIONS TO ASK AND WHY

- Is the airway compromised?
  —The first and most important question to ask relates to the presence of airway compromise, since it demands immediate attention if present. Airway compromise may result from intrinsic occlusion or extrinsic compression of the airway. Airway edema may result from swelling caused by trauma or allergic reaction. Neck masses may also be associated with intra-thoracic masses that can cause respiratory distress.

- Are there systemic signs of illness?
  —Other questions that help with the differential diagnosis process are the presence or absence of systemic signs, such as fever, weight loss, anorexia, night sweats, lethargy, or fatigue. Some elements of the differential diagnosis are associated with these systemic findings, such as malignancy, and others are clearly more localized.

- Is there history of or clinical concern for trauma?
  —This question will help identify acute causes of neck swelling that may require surgical intervention, such as rapidly expanding hematoma. Acute bleeding prompts immediate identification of the source of bleeding and subsequent hemostasis.

TABLE 13-1. | **Differential diagnosis of neck mass by etiology.**

Category	Causes	Category	Causes
Congenital	Thyroglossal duct cyst Branchial cleft cyst Cystic hygroma (lymphangioma) Squamous epithelial cyst (congenital or posttraumatic) Pilomatrixoma (Malherbe calcifying epithelioma) Hemangioma Dermoid cyst Cervical rib	"Antigen"-mediated (Cont.)	Rosai-Dorfman disease (sinus histiocytosis with massive lymphadenopathy) Sarcoidosis Caffey-Silverman syndrome (infantile hyperostosis)
Inflammatory		**Trauma**	Hematoma Sternocleidomastoid tumor of infancy (fibromatosis colli) Subcutaneous emphysema Acute bleeding Arteriovenous fistula Foreign body Cervical spine fracture
Infection	Lymphadenopathy—secondary to local head and neck infection Lymphadenopathy—secondary to systemic infection—infectious mononucleosis, cytomegalovirus, HIV, toxoplasmosis, others Lymphadenitis—streptococcal, staphylococcal, fungal, mycobacterial, cat-scratch disease, tularemia Focal myositis—inflammatory muscular pseudotumor Lemierre syndrome	**Neoplasm**	
		Benign	Epidermoid Lipoma, fibroma, neurofibroma Keloid Goiter (with or without thyroid hormone disturbance) Osteochondroma Teratoma (may be malignant) "Normal" anatomy or variant
"Antigen"-mediated	Local hypersensitivity reaction (sting/bite) Serum sickness, autoimmune disease Pseudolymphoma (secondary to phenytoin) Kawasaki disease	Malignant	Lymphoma—Hodgkin disease or non-Hodgkin lymphoma Leukemia Rhabdomyosarcoma Neuroblastoma Histiocytosis X Nasopharyngeal squamous cell carcinoma Thyroid or salivary gland tumor

TABLE 13-2. | **Life-threatening causes of neck mass.**

Hematoma secondary to trauma
Cervical spine injury
Vascular compromise or acute bleeding
Late arteriovenous fistula

Subcutaneous emphysema with associated airway or pulmonary injury

Local hypersensitivity reaction (sting/bite) with airway edema

Airway compromise with epiglottitis, tonsillar abscess, or infection of floor of mouth or retropharyngeal space

Bacteremia/sepsis associated with local infection of cyst (cystic hygroma, thyroglossal, or branchial cleft)

Lymphoma with mediastinal mass and airway compromise

Tumor-leukemia, rhabdomyosarcoma, histiocytosis

Thyroid storm from thyroid mass

Mucocutaneous lymph node syndrome with coronary vasculitis

TABLE 13-3.	Differential diagnosis of neck mass by location.
Location	*Causes*
Parotid	Lymphadenitis, cystic hygroma, hemangioma, parotitis, Sjögren, Caffey-Silverman syndrome, lymphoma parotid tumor
Postauricular	Lymphadenitis, branchial cleft cyst (1st), squamous epithelial cyst
Submental	Lymphadenitis, cystic hygroma, thyroglossal duct cyst, dermoid, sialadenitis
Submandibular	Lymphadenitis, cystic hygroma, sialadenitis tumor, cystic fibrosis
Jugulodiagastric	Lymphadenitis, squamous epithelial cyst, branchial cleft cyst (1st), parotid tumor; normal: transverse process C2, styloid process
Midline Neck	Lymphadenitis, thyroglossal duct cyst, dermoid, laryngocele; normal: hyoid bone, thyroid
Sternomastoid (anterior)	Lymphadenitis, branchial cleft cyst (2nd, 3rd), pilomatrixoma, rare tumors
Spinal Accessory	Lymphadenitis, lymphoma, metastasis (from nasopharynx)
Paratracheal	Thyroid, parathyroid, esophageal diverticular
Supraclavicular	Lymphadenitis, cystic hygroma, lipoma, lymphoma, metastasis; normal: fat pad, pneumatocele of upper lobe of lung
Suprasternal	Thyroid, lipoma, dermoid, thymus, mediastinal mass

In addition, any trauma to the cervical spine requires stabilization of the cervical spine and evaluation.

- Is the swelling due to lymphadenitis or lymphadenopathy?
  —This question will help elucidate whether there are signs of active infection (i.e., lymphadenitis) as opposed to enlargement without infection (i.e., lymphadenopathy). Signs of lymphadenitis include swelling, redness, warmth, and tenderness. Signs of lymphadenopathy may include swelling and no or mild tenderness, but the absence of significant overlying erythema, warmth, or tenderness.

- Is the swelling acute, subacute, or chronic?
  —This question provides insight into possible causes of the neck swelling. Bacterial infections are usually acute and progressive. Other infections are more subacute, including Epstein-Barr virus (EBV) infection, cat-scratch disease, or tuberculosis. Congenital defects may be more chronic, with perhaps an acute superinfection that brings them to medical attention. A tumor may progressively increase in size over a variable time course depending on its histologic characteristic.

SUGGESTED READINGS

1. Pruden CM, McAneney CM. Neck mass. In: Fleisher GR, Ludwig S, Bachur RG, Gorelick MH, Ruddy RM, Shaw KN, eds. *Textbook of Pediatric Emergency Medicine.* 6th ed. Philadelphia: Lippincott Williams & Wilkins; 2010:385-391.
2. Friedman AM. Evaluation and management of lymphadenopathy in children. *Pediatr Rev.* 2008;29:53-59.
3. Leung AK, Davies HD. Cervical lymphadenitis: etiology, diagnosis and management. *Curr Inf Dis Rep.* 2009;11:183-189.
4. Nield LS, Kamat D. Lymphadenopathy in children: when and how to evaluate. *Clin Pediatr.* 2004;43:25-33.
5. Kandom N, Lee EY: Neck masses in children: current imaging guidelines and imaging findings. *Semin Roentgenol.* 2012;47:7-20.

CASE 13-1

Six-Year-Old Girl

STEPHEN LUDWIG

BRANDON C. KU

HISTORY OF PRESENT ILLNESS

The patient is a 6-year-old girl who was well until 2 weeks ago when she began to complain of tenderness on the right side of her neck. This continued for 1 week, after which the parents noticed swelling on the right side of her neck. The swelling and tenderness increased and the patient developed decreased range of neck motion. There was no dysphagia and no upper respiratory infection symptoms. The patient did not have antecedent trauma. She frequently played with the neighbor's cat but had no known exposure to other animals such as rabbits. A tuberculin skin test, performed 1 week ago, was negative; an anergy panel had not been placed.

MEDICAL HISTORY

The patient had chicken pox 1 month ago. There are no known allergies. She did not receive any prescribed medications. There had been no recent travel.

PHYSICAL EXAMINATION

T 37.8°C; HR 96 bpm; RR 20; BP 106/69 mmHg; Weight 23 kg (75%-90%); Height 44.5 cm (25%-50%)

On general examination, the patient was alert and in no acute distress. She was normocephalic; optic discs were sharp; pupils were equal, round and reactive to light; extraocular muscles were intact; tympanic membranes were gray bilaterally, mobile; nose was without discharge; mouth was without lesions, but mucous membranes were notable for pallor, few petechiae of posterior pharynx. Neck on left side was supple with no prominent adenopathy. There was erythema and swelling that was midline and more prominent just to the left of the midline (Figure 13-1) that was tender to palpation and moved with swallowing.

There was no movement with tongue thrust and the mass had well-defined borders. The following were also noted. Lungs: clear lung fields with decreased breath sounds at bases but no rales. Cardiac: regular rate and rhythm; II/IV systolic murmur, no gallop, no rub. Abdomen: soft, nontender, nondistended; positive bowel sounds × 4; no hepatosplenomegaly. Nodes: no prominent adenopathy. Skin: no rash. Neurologic examination: CN II-XII intact; motor 5/5 throughout; DTR 2+ bilateral on upper extremities and lower extremities; proprioception intact.

DIAGNOSTIC STUDIES

WBC count, 9100/mm³ (56% segmented neutrophils, 34% lymphocytes, 5% eosinophils, 5% monocytes);

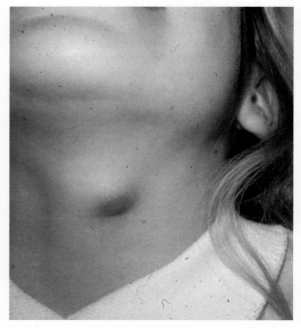

FIGURE 13-1. Neck mass in the patient (Case 13-1).

hemoglobin, 11.2 mg/dL; platelets, 565000/mm³; ESR, 45 mm/h; PT/PTT, 11.6/24.6 seconds; *Bartonella henselae* antibody titers, 1:32; T3, 1.6; TSH, 4.3.

COURSE OF ILLNESS

The patient had evidence of an acute infection. There was tenderness, swelling, and limitation of range of motion. Because of the acute nature of this illness, the size of the mass (>3 cm), and the progression of neck swelling, hospitalization was indicated.

DISCUSSION CASE 13-1

DIFFERENTIAL DIAGNOSIS

The differential diagnosis in this case included an infected thyroglossal duct cyst. Lymphadenitis was possible, although the location was unusual. Bacteria that typically cause cervical lymphadenitis include *Staphylococcus aureus*, group A beta-hemolytic *Streptococcus*, *Bartonella henselae*, actinomycosis, and oral anaerobes. Cat-scratch lymphadenitis was less likely. The indirect fluorescent antibody (IFA) test has high sensitivity (>95%) and specificity (>98%) for the diagnosis of cat-scratch disease for patients who meet the classic case definition of CSD. Enzyme immunoassay (EIA) testing for IgM and IgG antibodies to *B. henselae* is also commercially available. A high antibody titer (>1:64) is suggestive of recent infection. However, 2%-6% of asymptomatic cat owners have a low-level positive antibody titer (~1:16 or 1:32). In such cases, paired serologic studies (antibody studies repeated 2 weeks later and performed at the same time as a sample of the serum from the initial test) to detect an increase in the antibody titer may be helpful to confirm the disease; those without any change in the antibody titer when repeated 2 weeks later are unlikely to have an acute infection with *B. henselae*. The low-level positive in this case was thought to be unrelated to the child's symptoms.

In the location of this neck swelling, one must also consider thyroid-related masses such as tumors arising from the thyroid or aberrant thyroid gland. Thyroid function studies were normal. The CT scan showed a mass that was larger than clinically appreciated. There was also minimal tracheal deviation that was suggestive of a thyroid nodule. Thus, it was determined that a tissue diagnosis was required without delay.

DIAGNOSIS

A neck CT scan revealed a 4 × 5 cm solid neck mass with minimal tracheal deviation. Biopsy of the mass did not reveal lymph node or thyroid tissues; fibrotic changes along with numerous neutrophils, lymphocytes, and monocytes were consistent with an inflammatory process. Bacterial cultures from the mass obtained during a needle biopsy were positive for *Eikenella corrodens*; smears for acid-fast bacilli (AFB) were negative. **The diagnosis was that of a thyroglossal duct cyst that was infected with** *Eikenella corrodens*.

INCIDENCE AND EPIDEMIOLOGY OF THYROGLOSSAL DUCT CYST

Thyroglossal duct cysts are congenital remnants that occur when one thyroid migrates from the base of the tongue to its position in the neck. It occurs anywhere from the base of the tongue through the hyoid bone to just above the thyroid cartilage. Although asymptomatic while dormant, they may become symptomatic when infected.

CLINICAL PRESENTATION

Thyroglossal duct cysts may be evident at birth or may be dormant for many years until they become infected producing redness, swelling, and pain. The mass of a thyroglossal duct cyst may enlarge to the point of respiratory compromise. *Eikenella corrodens* is a slow growing organism that has been reported to cause a variety of clinical infections from infected neck masses to brain abscesses, lung infection, bite wound infection, and bone and joint space infections.

DIAGNOSTIC APPROACH

The diagnosis is suspected clinically by position and movement with swallowing or protrusion of the tongue. Ultrasound is the preferred imaging modality though CT scan may further delineate the size and location of the mass. The possibility of an aberrant thyroid must be ruled out. A diagnostic clue to the thyroglossal duct cyst is that it moves when the patient is asked to swallow. The cyst may contain elements of thyroid tissue; thus, if the cyst shows solid elements they should be identified with a nuclear scan prior to surgery, lest they be inadvertently removed. Thyroglossal duct cysts are the most common midline lesions.

Eikenella corrodens was isolated in this case. It is an unusual organism but one that should be considered if the patient has active periodontal disease or deteriorated oral health. It is also more common in individuals who are immunocompromised although that was not the circumstance in our patient. Excisional biopsy is the usual method to confirm the diagnosis; the excisional biopsy is typically performed after resolution of the acute superinfection.

TREATMENT

The ultimate treatment is surgical. Removal of the cyst and the other remnants of the migration tract are important. This is difficult and detailed surgery that involves surgery in the field of many other important vital structures. Prior to surgery, antibiotic therapy may be helpful in lessening

the inflammation and aiding in the postoperative healing process. Antibiotics to cover Gram-positive organism are customary. *Eikenella corrodens* is a usual Gram-negative organism that probably derives from active periodontal disease. Treatment may be effective with a wide range of antibiotics, however, usually the combination of antimicrobial therapy and surgical draining is required to effect complete recovery.

SUGGESTED READINGS

1. Paul K, Patel SS. *Eikenella corrodens* infections in children and adolescents: case reports and review of the literature. *Clin Infec Dis.* 2001;33:545-61.
2. Marra S, Hotaling AJ. Deep neck infections. *Am J Otolaryngol.* 1996;17:287-298.
3. Sheng WS, Hsueh PR, Hung CC, et al. Clinical features of patients with invasive *Eikenella corrodens* infections and microbiological characteristics of the causative isolates. *Euro J Clin Microbiol Infect Dis.* 2001;20:231-236.
4. Cheng AF, Man DW, French GL. Thyroid abscess caused by Eikenella corrodens. *J Infect.* 1988;16:181-185.
5. LaRiviere CA, Waldhausen JH. Congenital cervical cysts, sinuses and fistulae in pediatric surgery. *Surg Clin North Am.* 2012;92:583-597.
6. Goff CJ, Allred C, Glade RS. Current management of congenital cysts sinuses and fistulae. *Curr Opin Otolarygol Head Neck Surg.* 2012;20:533-539.

CASE 13-2

Two-Year-Old Girl

STEPHEN LUDWIG

BRANDON C. KU

HISTORY OF PRESENT ILLNESS

The patient is a 2-year-old Vietnamese girl who has been well until her mother noted a bump under her jaw a few days ago. She has not had any fever or upper respiratory tract symptoms (cough, rhinorrhea), or sore throat. She has been acting well. The bump does not hurt, is not red, but during the last 2-3 days it has increased in size from pea-sized to 4-5 cm, and it now looks purple. She had normal oral intake and urine output. There was no vomiting, diarrhea, or rash. The patient

sweats at night, but this is not new. There has been no weight loss or change in appetite. Sleep pattern is normal. There was no history of animal bites. There was no dyspnea or wheezing.

MEDICAL HISTORY

The girl was born at term by spontaneous vaginal delivery without complications. She had pyelonephritis twice, once at 14 months of age and again at 16 months of age. A voiding cystourethrogram performed after the second episode of pyelonephritis revealed grade 3 vesicoureteral reflux. She did not have frequent upper respiratory infections, otitis media, or pneumonia. She has not had any skin or soft tissues infections. Her only medication was trimethoprim-sulfamethoxazole which she received as prophylaxis against urinary tract infections. She has received her routinely recommended immunizations, including measles, mumps, rubella, and varicella vaccination at 15 months of age. She has no known allergies. There is no family history of recurrent infections, immune dysfunction or autoimmune disease. The patient lives with parents in a semi-rural area of New York state. Her maternal grandmother assists with childcare. No family members or recent visitors have been incarcerated or live or work in nursing homes or other chronic care facilities. The family does not have any pets. The only animal with whom the child interacts is an older cat owned by a maternal aunt who lives nearby.

PHYSICAL EXAMINATION

T 36.0°C axillary; HR 108; RR 22; BP 121/60; Weight 12.8 kg (30th percentile); Height 91 cm (30th percentile); Head Circumference 48.1 cm (25th percentile)

On general examination, the patient was alert, well nourished, and well developed. She cooperated with the examination in a manner appropriate for her age. She had a 3 × 2 cm firm nodule with purplish hue of overlying skin at the angle of the right mandible (Figure 13-2). It was not tender. There was no overlying warmth or discharge. There were no cardiac murmurs or rubs. The lungs were clear to auscultation bilaterally. With the exception of the neck, there were no masses or enlarged lymph nodes elsewhere.

DIAGNOSTIC STUDIES

Hemoglobin, 13 g/dL; platelets, 210 000/mm³; WBC count, 6400/mm³ (45 segmented neutrophils, 46 lymphocytes, 8 monocytes); sodium, 139 mEq/L; chloride, 100 mEq/L; blood urea nitrogen, 17 mg/dL; glucose, 84 mg/dL; PT, 12.8; PTT, 31.9 seconds; phosphorous, 4.5 mg/dL; calcium, 8.2 mg/dL; magnesium, 1.6 mg/dL; cat-scratch titers, <1:32.

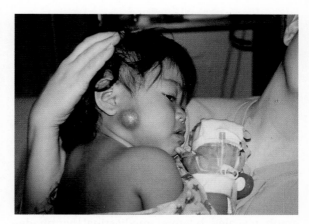

FIGURE 13-2. Neck mass in the patient (Case 13-2).

COURSE OF ILLNESS

The primary pediatrician initiated treatment with oral amoxicillin-clavulanate with an increase in the size of the mass over 2 weeks. Therefore, the antibiotic regimen was changed to clindamycin without any substantive change in the lymph node after 1 week. Tuberculin skin testing by purified protein derivative resulted in a 10-mm area of induration. A chest X-ray (Figure 13-3) revealed

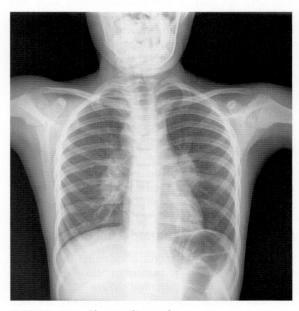

FIGURE 13-3. Chest radiograph.

additional findings that prompted an excisional biopsy of the lymph node and bronchoscopy.

DISCUSSION CASE 13-2

DIFFERENTIAL DIAGNOSIS

The patient was characterized by having an increased neck mass. The mass in this case did not hurt. This differential is from an acute adenoiditis with a usual bacterial organism. The location of the mass was over the mandible in a position typical for a lymph node. The patient was treated with antibiotics without response. The chest radiograph revealed bilateral mediastinal lymphadenopathy (Figure 13-3). A chest CT confirmed hilar lymphadenopathy but did not identify any focal lung abnormalities. She was admitted for excisional biopsy of the lymph nodes of the neck and bronchoscopy.

Lymph node pathology revealed necrotizing granulomas consistent with atypical mycobacterial infection. In addition, there were two other findings of importance, a positive PPD and positive chest radiograph. These findings required that a tissue diagnosis be made and so the patient was sent for biopsy and bronchoscopy after less invasive diagnostic studies failed to reveal an etiology. The pathology showed a pattern consistent with atypical mycobacterial infection. This was also consistent with the child's course of an acute enlargement of a lymph node but not the signs of an acute bacterial infection. There was no history of trauma. The location of the mass was not usual for a congenital lesion.

DIAGNOSIS

Nontuberculous mycobacterial infection causing adenitis in neck and mediastinum. There was no underlying immunodeficiency found in this patient.

INCIDENCE AND EPIDEMIOLOGY OF ADENITIS

Most cases of mycobacterial adenitis in children are usually caused by nontuberculosis mycobacteria rather than *Mycobacterium tuberculosis*. Nontuberculous mycobacteria typically include *M. abscessus, M. chelonae, M. fortuitum, M. avium* complex, and *M. kansasii*. They are typically found in soil and water, including natural and treated water sources.

CLINICAL MANIFESTATIONS

Cervical or submandibular adenitis most commonly occurs in otherwise healthy children 1-5 years of age. The likely mechanism is ingestion of contaminated sources such as soil. *Mycobacterium avium* complex is identified most often. The presentation is protracted lymphadenopathy; the affected lymph nodes are usually unilateral and nontender. In the absence of effective therapy, the affected lymph nodes may resolve or progression to liquefaction with violaceous discoloration of the overlying skin, followed by spontaneous and prolonged drainage from a cutaneous fistula. Nontuberculous mycobacteria may also involve other lymph node groups, including the mediastinal lymph nodes as in this case. In the chest, the findings are relatively silent and relate primarily to enlargement of paratracheal lymph nodes.

DIAGNOSTIC APPROACH

In this case, the diagnosis was strengthened by findings of enlarged mediastinal nodes and the notation of a positive PPD.

Tuberculin skin testing. Tuberculin skin tests (i.e., purified protein derivative) may be negative or positive. Many children have intermediate induration (5-10 mm) though up to one-third of affected children may have induration more than 10 mm. In this case, although there was strong suspicion for nontuberculous mycobacteria, there was the need to confirm the diagnosis with biopsy or bronchoscopy findings.

Biopsy. As much material as possible is required; swabs typically have poor yield. The specimens should be placed in both broth and solid media. Cultures in broth media have a higher yield and tend to produce more rapid results than specimens plated on solid media; solid media, however, permit observation of colony morphology and recognition of multiple mycobacterial species. Excisional biopsy is often performed for simultaneous diagnosis and treatment.

TREATMENT

The treatment in cases of atypical mycobacteria is lymph node excision. Many nodes may regress on their own if untreated. However, the need to establish a diagnosis usually prompts excision. If excision is not possible because of location (e.g., facial nerve injury may occur with excision of preauricular lymph nodes), antimicrobial therapy may be beneficial. Treatment depends on the nontuberculous mycobacteria isolated. Treatment typically involves at least two effective drugs. Empiric therapy, while awaiting culture and susceptibility results, often includes clarithromycin in combination with rifabutin, rifampin, ciprofloxacin, or ethambutol. A randomized trial compared a "wait-and-see" approach with 12-weeks of clarithromycin plus rifabutin; eligible patients all had red, fluctuant lymphadenitis. The median time to resolution of disease (defined as a 75% or greater reduction in lymph node size with cured fistula and total skin closure without recurrence) was 36 weeks for the treated group and 40 weeks for the "wait-and-see" group.

SUGGESTED READINGS

1. Altman RP, Margileth AM. Cervical lymphadenopathy from atypical mycobacteria: diagnosis and surgical treatment. *J Pediatr Surg.* 1975;10:419-422.

2. Dhooge I, Dhooge C, DeBaets F, et al. Diagnostic and therapeutic management of atypical mycobacterial infections in children. *Euro Arch Oto-Rhin-Laryngol.* 1993;250:387-391.

3. Benson-Mitchell R, Buchanan G. Cervical lymphadenopathy secondary to atypical mycobacterial in children. *J Laryngol Otolo.* 1996;110:48-51.

4. Danielides V, Patrikakos G, Moerman M, et al. Diagnosis, management and surgical treatment of nontuberculous mycobacterial head and neck infection in children. *J Oto-Rhino-Laryngol.* 2002;64:284-289.

5. Scott CA, Atkinson SH, Sodha A, et al. Management of lymphadenitis due to non-tuberculous mycobacterial infection in children. *Pediatr Surg Int.* 2012;28:461-466.

6. Tortoli E. Clinical manifestations of nontuberculous mycobacteria infections. *Clin Microbiol Infect.* 2009;15:906-910.

7. Clark JE. Nontuberculous lymphadenopathy in children: using evidence to plan optimal management. *Adv Exp Med Biol.* 2011;719:117-121.

8. Griffith DE, Aksamit T, Brown-Elliott BA, et al. An official ATS/IDSA statement: diagnosis, treatment, and prevention of nontuberculous mycobacterial disease. *Am J Resp Crit Care Med.* 2007;175:367-416.

9. Hazra R, Robson CD, Perez-Atayde AR, Husson RN. Lymphadenitis due to nontuberculous mycobacteria in children: presentation and response to therapy. *Clin Infect Dis.* 1999;28:123-129.

10. Lindeboom JA. Conservative wait-and-see therapy versus antibiotic treatment for nontuberculous mycobacterial cervicofacial lymphadenitis in children. *Clin Infect Dis.* 2011;52:180-184.

CASE 13-3

Two-Month-Old Boy

PAUL L. ARONSON

HISTORY OF PRESENT ILLNESS

A 2-month-old male presented with a 3-day history of neck swelling and 1 day of neck redness. The parents did not notice any swelling prior to the past 3 days. He has had a fever at home for 1 day. His oral intake has been adequate. The patient had no emesis, diarrhea, respiratory symptoms, or rash elsewhere on the body. There was no cat or TB exposure.

MEDICAL HISTORY

The patient was born at term during an uncomplicated delivery. There have been no hospitalizations. The patient had not yet received any immunizations. There were no known allergies and the patient had not received any medications. Family history is notable for no significant illnesses. The mother and father had arrived from West Africa 6 months ago.

PHYSICAL EXAMINATION

T 38.5°C; HR 176 bpm; RR 44/min; BP 112/76 mmHg; SpO$_2$ 97% in room air; Weight 6.2 kg (75th-90th percentile); Length 60 cm (90th percentile); Head Circumference 41 cm (90th percentile)

The infant was not in any distress. The head was normocephalic and the anterior fontanelle was open and flat. The oropharynx was clear. A tender, mildly indurated erythematous mass arose in the superior portion of the neck at the angle of the jaw. There was no fluctuance. The lung and heart sounds were normal. There was no hepatomegaly, and no axillary or inguinal lymphadenopathy.

DIAGNOSTIC STUDIES

The complete blood count revealed the following: 15 300 WBCs/mm³ (9% band forms, 65% segmented neutrophils, and 26% lymphocytes); hemoglobin, 11.7 g/dL; platelets, 296 000/mm³. Serum electrolytes revealed the following: sodium, 135 mEq/L; potassium, 5.3 mEq/L; chloride, 103 mEq/L; bicarbonate, 24 mEq/L; blood urea nitrogen, 4 mg/dL; creatinine, 0.2 mg/dL; and glucose, 113 mg/dL. Cerebrospinal fluid examination revealed 1 WBC, no RBCs, and a glucose of 68 mg/dL. There were no bacteria on gram stain. Blood, cerebrospinal fluid, and urine cultures were obtained. CT scan of neck with intravenous contrast was obtained (Figure 13-4).

COURSE OF ILLNESS

The patient was admitted to receive broad-spectrum intravenous antibiotics. On day 2 of hospitalization there was significant drainage from the lesion on the neck. The patient underwent operative drainage of the mass on hospital day 3.

DISCUSSION CASE 13-3

DIFFERENTIAL DIAGNOSIS

The causes of neck masses in infants are summarized in Table 13-4. The early age of onset in this case indicated that the mass was likely congenital in origin. Congenital causes of neck masses include thyroglossal duct cyst, branchial cleft cyst, cystic

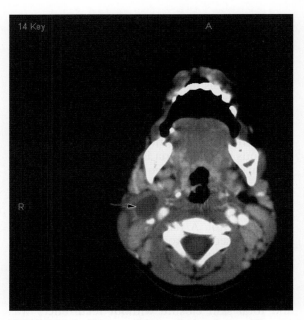

FIGURE 13-4. CT scan of the neck showing a well-circumscribed lesion with a nonenhancing area of hypoattenuation posterior to the angle of the mandible (arrow) on the right side.

TABLE 13-4.	Differential diagnosis of neck swelling in infants.
Mechanism	*Examples*
Congenital	Thyroglossal duct cyst Branchial cleft cyst Cystic hygroma Hemangioma Dermoid cyst
Infectious	Lymphadenitis Retropharyngeal abscess Superinfected congenital lesions Reactive lymphadenopathy due to viral infection
Oncologic	Lymphoma Leukemia Metastasis Other (teratoma, neuroblastoma, sarcoma)
Other	Neonatal torticollis Hematoma

hygroma, and hemangioma. An important distinguishing feature between branchial cleft cysts and thyroglossal duct cysts is the location in the neck; thyroglossal duct cysts are midline while branchial cleft cysts are lateral in the neck, usually at the anterior border of the sternocleidomastoid muscle near the angle of the mandible. The mass in this case was adjacent to the angle of the jaw, suggesting a branchial cleft cyst. In addition to the fever, the mass was warm, erythematous and increasing in size, indicating that an infection had complicated the anomaly (Figure 13-5). Other possible lateral lesions besides a branchial cleft cyst would include cystic hygroma or hemangioma. Cystic hygromas, or lymphangiomas, can be very large, and present similarly to this patient. However, they usually arise in the submental, submandibular, or supraclavicular areas and are usually nontender, although they can uncommonly be superinfected. Hemiangiomas are also often erythematous and can increase in size during early infancy, but do so more slowly. In addition, hemangiomas are vascular, nontender often raised lesions (Figure 13-6), and a hemangioma would not be expected to cause a fever. Neonatal torticollis can cause a firm, often calcified consistency lesion in the sternocleidomastoid muscle. However, redness and increasing size of the lesion do not occur; the infant's head will be tilted toward the mass with the chin pointed

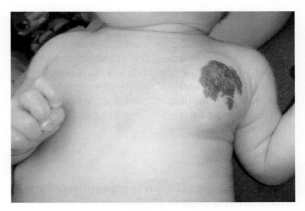

FIGURE 13-6. Hemangioma of the chest.

opposite, and neonatal torticollis usually presents in the first 3 weeks of life. A tumor is possible but less likely in this age range. Also, a tumor would not usually have the inflammatory signs that were evident in this child. Bacterial lymphadenitis can present similarly to an infected branchial cleft cyst, with fever, erythema, swelling, and often fluctuance (Figure 13-7).

DIAGNOSTIC TESTS

The fever in this 2-month-old boy necessitated a full sepsis workup to evaluate for serious bacterial illness, including blood, urine, and cerebrospinal fluid

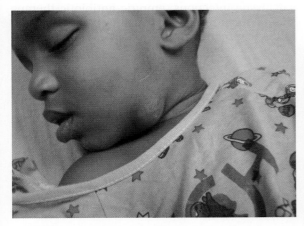

FIGURE 13-5. Superinfected branchial cleft cyst located on the anterior border of the sternocleidomastoid muscle.

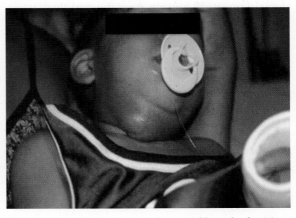

FIGURE 13-7. Acute bacterial cervical lymphadenitis.

cultures. For a neck mass, ultrasound is often the first line imaging modality to characterize the lesion. CT scan with intravenous contrast is obtained with concern for deeper infections of the neck, as in this case, or when ultrasound is unable to assess the full extent of the mass. For large neck masses without signs of infection, magnetic resonance imaging may be used due to the lack of ionizing radiation with this modality.

DIAGNOSIS

The diagnosis on CT scan is superinfected branchial cleft cyst (Figure 13-4).

INCIDENCE AND ETIOLOGY OF BRANCHIAL CLEFT CYST

Branchial cleft cysts are the most common congenital lesions presenting with neck infection. The branchial arches develop in utero, with clefts in between the arches. Branchial cleft cysts are remnants of the branchial arches and clefts that fail to involute during embryonic development, and can arise from any of the five arches. Second branchial cleft cysts, as this patient had, are the most common type of branchial arch anomaly, occurring in up to 95% of cases. These cysts usually present as masses at the anterior border of the sternocleidomastoid muscle or at the angle of the mandible. First branchial cleft cysts occur in the parotid or postauricular areas. Third branchial cleft cysts occur at the anterior border of the sternocleidomastoid muscle, near the middle to lower part of the neck, while fourth branchial cleft cysts occur in the lower neck area.

TYPICAL PRESENTATION

The most common presentation of a branchial cleft cyst is a painless mass in the lateral neck of a child, along the anteromedial border of the sternocleidomastoid muscle. Occasionally, a patient may present due to compressive symptoms such as respiratory or feeding difficulty from local mass effect. Presentation may occur when the previously undiagnosed cyst becomes secondarily infected, as in this case. Signs of infection include fever, redness, tenderness, and increasing swelling of the neck. Sinus tracts may also occur, with resultant purulent drainage from the mass. The clinical presentation depends on the location as noted above and state of infection of the cyst.

DIAGNOSTIC RATIONALE

Ultrasound is often the first imaging study obtained, although CT scan with intravenous contrast is often used and is recommended to assess for deep neck infection. Magnetic resonance imaging may be utilized for preoperative planning.

TREATMENT

Branchial cleft cysts are treated with surgical excision. Removing the entire cyst is often difficult and recurrences do occur if remnants are left in situ. Antibiotic treatment is used with bacterial superinfection to decrease the acute inflammatory response prior to surgery, often for 4-6 weeks prior to excision; antibiotics with activity against Gram-positive skin flora and oral anaerobes. Reasonable options include ampicillin-sulbactam, amoxicillin-clavulanate, and clindamycin. If the patient or a family member is known to be colonized with methicillin-resistant *Staphylococcus aureus* (MRSA) or to have recurrent skin and soft tissue infections, empiric antibiotic therapy should include agents usually effective against MRSA (e.g., clindamycin).

SUGGESTED READINGS

1. Pruden CM, McAneney CM. Neck mass. In: Fleisher GR, Ludwig S, Bachur RG, Gorelick MH, Ruddy RM, Shaw KN, eds. *Textbook of Pediatric Emergency Medicine.* 6th ed. Philadelphia: Lippincott Williams & Wilkins; 2010:385-391.
2. Nour YA, Hassan MH, Gaafar A, Eldaly A. Deep neck infections of congenital causes. *Otolaryngol Head Neck Surg.* 2011;144(3):365-371.
3. Rosa PA, Hirsch DL, Dierks EJ. Congenital neck masses. *Oral Maxillofac Surg Clin North Am.* 2008;20(3):339-352.

CASE 13-4

Two-Year-Old Boy

HEIDI C. WERNER

HISTORY OF PRESENT ILLNESS

A 2-year-old American-African male was brought to the emergency department by his mother for evaluation of swelling under his chin. His mother had noted the swelling 2 days prior and he complained of difficulty swallowing prior to coming to the emergency department. He had no history of fever, difficulty breathing, increased snoring, rash, night-sweats, or weight loss.

MEDICAL HISTORY

The patient was born at 32 weeks gestation with a birth weight of 1300 g and was hospitalized for 2-3 months. His perinatal course was complicated by episodes of central apnea which warranted a home apnea monitor until the age of 4 months. He had an inguinal hernia repaired prior to discharge from the hospital. The mother had been treated with rifampin due to a positive tuberculin skin test. Her chest radiograph was reportedly normal. The child had never received a tuberculin skin test.

PHYSICAL EXAMINATION

T 38.1°C; HR 113 bpm; RR 24/min; BP 103/73 mmHg; Weight 12.9 kg

In general, the child was alert and watchful in no acute distress. The tympanic membranes were normal in appearance and mobility. There was no nasal discharge. The neck was supple with a full range of motion. There was a 2 × 2 cm mobile lymph node in the right submandibular area. It was not erythematous or tender. There were also 2 × 4 cm mobile, nontender postcervical, and postauricular nodes. There was shotty axillary, anterior cervical and inguinal adenopathy. The chest was clear to auscultation. There were two small subcentimeter hyperpigmented macules on the upper back. There were no other skin lesions.

DIAGNOSTIC STUDIES

The WBC count was 7600/mm³ with 22% segmented neutrophils, 2% eosinophils, 66% lymphocytes, and 10% monocytes. The hemoglobin and platelet counts were normal. The total bilirubin was 0.4 mg/dL. AST and ALT were 40 U/L and 21 U/L, respectively. Erythrocyte sedimentation rate was 1 mm/h. Epstein-Barr virus titers revealed undetectable levels of viral capsid antigen (VCA) IgM, VCA IgG, and Epstein-Barr nuclear antigen antibody, consistent with no previous or current evidence of Epstein-Barr virus infection. A tuberculin skin test using purified protein derivative (PPD) and anergy panel were placed.

COURSE OF ILLNESS

The patient was discharged to home with a presumptive diagnosis of lymphadenitis caused by nontuberculous mycobacteria. He saw his pediatrician because of progressive cervical lymphadenopathy, which was now bilateral. His erythrocyte sedimentation rate increased to 67 mm/h. During the course of his evaluation, the patient had negative titers for toxoplasmosis, cat-scratch disease, and cytomegalovirus. A neck CT (Figure 13-8) prompted consideration of a diagnosis that was confirmed by lymph node biopsy.

DISCUSSION CASE 13-4

DIFFERENTIAL DIAGNOSIS

Lymph node enlargement, in the acute setting, has a broad differential diagnosis (Table 13-5) with infectious etiologies being the most common. With progressive and massive lymph node enlargement (Figure 13-8), lack of fever and negative infectious testing, oncologic diagnoses become more likely and biopsy is indicated. Rosai-Dorfman disease is a unique entity that is characterized by self-limited proliferation of the histiocytes.

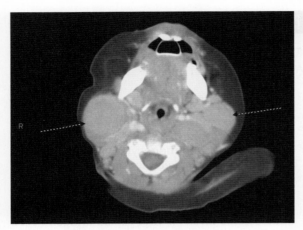

FIGURE 13-8. Neck CT reveals multiple markedly enlarged lymph nodes along the internal jugular chains bilaterally, most prominent at the bilateral jugulodigastric regions. The largest lymph node measures 3.1 cm by 2.6 cm on the right, 2.6 cm by 2.7 cm on the left. There are also prominent lymph nodes along the spinal accessory chains, supraclavicular regions, and superior mediastinum.

DIAGNOSIS

The progression of this child's neck mass and the elimination of the other causes of massive neck swelling prompted the biopsy of the lymph nodes. The lymph node biopsy revealed an infiltration of histiocytes filling the sinus of the lymph nodes as well as positive staining for S-100. **This finding in the context of the clinical presentation confirmed the diagnosis of sinus histiocytosis with massive lymph adenopathy (SHML) or Rosai-Dorfman disease.** This disease, first described in 1969, is thought to be caused by a massive over response of the immune system with production of histocytes in response to a viral trigger. The lymph nodes become greatly enlarged and then regresses spontaneously.

INCIDENCE AND EPIDEMIOLOGY OF ROSAI-DORFMAN DISEASE

The incidence of this condition is unknown and presumed to be rare. No single etiologic agent has been determined. There is a male predominance in both Caucasian and African American children.

TABLE 13-5.	Causes of peripheral lymphadenopathy in children.
Infectious (Bacterial)	
Group A beta-hemolytic *Streptococcus*	
Staphylococcus aureus	
Francisella tularensis (tularemia)	
Bartonella henselae (cat-scratch disease)	
Diphtheria	
Infectious (Viral)	
Epstein-Barr virus	
Herpes simplex virus	
Cytomegalovirus	
Mumps	
Measles	
Hepatitis viruses	
Human immunodeficiency virus	
Infectious (Other)	
Mycobacterium tuberculosis	
Nontuberculous mycobacteria	
Histoplasmosis	
Coccidioidomycosis	
Cryptococcosis	
Toxoplasmosis	
Secondary syphilis	
Borrelia burgdorferi (Lyme disease)	
Malignancy	
Lymphoma	
Leukemia	
Neuroblastoma	
Rhabdomyosarcoma	
Thyroid cancer	
Lymphoproliferative	
Rosai-Dorfman disease	
Hemophagocytic lymphohistiocytosis	
Autoimmune lymphoproliferative disease	
Immunologic	
Serum sickness	
Drug reaction (phenytoin, carbamazepine)	
Miscellaneous	
Sarcoidosis	
Kawasaki disease	
PFAPA	
Castleman disease	
Kikuchi disease[a]	
Churg-Strauss syndrome	
Systemic lupus erythematosus	
Rheumatoid arthritis	

[a]Also called Kikuchi-Fujimoto disease

Most cases have been described in children although there are reports across the age spectrum.

CLINICAL PRESENTATION

Clinical presentation is usually that of *painless* bilateral cervical adenopathy that continues to increase in size despite attempted therapies (87% of cases). Other nodal sites include the mediastinum, retroperitoneal, axillary, and inguinal areas. There are also reports of extra-nodal involvement in nasal cavity, salivary glands, sinuses, tonsils, trachea, eyes, and orbit. Leukocytosis, hypochromic, normocytic anemia, and elevated ESR are common laboratory findings.

DIAGNOSTIC APPROACH

Lymph node histology. The diagnosis is based on histologic findings on biopsy. Histiocytes with benign cytologic characteristics fill the sinus of the affected lymph nodes. The histiocytes contain normal appearing lymphocytes within their cytoplasm. This finding is termed lymphophagocytosis or emperipolesis. In contrast to typical histiocytes, the histiocytes in Rosai-Dorfman also strongly express S-100 protein, a family of proteins that regulate intracellular processes such as cell growth and motility, cell cycle regulation, transcription, and differentiation.

Radiologic studies. Lymphadenopathy in children with Rosai-Dorfman disease typically involves the cervical nodes. Lymph node enlargement is massive and bilateral; the enlarged lymph nodes are not tender. These enlarged lymph nodes can be easily visualized on CT, ultrasound, and MRI, though no specific imaging characteristics allow differentiation of lymphadenopathy in Rosai-Dorfman

disease from other disease processes causing lymph adenopathy.

TREATMENT

Treatment is primarily supportive and spontaneous resolute is frequently observed. Yet, lymphadenopathy may increase and lead to airway compromise necessitating artificial airway support. Surgery may be required for lymph node debulking when they compress the airway or vital organs. There are anecdotal reports of varying degrees of improvement with corticosteroids, methotrexate, or mercaptopurine.

SUGGESTED READINGS

1. Rosai J, Dorfman FR. Sinus histiocytosis with massive lymphadenopathy: a pseudolymphomatous benign disorder. *Cancer*. 1972;30:1174-1188.
2. Faucar E, Rosai J, Dorfman RF. Sinus histiocytosis with massive lymphadenopathy (Rosai-Dorfman disease): review of the entity. *Semin Diagn Pathol*. 1990;7:19-73.
3. Ünal ÖF, Köyba S, Kaya S. Sinus histiocytosis with massive lymphadenopathy (Rosai-Dorfman disease). *Internat J Pediatr Otorhinolaryn*. 1998;44:173-176.
4. Ahsan SF, Madgy DN, Poulik J. Otolaryngologic manifestations of Rosai-Dorfman disease. *Internat J Pediatr Otorhinolaryn*. 2001;59:221-227.
5. McGill TJI, Wu CL. Weekly clinicopathological exercises: case 19-2002: a 13-year-old girl with a mass in the left parotid gland and regional lymph nodes. *N Engl J Med*. 2002;346:1989-1996.

CASE 13-5

Two-and-a Half-Year-Old Boy

STEPHEN LUDWIG

BRANDON C. KU

HISTORY OF PRESENT ILLNESS

Patient is a 2.5-year-old white male who presented to the emergency department with a 4-day history of fever and 2 days prior awoke with his head twisted to the left and an estimated 3 cm swollen lymph node in the right cervical region. He was brought to his primary physician who prescribed

amoxicillin-clavulanate for suspected bacterial lymphadenitis. On the day prior to admission, his fevers continued. Two days prior to these symptoms he was at a friend's house where he was exposed to several cats, but there was no cat-scratch noted. During the past 2 days the parents noticed increased irritability, fevers, chills, and night sweats. The child also had decreased oral

intake during the past 3 days. There was no diarrhea or emesis. There was no joint swelling.

MEDICAL HISTORY

Patient was a full-term infant of spontaneous vaginal delivery with no complications. The medical
history is notable for beta-thalassemia minor diagnosed at 9 months of age on a screening complete
blood count. He had no prior hospital admissions.
There were no known allergies, and immunizations are up-to-date. The amoxicillin-clavulanate
was the patient's only medication. The family history is notable for beta-thalassemia in the mother,
juvenile polyps in the father, and systemic lupus
erythematosus in the paternal grandmother. The
boy lives with his parents and a healthy 5-month-
old sister.

PHYSICAL EXAMINATION

   T 40.0°C; HR 153 bpm; RR 26 min; BP 135/77;
   Weight 12.2 kg (10th percentile)

On general examination, the patient was irritable.
His tympanic membranes were mildly erythematous but had normal movement with insufflation. He
had mild bulbar and palpebral conjunctival injection. His lips were dry and cracked (Figure 13-9A).
His pharynx was erythematous but without exudate.
There was a 1.5 × 3 cm right cervical lymph node;
it was not tender. His lungs were clear to auscultation and there was no murmur. He had mild right
upper quadrant tenderness and his liver edge was
palpable 1.5 cm below the right costal margin. The
spleen was not palpable. His hands looked swollen
(Figure 13-9B).

DIAGNOSTIC STUDIES

WBCs, 14 900/mm³ (11 basophils, 75 segmented
neutrophils, 9 lymphocytes, 5 monocytes); hemoglobin, 8.8 g/dL—MCV 57.2; RDW 16.2; platelets,
410 000/mm³; ESR, 65; total bilirubin, 0.9; albumin, 3.4; AP, 282; ALT, 205; AST, 136; ALT, 205; GGT,
176; amylase, <30 lipase, 63.
   A chest radiograph revealed normal heart size.
There are no areas of consolidation.
   Viral PCR panel on nasopharyngeal aspirates:
negative for respiratory syncytial virus, adenovirus,

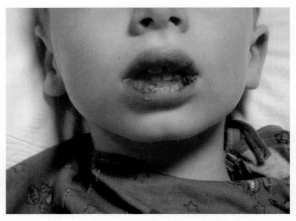

A

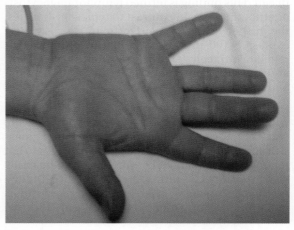

B

FIGURE 13-9. Photographs of the patient's: **A.** Lips.
B. Hands.

influenza A/B, parainfluenza virus 1, 2, and 3, and
human metapneumovirus.
   Blood culture negative. Urinalysis, negative
nitrite, moderate leukocytes; 0-2 RBCs; 15-20 WBCs.

COURSE OF ILLNESS

During the next 1-2 days he developed more
prominent conjunctival injection and an erythematous rask on his trunk and extremities; the rash
consisted of 0.5-2 cm nonconvalescent maculopapular lesions. No lesions were apparent on his
hands or feet. There were no oral lesions but one
examiner noted strawberry tongue.

DISCUSSION CASE 13-5

DIFFERENTIAL DIAGNOSIS

This child was evaluated for a number of causes of acute lymph node enlargement including group A beta-hemolytic *Streptococcus*, mononucleosis, cat-scratch disease, hepatitis, cytomegalovirus, adenovirus, and other infectious causes. All of those infections are in the differential diagnosis. The adenopathy was not progressive to a suppurative state but was more subacute in its course. Other considerations would be tuberculosis and atypical mycobacterium.

DIAGNOSIS

The boy's lips were red, dry, and cracked (Figure 13-9A). He had palmar erythema and his fingers were (Figure 13-9B) swollen and "sausage-like." **The final constellation of symptoms and clinical course best fit the diagnosis of Kawasaki disease.** The findings of decreased shortening fraction on echocardiograph also supported the diagnosis. The child was treated with intravenous immune globulin (IVIG) and aspirin. His fevers resolved within 16 hours of starting the IVIG infusion.

INCIDENCE AND EPIDEMIOLOGY OF KAWASAKI DISEASE

The peak incidence is in early childhood. The median age for Kawasaki disease is 2 years; more than 80% of children are under 4 years of age. It is extremely rare beyond 8 years of age. Children of Japanese and Korean descent are at highest risk, and even for children of Asian descent living in the United States. The incidence in Japan and Korea is 50-100/100000 in less than 5 year olds. In the United States, the incidence by ethnic background is 5/100000 in Asians, 1.5/100000 in African Americans, and less than 1/100000 in Europeans and Hispanics. Kawasaki disease is more prevalent in the winter and spring.

CLINICAL PRESENTATION

The criterion for the diagnosis is to identify the common clinical presentations. This includes fever higher than 38.2°C for more than 5 days, and four of the five clinical criteria: (1) nonpurulent conjunctivus, (2) polymorphous rash, (3) mucous membrane changes, particularly cracked red lips and strawberry tongue, (4) enlarged lymph node that measures greater than 1.5-2 cm (a single enlarged lymph node as opposed to multiple enlarged lymph nodes), and (5) extremity changes usually swelling of the hands and feet. Despite this set of clinical criteria there are many other potential manifestations including cardiac disease, vasculitis symptoms, aseptic meningitis, hydrops of the gall bladder, hepatic dysfunction, urethritis, uveitis, and arthritis/arthralgia. Young children with this disease are often extremely irritable, and the irritability and fever often abruptly resolve with treatment. Children less than 1 year of age often do not meet all the diagnostic criteria and are often considered to have "atypical" or "incomplete" Kawasaki disease. Many authors have described the clinical manifestations in terms of three phases: acute, subacute, and convalescent.

DIAGNOSTIC APPROACH

The diagnosis is not based on any single laboratory test but on a confluence of the clinical findings. Beyond documentation of the findings there may be suggestive laboratory evidence.

Complete blood count. The WBC count may be normal but more than 50% of affected children have a WBC count more than $15000/mm^3$. A normocytic anemia is often present. Thrombocytosis is virtually always present after the first week of fever.

Inflammatory markers. Most patients have an elevated erythrocyte sedimentation rate (ESR) and C-reactive protein (CRP). While these test abnormalities are nonspecific, a normal ESR or CRP makes the diagnosis of Kawasaki disease unlikely.

Hepatic function tests. The alanine aminotransferase and aspartate aminotransferase values are mildly elevated. There may also be elevations in the gamma glutamyl transferase and bilirubin. Approximately half the patients with Kawasaki disease have at least one abnormality in the tests of hepatic "function."

Lumbar puncture. A lumbar puncture is not routinely required but may be performed to diagnose or exclude bacterial meningitis in an irritable child. Among those undergoing lumbar puncture, cerebrospinal fluid white blood cell count is elevated in 25%-50%; the CSF pleocytosis is mild and lymphocytes predominate.

Urinalysis and urine culture. Urethritis leads to sterile pyuria from a clean catch sample; bladder catheterization may not reliably permit detection of pyuria attributable to urethritis.

Slit lamp examination. Uveitis is present in up to 85% of children with Kawasaki disease. While the absence of uveitis does not exclude the possibility of Kawasaki disease, the presence of uveitis makes other conditions in the differential diagnosis, particularly systemic juvenile idiopathic arthritis, unlikely.

Electrocardiogram (ECG). An ECG may demonstrate arrhythmia, ischemia, or low voltage.

Echocardiogram. An echocardiogram should never be performed to "rule out" Kawasaki disease as abnormalities typically develop after 10 or more days of symptoms. An echocardiogram is important to document the presence or absence of findings such as coronary artery ectasia or aneurysms, pericardial effusions, valvular abnormalities, and diminished ventricular function that may warrant additional treatment or monitoring.

TREATMENT

Initial treatment is IVIG, 2 g/kg infused over 12 h. Often aspirin is prescribed for its antiplatelet adherence effects. The role of corticosteroids remains controversial. A randomized, placebo-controlled trial found no difference in clinical outcomes between children treated with IVIG and 30 mg/kg methylprednisolone (administered as a single dose) and those treated with IVIG alone. Patients will also require supportive care depending on their symptom complex. Regular follow-up care with a pediatric cardiologist is indicated.

SUGGESTED READINGS

1. Shulman ST, Inocencio J, Hirsh R. Kawasaki's disease. *Pediatr Clin North Amer.* 1995;42:1205-1222.
2. Newburger JW, Takahashi M, Beiser AS, et al. A single intravenous infusion of gamma globulin as compared with four infusions in the treatment of acute Kawasaki syndrome. *N Engl J Med.* 1991;324:1633-1639.
3. Mori M, Imagawa T, Yasui K, et al. Predictors of coronary artery lesions after intravenous [gamma]-globulin treatment in Kawasaki disease. *J Pediatr.* 2000;137:177-180.
4. Shinohara T, Tanihira Y. A patient with Kawasaki disease showing severe tricuspid regurgitation and left ventricular dysfunction in the acute phase. *Pediatr Cardiol.* 2003;24:60-63.
5. Kanegaye JT, Van Cott E, Tremoulet AH, et al. Lymph node first presentation of Kawasaki disease compared with bacterial cervical adenitis and typical Kawasaki disease. *J Pediatr.* 2013 [epub ahead of print].
6. Dominquez SR, Anderson MS. Advances in the treatment of Kawasaki disease. *Curr Opin Pediatr.* 2013; 25:103-109.
7. Newburger JW, Sleeper LA, McCrindle BW, et al. and the Pediatric Heart Network Investigators. Randomized trial of pulsed corticosteroid therapy for primary treatment of Kawasaki disease. *N Engl J Med.* 2007;356: 663-675.

CASE 13-6

Sixteen-Year-Old Boy

PRATICHI K. GOENKA

HISTORY OF PRESENT ILLNESS

A 16-year-old male was transferred from a referral hospital for management of evolving respiratory failure. He was in his usual state of good health until 1 week prior to admission. He had been helping friends renovate a house and developed sore throat, swollen glands in his neck, malaise, occasional vomiting, and fever to 102°F. His mother noted changes in his voice that this time. He went to his primary physician who noted "kissing tonsils" and a pharyngeal exudate and diagnosed mononucleosis. He was started on oral prednisone and sent home with follow-up the next day. The next day, his voice was improved, and the regimen was continued.

He was seen in the emergency room at a community hospital 1 day prior to admission because of ongoing swelling of his glands and the development of chest pains and trouble sleeping (increased pain while lying down). A chest radiograph was initially reported as negative, but the family was called the next day because the reviewing radiologist felt that there was cardiomegaly. The patient returned to his primary physician and was referred for evaluation of chest pain, shortness of breath, orthopnea, fever, chills, and diaphoresis. In the emergency room, his respiratory rate was 40/minute and his SpO_2 = 83% in room air. He had scattered petechiae on his trunk, face, and extremities. Echocardiogram showed mildly enlarged heart, small pericardial effusion, no vegetations. Blood urine and pleural fluid cultures were sent, and he was started on levofloxacin, ceftriaxone, vancomycin, and doxycycline. The patient continued to deteriorate and required endotracheal intubation.

MEDICAL HISTORY

Immunizations were not up-to-date. He had not received his tetanus booster or the hepatitis B vaccine series. There were no pets in the home but the patient had exposure to friends' cats and dogs. There were no known tick exposures. The patient lived with his mother and three brothers. The only ill contact was his mother who had a sore throat.

PHYSICAL EXAMINATION

T 39°C; HR 110 bpm; RR 20/min (ventilator rate); BP 110/70 mmHg

On examination the patient was intubated and sedated. There were multiple 1-2 cm submandibular lymph nodes and generalized swelling of neck and face. There was no hepatosplenomegaly. The scrotum and extremities were very edematous. A foley catheter was in place. There were no splinter hemorrhages or subcutaneous nodules on the extremities. There were a few scattered petechiae on trunk.

DIAGNOSTIC STUDIES

The WBC count was 25 600/mm^3 (31% band forms, 50% segmented neutrophils, and 16% lymphocytes). The hemoglobin was normal but the platelet count was 33 000/mm^3. Serum electrolytes were consistent with mild acute renal failure. ALT and AST were 99 U/L and 81 U/L, respectively. There was mild PT and PTT prolongation.

COURSE OF ILLNESS

CT of the chest (Figure 13-10) suggested a likely cause, especially in the context of constellation of pharyngitis, neck pain, and clinical deterioration accompanied by face and neck swelling.

DISCUSSION CASE 13-6

DIFFERENTIAL DIAGNOSIS

This case was remarkable in that what started as a simple febrile illness with generalized adenopathy and neck swelling rapidly advanced to pneumonia, pneumothoracic pleural effusion, and respiratory failure. One of the initial questions in the evaluation of any neck mass should be "Is there evidence for airway compromise?" In this case, pursuing those questions and the rapid deterioration of the patient led to the appropriate diagnosis. In assessing the neck swelling it may be important to assess other sites in the pulmonary system including airways and lungs. At the beginning of the course, the differential diagnosis included streptococcal pharyngitis, mononucleosis, adenovirus, CMV, and other mono-like virus illness. As the process advanced and as a pulmonary component was identified, other organisms both viral and bacterial (aerobic and anaerobic) were considered. The presence of pleural fluid prompted its research to identify the organism. *Fusobacterium necrophorum* was eventually isolated.

DIAGNOSIS

The CT revealed a filling defect in the left internal jugular vein (Figures 13-10A and 13-10B). The filling defect is initially visualized in Figure 13-10A and completely visualized in Figure 13-10B. This finding was consistent with an internal jugular vein thrombus causing partial venous obstruction. There were

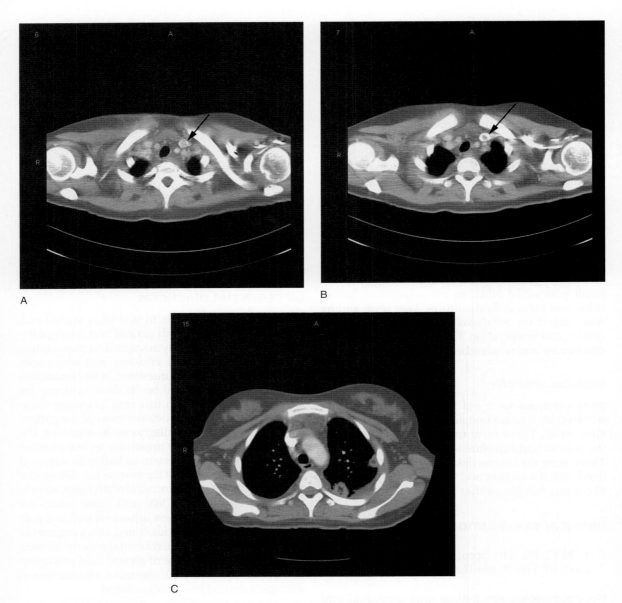

FIGURE 13-10. CT of the neck and chest showing: **A.** An initial filling defect in the left internal jugular vein (arrow). **B.** More complete filling defect of the left internal jugular vein (arrow). **C.** Pulmonary nodules with central cavitation.

also multiple, ill-defined peripheral, many with central cavitation and a small left pleural effusion (Figure 13-10C). The lung nodules were consistent with septic emboli. **The patient was diagnosed with Lemierre syndrome.** Isolation of a *Fusobacterium*

species from the pleural fluid further suggested the diagnosis of Lemierre syndrome or septic thrombophlebitis of the internal jugular vein.

Lemierre syndrome consists of acute tonsillo-pharyngeal adenopathy, neck pain, fever, and the development of supportive thrombophlebitis of the internal jugular vein. Neck swelling may be moderate to more severe and accompanied by severe neck pain. Patients may also develop septic pulmonary emboli as the patient in this case. The organism that typically causes this syndrome is *Fusobacterium*; an obligatory anaerobic Gram-negative bacillus that can be part of normal oral or gastrointestinal flora. Other reported causes of septic thrombophlebitis include *Staphylococcus aureus, Streptococcus pyogenes,* and *Streptococcus milleri* group bacteria (e.g., *Staphylococcus intermedius*). Other infections caused by *Fusobacterium* spp. include bacteremia, otitis media, mastoiditis, peritonsillar abscess, and less commonly, septic arthritis and meningitis. Neurologic manifestations of Lemierre syndrome occur as a consequence of intracranial infection or lateral sinus thrombosis complicating mastoiditis; this complication is related to the anatomical proximity and the thin bone that separates the mastoid from the lateral sinus.

INCIDENCE AND EPIDEMIOLOGY OF LEMIERRE SYNDROME

This is a rare condition that appears in only isolated case reports in the literature. The condition occurs in adolescents and young adults.

CLINICAL MANIFESTATIONS

The infection begins as a simple tonsillopharyngeal infection and then advances. Neck swelling and pain are localized to enlarge submandibular nodes at first and then become more generalized. The course often evolves to pulmonary involvement. Septic emboli may develop and be showered to other body sites causing symptoms in the central nervous system and elsewhere. The syndrome had been uniformly fatal. However, with early detection by CT scan and aggressive antibiotic therapy, good results have been reported.

DIAGNOSTIC APPROACH

When the specific origin of neck swelling cannot be determined a CT scan or MRI of the neck is indicated to determine the location and nature of the swelling. In Lemierre syndrome, the findings of suppurative thrombophlebitis are central to the diagnosis. CT or MRI images may demonstrate a filling defect in the involved vessel (as seen in Figures 13-10A and B) or inflammatory changes in and surrounding the vessel itself. CT scanning may also reveal septic emboli to the CNS, lungs, or elsewhere (Figure 13-10C demonstrates lung nodules consistent with pulmonary septic emboli). Recovery of the organism from abscess drainage or from pleural fluid will confirm the *Fusobacterium* isolate. A positive blood culture along with imaging findings consistent with thrombophlebitis cinches the diagnosis of Lemierre syndrome.

TREATMENT

Antibiotic treatment for Lemierre ultimately depends on the causative bacterium. Fusobacterim spp. are typically susceptible to penicillin, metronidazole, and clindamycin. Piperacillin-tazobactam or ampicillin-sulbactam is used when broader therapy is required empirically while awaiting identification of the organism. Surgical debridement of necrotic tissues and drainage of pleural empyema may be required. Children with ongoing development of pulmonary septic emboli may require placement of an inferior vena cava filter (e.g., Greenfield filter). The role of routine anticoagulation therapy in internal jugular venous thrombosis is controversial. Potential indications for anticoagulation include cerebral infarction or sinus venous thrombosis. Treatment may need to be prolonged over several weeks. There have not been any large case series or clinical trials to determine the best course of therapies. Mortality is relatively uncommon, occurring in fewer than 5% of affected patients.

SUGGESTED READINGS

1. Alvarez A, Schreiber JR. Lemierre's syndrome in adolescent children—anaerobic sepsis with internal jugular vein thrombophlebitis following pharyngitis. *Pediatr.* 1995;96:354-359.
2. Weesner CL, Cisek JE. Lemierre syndrome: the forgotten disease. *Ann Emerg Med.* 1993;22:256-258.
3. Moreno S, Garcia AJ, Pinilla B, et al. Lemierre's disease: postanginal bacteremia and pulmonary involvement caused by Fusobacterium necrophorum. *Rev Infec Dis.* 1989;11:319-324.

4. DeSena S, Rosenfeld DL, Santos S, et al. Jugular thrombophlebitis complicating bacterial pharyngitis (Lemierre's syndrome). *Pediatr Radiol.* 1996;26:141-144.
5. Sinave CP, Hardy GJ, Fardy PW. The Lemierre syndrome: suppurative thrombophlebitis of the internal jugular vein secondary to oropharyngeal infection. *Medicine (Baltimore).* 1989;68:85-94.
6. Megged O, Assous MB, Miskin H, Peleg U, Schlesinger Y. Neurologic manifestations of Fusobacterium infections in children. *Eur J Pediatr.* 2013;172:77-83.

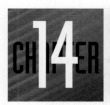

CH 14 ER CHEST PAIN

DEBRA BOYER

LIANNE KOPEL

DEFINITION OF THE COMPLAINT

Chest pain is a relatively common complaint in children with a frequency of 0.6% of pediatric emergency room visits. It occurs equally in boys and girls with a median age at presentation of 12 years. The most common causes of chest pain in children are generally benign but this complaint causes much anxiety among parents and patients due to concern for a cardiac etiology (Table 14-1).

In understanding the multiple causes for chest pain, one must consider the various innervation patterns that occur throughout the chest. Musculoskeletal pain is transmitted via intercostal nerves while the vagus nerve innervates the large bronchi and trachea. Pain fibers from the parietal pleura travel via intercostal nerves while the visceral pleura lacks pain fibers. Peripheral diaphragmatic disease is transmitted through intercostal fibers, and therefore can cause referred pain in the chest wall. This is in contrast to the central diaphragm, innervated by the phrenic nerve, which results in pain referred to the shoulder. The pericardium has multiple innervations including the phrenic, vagal, and recurrent laryngeal nerves, as well as the esophageal plexus. Thus, pericardial disease can present with diverse sensations and can be difficult to diagnose. Finally, cardiac pain itself transmits via the thoracic sympathetic chain and other cardiac nerves. Chest pain, therefore, is a very general term that can describe a variety of symptoms and etiologies. Only by a very careful history and physical examination can one accurately determine the cause of the patient's discomfort.

COMPLAINT BY CAUSE AND FREQUENCY

Causes of chest pain in children can be separated by age (Table 14-2) or etiology (Table 14-3). Chest pain is classified as idiopathic in 20%-61% of cases. In terms of organic etiology, 7%-69% of cases are determined to be musculoskeletal, 13%-24% of cases are respiratory (including asthma), less than 10% of cases are psychogenic and gastrointestinal in origin, and cardiac causes are found in 5% of cases or less. Children younger than 12 years of age are more likely to have a cardiac or respiratory etiology, whereas children older than 12 years of age will more often have psychogenic causes for their chest pain. In one study, most children presented with pain duration of less than 24 hours. However, children with a nonorganic cause are more likely to have pain lasting over 6 months.

CLARIFYING QUESTIONS

A complete history and physical examination will often reveal the diagnosis in a patient with chest pain. It is essential to have the patient describe the pain in detail: time of onset, duration, frequency, intensity, location, radiation, precipitating, and relieving factors. The patient's activity at the time of diagnosis can often provide valuable information. The following questions may provide clues to the diagnosis:

- Is the chest pain associated with exertion, syncope, or palpitations?
  —Chest pain associated with exertion, syncope, or palpitations is more concerning for

TABLE 14-1.	Common causes of chest pain in children.
Musculoskeletal	*Asthma*
Cough	Psychogenic
Pneumonia	Costochondritis
Idiopathic	Gastroesophageal reflux

cardiopulmonary disease and warrants further investigation. Chest pain with exertion may indicate exercise-induced asthma. Hypertrophic cardiomyopathy and aortic stenosis should always be considered in children presenting with chest pain on exertion. In children with anomalous coronary arteries, there may be insufficient coronary blood flow during exercise,

TABLE 14-2.	Causes of chest pain in childhood by age.				
Disease Prevalence	*School Age*	*Adolescent*	*Disease Prevalence*	*School Age*	*Adolescent*
Common	Idiopathic	Idiopathic	**Rare (Cont.)**	—Coronary artery disease (anomalous coronary artery, Kawasaki disease, long-standing diabetes mellitus)	—Coronary artery disease (anomalous coronary artery, Kawasaki disease, long-standing diabetes mellitus)
	Cough	Psychogenic			—Congenital heart disease
	Asthma	Cough		—Congenital heart disease	—Myocarditis
	Pneumonia	Asthma		—Myocarditis	—Pericarditis
	Musculoskeletal causes —Muscle strain —Trauma —Costochondritis	Musculoskeletal causes —Muscle strain —Trauma —Costochondritis		—Pericarditis —Arrhythmias	—Arrhythmias
		Pneumonia		Sickle cell disease	Sickle cell disease
Less Common	Gastroesophageal reflux	Trauma		Pulmonary embolism	Pulmonary embolism
	Pneumothorax	Cocaine/tobacco use		Esophageal foreign body	Esophageal foreign body
	Pneumomedias-tinum	Methamphetamine use		Pleurodynia (Coxsackievirus)	Pleurodynia (Coxsackievirus)
	Pleural effusion	Gastroesophageal reflux		Tietze syndrome	Tietze syndrome
		Pleural effusion		Slipping rib syndrome	Slipping rib syndrome
		Pneumothorax		Precordial catch syndrome	Precordial catch syndrome
		Pneumomediastinum		Peptic ulcer disease	Fitz-Hugh-Curtis syndrome
		Gynecomastia			Shingles
		Pubertal breast development			Chest wall tumors
		Fibrocystic breast disease			Cholecystitis
Rare	Cardiovascular —Structural (aortic/pulmonic stenosis, hypertrophic cardiomyopathy, mitral valve prolapse)	Cardiovascular —Structural (aortic/pulmonic stenosis, hypertrophic cardiomyopathy, mitral valve prolapse)			Pancreatitis
					Aortic aneurysm
					Peptic ulcer disease

TABLE 14-3. | **Causes of chest pain in childhood by etiology.**

Musculoskeletal/ Chest Wall	Muscle strain	**Cardiac**	Structural —Aortic/Pulmonic stenosis —Hypertrophic cardiomyopathy —Mitral valve prolapse
	Costochondritis		Coronary artery disease/myocardial infarction —Anomalous coronary artery —Kawasaki disease —Long-standing diabetes mellitus
	Cough		
	Tietze syndrome		
	Slipping rib syndrome		
	Precordial catch syndrome		
	Pleurodynia		Myocarditis
	Trauma		Pericarditis
	Herpes zoster		Arrhythmias —SVT —VT
Pulmonary	Asthma		
	Pneumothorax/pneumomediastinum	**Psychiatric**	Panic attack
	Pneumonia		Conversion reaction
	Pleural effusion	**Miscellaneous**	Sickle cell disease —Vasoocclusive crisis —Acute chest syndrome
	Pleuritis		
	Pulmonary embolism		
Gastrointestinal	Gastroesophageal reflux		Aortic aneurysm or dissection (Marfan syndrome/Ehlers-Danlos syndrome/Turner syndrome)
	Esophageal foreign body		
	Esophagitis —Eosinophilic esophagitis —Esophagitis secondary to bulimia —Pill esophagitis (e.g., iron, tetracyclines, NSAIDs)		Cocaine, tobacco, methamphetamine use
			Breast —Gynecomastia —Fibrocystic disease —Adolescent breast development —Infectious (mastitis)
	Esophageal Rupture (Boerhaave syndrome)		
	Peptic ulcer disease		
	Cholecystitis		
	Pancreatitis		
	Fitz-Hugh-Curtis syndrome		

causing symptoms to manifest at this time. In some cases, syncope may also occur. Palpitations may indicate an underlying arrhythmia such as supraventricular tachycardia or ventricular tachycardia.

- How is the pain characterized?
  —Pain that is worse on inspiration or coughing but is poorly localized may indicate pleural or pulmonary pathology, whereas similar pain that is well localized and elicited on palpation is usually related to a chest wall etiology. Cardiac pain

may be described as squeezing or pressure-like in quality, and may radiate to the left arm or neck. Midsternal pain may come from the esophagus, particularly if it worsens when supine. Kehr sign, or acute pain felt in the shoulder, may represent blood in the peritoneal cavity. Finally, psychogenic pain may be nonspecific in location and vague in quality.

- Is there a family history of sudden death?
  —Hypertrophic cardiomyopathy is inherited in an autosomal dominant fashion, so there may be

a family history of sudden death. These patients may have a murmur that is augmented with standing or a Valsalva maneuver. Furthermore, their chest pain may be most severe with exercise. In congenital hyperlipidemia, patients may present at a young age with myocardial infarction and have a family history of sudden death.

- Is the pain relieved with changes in position?
  —Patients with pericarditis often have stabbing precordial pain that worsens while lying down and improves with sitting and leaning forward. These patients are often febrile, have a friction rub that is best heard while the patient leans forward, and may also have distant heart sounds, jugular venous distension, and pulsus paradoxus.

- Is there a history of precipitating trauma?
  —In the trauma patient, tachycardia and hypotension may be secondary to a hemothorax or other vascular injury. In patients with poor perfusion and decreased cardiac output, one should consider myocardial contusion, tension pneumothorax, and cardiac tamponade.

- Is there a prior history of cardiorespiratory disease?
  —Patients with a history of asthma, cystic fibrosis, and connective tissue disorders have an increased risk of pneumothorax and pneumomediastinum.

- Can the pain be reproduced on physical examination?
  —Musculoskeletal pain generally can be elicited by palpation of the chest wall. Costochondritis, most commonly seen in teenage girls, is associated with palpable pain over the costal cartilage. Muscle strain, which may result from cough or new/vigorous physical activity, will generally have palpable pain over the affected muscle.

- Does the child have fever?
  —Fever is a nonspecific sign that may be present with pneumonia, pericarditis, myocarditis, endocarditis, or pleurodynia (most often caused by infection with coxsackievirus B).

- Is the child taking any medications?
  —Oral contraceptives increase the risk of pulmonary embolism. Steroids and nonsteroidal antiinflammatory medications increase the risk for gastritis. Iron, tetracyclines, and nonsteroidal antiinflammatory agents among others may cause pill esophagitis.

- Does the pain relate to meals?
  —Chest pain from gastroesophageal reflux commonly occurs after meals.

- Have there been any recent stressors in the patient's life?
  —Psychogenic chest pain may occur in patients with recent major stressful events in their lives. These patients often have multiple somatic complaints in addition to chest pain. A family history of depression or a somatization disorder increases the likelihood that a child will develop psychogenic pain.

- Does the pain wake the child from sleep?
  —Children who awake from sleep secondary to chest pain are more likely to have an organic etiology.

- Is there a history of substance use or abuse?
  —Tobacco use may be associated with a chronic cough and chest pain. Cocaine and methamphetamine abuse may lead to coronary artery vasospasm and ischemic chest pain.

SUGGESTED READINGS

1. Byer RL. Pain-chest. In: Fleisher GR, Ludwig S, eds. *Textbook of Pediatric Emergency Medicine*. 6th ed. Philadelphia: Wolters Kluwer Health/Lippincott Williams & Wilkins; 2010:434-442.
2. Thull-Freedman J. Evaluation of chest pain in the pediatric patient. *Med Clin North Am*. 2010;94(2):327-347.
3. Tunnessen WW. Chest pain. In: Tunnessen WW, Roberts KB, eds. *Signs and Symptoms in Pediatrics*. 3rd ed. Philadelphia: Lippincott Williams & Wilkins; 1999:361-369.
4. Kocis KC. Chest pain in pediatrics. *Pediatr Clin North Am*. 1999;46(2):189-203.
5. Lin CH, Lin WC, Ho YJ, Chang JS. Children with chest pain visiting the emergency department. *Pediatr Neonatol*. 2008;49(2):26-29.

CASE 14-1

Seventeen-Year-Old Boy

DEBRA BOYER

PHUONG VO

HISTORY OF PRESENT ILLNESS

The patient is a 17-year-old boy who was in good health until 3 days prior to his admission. At that time, he fell while playing basketball and noted some pain in his right thigh. He also complained of shortness of breath and chest discomfort when lying flat. He denied fever, rash, joint pains, and cough.

MEDICAL HISTORY

Bilateral inguinal hernia repairs were performed in infancy, but he has no history of other hospitalizations. He was not taking any medications. A paternal uncle required a renal transplant at 43 years of age for an unknown diagnosis. A maternal grandmother has systemic lupus erythematosus.

PHYSICAL EXAMINATION

T 37.2°C; HR 92 bpm; RR 20/min; BP 151/66 mmHg; SpO$_2$ 100% in room air

Weight 50th percentile; Height 75th percentile

Initial examination revealed a teenage boy who was awake and alert and in no respiratory distress. A rash was distributed across his nose and cheeks. The rash consisted of erythematous patches with keratotic scaling (Figure 14-1). His chest examination demonstrated decreased breath sounds at the right base. No wheezes or rales were noted. His cardiac examination was significant for slightly diminished heart sounds but no murmurs or rubs. His right thigh was swollen with a circumference 6 cm greater than the left thigh. He also had swelling of his right calf, which was 2 cm greater than the left calf. Flexion of the right knee was limited and there was mild calf pain with dorsiflexion of the right foot. The remainder of his physical examination was normal.

DIAGNOSTIC STUDIES

Laboratory analysis revealed a peripheral blood count with 6000 WBCs/mm^3 with 79% segmented neutrophils and 14% lymphocytes. Hemoglobin was 12.9 g/dL and the platelet count was 156000/mm^3. An erythrocyte sedimentation rate was elevated at 101 mm/h. Prothrombin and partial thromboplastin times were 13.6 and 31.9 seconds, respectively. Urinalysis revealed large blood and 3+ protein. A Doppler ultrasound of the right lower extremity revealed a thrombus extending from the superficial femoral vein to the calf vein.

COURSE OF ILLNESS

The patient was admitted and treated with intravenous heparin at 20 units/kg/h for his deep vein thrombosis (DVT) and with furosemide for his hypertension. A chest roentgenogram in conjunction with further laboratory work suggested an underlying condition that predisposed to this presentation (Figure 14-2).

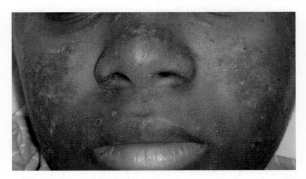

FIGURE 14-1. Rash on the face.

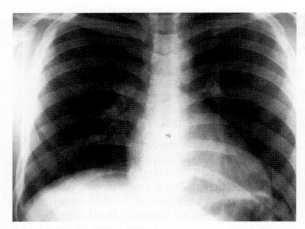

FIGURE 14-2. Chest radiograph.

DISCUSSION CASE 14-1

DIFFERENTIAL DIAGNOSIS

Chest pain in children and adolescents is rarely life-threatening. The majority of cases of chest pain in these age groups are classified as idiopathic. Among adolescents, the most common nonidiopathic etiologies include psychogenic, cough, asthma, pneumonia, and musculoskeletal pain. Less common etiologies include trauma, drug use or abuse, gastroesophageal reflux, and pneumothorax. Cardiac etiologies are exceedingly uncommon, but should be considered in certain clinical situations, such as patients with syncope and exertional or positional symptoms.

This patient has many physical and laboratory findings that warrant further evaluation. The two most worrisome findings include his chest pain when supine and his deep venous thrombosis. Shortness of breath and chest pain that worsens while lying supine suggests possible pericardial disease. The development of deep venous thrombosis in an otherwise healthy adolescent is extremely uncommon. In this situation one should suspect underlying hypercoagulable disorders. Finally, this DVT in conjunction with shortness of breath and chest pain suggest a pulmonary embolus as a possible diagnosis.

DIAGNOSIS

The chest roentgenogram revealed blunting of the right costophrenic angle, suggesting a small right pleural effusion, and cardiomegaly (Figure 14-1). An echocardiogram demonstrated a small-to-moderate-sized pericardial effusion that accounted for the finding of cardiomegaly on the chest radiograph. A ventilation-perfusion (VQ) scan suggested a low probability of pulmonary embolus.

As his hospitalization progressed, his hemoglobin dropped acutely to 10.3 g/dL and Coombs positive warm antibodies were demonstrated. A 24-hour urine collection demonstrated 8.5 g protein/day. Antinuclear antibody titer was elevated at 1:1280 and complement C3 and C4 were decreased. Autoantibody studies were positive including anti-Smith, anti-RNP, anti-SSA, anti-SSB, anti-SCL 70, and anti-JO 30. As part of his hypercoagulable work up, he was found to have anticardiolipin antibodies and antiphospholipid antibodies.

These laboratory values along with his clinical picture, including the rash, suggested the underlying diagnosis of systemic lupus erythematosus (SLE). He was treated with prednisone for his nephritis. After a period of time, his anticoagulation was changed to low-molecular weight heparin and he was discharged home on the tenth day of hospitalization.

INCIDENCE AND EPIDEMIOLOGY

SLE is a multisystemic autoimmune disorder that can present in children and adolescents. Determining the incidence of SLE in children is difficult with minimal data. However, national registries in Canada and Finland have suggested a mean annual incidence of 0.36/100 000 and 0.37/100 000, respectively. Studies in the United States have suggested an annual incidence of 0.53-0.60/100 000.

SLE rarely develops before the age of 5, and most commonly has its onset during adolescence. Girls are more commonly affected than boys with a ratio of approximately 5:1. There is a suggestion of a higher incidence in African-Americans followed by Hispanic children/adolescents.

CLINICAL PRESENTATION

SLE has a quite variable presentation, with children often having more severe presentations than adults. The most common presenting signs and symptoms overall include fever, arthralgias or arthritis, rashes, lymphadenopathy, hepatosplenomegaly, malaise, and weight loss. However, almost all organ systems have the potential for involvement.

Constitutional symptoms are common at diagnosis and with disease flares. Cutaneous findings may include the classic butterfly rash, discoid rash, or even mucosal ulcerations. Arthralgias and arthritis as well as aseptic necrosis of the femoral head may occur. Classic cardiac findings may include pericarditis, pericardial effusions, myocarditis, and Libman-Sacks endocarditis. Pulmonary manifestations occur in approximately 50% of patients. Both pleural and parenchymal involvement can occur with pleuritis and pneumonitis most often seen. Neurologic findings include seizures, psychosis, cerebrovascular accidents, peripheral neuropathies, and pseudotumor cerebri. Ocular findings includes papilledema and retinopathy. From a hematologic standpoint, patients with SLE are at a higher risk for the development of the antiphospholipid syndrome placing them at high risk of thromboembolic events. Finally, renal disease is also common with the development of glomerulonephritis, nephrotic syndrome and hypertension. These renal manifestations are probably the major prognostic factors in patients with SLE.

DIAGNOSTIC APPROACH

With such a variable presentation, attempts have been made to provide criteria for the diagnosis of SLE. The American College of Rheumatology updated the criteria for the diagnosis of SLE in 1997 (Table 14-4).

In general, patients with a minimum of 4 of the 11 criteria are diagnosed with SLE. The criteria can present serially or simultaneously and during any interval of observation. In childhood, this has a sensitivity of 96% and a specificity of 100%.

Acute-phase reactants. Most acute-phase reactants will be elevated in lupus exacerbations, including erythrocyte sedimentation rate, serum ferritin levels, and a hypergammaglobulinemia.

Hematologic studies. Approximately 50% of children with SLE will have anemia of chronic disease.

Other findings include an acute hemolytic anemia, leukopenia and thrombocytopenia. As mentioned previously, a high proportion of SLE patients will have a hypercoagulable state with the presence of antiphospholipid antibodies.

Autoantibodies. The majority of SLE patients will have detectable antinuclear antibodies. Those antinuclear antibodies that can be seen in SLE include anti-dsDNA, anti-DNP, anti-Ro (SS/A), anti-La (SS/B), anti-Sm and anti-histone antibodies. Various other autoantibodies include antierythrocyte, antilymphocytotoxic, antitissue specific, antiphospholipid antibodies as well as rheumatoid factors. In terms of diagnosis, antibodies against dsDNA are considered pathognomonic of SLE.

Complement levels. Decreased complement levels are particular indicators of active disease in SLE. One can measure either complement components C3 and C4 or total hemolytic complement, as measured by CH_{50} (ability of a test sample to hemolyze 50% of antibody coated erythrocytes).

Urinalysis. The most common abnormality on a urinalysis in SLE is proteinuria. Hematuria and RBC casts also occur. Further tests to evaluate for lupus nephritis include creatinine clearance, glomerular filtration rate studies, renal ultrasonography, and biopsy.

TREATMENT

There is no standard protocol to treat patients with SLE, as each child has a variable presentation. The primary goal is to prevent exacerbations, rather than treat each flare episodically. Certain recommendations are universal including the need to avoid exposure to excessive sunlight.

A variety of pharmacologic agents are available to treat symptoms of SLE. Nonsteroidal antiinflammatory agents are typically used for the treatment of musculoskeletal complaints. Patients with anticardiolipin antibodies often receive low-dose aspirin to decrease the risk of thromboembolisms. Hydroxychloroquine can be very effective in conjunction with glucocorticoids to minimize disease exacerbations. However, these agents may not always be effective in controlling the disease and other immunosuppressive agents

TABLE 14-4.	American College of Rheumatology diagnostic criteria for systemic lupus erythematosus.[4]
Criterion*	**Definition**
Malar Rash	Fixed erythema, flat or raised, over the malar eminences, often sparing the nasolabial folds
Discoid Rash	Erythematous raised patches with adherent keratotic scaling and follicular plugging. Older lesions may scar and appear atrophic
Photosensitivity	Skin rash as a result of unusual reaction to sunlight, by patient history or physician observation
Oral Ulcers	Oral or nasopharyngeal ulceration, usually painless, observed by a physician
Nonerosive Arthritis	Nonerosive arthritis involving ≥2 peripheral joints, characterized by tenderness, swelling, or effusion
Serositis	a) Pleuritis: History of pleuritic pain or rub heard by a physician or evidence of pleural effusion or b) Pericarditis: Documented by ECG or rub or evidence of pericardial effusion
Renal Disorder	a) Persistent proteinuria >0.5 g/d or >3+ if quantitation not performed or b) Cellular casts: May be red blood cell, hemoglobin, granular, tubular, or mixed
Neurologic Disorder	a) Seizures: In the absence of offending drugs or known metabolic derangements (e.g., uremia, ketoacidosis, electrolyte imbalance) or b) Psychosis: In the absence of offending drugs or known metabolic derangements (e.g., uremia, ketoacidosis, electrolyte imbalance)
Hematologic Disorder	a) Hemolytic anemia: With reticulocytosis or b) Leukopenia: <4000/mm³ total on ≥2 occasions or c) Lymphopenia: <1500/mm³ on ≥2 occasions or d) Thrombocytopenia: <100 000/mm³ in the absence of offending drugs
Immunologic Disorder	a) Anti-DNA: Antibody to native DNA in abnormal titer or b) Anti-Sm: Presence of antibody to Sm nuclear antigen or c) Positive finding of antiphospholipid antibodies based on (1) an abnormal serum level of IgG or IgM anticardiolipin antibodies, (2) a positive test result for lupus anticoagulant using a standard method, or (3) a false-positive serologic test for syphilis known to be positive for at least 6 months and confirmed by *Treponema pallidum* immobilization or fluorescent treponemal antibody absorption tests
Antinuclear Antibody	An abnormal titer of antinuclear antibody by immunofluorescence or an equivalent assay at any point in time and in the absence of drugs known to be associated with drug-induced lupus syndrome

*Diagnostic for systemic lupus erythematosus if four or more criteria are present

such as azathioprine, cyclophosphamide, and methotrexate may be needed.

SUGGESTED READINGS

1. Hiraki LT, Benseler SM, Tyrrell PN, Hebert D, Harvey E, Silverman ED. Clinical and laboratory characteristics and long-term outcomes of pediatric systemic lupus erythematosus: a longitudinal study. *J Pediatr.* 2008;152:550-556.
2. Lawrence EC. Systemic lupus erythematosus and the lung. In: Lahita RG, ed. *Systemic Lupus Erythematosus.* New York: Academic Press; 1987:691-708.
3. Petty RE, Cassidy JT. Systemic lupus erythematosus. In: Cassidy JT, Petty RE, eds. *Textbook of Pediatric Rheumatology.* 4th ed. Philadelphia: WB Saunders, 2001:396-438.
4. Tucker LB. Caring for the adolescent with systemic lupus erythematosus. *Adol Med: State of the Art Reviews.* 1998;9:59-67.
5. Tan EM, Cohen AS, Fries JF, Masi AT, McShane DJ, Rothfield NF, et al. The 1982 revised criteria for the classification of systemic lupus erythematosus. *Arthritis Rheum.* 1982;25:1271-1277.
6. Hochberg MC. Updating the American College of Rheumatology revised criteria for the classification of systemic lupus erythematosus [letter]. *Arthritis Rheum.* 1997;40:1725.

CASE 14-2

Fifteen-Year-Old Boy

PRATICHI K. GOENKA

HISTORY OF PRESENT ILLNESS

The patient, a 15-year-old boy, was well until 1 week ago. At that time, he developed the acute onset of chest pain accompanied by fever and chills. He described the pain as sharp and intermittent. It was mid-sternal and did not radiate. The pain did not increase with exertion, but was worse while lying supine or with subtle movement. He denied any syncope, shortness of breath, or diaphoresis. He did not have night sweats, cough, or weight loss.

MEDICAL HISTORY

The boy had no significant medical history. He emigrated from Liberia 6 weeks prior to his presentation. He had received bacille Calmette-Guerin immunization 5 years prior and was noted to have a 12 mm induration after tuberculin skin testing (purified protein derivative; PPD) on arrival in the United States.

PHYSICAL EXAMINATION

T 36.8°C; HR 80 bpm; RR 24/min; BP 111/64 mmHg

Weight 25th to 50th percentile

In general, he was a lean boy in no acute distress. His cardiac examination revealed a normal S1 and S2 with a regular rate and rhythm. No cardiac murmur was appreciated. His chest examination demonstrated clear breath sounds bilaterally. His liver edge was minimally palpated just below his right costal margin. The remainder of his physical examination was within normal limits.

DIAGNOSTIC STUDIES

The complete blood count revealed a WBC count of 6800 cells/mm³. The hemoglobin was 12.8 gm/dL and the platelet count was 426 000/mm³. Serum electrolytes, blood urea nitrogen, and creatinine were normal. Calcium, albumin, AST, alkaline phosphatase, total bilirubin and prothrombin and partial thromboplastin times were also normal. Lactate dehydrogenase was elevated at 904 U/L. A chest roentgenogram (Figure 14-3A) was initially interpreted as normal.

COURSE OF ILLNESS

The patient was then discharged home with ibuprofen for his chest pain. The chest roentgenogram (Figure 14-3A) was reviewed the following day and the interpretation revised. Computed tomography of the chest also revealed significant abnormalities (Figure 14-3B).

DISCUSSION CASE 14-2

DIFFERENTIAL DIAGNOSIS

Chest pain in an adolescent boy is rarely life-threatening. However, a careful history and physical examination must be undertaken to determine which cases require further investigations.

The majority of cases of chest pain in childhood are classified as idiopathic. Adolescents are more likely to have psychogenic causes for their chest pain than younger children, with this diagnosis being more common in girls. Musculoskeletal causes are quite common, including muscle strain, trauma, and costochondritis. Other common etiologies can include cough, asthma, and pneumonia. Less commonly, chest pain in adolescents is caused by gastroesophageal reflux, pneumothorax, pneumomediastinum, or pleural effusion. In an adolescent with chest pain, it is important to inquire about tobacco, cocaine, and methamphetamine use as these all can be associated with chest pain. In adolescent girls, one should consider pubertal breast development or fibrocystic breast disease, and in boys gynecomastia. Rarely, but importantly, one should consider cardiovascular causes of chest pain including structural diseases (e.g., idiopathic

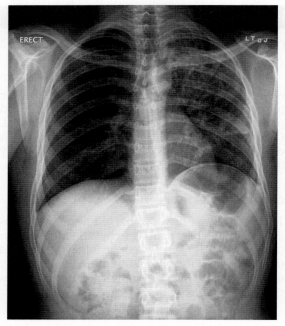

A

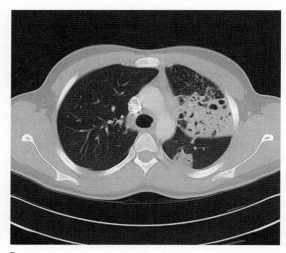

B

FIGURE 14-3. **A.** Chest radiograph. **B.** Chest CT.

hypertrophic cardiomyopathy), coronary artery disease, myocarditis, pericarditis, and arrhythmias.

The features of this case that warrant further evaluation include the acute onset of chest pain as well as variability with positional changes.

DIAGNOSIS

The chest roentgenogram revealed numerous small cystic spaces with increased interstitial and air space opacities in the left upper lobe (Figure 14-3A). The chest CT revealed dense consolidation in the left upper lobe containing cavitary lesions and air bronchograms (Figure 14-3B); an additional focus of consolidation is seen in the left lower lobe. An echocardiogram performed demonstrated a 10 mm circumferential pericardial effusion with nodular areas noted alongside the myocardial surface. Electrocardiogram revealed ST elevation. A repeat PPD demonstrated a 19 mm area of induration. The patient underwent pericardial window placement with pericardial biopsy. Stains of pericardial fluid were negative for acid-fast bacilli but microscopic examination of the pericardial tissue revealed numerous granulomas and acid-fast smear of the tissue demonstrated organisms. *Mycobacterium tuberculosis* was detected from culture of the pericardial tissue 12 days after inoculation. **The diagnosis is tuberculosis complicated by tuberculous pericarditis.** He was treated with isoniazid, rifampin, pyrazinamide, and ethambutol.

Sputum was acid-fast stain and acid-fast culture was negative. His family refused human immunodeficiency virus (HIV) testing. He was ultimately discharged home to complete his treatment under directly observed therapy.

INCIDENCE AND EPIDEMIOLOGY

Mycobacterium tuberculosis infections are the most frequent cause of death worldwide due to a single infectious organism. Approximately one-third of the world's population has been infected with *M. tuberculosis*. Generally, infection occurs through inhalation of droplet nuclei and cause pulmonary infections. The HIV epidemic has significantly increased the infection rate worldwide.

Pericarditis may be due to infectious or noninfectious causes (Table 14-5). Pericarditis, an uncommon complication of tuberculosis infection, can be fatal even with proper diagnosis and treatment. Tuberculous pericarditis occurs by extension of an adjacent focus of infection. This may include mediastinal or hilar nodes, lung,

TABLE 14-5.	Most common causes of pericarditis.
Infectious	
Bacteria	*Streptococcus pneumoniae*
	Staphylococcus aureus
	Neisseria meningitidis
	Haemophilus influenzae
	Mycobacterium tuberculosis
	Peptostreptococcus species
	Prevotella species
Viruses	Coxsackie viruses
	Echoviruses
	Adenovirus
	Influenza
	Epstein-Barr virus
Fungi	Histoplasma capsulatum
	Cryptococcus neoformans
	Candida albicans
Parasites	Toxoplasma gondii
	Entamoeba histolytica
Noninfectious	
Cardiac Injury	Acute myocardial infarction
	Blunt or penetrating trauma
	Irradiation
Malignancy	Primary
	Metastatic
Collagen Vascular Disease	Systemic lupus erythematosus
	Rheumatic fever
Drug-induced	Dantrolene, Doxorubicin, Isoniazid, Mesalamine, Phenytoin
Idiopathic	

spine, or sternum. It occurs less commonly in association with miliary tuberculosis.

Tuberculous pericarditis is believed to occur in 0.4%-4% of children with tuberculosis. The prevalence of tuberculosis varies among geographic regions. Certainly, its relationship to HIV disease is well known. In many African countries where tuberculosis and HIV are endemic, pericarditis in an HIV-positive patient is tuberculosis until proven otherwise.

CLINICAL PRESENTATION

The presentation of pericarditis varies depending on the cause. The pain associated with pericarditis is often retrosternal, radiating to the shoulder and neck. The pain is typically worsened by deep breathing, swallowing, and supine positioning. Tuberculosis pericarditis can have both acute and insidious presentations. The most common symptoms include cough, dyspnea, and chest pain, as described earlier. Other associated symptoms may include night sweats, orthopnea, weight loss, and edema. Physical examination may reveal fever, tachycardia, and pericardial rub. Pulsus paradoxus, hepatomegaly, pleural effusions, and muffled heart sounds are often associated with the condition.

DIAGNOSTIC APPROACH

The diagnosis of pericarditis is straightforward but establishing *M. tuberculosis* as the etiologic agent is more challenging.

Tuberculin skin test. A positive skin test increases the suspicion for tuberculosis pericarditis, but a negative skin test does not eliminate the diagnosis.

Chest imaging. Chest radiograph will generally reveal cardiomegaly due to pericarditis and pericardial effusions. Approximately 40% of patients with tuberculous pericarditis will have an associated pleural effusion. Patients with tuberculous pericarditis may also have findings suggestive of pulmonary or miliary tuberculosis.

Electrocardiogram. Electrocardiogram is abnormal in most cases of pericarditis, reflecting pericardial inflammation. ST-segment elevations develop early in the illness. Large pericardial effusions are associated with reduced QRS voltage. Other ECG findings include PR depression or electrical alternans if pericardial effusion is also present.

Echocardiogram. Echocardiogram detects associated pericardial effusions and pericardial thickening. Patients with tuberculous pericarditis may have nodular densities along the pericardium.

Pericardiocentesis and pericardial biopsy. Acid-fast stains of pericardial fluid are often negative, however, pericardial fluid cultures are positive for *M. tuberculosis* in approximately 50% of cases.

Polymerase chain reaction testing to detect *M. tuberculosis* has been attempted but the reliability of this test in pericardial fluid specimens is not clear. Granulomas detected on microscopic examination of pericardial tissue strongly suggest the diagnosis of tuberculous pericarditis. Pericardial tissue is usually acid-fast stain and culture positive and is considered critical to confirming the diagnosis. This will yield the most accurate results if the pericardial tissue is obtained prior to the start of antituberculous therapy.

HIV test. Due to the close association of HIV and tuberculous pericarditis, HIV testing should be performed in all patients diagnosed with tuberculous pericarditis.

TREATMENT

If the patient has hemodynamic compromise, pericardiocentesis is indicated. Certainly, in cases of tamponade this is necessary. A second option for drainage is an open surgical procedure, which allows for removal of the pericardial fluid as well as obtaining pericardial tissue for culture and histopathologic study. Controversy does exist as to whether in uncomplicated cases, pericardiocentesis versus open drainage should be the procedure of choice in suspected tuberculous pericarditis.

Either way, one must strive to prevent the formation of a constrictive pericarditis.

Antibiotic therapy consists of the same regimens as for pulmonary tuberculosis. Adjuvant corticosteroid therapy appears to decrease the amount of effusion and reaccumulation of pericardial fluid, reducing the need for repeated interventions. Long-term complications of tuberculous pericarditis include constrictive pericarditis.

SUGGESTED READINGS

1. Dooley DP, Carpenter JL, Rademacher S. Adjunctive corticosteroid therapy for tuberculosis: a critical reappraisal of the literature. *Clin Infect Dis.* 1997;25:872-877.
2. Gewitz MH, Vetter VL. Cardiac emergencies. In: Fleisher GR, Ludwig S, eds. *Textbook of Pediatric Emergency Medicine.* 4th ed. Baltimore, Maryland: Lippincott Williams &Wilkins; 2000:659-700.
3. Haas DW. *Mycobacterium tuberculosis.* In: Mandell GL, Bennett JE, Dolin R, eds. *Mandell, Douglas, and Bennett's Principles and Practice of Infectious Diseases.* 5th ed. Philadelphia: Churchill Livingstone; 2000:2576-2604.
4. Starke JR. Tuberculosis. In: McMillan JA, DeAngelis CD, Feigin RD, Warshaw JB, eds. *Oski's Pediatrics: Principles and Practice.* 3rd ed. Philadelphia: Lippincott Williams & Wilkins; 1999:1026-1039.
5. Trautner BW, Darouiche RO. Tuberculous pericarditis: optimal diagnosis and management. *Clin Infect Dis.* 2001;33:954-961.

CASE 14-3

Twenty-Year-Old Boy

DEBRA BOYER

ALICIA CASEY

HISTORY OF PRESENT ILLNESS

The patient is a 20-year-old boy with a history of spina bifida. Six days prior to admission he reported fatigue and was unable to leave his house. During the next few days, he developed a fever, sore throat, and myalgias. Two days prior to admission, he noted increasing shortness of breath which was worse while lying supine. He described a "pounding" discomfort in his chest.

MEDICAL HISTORY

The boy was born at full term and found to have a meningomyelocele at birth. His spinal defect was at L3 and he underwent surgical correction when he was 4 days old. A ventriculoperitoneal (VP) shunt was placed in the first weeks of life. He has required several shunt revisions due to obstruction. The last revision was 6 years ago. He also has a history of bilateral club feet. Four months prior to admission he was diagnosed with pelvic osteomyelitis related to extension of a gluteal ulcer. He was treated with surgical debridement and 3 months of intravenous antibiotics.

He is able to walk with a brace and has a mild intellectual disability. At the time of presentation, he was not taking any medication. He had a tattoo drawn on his arm 2 weeks prior. There is a family history of asthma in his mother, and his father died at age 40 of a myocardial infarction.

PHYSICAL EXAMINATION

T 41.3°C; HR 138 bpm; RR 20/min; BP 113/80 mmHg; Oxygen saturation, 98% in room air

In general, he was an obese young boy in moderate respiratory distress. His oropharyngeal examination revealed an exudative pharyngitis. His cardiac examination revealed a normal S1 and S2 without murmur, rub, or gallop. His physical examination was otherwise unremarkable.

DIAGNOSTIC STUDIES

The complete blood count revealed a WBC count of 13 500 cells/mm³ with 42% segmented neutrophils, 26% lymphocytes, 18% atypical lymphocytes, and 1% monocytes. The hemoglobin was 11.3 gm/dL, and his platelets were 133 000/mm³. Electrolytes, blood urea nitrogen, and glucose were within normal limits. A serum creatinine was slightly elevated at 1.1 mg/dL. Total bilirubin was elevated at 4.0 mg/dL with an unconjugated fraction of 2.3 mg/dL. Aspartate aminotransferase and alanine aminotransferase were 246 U/L and 130 U/L, respectively. Erythrocyte sedimentation rate was mildly elevated at 44 mm/h. A chest roentgenogram revealed normal heart size and no pulmonary infiltrates.

COURSE OF ILLNESS

Prior to his arrival at the hospital, the patient was administered adenosine twice for tachycardia with heart rate above 160 bpm. This did not have any significant effect. On arrival in the emergency department, his chest pain resolved and his electrocardiogram abnormalities resolved. An echocardiogram demonstrated a shortening fraction of 28% and no wall motion abnormalities.

The boy was evaluated for a possible myocardial infarction, given his family history. His cardiac enzymes remained normal. He developed bilious emesis believed to be secondary to his hepatitis. He had a repeat electrocardiogram (Figure 14-4) and echocardiogram on arrival in the intensive care unit. The electrocardiogram suggested a diagnostic category and the specific cause was suggested by the initial laboratory testing and confirmed later by serologic testing.

DISCUSSION CASE 14-3

DIFFERENTIAL DIAGNOSIS

The most common causes of chest pain in children and adolescents include musculoskeletal/chest wall pain, pulmonary causes, GI causes, and miscellaneous causes including psychogenic etiologies and hyperventilation. Chest pain due to cardiac conditions is rare, but warrants a high index of suspicion given the potential morbidity and mortality.

The concerning factors in this patient are his positional shortness of breath, his early family history of myocardial infarction, and his abnormal electrocardiogram. On presentation, he was tachycardic and febrile. Concern for a possible cardiac etiology should be raised in any child or adolescent with chest pain on exertion, palpitations, syncope, abnormal cardiac findings on examination or electrocardiogram, history of cardiac disorder, or with a family history of significant cardiac illness.

Cardiac etiologies for chest pain in the pediatric population include structural lesions causing left ventricular outflow tract obstruction, such as aortic stenosis, aortic dissection, rupture of aortic aneurysm, coronary artery abnormalities, pericarditis, myocarditis, cardiomyopathy, pulmonary hypertension, mitral valve prolapse, atrial myxomas, cardiac device complications, and drugs. A thorough history and physical examination will help to identify any findings concerning cardiac causes of chest pain. The complaint of chest pain may be the first indication that there is a cardiac issue in a pediatric patient. Patients with left ventricular outflow tract obstruction may have pain associated with dizziness and fatigue. Patients with hypertropic or dilated cardiomyopathy may present with chest pain, exercise intolerance, or

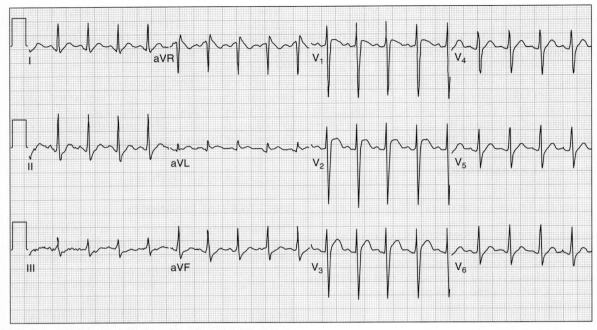

FIGURE 14-4. Electrocardiogram.

fatigue. Chest pain occurs in patients with coronary artery disease due to myocardial ischemia. Unfortunately, these disorders may present with sudden death. In children, coronary artery disease can be the result of congenital abnormalities of the coronary arteries, secondary to hypertrophic cardiomyopathy, a result of Kawasaki disease, due to postcardiac surgical complications, or secondary to familial hypercholesterolemia. Patients with either corrected or uncorrected congenital heart disease, or with a history of cardiac transplantation, may complain of chest pain. In this population, chest pain must be carefully evaluated. Arrhythmias, such as supraventricular tachycardia and ventricular tachycardia, can also present with chest pain and palpitations. Finally, inflammatory/infectious causes, such as myocarditis and pericarditis, may also present with chest pain, often with a history of recent infection.

DIAGNOSIS

Repeat electrocardiogram showed sinus tachycardia at 139 bpm with 2 mm ST segment elevations in leads V2 and V3 (Figure 14-4). Repeat echocardiogram revealed a left ventricular ejection fraction of 25% with dilated left and right ventricles. Cardiac catheterization demonstrated a left ventricle end-diastolic pressure of 16 mmHg and a cardiac index of 4.4 L/min. Soon after admission, he developed congestive heart failure with respiratory distress, diaphoresis, somnolence, and hypotension. He was ultimately treated with dopamine and dobutamine. To help determine the etiology of his myocarditis, Epstein-Barr virus (EBV) studies were sent. Monospot testing was positive. His course was also complicated by hepatitis, thrombocytopenia, and an atypical lymphocytosis. EBV viral capsid IgG (VCA) was 1:640; early antigen IgG (EA), 1:80; and Epstein-Barr nuclear antigen (ENBA) IgG, undetectable. **He was diagnosed with probable acute EBV myocarditis.**

INCIDENCE, EPIDEMIOLOGY, AND ETIOLOGY

EBV is a member of the herpes virus family and is also known as Human Herpes Virus 4. It is a relatively common infectious organism, causing a clinical syndrome of infectious mononucleosis. This syndrome is most frequently seen in adolescents and young adults. Boys and girls are affected equally, and approximately 90% of adults have evidence of past infection. There is no seasonal pattern to infections.

EBV believed to have low contagiousness and transmission generally requires close personal contact between individuals. This is why infectious mononucleosis has been termed "the kissing disease." The virus is viable in saliva outside of the body for several hours. Intermittent excretion of the virus in saliva may persist lifelong.

The classical clinical syndrome consists of fever, pharyngitis with petichiae and exudate, lymphadenopathy, atypical lymphocytosis, and fatigue developing after an incubation period of 30-50 days. Hepatosplenomegaly and rash are frequently observed with a morbilliform rash occurring more commonly in patients treated with antibiotics in the penicillin family. Most cases of EBV infection are self-limited, although rare complications can be seen. These complications can be multisystemic and include hematologic, hepatorenal, splenic, dermatologic, immunologic, central nervous system, and cardiopulmonary complications. Lymphomas can occur after EBV infection in immunocompetent persons, as well as those with defects of cellular immunity.

Myocarditis in EBV infection is a rare, but well-described complication of EBV infection. In children and adolescents, myocarditis is an uncommon illness that can be associated with significant morbidity and mortality. Viruses are thought to be the most common etiologic agents causing acute lymphocytic myocarditis in both children and adults. Common viruses causing myocarditis include adenovirus, enterovirus (including coxsackie B and rhinovirus), parvovirus, cytomegalovirus, EBV, human herpesvirus 6, influenza, human metapneumovirus, respiratory syncytial virus, and HIV. Several patients with viral infections who will go on to develop myocarditis is unknown. Less commonly, myocarditis can occur as a complication of other nonviral infectious agents, such as *Mycoplasma pneumoniae*, *Chlamydophila pneumonia*, *Borrelia burgdorferi*, *Lysteria monocytogenes*, *Clostridium perfringens*, Staphylococcus, Streptococcus, Meningococcus, Diptheria, and *Trypanosomacruzi*. Also rare are noninfectious etiologies, such as drugs, hypersensitivity reactions, autoimmune diseases, vaccinations, and cancer.

CLINICAL PRESENTATION

Acute myocarditis in children presents with a wide range of signs and symptoms and because of the variable presentation it is often misdiagnosed. Often there is a recent history of respiratory or gastrointestinal illness prior to presentation. Presentation may include chest pain, respiratory symptoms, fevers, gastrointestinal complaints, cardiogenic shock, and sudden death. Some pediatric patients may present with acute fulminant myocarditis and some may present without obvious cardiac-related symptoms. Myocarditis is often more fulminant in children in comparison to adults. Newborns and infants with myocarditis may present with a decreased appetite, fever, irritability, and diaphoresis. Older children may complain of chest pain, shortness of breath, positional dyspnea, fatigue, fever, pallor, diaphoresis, palpitations, rashes, and decreased exercise tolerance. Physical examination is often nonspecific and may include tachycardia and tachypnea. With the development of congestive heart failure there may be jugular venous distention, hepatomegaly, and rales on pulmonary examination. As the disease progresses, respiratory distress can become more prominent. Arrhythmias can develop including ventricular tachycardia and conduction delays.

DIAGNOSTIC APPROACH

Acute myocarditis is a difficult diagnosis to make and it is appropriate to have a high index of suspicion for this in the appropriate setting. If EBV is suspected as a possible cause of myocarditis, studies should be sent to confirm this diagnosis.

MYOCARDITIS DIAGNOSIS

Laboratory investigations. Measurement of cardiac enzymes and inflammatory markers are often obtained during the work up for myocarditis. Troponin levels are not elevated in all patients with myocarditis, but this is a sensitive marker of myocardial damage. Patients with myocarditis may have elevation of inflammatory mediators, but this is also nonspecific.

Electrocardiogram (ECG). Patients with myocarditis may develop nonspecific ECG changes including sinus tachycardia, low-voltage QRS complexes, T waves abnormalities, ST-segment changes, abnormal axis, heart block, ventricular hypertrophy, and atrial enlargement. Findings indicative myocardial infarction may be found.

Echocardiogram. When myocarditis is suspected, echocardiographic evaluation is essential. Findings include atrial dilation, atrioventricular valve regurgitation, and evidence of systolic dysfunction. This may be accompanied by pericardial effusion and possibly tamponade.

Chest roentgenogram. With myocarditis, the chest roentgenogram may reveal cardiomegaly, pulmonary congestion, and pleural effusions.

Endomyocardial biopsy. This remains the gold standard for diagnosis. The histologic criteria for diagnosis included inflammatory cell infiltrate and cardiac myocyte necrosis. Because tissue involvement is patchy and it is risky and difficult to obtain samples, endomyocardial biopsy is only recommended in specific cases.

Cardiac magnetic resonance imaging (MRI). In adults this is known to be a useful noninvasive technique for the diagnosis of myocarditis. Patchy subepicardial tissue involvement with edema, inflammation, and scarring is seen. There is not sufficient experience in making the diagnosis of myocarditis using cardiac MRI in pediatric patients, but further studies are ongoing.

EBV DIAGNOSIS

Complete blood count. In the setting of acute EBV infection, one will generally see a lymphocytosis. Classically, the patient will have more than 10% atypical lymphocytes.

Monospot. This tests for the presence of heterophile antibodies which are found in approximately 85% of older children and adults with EBV infection. This antibody appears during the first 2 weeks of infection and gradually disappears over 6 months. It is important to know that the heterophile antibody test will often be negative in children younger than 4 years of age.

EBV-specific antibodies. Antibody testing to EBV antigens is useful in the diagnosis when evaluating patients with negative heterophile antibody testing. EBV viral capsid antigen (VCA) testing is most commonly performed to evaluate for EBV infection. EBV VCA IgG rises high early in the illness and persist for life, so this testing is not useful for the diagnosis of acute infection. Testing for EBV VCA IgM and EBV early antigen (EA) is useful to identify active and recent infections. Antibody to EBV nuclear antigen (NA) is not present until several weeks to months postinfection. The presence of EBV VCA IgM and absence of NA antibodies is considered diagnostic of acute EBV infection.

EBV viral isolation/detection. Isolation of EBV from oral secretions is possible, but difficult and does not indicate acute infection. Testing for the presence EBV DNA by PCR, or RNA by RT-PCR on blood or tissue specimens may be useful in selected cases including patients with immune dysfunction.

Liver function tests. Many patients will develop hepatitis from an EBV infection, with elevated aspartate aminotransferase, alanine aminotransferase, and lactic dehydrogenase. Patients may also develop hyperbilirubinemia.

TREATMENT

Patients who present with myocarditis should be treated supportively. Therapy may include observation, medications for heart failure, and cardiogenic shock including inotropes, afterload reducers, diuretics and antiarrhythmics, mechanical ventilation, temporary cardiac pacing, and mechanical circulatory support. The use of immunomodulatory therapy for treatment of acute myocarditis is not routinely recommended, but may be considered in certain groups of patients. Restriction of activity following acute myocarditis is generally recommended, although the effect of exercise on patients with myocarditis has not been studied.

The use of steroids for the treatment of EBV myocarditis is recommended as in other cases of complicated EBV infection. The combination of steroids and antiviral agents for the treatment of complicated EBV in immunocompetent individuals has been debated and is described in several case reports/case series. However, this combination has not been rigorously studied as the disease entity is relatively rare. In the presence of severe complications this combination could be considered.

SUGGESTED READINGS

1. Reddy S, Singh H. Chest pain in children and adolescents. *Pediatr Rev.* 2010;31(1):e1-e9.

2. American Academy of Pediatrics. *Red Book: 2012 Report of the Committee on Infectious Diseases.* Pickering LK, ed. 29th ed. Elk Grove Village, IL: American Academy of Pediatrics; 2012.

3. Sagar S, Liu P, Copper L. Myocarditis. *Lancet.* 2012; 379(9817):738-747. [Epub Dec 18, 2011.]

4. Rafailidis P, Mavros M, Kapaskelis A, Falagas M. Antiviral treatment for severe EBV infections in apparently immunocompetent patients. *J Clin Virol.* 2010;49(3):151-157. [Epub Aug 24, 2010].

5. Simpson K, Canter C. Acute myocarditis in children. *Expert Rev Cardiovasc Ther.* 2011;9(6):771-783.

CASE 14-4

Seventeen-Year-Old Boy

DEBRA BOYER

PHUONG VO

HISTORY OF PRESENT ILLNESS

The patient is a 17-year-old boy who presented with left-sided chest pain. He was well until 8 days prior to presentation when he developed left axillary and shoulder pain. The pain was worse with inspiration. He denied fever, nausea, vomiting, or diarrhea. He reported rhinorrhea and a dry cough 2 weeks prior. He had mild shortness of breath with exercise. He had no history of trauma.

MEDICAL HISTORY

The boy had a history of depression with no history of suicide attempts. He denied a history of asthma or other chronic illnesses. His family and social histories are noncontributory. He denied any drug use, but did admit to having smoked cigarettes in the past.

PHYSICAL EXAMINATION

T 36.6°C; HR 108 bpm; RR 18-20/min; BP 120/60 mmHg; SpO$_2$ 95% in room air

Weight 50th percentile-75%; Height 75th-90th percentile

In general, he was in no acute respiratory distress. His chest examination revealed no chest wall deformity and was nontender to palpation. Breath sounds were decreased at the bases, left greater than right. No wheezes or rales were appreciated. His cardiac examination revealed normal S1 and S2 with no murmurs, rubs, or gallops heard. The remainder of his physical examination was normal.

DIAGNOSTIC STUDIES

A complete blood count revealed a WBC count of 5600 cells/mm^3 with 55% segmented neutrophils, 31% lymphocytes, 11% monocytes, and 3% eosinophils. Electrolytes were normal.

COURSE OF ILLNESS

A chest roentgenogram was considered diagnostic (Figure 14-5).

DISCUSSION CASE 14-4

DIFFERENTIAL DIAGNOSIS

The differential diagnosis for chest pain in this adolescent boy should focus on the acute nature of his pain. In general, the most common etiologies for chest pain in the adolescent age group include psychogenic, cough, asthma, musculoskeletal pain,

pneumomediastinum commonly present with the acute onset of chest pain. Some abdominal processes, such as pancreatitis or cholecystitis, may present with acute chest pain. Cardiovascular causes are less common but are life-threatening. With acute chest pain, one should consider coronary artery disease, arrhythmias, structural cardiac defects, and infections.

DIAGNOSIS

A chest roentgenogram revealed a left pneumothorax (Figure 14-5). **The diagnosis is left spontaneous pneumothorax.**

INCIDENCE, EPIDEMIOLOGY, AND PATHOPHYSIOLOGY

Pneumothoraces are divided into three groups: spontaneous, traumatic, and iatrogenic. Within spontaneous pneumothoraces, one can have either a primary or secondary event. A primary spontaneous pneumothorax occurs when there is no underlying lung disease and a secondary spontaneous pneumothorax occurs in patients with underlying lung pathology.

The incidence of primary spontaneous pneumothorax ranges between 7.4 and 18 cases per 100000 men and between 1.2 and 6 cases per 100000 women. It is most common in tall, lean boys between 10 and 30 years of age. Cigarette smoking increases the risk of developing a primary spontaneous pneumothorax in a dose-dependent fashion.

Secondary spontaneous pneumothoraces occur in patients with underlying lung disease. The major causes include airway disease (e.g., cystic fibrosis), infection (e.g., pneumocystis carinii pneumonia), interstitial lung disease, connective-tissue disease, malignancy, and thoracic endometriosis. The incidence of secondary spontaneous pneumothorax is 6.3 cases per 100000 men and 2 cases per 100000 women. Secondary spontaneous pneumothoraces have a later peak incidence at 60-65 years of age.

Subpleural bullae are seen in 76%-100% of children who are taken to video-assisted thoracoscopic surgery. There is some speculation as to the mechanism of bullae formation. It is likely that elastic fibers are degraded in the lung, which ultimately leads to an imbalance in the protease/antiprotease

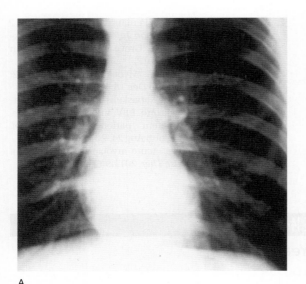

A

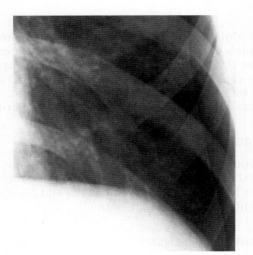

B

FIGURE 14-5. A. Chest radiograph. **B.** Chest radiograph close-up.

and pneumonia. These causes most often produce a subacute and subtle type of chest pain.

Thus, the acute onset of chest pain in this boy should focus on the differential diagnosis of a number of other causes. Certainly, tobacco use or the abuse of cocaine or methamphetamine may cause the acute onset of chest pain secondary to vasospasm of the coronary arteries. Pneumothorax or

system and the development of bullae. A pneumothorax then develops as alveolar pressure increases with air subsequently leaking into the interstitium.

Traumatic pneumothoraces occur secondary to blunt, crush, or penetrating trauma to the chest, as a result of mechanical ventilation, or by injury from a diagnostic or therapeutic procedure.

CLINICAL PRESENTATION

Primary spontaneous pneumothorax usually develops while the patient is at rest. Patients describe pleuritic ipsilateral chest pain and dyspnea. With a small pneumothorax, the physical examination may be completely normal. Tachycardia may be noted. In patients with a large pneumothorax, one may see poor chest wall movement, a hyperresonant chest, and decreased breath sounds on the side with the pneumothorax. Tachycardia and hypotension indicate that the patient has developed tension physiology and requires emergent intervention.

With a large pneumothorax, the patient develops a decreased vital capacity and an increased alveolar-arterial oxygen gradient. In patients with primary spontaneous pneumothoraces, their underlying lung function is normal and, therefore, they do not develop hypercapnia. In contrast, patients with secondary spontaneous pneumothoraces by definition have underlying lung disease and are more likely to develop hypercapnia.

DIAGNOSTIC APPROACH

Chest roentgenogram. A posterior-anterior chest roentgenogram reveals the presence of a pneumothorax. Small apical pneumothoraces may be difficult to detect in this fashion, and on occasion an expiratory roentgenogram will be necessary.

Chest computed tomography (CT). A chest CT may be necessary to differentiate a bulla from a pneumothorax.

TREATMENT

A variety of treatment options exist when managing a pneumothorax. They range from observation, simple aspiration with a catheter, chest tube insertion, pleurodesis, thoracoscopy with video-assisted thoracoscopic surgery, and thoracotomy.

Patients with small primary spontaneous pneumothoraces may be observed without intervention if there is no respiratory distress. They may be treated with supplemental oxygen to hasten the reabsorption of air. With supplemental oxygen, the air is reabsorbed at a rate of 2% per day. With larger primary spontaneous pneumothoraces, needle aspiration or chest tube insertion are required. Secondary spontaneous pneumothoraces generally require intervention as patients are usually ill due to their underlying lung disease.

The main debate with spontaneous pneumothoraces is the ability to prevent recurrences. With a primary spontaneous pneumothorax, the recurrence rate is around 30% and most will recur 6 months to 2 years after the initial event. Smoking and younger age are risk factors for recurrent disease. The recurrence rate with secondary spontaneous pneumothoraces is similar at 39%-47%.

The general consensus is to recommend preventative therapy after the second ipsilateral pneumothorax. However, patients who participate in risky activities such as scuba diving and flying should be considered for intervention after their first spontaneous pneumothorax. Options for recurrence prevention include the instillation of sclerosing agents through a chest tube and mechanical pleurodesis. With video-assisted thoracoscopic procedures, blebs can also be identified and oversewn.

SUGGESTED READINGS

1. Baumann MH, Strange C, Heffner JE, et al. Management of spontaneous pneumothorax: an American College of Chest Physicians Delphi Consensus Statement. *Chest.* 2001;119:590-602.
2. Sahn SA, Heffner JE. Spontaneous pneumothorax. *N Engl J Med.* 2000;342:868-874.
3. Weissberg D, Refaely Y. Pneumothorax: experience with 1,199 patients. *Chest.* 2000;117:1279-1285.
4. Montgomery M. Air and liquid in the pleural space. In: Chernick V, Boat TF, eds. *Kendig's Disorders of the Respiratory Tract in Children.* Philadelphia, PA: W.B. Saunders Company; 1998:403-409.

CASE 14-5

Three-Year-Old Girl

DEBRA BOYER

TREGONY SIMONEAU

HISTORY OF PRESENT ILLNESS

The patient is a 3-year-old girl who was brought to the emergency department crying and clutching her chest. She was extremely difficult to console. She had poor oral intake during the last day with decreased urine output. On the evening of admission, she was found sitting in bed whimpering and holding her chest. She did not have a history of vomiting or diarrhea. Her temperature had not been measured but she did not feel subjectively warm.

MEDICAL HISTORY

The girl had been seen in the emergency department 3 weeks prior and diagnosed with viral stomatitis. Culture of the lesions grew HSV I and the lesions had resolved by the time of this presentation. She had only been taking ibuprofen at home. The remainder of her medical history was unremarkable.

PHYSICAL EXAMINATION

T 38.2°C; HR 130 bpm; RR 30/min; BP 98/60 mmHg; Oxygen saturation, 95% in room air

Weight 75th to 90th percentile

In general, she was crying and difficult to examine, holding her chest with both arms. She was not in significant respiratory distress. Her chest examination revealed no apparent bony tenderness over her sternum or ribs. She had decreased aeration at the left base with no wheezes or rales appreciated. Her eyes were slightly sunken and she had some crusty nasal discharge. Her lips and other mucous membranes were dry. The remainder of her physical examination was normal.

DIAGNOSTIC STUDIES

The girl's complete blood count revealed 19 000 WBCs/mm^3 (8% band forms, 81% segmented neutrophils, 11% lymphocytes). Hemoglobin was 12.8 g/dL and platelet count was 402 000/mm^3. Electrolytes and liver function tests were normal.

COURSE OF ILLNESS

The girl was given a 40 mL/kg normal saline fluid bolus. She refused to drink and was therefore placed on maintenance intravenous fluids. A chest roentgenogram revealed the diagnosis (Figure 14-6).

DISCUSSION CASE 14-5

DIFFERENTIAL DIAGNOSIS

As with adolescents, chest pain in the school-aged child is very rarely a life-threatening condition. Common causes of chest pain in this age group include asthma, pneumonia, and musculoskeletal (muscle strain, trauma, costochondritis). It is also

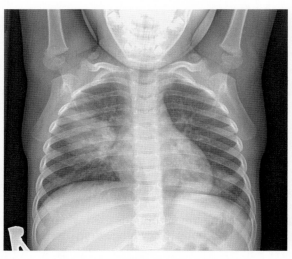

FIGURE 14-6. Chest radiograph.

quite common for chest pain to be deemed idiopathic. Less commonly, one may see a child with gastroesophageal reflux, pneumothorax, pneumomediastinum, or pleural effusion present with chest pain. As with the older child, the history and physical examination are crucial in guiding the appropriate work up.

Rarely, one will see a child with chest pain and cardiovascular disease. However, one must remember that this is the diagnosis that most families will be concerned about. Thus, it must be addressed, if even to reassure the family and child that it is not a concern. Certainly, children with palpitations, syncope, or chest pain with exertion should have a thorough evaluation for any cardiovascular disease. Finally, toddlers are always at risk for foreign body ingestion. While aspirated foreign bodies are not likely to give chest pain, esophageal foreign bodies may commonly present with chest pain.

DIAGNOSIS

The chest roentgenogram revealed round airspace opacities in the apical segment of the right lower lobe and the posterior basal segment of the left lower lobe (Figure 14-6). **The diagnosis is pneumonia.**

INCIDENCE AND EPIDEMIOLOGY

In children younger than 5 years of age, the yearly incidence of community-acquired pneumonia is 36-40/1000, and for 5-14 year olds, the incidence is 11-16/1000. In the United States, 1-4/1000 children are hospitalized every year with a lower respiratory tract infection. It is fairly difficult to develop a consensus definition of a case of pneumonia. Some define it based on an abnormal chest roentgenogram, while others require only the presence of clinical symptoms.

There are a large number of organisms that can cause community-acquired pneumonia in children. The most common causes include viruses (respiratory syncytial virus, influenza A and B, parainfluenzae, human metapneumovirus, adenovirus, and rhinovirus) *Mycoplasma pneumoniae, Chlamydia species* (*C. trachomatis* and *C. pneumoniae*) bacteria (*Streptococcus pneumoniae, Mycobacterium tuberculosis, Staphylococcus aureus, Hae-*

mophilus influenzae type B, and nontypeable *H. influenzae*). Less common etiologies include other viruses (varicella, enteroviruses, cytomegalovirus, and Epstein-Barr virus), *Chlamydia psittaci,* less common bacteria (*Streptococcus pyogenes,* anaerobic mouth flora, *Bordetella pertussis, Klebsiella pneumoniae,* and *Legionella*), and fungi (*Coccidioides immitis, Histoplasma capsulatum,* and *Blastomyces dermatitidis*).

Often, the difficulty is in differentiating a bacterial from a nonbacterial pneumonia. Classically, lobar infiltrates, cavitary lesions, and large pleural effusions suggest either bacterial or mycobacterial infections. Viral pneumonias typically present with diffuse radiographic involvement, but focal infiltrates can be seen. Laboratory data has been used in an attempt to differentiate viral from bacterial pneumonia, with C-reactive protein and white blood cell counts more significantly elevated in bacterial pneumonias. Ultimately, when attempting to determine the etiologic agent for pneumonia, one must consider the underlying immunologic function of the patient. Certainly, immunocompromised patients are susceptible to several other infectious etiologies that may be life-threatening.

One must also consider that some noninfectious processes may cause a similar clinical picture. These would include gastroesophageal reflux, chemical aspiration, asthma, hypersensitivity pneumonitis, and pulmonary hemosiderosis.

CLINICAL PRESENTATION

Generally, viral pneumonia will commence with upper respiratory tract infection symptoms, fever, rhinorrhea, and cough. Respiratory symptoms may be insidious. This is in contrast to most bacterial pneumonias where there is often an acute onset with fever, cough, and chest pain.

On physical examination, patients may have signs that are suggestive of consolidation (dullness to percussion, bronchial breath sounds, and egophony). This is more suggestive of a bacterial process. In contrast, patients with *Mycoplasma* or viral infections may have unimpressive physical examinations, but have very distinct infiltrates noted on their chest roentgenograms. Furthermore, patients with *Mycoplasma* may have a concurrent bullous myringitis.

DIAGNOSTIC APPROACH

Chest roentgenogram. As mentioned previously, the difficulty in diagnosing a pneumonia is differentiating a bacterial from a viral process. Lobar consolidation, cavitation, and large pleural effusions suggest a bacterial or mycobacterial process. Small, bilateral pleural effusions are present in approximately 20% of children with *M. pneumoniae* pneumonia. Pneumococcal pneumonia is the most common bacterial cause of lobar consolidation. However, approximately 10% of cases of *Mycoplasma* pneumonia present with lobar consolidation. Pneumatoceles are detected in two-thirds of children with pneumonia due to *S. aureus* (Figure 14-7). Viral pneumonias typically have a diffuse appearance that may be either interstitial or alveolar. Disease confined to the lower lobes, or the upper lobes in supine patients may suggest aspiration pneumonia.

Chest computed tomography (CT) or ultrasound. For an uncomplicated pneumonia, chest CT or ultrasound is not necessary. However, chest CT is useful in cases of recurrent pneumonia or in recalcitrant cases. Furthermore, in the immunocompromised patient, a chest CT may reveal subtle parenchymal disease. In children with a unilateral pleural effusion, chest CT and chest ultrasound can detect loculations and distinguish pleural effusions from anatomic abnormalities such as pulmonary lobe sequestration.

Sputum examination. Sputum culture may help identify the bacterial cause of pneumonia in adolescents but is not commonly predictive of the cause of pneumonia in younger children due to the difficulty in obtaining an adequate sputum sample. In addition, real-time PCR can be performed to detect the presence of viral products. PCR can also be used to detect *M. pneumoniae*. A nasopharyngeal wash or aspirate is the most sensitive specimen for these studies.

Bronchoscopy. As with chest CT, a bronchoscopy is not necessary in the uncomplicated pneumonia. However, a pneumonia that does not respond to appropriate antibiotic therapy may require bronchoscopy to obtain appropriate samples for culture. With this technique, a bronchoalveolar lavage is performed which can be analyzed for the causative organisms via gram stain, culture, and viral studies. Bronchoscopy is often indicated in immunocompromised patients who are at risk for opportunistic infections in addition to common bacterial and viral etiologies.

TREATMENT

In the majority of cases, the causative organism is hypothesized but not verified. Therefore, therapy must be empiric. Table 14-6 summarizes the common organisms and recommended therapy by age group. In the newborn period, the most common organisms include group B streptococci, enteric Gram-negative bacteria (particularly *Escherichia coli* and *Klebsiella* species), and *Listeria monocytogenes*. Thus, a combination of ampicillin and either gentamicin or cefotaxime is often used. There is no consensus as to when the newborn period is over, but after 3 weeks of age, the causative organisms tend to switch to *Chlamydia trachomatis*, viruses, *Streptococcus pneumoniae*, *Bordetella pertussis*, and *S. aureus*. Currently, the prevailing opinion is to treat these children (generally 3 week to 3 month age group) with amoxicillin, ampicillin, or cefotaxime.

From 3 months to approximately 5 years of age, the causative organisms tend to include

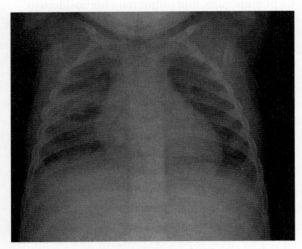

FIGURE 14-7. Chest radiograph showing round lucencies within the right upper lobe indicating pneumatocele formation.

TABLE 14-6.	Common microbial causes and recommended empiric treatment for the hospitalized patient with community-acquired pneumonia.	
Age	**Common Organisms**	**Common Treatment**
0-3 weeks	Group B streptococcus *Escherichia coli* *Klebsiella* species *Listeria monocytogenes*	Ampicillin and cefotaxime
3 weeks to 3 months	*Chlamydia trachomatis* *Streptococcus pneumoniae* *Bordetella pertussis* Respiratory syncytial virus (RSV) and parainfluenza viruses (PIV)	Ampicillin +/– azithromycin

3 months to 5 years	RSV, PIV, influenza, human
	  metapneumovirus, adenovirus,
	  rhinovirus
	Streptococcus pneumoniae
	Haemophilus influenzae
	Staphylococcus aureus
	Mycoplasma pneumoniae
		Ampicillin +/– azithromycin

5-15 years	*Mycoplasma pneumoniae* *Chlamydia pneumonia* *Streptococcus pneumonia*	Ampicillin and amoxicillin are first line; use azithromycin in addition to beta-lactam therapy if atypical bacteria are significant considerations and instead of beta-lactam theapy if findings are characteristic of atypical infections. Levofloxacin and doxycycline (age >7 years) also provide coverage against atypical bacteria

viruses, *S. pneumoniae, H. influenzae, M. pneumoniae,* and *M. tuberculosis.* In a study of 3475 *S. pneumoniae* isolates by Whitney and colleagues, ampicillin was effective against 98% of isolates with intermediate sensitivity against penicillin while erythromycin and second-generation cephalosporin antibiotics were effective against only 65% of those same isolates. For these reasons, the Pediatric Infectious Disease Society (PIDS) and the Infectious Diseases Society of America (IDSA) clinical practice guidelines recommend either amoxicillin or ampicillin for the treatment of uncomplicated lobar pneumonia. Children allergic to aminopenicillins can receive either clindamycin or second- or third-generation cephalosporin-class antibiotics. Children with antecedent influenza infection are at higher risk for pneumonia due to *S. aureus.* For these children, an agent with activity against both *S. pneumoniae* and *S. aureus,* such as amoxicillin-clavulanate, clindamycin, or azithromycin, is preferred to treat pneumonia in the child with influenza. If methicillin-resistant staph aureus (MRSA) is suspected, clindamycin or vancomycin can be added to the regimen.

Finally, in the 5-15-year age group, *Mycoplasma* and *Chlamydophila* pneumoniae are more common than other etiologies including *S. pneumoniae. Mycoplasma* pneumonia has been shown in some studies to cause greater than 40% of community-acquired pneumonias in this age group. The PIDS/IDSA guidelines recommend ampicillin or amoxicillin as first-line therapy for suspected bacterial pneumonia. A macrolide can be used in addition to beta-lactam therapy if atypical bacteria, such as Mycoplsama, are significant considerations and instead of beta-lactam therapy if findings are characteristic of an atypical infection. Macrolides provide coverage for atypical bacteria but provide suboptimal coverage for pneumococcus. Treatment failure and breakthrough infections have occurred when macrolides, such as azithromycin, were used to treat serious pneumococcal infections. Certainly, in any age range, one should pursue the diagnosis of *M. tuberculosis* if it is at all clinically suspected.

SUGGESTED READINGS

1. Bradley JS, Byington CL, Shah SS, et al. The management of community-acquired pneumonia in infants and children older than 3 months of age: clinical practice guidelines by the Pediatric Infectious Diseases Society and the Infectious Diseases Society of America. *Clin Infect Dis.* 2011;53:e25-e76.
2. Byer RL. Pain—chest. In: Fleisher GR, Ludwig S, eds. *Textbook of Pediatric Emergency Medicine*, 6th ed. Philadelphia: Lippincott Williams & Wilkins; 2010: 434-442.
3. Mani CS, Murray DL. Acute pneumonia and its complications. In: Long SS, Pickering LK, Prober CG, eds. *Principles and Practice of Pediatric Infectious Diseases.* 3rd ed. Philadelphia: Elsevier; 2008:245-257.
4. McIntosh K. Community-acquired pneumonia in children. *N Engl J Med.* 2002;346:429-437.
5. Ferwerda A, Moll HA, de Groot R. Respiratory tract infections by *Mycoplasma pneumoniae* in children: a review of diagnostic and therapeutic measures. *Eur J Pediatr.* 2001;160:483-491.
6. Franquet T. Imaging of pneumonia: trends and algorithms. *Eur Resp J.* 2001;18:196-208.
7. Whitney CG, Farley MM, Hadler J, et al. Increasing prevalence of multidrug-resistant *Streptococcus pneumoniae* in the United States. *N Engl J Med.* 2000;343:1917-1924.

CASE 14-6

Fifteen-Year-Old Boy

DEBRA BOYER

TREGONY SIMONEAU

HISTORY OF PRESENT ILLNESS

The patient is a 15-year-old boy with a history of asthma and chronic sinusitis who presented with a 2-day history of shortness of breath and chest pain. He described the pain as an ache with an occasional squeezing feeling. He developed wheezing which required increasing use of his Albuterol inhaler. However, this did not relieve his symptoms. He also developed a productive cough. His mother believed that he had increasing fatigue since the morning of his presentation, as well as a decreased appetite. He denied fever, vomiting, or diarrhea.

MEDICAL HISTORY

The boy had asthma diagnosed at the age of 7 years, requiring multiple emergency department visits and hospitalizations. Two years prior he had one asthma admission which lasted for 1 week. He has never required endotracheal intubation or intensive care unit hospitalization. He had recently been started on a leukotriene inhibitor for his asthma. Many of his prior admissions for asthma exacerbations have included cardiology evaluations for chest pain. He also has a history of chronic sinusitis requiring six sinus surgeries during the last 3 years, as well as a somatization disorder diagnosed by psychiatry. His daily medications included montelukast and inhaled fluticasone and albuterol as needed.

The patient was recently admitted to the hospital for an asthma exacerbation and gastroenteritis. During that admission, he was seen by cardiology for bradycardia and chest pain. An echocardiogram at that time revealed a shortening fraction of 26% and a left ventricular end-diastolic pressure of 5.5 mmHg. A Holter monitor and exercise test were both normal.

PHYSICAL EXAMINATION

T 37.0°C; HR 110/min; RR 26/min; BP 85/60 mmHg; Oxygen saturation, 91% in room air

In general, he was an uncomfortable boy in moderate respiratory distress. He was short of breath and only able to speak in fragmented sentences. He was sitting up for comfort. His oropharynx was dry. His chest examination revealed that he had diffuse rales and wheezes with fair aeration throughout. His cardiac examination indicated an active precordium, tachycardia with regular rhythm. There were no murmurs or rubs noted. An intermittent gallop was appreciated. His liver was palpable 3 cm below the right costal margin. His extremities were cool with weak pulses and slightly delayed capillary refill.

DIAGNOSTIC STUDIES

Laboratory analysis revealed 7500 WBCs/mm^3. Electrolytes, blood urea nitrogen, creatinine, and liver function tests were all within normal limits. Electrocardiogram revealed a normal sinus rhythm at a rate of 100 bpm. There was possible right atrial enlargement and some ST segment depression.

COURSE OF ILLNESS

A chest roentgenogram suggested the diagnosis (Figure 14-8).

DISCUSSION CASE 14-6

DIFFERENTIAL DIAGNOSIS

The most common causes for chest pain in the adolescent age group are cough, asthma, pneumonia, musculoskeletal, and idiopathic. With this

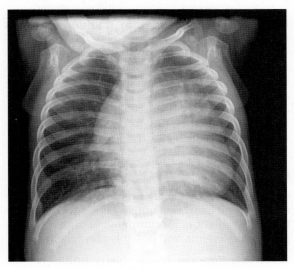

FIGURE 14-8. Chest radiograph revealing cardiomegaly and pulmonary edema.

patient's medical history of asthma, it is natural for asthma to be the initial focus of concern. However, the patient's physical examination was not consistent with an asthma exacerbation, and therefore, other diagnoses were appropriately considered.

The concerning features on this patient's physical examination included signs of congestive heart failure: bilateral rales, a gallop, and a palpable liver edge 3 cm below the right costal margin. Furthermore, his shortness of breath was significantly worse while lying down. Dyspnea with an asthma exacerbation is not generally positional in nature to this extent.

Thus, the differential diagnosis for heart failure in this adolescent would include (1) congenital heart disease from pressure overload (e.g., aortic stenosis), or volume overload (e.g., aortic regurgitation, arrhythmias), (2) acquired heart disease (e.g., myocarditis, cardiomyopathy, (3) pericarditis, (4) cor pulmonale, endocarditis), (5) hypoglycemia, (6) storage diseases, and (7) ingestions such as cardiac toxins (e.g., digitalis) and arrythmogenic drugs (e.g., tricyclic antidepressants).

DIAGNOSIS

The boy's chest roentgenogram revealed pulmonary edema with massive cardiomegaly (Figure 14-8). An echocardiogram was performed and demonstrated a shortening fraction of less than 20% with left-ventricular end diastolic pressure of 6.4 cm. The left ventricle was noted to be dilated. **The diagnosis is a dilated cardiomyopathy.** He was initially treated with intravenous furosimide. He was then started on a milrinone infusion. Multiple laboratory studies were sent including infectious serologies and thyroid function tests which did not reveal an etiology for his cardiomyopathy. Ultimately, a cardiac catheterization was performed which revealed a cardiac index of 2.81 and superior vena cava saturation of 75%. An endomyocardial biopsy was performed which demonstrated an eosinophilic and monocytic infiltrate.

INCIDENCE AND EPIDEMIOLOGY

By definition, cardiomyopathy is a structural or functional abnormality of the ventricular myocardium which does not involve coronary artery disease, hypertension, valvular, or congenital heart disease. Cardiomyopathy in children can be divided into primary and secondary forms. Primary cardiomyopathies are either dilated, hypertrophic, restrictive, or arrhythmogenic. Dilated cardiomyopathy occurs in 40/100000 people. Secondary cardiomyopathies can occur as a result of multiple etiologies including infection, metabolic disorders, general systemic diseases, hereditary forms, and toxins. Table 14-7 summarizes the known causes of dilated cardiomyopathy.

This patient presented with a dilated cardiomyopathy with no definitive etiology. Two-thirds of children with primary dilated cardiomyopathy have

an idiopathic etiology. For patients with dilated cardiomyopathy, the 1-year risk of death or transplantation is approximately 30% and the 5-year risk is approximately 40%. Aside from idiopathic, the most common causes of dilated cardiomyopathy in children include myocarditis and neuromuscular diseases.

CLINICAL PRESENTATION

Patients with a dilated cardiomyopathy will most commonly have an insidious onset to their symptoms. The most common complaints in adolescents include shortness of breath and poor exercise tolerance which are the result of decreased cardiac output and pulmonary edema. It is important to note that infants will not be able to complain of these same symptoms. Thus, their presentation will often include more subtle symptoms including tachypnea, irritability, and difficulty with feeding. Seventy-one percent of children with dilated cardiomyopathy present with congestive heart failure at diagnosis.

Patients will often be tachycardic, tachypneic, and nervous. Hypotension may be seen with poor cardiac output and fever may indicate an infection that has brought the patient to medical attention. Quite often, patients will have orthopnea, preferring to remain in the upright position. With pulmonary edema, many patients will wheeze, but will be unresponsive to traditional asthma therapies.

On chest wall palpation, one may find a laterally displaced point of maximal impulse. With auscultation of the cardiac sounds, one may appreciate a prominent pulmonic segment of the second heart sound and/or a gallop. With congestive heart failure, many patients will have a liver edge that is abnormally below the right costal margin.

DIAGNOSTIC APPROACH

Chest roentgenogram. Patients will generally have an increased heart size noted. This is secondary to left-sided dilation. Accompanying signs include pulmonary edema and possibly pleural effusions.

Electrocardiogram. Sinus tachycardia is the most common finding, with supraventricular or ventricular tachycardia possible as well. Signs of

TABLE 14-7.	Known causes of dilated cardiomyopathies.
Category	*Etiology*
Infectious	Viral Bacterial Fungal Parasitic Rickettsial Mycobacterial
Inflammatory	Juvenile inflammatory arthritis Lupus erythematosus Dermatomyositis Reye syndrome Sarcoidosis Scleroderma Kawasaki disease
Toxic	Alcohol Chemotherapeutic agents (anthracyclines) Cobalt Hemochromatosis Lead Other medications (antiretrovirals, chloramphenicol)
Familial Cardiomyopathies	
Neuromuscular	Muscular dystrophy (DuchenneBecker) Friedreich ataxia Polymyositis Myotonic dystrophy Mitochondrial (Kearns-Sayre, MELAS)
Metabolic	Thiamine deficiency Hypothyroidism Thyrotoxicosis Cushing disease Pheochromocytoma Inborn errors of metabolism

left ventricular hypertrophy and nonspecific ST-segment and T-wave abnormalities may also be seen.

Echocardiogram. The left atrium and left ventricle are generally noted to be enlarged. There may be increased end-diastolic and systolic volumes. Poor wall movement may be seen secondary to ischemic injury. With this imaging modality, pericardial, and pleural effusions may also be noted.

Cardiac catheterization. One can obtain hemodynamic data on pressures in the aorta, left ventricle, pulmonary capillary wedge, and pulmonary artery. The cardiac output can be calculated and will be decreased. An endomyocardial biopsy can be performed and may be useful to determine the etiology for the cardiomyopathy.

TREATMENT

Inotropic agents such as the sympathomimetic drugs dopamine, dobutamine, and epinephrine are often required to support the poor cardiac output. Milrinone and amrinone are inotropes as well that can be used to treat patients with signs of congestive heart failure. Digoxin is used for long-term therapy and increased cardiac contractility.

Since fluid overload is quite common in this clinical scenario, diuretics such as furosemide are often necessary. Peripheral vasodilators including nitroprusside and hydralazine may be used to decrease afterload and thus increase cardiac output. ACE inhibitors can have similar effects to reduce afterload.

With dilation of the cardiac chambers, the patient is at risk for thrombus formation. Anticoagulation or antiplatelet drugs should be considered. Certainly, if the underlying etiology of the cardiomyopathy is determined, a more specific therapy may be warranted.

Finally, in severe cases, cardiac transplantation is required. It is difficult to determine which children/adolescents should be considered for transplantation. Certainly, those children who are still quite ill despite maximal intervention should have this option explored.

SUGGESTED READINGS

1. Gewitz MH, Woolf PK. Cardiac emergencies. In: Fleisher GR, Ludwig S, eds. *Textbook of Pediatric Emergency Medicine*. 6th ed. Philadelphia: Lippincott Williams & Wilkins; 2010:690-729.
2. Spencer CT. Dilated cardiomyopathy and myocarditis. In: Lai WW, Mertens LL, Cohen MS, Geva T, eds. *Echocardiography in Pediatric and Congenital Heart Disease: From Fetus to Adult*. Hoboken: Wiley-Blackwell; 2009:558-580.
3. Towbin JA, Bowles NE. Cardiomyopathy. In: McMillan JA ed. *Oski's Pediatrics* 4th ed. Philadelphia: Lippincott Williams & Wilkins; 2006:1606-1614.
4. Olson TM, Hoffman TM, Chan DP. Dilated congestive cardiomyopathy. In: Driscoll DJ, eds. *Moss and Adams' Heart Disease in Infants, Children, and Adolescents*. 7th ed. Philadelphia: Lippincott Williams & Wilkins; 2008:1195-1206.
5. Wilkinson JD, Landy DC, Colan SD, et al. The Pediatric cardiomyopathy registry and heart failure: key results from the first 15 years. *Heart Fail Clin*. 2010;6(4):401-413.

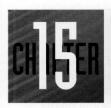

CHAPTER 15

JAUNDICE

STACEY R. ROSE

DEFINITION

Jaundice is the yellow discoloration of the skin, mucous membranes, and sclerae caused by elevated serum levels of bilirubin, a by-product of heme breakdown. Bilirubin is a lipophilic pigment and must bind to plasma albumin to be transported to the liver. It is then taken up by hepatocytes for conjugation with solubilizing sugars to form bilirubin diglucuronides (and, less commonly, monoglucuronides), which can be excreted into bile. Several factors can cause jaundice. While many of these processes are pathologic, physiologic jaundice in neonates, a benign process, accounts for the vast majority of clinically encountered jaundice in pediatrics.

CAUSE AND FREQUENCY

Jaundice may be secondary to an unconjugated or conjugated hyperbilirubinemia (Table 15-1). In general, unconjugated hyperbilirubinemia results from overproduction of bilirubin, impaired uptake of bilirubin by hepatocytes, or impaired conjugation. A primary cause of overproduction is hemolysis, which is usually associated with other laboratory abnormalities including anemia, elevated LDH, low haptoglobin, and increased reticulocyte count. Reduced uptake of bilirubin can be due to poor blood flow to the liver, certain drugs, and various inherited diseases. Impaired bilirubin conjugation is usually due to various inherited disorders, such as Gilbert syndrome or Crigler-Najjar, where the enzymes needed for conjugation are deficient.

Conjugated hyperbilirubinemia occurs secondary to cholestatic conditions or direct hepatocellular injury. Cholestasis results from intra- or extrahepatic impairments in bile flow, and is accompanied by elevations in alkaline phosphatase and/or gamma-glutamyl transpeptidase (GGT). The differential diagnosis of cholestatic jaundice in the older child differs from diseases that present early in life. Young infants are more likely to have congenital anatomic anomalies, such as biliary atresia, or inborn metabolic disorders such as galactosemia. In contrast, older children are more likely to experience acquired or secondary liver diseases, such as cholelithiasis or sclerosing cholangitis. There is often an overlap between syndromes causing cholestasis and those resulting in hepatocellular injury. Generally, hepatocellular injury is accompanied by elevations in the transaminases (AST and ALT). Additionally, synthetic liver dysfunction, evidenced by hypoalbuminemia as well as prolonged coagulation measurements, may also be present. There are many causes of hepatocellular injury including infectious, autoimmune or toxic hepatitis, or metabolic processes such as alpha-1 antitrypsin deficiency.

QUESTIONS TO ASK AND WHY

- Is the elevated bilirubin level all unconjugated? Is the process a conjugated hyperbilirubinemia?
  —Separating a total bilirubin measurement into its conjugated and unconjugated components is a critical step in the evaluation of hyperbilirubinemia in a child. Conjugated hyperbilirubinemia

TABLE 15-1.	Common causes of jaundice in infants and children.

Unconjugated	*Conjugated*

Bilirubin Overproduction
• Hemolysis
  ◦ Isoimmune hemolytic disease
  ◦ Hemoglobinopathies or RBC membrane defects
  ◦ G6PD deficiency
• Cephalohematoma or significant bruising
• Polycythemia
	Intrahepatic Processes
	• Obstruction
	  ◦ Alagille syndrome
	• Metabolic disorders
	  ◦ Galactosemia
	  ◦ Tyrosinemia
	  ◦ Endocrinopathies
	  ◦ Zellweger syndrome
	• Inherited disorders
	  ◦ Dubin-Johnson syndrome
	  ◦ Rotor syndrome
	  ◦ Progressive familial intrahepatic cholestasis (PFIC), types I (Byler syndrome), II, III
	  ◦ Cystic fibrosis
	• Other
	  ◦ Total parenteral nutrition

Impaired Bilirubin Uptake
• Increased enterohepatic circulation
  ◦ Breastfeeding jaundice
  ◦ Intestinal obstruction
  ◦ Ileus
• Poor blood flow
  ◦ Sepsis
  ◦ Congestive heart failure
	Extrahepatic Obstruction
	• Biliary atresia
	• Choledochal cyst
	• Cholelithiasis
	• Primary sclerosing cholangitis
	• Primary biliary cirrhosis

Impaired Bilirubin Conjugation
• Crigler-Najjar types I and II
• Gilbert syndrome
• Breastmilk jaundice
	Hepatocellular Injury
	• Infectious
	  ◦ TORCH
	  ◦ Viral, bacterial, parasitic hepatitis
	  ◦ Sepsis
	• Metabolic
	  ◦ Alpha 1 antitrypsin deficiency
	  ◦ Wilson disease
	  ◦ Neonatal hemochromatosis
	• Toxic
	  ◦ Alcohol
	  ◦ Drugs/medications
	• Immunologic/other
	  ◦ Idiopathic neonatal hepatitis
	  ◦ Autoimmune hepatitis
	  ◦ Hepatitis secondary to inflammatory bowel disease

is present when the conjugated fraction is at least 1.5 mg/dL or accounts for greater than 15% of the total bilirubin measurement. Conjugated hyperbilirubinemia is abnormal and merits prompt evaluation, particularly in infants, since diseases like biliary atresia require urgent therapy. An increased unconjugated bilirubin level suggests a very different differential diagnosis and may also be a medical emergency when levels are very high since unconjugated bilirubin is able to cross the blood-brain barrier and directly injures the brain.

Sometimes the terms "direct" and "indirect" bilirubin are used interchangeably with the terms "conjugated" and "unconjugated." The former terms derive from the van den Bergh reaction in which the conjugated bilirubin component is measured *directly* (by colorimetric analysis after reaction with a diazo compound). In the van den Bergh assay's next step, the addition of methanol allows for a measurement of total bilirubin; the unconjugated fraction is then determined—*indirectly*—by subtracting the conjugated bilirubin level from the total bilirubin level. Of note, measurement of the direct bilirubin fraction detects not only bilirubin di- and mono-glucuronides, but also "delta" bilirubin, which forms when conjugated bilirubin seeps retrograde into the serum and binds covalently to albumin. Because of the delta component's long half-life, the "direct fraction" can remain deceptively elevated even as a conjugated hyperbilirubinemia improves.

• Does the jaundiced baby have other concerning physical findings?
—A significant unconjugated hyperbilirubinemia can result from the accelerated breakdown of red blood cells secondary to a cephalohematoma or extensive bruising. A newborn afflicted with a TORCH infection might have microcephaly, growth retardation, hepatosplenomegaly, chorioretinitis, or rash. A heart murmur is often heard in children with Alagille syndrome, while a baby with Zellweger syndrome will be hypotonic and dysmorphic. Additionally, the presence of hypotonia, opsithotonus (backward arching of the trunk), or retrocollis (backward arching of the neck) on neurologic examination should raise immediate concerns for acute bilirubin encephalopathy or kernicterus.

- Is there a family history of jaundice?
  —Many of the disorders that present with jaundice are heritable. Alpha-1-antitrypsin deficiency, Crigler-Najjar syndromes type I and II, galactosemia, and tyrosinemia are just a few of the autosomal recessive diseases associated with neonatal jaundice. However, Alagille syndrome is an autosomal dominant disorder (but with variable reentrance and expressivity). The inheritance of glucose-6-phosphate (G6PD) deficiency is X-linked but so highly polymorphic that it should be considered in the evaluation of boys and girls alike.

- Were there changes in the child's diet, or other new "exposures," that preceded the onset of jaundice?
  —Deficiencies in the metabolism of galactose or fructose can lead to jaundice in infants. Likewise, children with G6PD deficiency can have hemolytic crises triggered by certain foods (e.g., fava beans), medications (e.g., sulfa drugs), and other compounds (e.g., mothballs).

- Does the baby have risk factors for severe neonatal hyperbilirubinemia?
  —Risk factors for neonatal jaundice include intrauterine and perinatal complications such as

gestational diabetes, prematurity, blood group incompatibility, or birth trauma resulting in extravascular blood collections. Other independent risk factors for the infant include ethnicity (East Asian, Native American, and others), polycythemia, acidosis, hypoalbuminemia, exclusive breastfeeding, urinary tract infection or sepsis, and a long, heterogeneous list of genetic disorders.

SUGGESTED READINGS

1. Abrams SH, Shulman RJ. Causes of neonatal cholestasis. UpToDate. www.uptodate.com/contents/causes-of-neonatal-cholestasis. Updated September 1, 2010. Accessed September 22, 2011.
2. American Academy of Pediatrics Subcommittee on Hyperbilirubinemia. American Academy of Pediatrics Clinical Practice Guideline: Management of hyperbilirubinemia in the newborn infant 35 or more weeks of gestation. *Pediatrics.* 2004;114:297-316.
3. Dennery PA, Seidman DS, Stevenson DK. Neonatal hyperbilirubinemia. *N Engl J Med.* 2001;344:581-590.
4. Maisels MJ. Neonatal jaundice. *Pediatr Rev.* 2006;27:443-453.
5. Maisels MJ, McDonagh AF. Phototherapy for neonatal jaundice. *N Engl J Med.* 2008;358:920-928.

CASE 15-1

One-Day-Old Girl

STACEY R. ROSE

HISTORY OF PRESENT ILLNESS

The patient is a 1-day-old girl in the newborn nursery. The baby was born the previous night at term by vaginal delivery. This morning, the nurses noted that she appeared jaundiced. She has some nasal congestion since birth but is otherwise doing well. She is bottle-feeding, taking 1-2 oz of formula every 2-3 hours with normal urine and stool patterns. She is afebrile.

MEDICAL HISTORY

The baby was born at 37 2/7 weeks by a precipitous vaginal delivery to a 20-year-old G5P3 mother. Apgar

scores at 1 and 5 minutes were 9 and 9, respectively. The patient's mother did not receive any prenatal care and all prenatal laboratories are unknown, except for her blood type which is A+. There were no known complications during pregnancy. Since the delivery was precipitous, she did not receive antibiotics prior to giving birth. She was afebrile at delivery and rupture of membranes occurred 4 hours prior.

PHYSICAL EXAMINATION

T 36.7°C; HR 146 bpm; RR 42/min; BP 89/46 mmHg; Pulse oximetry 100%; Weight 2.77 kg (10th percentile); Length 47 cm (10th percentile); Head Circumference 32 cm (5th percentile)

The patient is awake and alert. On HEENT examination, she has a flat, open anterior fontanelle, scleral icterus, and clear rhinorrhea. Her cardiac and lung examinations are within normal limits. Abdominal examination reveals a liver edge palpable 3 cm below the costal margin and a spleen palpable 1 cm below the costal margin. Her abdomen is otherwise soft, nontender, and nondistended with normoactive bowel sounds. The skin examination is significant for jaundice and erythematous peeling skin at her palms and soles but no other rash or petechiae. She has prominent axillary lymphadenopathy. While examining her extremities, she becomes irritable during palpation of her right arm and that she has little spontaneous movement of her arms or legs. However, there is no swelling or bruising along the extremities and she has full range of motion of all joints.

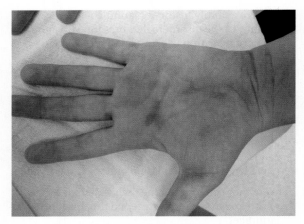

FIGURE 15-1. Rash on the hands of the patient's mother.

DIAGNOSTIC STUDIES

Complete blood count: WBCs, 29 000/mm³ (neutrophils 37%, bands 15%, lymphocytes 37%); hemoglobin, 12.7 g/dL; platelets, 48 000/mm³. Serum electrolytes: sodium, 136 mEq/L; potassium, 3.5 mEq/L; chloride, 105 mEq/L; bicarbonate, 22 mEq/L; blood urea nitrogen, 20 mg/dL; creatinine, 0.7 mg/dL; glucose, 72 mg/dL; calcium, 9.6 mg/dL. Liver function tests: total bilirubin, 4.1 mg/dL; direct bilirubin, 1.1 mg/dL; total protein, 7.1 mg/dL; albumin, 3.5 mg/dL; AST, 14 U/L; ALT, 47 U/L; alkaline phosphatase, 316 U/L.

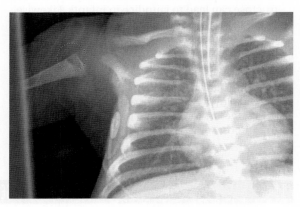

FIGURE 15-2. There are areas of metaphyseal lucency in the proximal humerus.

COURSE OF ILLNESS

During the assessment, a rash noted on the mothers hands strongly suggested the infant's diagnosis (Figure 15-1). Radiographs of the infant's humerus (Figure 15-2) and femur (Figure 15-3) were also consistent with the diagnosis. The infant was admitted to the neonatal intensive care unit for additional diagnostic testing and treatment.

DISCUSSION CASE 15-1

DIFFERENTIAL DIAGNOSIS

The patient had an unconjugated hyperbilirubinemia with otherwise normal liver function

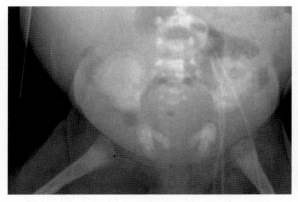

FIGURE 15-3. There are areas of metaphyseal lucency in the proximal femur.

tests. While many term infants develop physiologic jaundice within the first 24 hours of life, the presence of hepatosplenomegaly and thrombocytopenia should raise immediate concern for a pathologic process. Jaundice, hepatomegaly, and splenomegaly may be caused by congenital infections, often referred to as the TORCH infections; these infections can be acquired either in utero or during birth (Table 15-2). Given the lack of prenatal care, this patient is at particular risk for some of these conditions such as syphilis, HIV, and viral hepatitis. Sepsis and urinary tract infections can also cause an unconjugated hyperbilirubinemia, hepatomegaly, and thrombocytopenia and should be considered. Since the patient did not have a conjugated hyperbilirubinemia, anatomical or obstructive causes of hepatosplenomegaly, like biliary atresia, and metabolic processes, such as galactosemia, are less likely.

DIAGNOSIS

The mothers' hand revealed a pink, elliptical macules (Figure 15-1); the central area was darker than the periphery, which blended into the surrounding skin. The reddish hue, due to localized hyperemia, is characteristic of early secondary syphilis. Laboratory testing was significant for an RPR of 1:8 in the mother and 1:64 in the baby. These positive tests were confirmed with a positive *Treponema pallidum* particle agglutination (TP-PA) assay. The infant received a lumbar puncture to evaluate for neurosyphilis. CSF protein and cell count were normal and CSF Venereal Disease Research Laboratory (VDRL) test was 1:8. She had a liver ultrasound that showed a homogenous enlarged liver and spleen with a normal gallbladder. The chest radiograph was normal. However, long-bone radiographs revealed metaphyseal lucencies involving the proximal humerus (Figure 15-2) and femur (Figure 15-3) that were consistent with the diagnosis of congenital syphilis. Testing for other TORCH infections as well as hepatitis B and C and HIV was negative. Given the presence of a positive RPR and TP-PA in both the mother and baby, in conjunction with the clinical findings of lymphadenopathy, jaundice, hepatosplenomegaly, and metaphyseal dystrophy, the patient was diagnosed with **congenital syphilis**.

INCIDENCE AND EPIDEMIOLOGY

Syphilis is a sexually transmitted infection caused by the spirochete *Treponema pallidum*. Syphilis in children may be either acquired, usually due to sexual abuse, or congenital, resulting from transplacental transmission of the organism from an infected mother to her child. Rates of fetal transmission may occur at any stage of the disease and at any time during pregnancy but are highest when the mother is in the first and second stages

TABLE 15-2.	**TORCH infections.**
Infectious Agent	*Neonatal Clinical Manifestations*
Toxoplasma gondi	Chorioretinitis, hydrocephalus, intracranial calcifications, jaundice, hepatosplenomegaly, maculopapular rash, fever; often asymptomatic at birth
Syphilis (*Treponema pallidum*)	Rash, hepatosplenomegaly, jaundice, anemia, thrombocytopenia, snuffles, metaphyseal dystrophy, periostitis; may be asymptomatic at birth
Rubella	IUGR, deafness, cataracts, cardiac abnormalities, "blueberry muffin" rash, hepatosplenomegaly, jaundice, thrombocytopenia, microcephaly
Cytomegalovirus (CMV)	Deafness, IUGR, jaundice, hepatosplenomegaly, "blueberry muffin" rash, petechiae, anemia, thrombocytopenia, sepsis, periventricular calcifications, chorioretinitis, microcephaly; often asymptomatic at birth
Herpes Simplex Virus (HSV)	Skin, eyes, mouth disease— localized vesicular lesions CNS disease—lethargy, poor feeding, encephalitis, seizures Disseminated disease— multiorgan involvement— jaundice, hepatitis, DIC, hypotension, apnea
Human Immunodeficiency Virus (HIV)	Hepatosplenomegaly, failure to thrive, lymphadenopathy, recurrent infections, neurologic abnormalities; often asymptomatic at birth

of syphilis (60% to 90%) and lowest in late latent syphilis (<10%).

Rates of congenital syphilis parallel rates of syphilis in the adult population. There was a steep rise in the incidence of syphilis throughout the 1980s with a peak in congenital syphilis cases in 1991. Due in large part to enhanced screening, improved education for providers and increased awareness in communities with high rates of infection, syphilis rates fell precipitously through the 1990s, reaching a nadir in 2000, increasing again until 2008 with a slight decrease between 2009 and 2011. In 2011, there were 8.5 cases of congenital syphilis per 100 000 live births, resulting in 360 reported cases of congenital syphilis. Three states (Texas, California, and Florida) accounted for nearly one-half of all cases of congenital syphilis. Maternal risk factors associated with congenital syphilis include lack of, or poor prenatal care, unprotected sexual contact, trading of sex for drugs and cocaine abuse.

TABLE 15.3.	Clinical manifestations of congenital syphilis.
Early Disease	**Late Disease**
• Hepatosplenomegaly • Jaundice • Thrombocytopenia • Mucocutaneous rash, often involving the palms and soles • Condylomatous lesions • "Snuffles" (rhinitis) • Radiographic changes— periostitis and metaphyseal dystrophy • Osteochondritis and pseudoparalysis • Lymphadenopathy • Failure to thrive • Chorioretinitis • Renal abnormalities	• Prominence of forehead ("Olympian brow") • Scaphoid scapula • Tibial bowing ("saber shins") • Peg-shaped, notched teeth ("Hutchinson teeth") • Mulberry molars • Saddle nose • Rhagades (linear scars) • Painless arthritis of knees ("Clutton joints") • Interstitial keratitis (which may lead to blindness) • Eighth cranial nerve deafness • Juvenile paresis • Juvenile tabes

CLINICAL PRESENTATION

Transmission of syphilis during pregnancy can result in fetal or perinatal death, hydrops fetalis, intrauterine growth retardation, prematurity, or congenital abnormalities, which may occur early or late. Infants may be asymptomatic at birth but signs of early congenital syphilis usually present within the first few weeks of life. Late congenital syphilis results from chronic inflammation involving the bones, teeth, and CNS and appears after 2 years of age (Table 15-3).

The infant displayed many of the clinical features consistent with early congenital syphilis, including jaundice, hepatosplenomegaly, thrombocytopenia, rash, "snuffles," pseudoparalysis, and metaphyseal dystrophy of the humerus and femur.

DIAGNOSTIC APPROACH

Darkfield microscopy. Identification of spirochetes from moist lesions by darkfield microscopy is the quickest and most definitive way to diagnosis syphilis. However, this method requires special equipment, reagents, and trained personnel that may not be available in all clinical settings. As a result, serologic testing is much more widely used.

Treponemal and nontreponemal serologic testing. Two forms of serologic testing are available; nontreponemal and treponemal tests. Because each of these tests has several limitations with significant false-positive and false-negative result rates, a combination of tests is needed to establish the diagnosis of syphilis. Generally, a nontreponemal test, such as a VDRL or rapid plasma reagin (RPR), is used to screen for the disease and to follow response to treatment. If either of these tests is reactive, a confirmatory treponemal test, such as the fluorescent treponemal antibody absorption (FTA-ABS) or *T pallidum* particle agglutination (TP-PA), is performed.

Since maternal antibody may be passively transmitted to the fetus even after adequate treatment of syphilis in the mother, interpretation of serologic testing in the infant may be difficult. As in this case, congenital syphilis is confirmed when the infant's nontreponemal titers are at least four times greater than those of the mother. However, infants with titers less than fourfold their mothers' values may still be diagnosed with congenital syphilis based on the presence of other features. These include certain physical examination findings, serum and CSF laboratory values, radiologic studies, the presence of treponemes in the umbilical cord or placenta, and the treatment status of the mother. Given the complex algorithm used to diagnose and treat syphilis, please refer to the Centers for Disease Control and Prevention or the American Academy of Pediatrics for specific diagnostic and treatment algorithms and additional information.

Additional testing. The serologic status of the mother must be established before any newborn infant is discharged from the hospital. If maternal screening is positive and inadequately treated or untreated syphilis is suspected, or if the baby has any signs of congenital syphilis, the infant should undergo a (1) complete physical examination; (2) quantitative serum nontreponemal test; (3) complete blood count, including platelet count; (4) lumbar puncture with testing for CSF cell count, protein concentration, and a VDRL of the CSF; and (5) long-bone radiographs. Among infected infants, the CSF is abnormal in 50% of those with symptoms and 10% of those without symptoms. Additional testing such as a chest radiograph, liver function tests, ultrasonography, ophthalmologic examination and auditory brainstem response testing should be considered in the appropriate clinical setting. Infants evaluated for congenital syphilis should also be evaluated for other congenital infections.

TREATMENT

Infants with proven or highly probably congenital syphilis should be treated with aqueous crystalline penicillin G or penicillin G procaine for 10 days.

Nontreponemal titers should be followed closely to monitor response to treatment. If the initial CSF examination is abnormal, repeat lumbar punctures are recommended every 6 months until values normalize. Treatment failures are uncommon but treatment with an additional 10-day course of penicillin may be necessary if serum nontreponemal titers continue to rise or remain elevated, or, if the CSF evaluation remains abnormal. Infants with congenital syphilis should be examined and have quantitative nontreponemal tests every 2-3 months until nonreactivity is documented.

SUGGESTED READINGS

1. Azimi P. Syphilis (Treponema pallidum). In: Behrman RE, Kliegman RM, Arvin AR, eds. *Nelson's Textbook of Pediatrics*. 17th ed. Philadelphia, PA: WB Saunders Co.; 2004:978-982.
2. Centers for Disease Control and Prevention: 2011 sexually transmitted diseases surveillance. http://www.cdc.gov/std/stats11/syphilis.htm. Updated December 13, 2012. Accessed December 26, 2012.
3. Hyman EL: Syphilis. *Pediat Rev*. 2006;27:37-39.
4. Johnson KE. Overview of TORCH infections. UpToDate. www.uptodate.com/content/overview-of-torch-infections. Updated March 15, 2011. Accessed September 29, 2011.
5. Michelow IC, Wendel GD, Norgard MV, et al. Central nervous system infection in congenital syphilis. *New Eng J Med*. 2002;346:1792-1798.
6. American Academy of Pediatrics. Syphilis. In: Pickering LK, Baker CJ, Long SS, McMillan JA, eds. *Red Book: 2009 Report of the Committee on Infectious Diseases*. 28th ed. Elk Grove Village, IL: American Academy of Pediatrics; 2009:638-651.

CASE 15-2

Six-Week-Old Boy

STACEY R. ROSE

HISTORY OF PRESENT ILLNESS

A 6-week-old full-term boy was referred by his pediatrician for persistent jaundice and poor weight gain. The infant was seen by his pediatrician during the first week of life after the mother noted that he "looked yellow." At that time, he was otherwise doing well and the pediatrician diagnosed physiologic jaundice. He was brought to the pediatrician today for a well visit and it was noted that the patient was still jaundiced. Additionally, the patient has not gained any weight since his first visit at week 1 of life.

The infant is being fed a cow milk-based formula. The patient's mother reports that he has frequent episodes of emesis. She also reports that the infant has been increasingly fussy during feeds. She denies that the infant has had any diarrhea, fever, bleeding, or bruising.

MEDICAL HISTORY

The infant was born at 38 weeks gestation by vacuum-assisted vaginal delivery. His birth weight was 3.2 kg. Maternal prenatal labs were normal. His hospital stay was unremarkable and he was discharged home with her mother on his second day of life.

The infant has a healthy 3-year-old brother. There was no family history of jaundice, liver disease, anemia, or familial blood disorders.

PHYSICAL EXAMINATION

T 37.0°C; HR 136 bpm; RR 32/min; BP 88/60 mmHg; Weight 3.25 kg (<5th percentile); Length 52 cm (10th-25th percentile); Head Circumference 37 cm (10th-25th percentile)

On examination, the patient was fussy but consolable by his mother. He was jaundiced with an open, flat fontanelle. He did not have any dysmorphic features. Scleral icterus was present. The lung and cardiac examinations were normal. His abdomen was soft and nondistended with normoactive bowel sounds. A smooth, firm liver edge was palpable 2 cm below the costal margin. Additionally, there was a 4 cm soft, mobile nontender mass noted in the right upper quadrant. The genitourinary, extremity, and neurologic examinations were all normal.

DIAGNOSTIC STUDIES

Complete blood count: WBC, 6900/mm³ (neutrophils: 43%, lymphocytes: 48%); hemoglobin, 11.2 g/dL; platelets, 332 000/mm³. Liver function tests: total bilirubin, 9.5 mg/dL; direct bilirubin; 8.4 mg/dL; albumin, 3.2 mg/dL; ALT, 167 U/L; AST, 188 U/L; alkaline phosphatase, 641 U/L; gamma glutamyl transferase, 524 U/L. Serum electrolytes: normal. Urinalysis: normal.

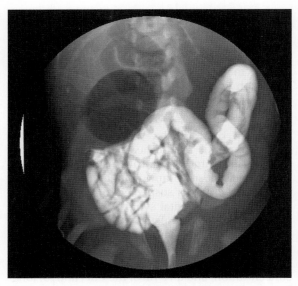

FIGURE 15-4. Gastrointestinal contrast series reveals a large lucent structure in the right upper quadrant with compression of the transverse colon.

COURSE OF ILLNESS

The patient underwent several imaging studies and was admitted for urgent evaluation of his abdominal mass and cholestatic jaundice. A contrast gastrointestinal series suggested the diagnosis (Figure 15-4).

DISCUSSION CASE 15-2

DIFFERENTIAL DIAGNOSIS

The presence of an abdominal mass requires urgent evaluation. Most abdominal masses in the neonatal period are renal in origin and include hydronephrosis, multicystic dysplastic kidneys, polycystic kidneys, or Wilm tumor. Other common causes include neuroblastomas, hepatomas, choledochal cysts, GI duplication cysts, pyloric stenosis (the "olive" of pyloric hypertrophy), ovarian cysts, or teratomas. Because this patient's mass was soft and mobile, it is most consistent with a nonretroperitoneal cystic structure.

TABLE 15-4.	**Causes of cholestatic jaundice in the neonate.**		
Obstructive	*Infectious*	*Metabolic*	*Iatrogenic/Other*
• Biliary atresia	• TORCH infections	• Alpha-1 antitrypsin disease	• Neonatal hepatitis
• Choledochal cyst	• Sepsis	• Hypothyroidism	• TPN
• Cholelithiasis	• UTI	• Galactosemia	• Intestinal obstruction
• Paucity of intrahepatic bile ducts (Alagille)		• Tyrosinemia	
		• Cystic fibrosis	
		• Neonatal hemochromatosis	
		• Zellweger syndrome	
		• Citrin deficiency	

Additionally, the patient has a persistent conjugated hyperbilirubinemia with elevations in alkaline phosphatase and gamma-glutamyl transferase consistent with neonatal cholestasis, a condition that results from accumulation of bile components in the blood due to impaired bile flow or excretion. There are a wide variety of causes, several of which require immediate intervention and hence prompt diagnosis and treatment are crucial.

Causes of neonatal cholestasis may be subdivided into various categories. Obstructive causes include biliary atresia, choledochal cyst, cholelithiasis, and paucity of intrahepatic bile ducts (Alagille syndrome). Though less common, some of the abdominal masses listed above, such as neuroblastomas, teratomas, or GI duplication cysts, can also cause cholestasis by compressing the biliary tree. Infectious, metabolic, or iatrogenic conditions may also be present, as outlined below (Table 15-4).

DIAGNOSIS

The patient had an abdominal ultrasound to assess the mass and hepatomegaly which revealed a 3.8 cm × 1.9 cm × 2.5 cm cystic structure inferior to the liver and adjacent to the right kidney, consistent with a **choledochal cyst**. Ultrasound also revealed a mildly enlarged liver and normal gallbladder. He had a hepatobiliary scan that failed to show tracer excretion into the small intestine. The gastrointestinal series showed a cystic structure in the right upper quadrant compressing the transverse colon (Figure 15-4). The structure was later identified as a choledochal cyst.

INCIDENCE AND ETIOLOGY

Choledochal, or biliary, cysts are cystic dilations in the biliary tree involving both intrahepatic and extrahepatic structures. They are a rare disorder, with an estimated incidence of 1:13 000 to 1 in 2 million. There is a 3:1 girl to boy predominance and some reports of familial occurrence. Incidence is highest in Asian countries, particularly Japan where more than half of the reported cases arise. Most cysts are thought to be congenital but some may be acquired. The pathophysiology remains unclear but leading theories suggest that they form due to the reflux of pancreatic enzymes into the common bile duct, which causes inflammation, weakness, and dilation of the duct. Other theories suggest an infectious cause related to fetal viral infection or abnormal in utero proliferation of biliary epithelial cells.

Biliary cysts have been divided into five subtypes (Table 15-5). Type I and IV cysts are the most common.

TABLE 15-5.	**Todani classification of biliary cysts.**
Type	*Features*
Type I	Dilatation of the common bile duct (most common)
Type II	Diverticulum of extrahepatic bile duct (rarest subtype)
Type III	Choledochocele—dilatation of intraduodenal portion of common bile duct
Type IV IV A IV B	Multiple cysts Intrahepatic and extrahepatic cysts Extrahepatic cysts only
Type V	Caroli disease—one or more intrahepatic biliary cysts

CLINICAL PRESENTATION

While choledochal cysts are most commonly seen in infants and children; an increasing number of patients are now diagnosed in adulthood. The classic pediatric presentation is a triad of abdominal pain, jaundice, and a palpable mass, though few patients present with all three symptoms in practice. Other common features in infants include failure to thrive, vomiting, and fever. Symptoms differ in older children and adults. An abdominal mass is rare and instead, many present with recurrent cholangitis, intermittent jaundice, and pancreatitis. If undetected, severe liver dysfunction, ascites, and coagulopathy may develop. Furthermore, there is a strong association between choledochal cysts and biliary malignancy, particularly in adult patients.

DIAGNOSTIC APPROACH

Abdominal ultrasound. Abdominal ultrasound is very effective in diagnosing choledochal cysts, particularly in infants or children and in adults if there is a high index of suspicion. Many cysts are now detected by prenatal ultrasound.

Direct cholangiography. The best method for definitive diagnosis of choledochal cyst or for delineating the precise cyst type and anatomy is by magnetic resonance cholangiopancreatography (MRCP) which has largely supplanted endoscopic retrograde cholangiopancreatography (ERCP) as the diagnostic test of choice because MRCP offers higher resolution of relevant anatomy. Less commonly used diagnostic options include percutaneous transhepatic cholangiography and intraoperative cholangiography. These techniques allow direct visualization of the involved biliary structures and help identify the presence of an anomalous pancreaticobiliary junction.

Other modalities. CT scanning may be used to delineate the cyst and its relationship to surrounding structures. Gastrointestinal contrast series, though performed in this case, are no longer routinely performed to diagnose choledochal cysts.

TREATMENT

The preferred treatment is surgical excision of the cyst and a roux-en-Y choledochojejunostomy. Complications from untreated cysts include recurrent cholangitis, pancreatitis, and biliary malignancy.

The infant was taken immediately to the operating room where he underwent direct cholangiography that revealed a choledochal cyst with dilation of the intrahepatic bile ducts and passage of contrast into the duodenum. The cyst was resected and a roux-en-Y hepatic jejunostomy was performed. The patient initially required parenteral nutrition but enteral feeds were slowly reintroduced as he recovered. One week after surgery, he was tolerating full feeds. His conjugated hyperbilirubinemia gradually improved and his direct bilirubin at the time of discharge had decreased to 2.6 mg/dL.

SUGGESTED READINGS

1. Lipsett PA, Pitt HA, Colombani PM, et al. Choledochal cyst disease: A changing pattern of presentation. *Ann Surg.* 1994;220:644-652.
2. Lipsett PA, Henry AP. Surgical treatment of choledochal cysts. *J Hepatobiliary Pancreat Sci.* 2003;10:352-359.
3. Suchy FJ. Cystic diseases of the biliary tract and liver. In: Behrman RE, Kliegman RM, Arvin AR, eds. *Nelson's Textbook of Pediatrics.* 17th ed. Philadelphia, PA: WB Saunders Co.; 2004:1343-1345.
4. Topazian M. Biliary cysts. UpToDate. http://www.uptodate.com/contents/biliary-cysts. Updated September 24, 2010. Accessed September 1, 2010.

CASE 15-3

Eight-Year-Old Girl

STACEY R. ROSE

HISTORY OF PRESENT ILLNESS

An 8-year-old girl presents with history of 2 days of headache, abdominal pain, vomiting, diarrhea, and 1 day of fever. Two days prior to admission, the patient developed a frontal headache that was relieved with acetaminophen. Shortly after, she started to complain of bilateral lower abdominal pain that soon spread to her left upper quadrant. The abdominal pain became more severe throughout the day and woke her from sleep. Overnight, she started having episodes of nonbloody, nonbilious emesis and nonbloody watery diarrhea. On the day of admission, she developed fever to 104°F and her parents noted that her eyes looked yellow so they brought her to the emergency room for evaluation.

The patient also reports recent fatigue and occasional chills but denies cough, rhinorrhea, congestion, sore throat, neck stiffness, joint pain, myalgias, or rash.

MEDICAL HISTORY

The patient was a full-term baby born in Malaysia with no complications. She moved to the U.S. at the age of 5 months. She has always been well and has had no prior hospitalizations or surgical procedures. She is up-to-date on all immunizations. She does not have any known allergies and was not taking any medications recently, other than acetaminophen for the headache. There is no family history of sickle cell disease, bleeding disorders, or liver disease. She lives at home with her parents and younger brother and is in second grade. The patient and her family report that they recently traveled to Pakistan to visit grandparents. They spent about 6 months there and returned about 2 weeks prior. They did not receive any specific vaccinations or medications prior to or during their travel.

PHYSICAL EXAMINATION

T 38.9°C; HR 96 bpm; RR 18/min; BP 97/65 mmHg; Weight 27.2 kg (50th-75th percentile)

On physical examination, the patient was awake, alert, smiling, and in no significant distress. HEENT examination was significant for mild scleral icterus and conjunctival pallor. Her oropharynx was clear, her neck was supple, and she had no cervical lymphadenopathy. Her lungs were clear to auscultation bilaterally. Cardiac examination revealed a regular rate and rhythm with a II/VI systolic ejection murmur at the right upper sternal border. On abdominal examination she was found to have a soft abdomen with normoactive bowel sounds. She was diffusely tender to palpation without guarding or rebound. Her liver was palpable about 2 cm below the costal margin and she had splenomegaly with the tip palpable about 3 cm below the left costal margin. The remainder of her examination was within normal limits.

DIAGNOSTIC STUDIES

Complete blood count: WBCs, 5800/mm^3 (neutrophils: 43%, lymphocytes: 45%, eosinophils: 5%); hemoglobin, 7.8 g/dL; mean corpuscular volume, 81.3 fL; platelets, 192 000/mm^3. Serum electrolytes: sodium, 140 mEq/L; potassium, 3.2 mEq/L; chloride, 103 mEq/L; bicarbonate, 19 mEq/L; blood urea nitrogen, 14 mg/dL; creatinine, 0.6 mg/dL; glucose, 112 mg/dL. Liver function tests: total bilirubin, 3.5 mg/dL; unconjugated bilirubin, 3.4 mg/dL; conjugated, 0.1 mg/dL; albumin, 4.4 mg/dL; ALT, 71 U/L; AST, 80 U/L; alkaline phosphatase, 240 U/L; GGT, 75 U/L. LDH, 410 U/L (elevated). Reticulocyte count, 3.1%. Urinalysis, small bilirubin, negative for RBCs or WBCs. CRP, 3.8 mg/dL; ESR, 98 mm/h; PT, 14.3 sec; PTT, 29.3 sec; INR, 1.22.

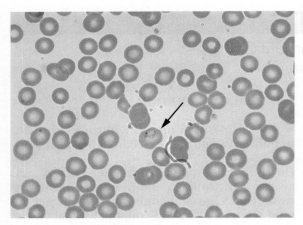

FIGURE 15-5. Blood smear.

COURSE OF ILLNESS

The patient was admitted to the hospital where a blood smear revealed the diagnosis (Figure 15-5).

DISCUSSION CASE 15-3

DIFFERENTIAL DIAGNOSIS

The patient has an unconjugated hyperbilirubinemia associated with splenomegaly, anemia, an elevated lactate dehydrogenase (LDH), and a reticulocytosis. These findings are consistent with hemolysis, which is the likely cause of jaundice in this patient. The presence of an underlying hemoglobinopathy, such as sickle cell disease, thalassemia, hereditary spherocytosis, or G6PD deficiency in the face of a viral or other infectious stressor, may precipitate an episode of hemolysis. Most of these conditions are detected by newborn screening but some may go undetected until late childhood or adulthood, particularly in this patient since she was born outside the United States and may not have had newborn screening. Other causes of hemolysis include autoimmune processes, drug reactions, transfusion reactions, hemolytic-uremic syndrome, sepsis with disseminated intravascular coagulation (DIC), and other infections.

In addition to hemolysis, the patient had hepatomegaly and mild elevations in transaminases, suggesting that hepatocellular injury may also be

TABLE 15-6.	Viral causes of hepatitis.

Common Viral Causes of Hepatitis

EBV
CMV
HSV
HHV-6
Adenovirus
Enterovirus
Influenza
HIV
Hepatitis A
Hepatitis B
Hepatitis C
Hepatitis D
Hepatitis E

contributing to the patient's jaundice. While there are various causes of hepatitis in this age group, the acute onset of symptoms and the presence of fever point to an infectious etiology. Viruses are seen very frequently and the most common of the extensive list of possible pathogens are listed below. Acute viral hepatitis is often accompanied by flu-like systemic symptoms such as headache, vomiting, and diarrhea seen in the patient (Table 15-6).

The differential diagnosis in this case must be expanded even further since the patient recently returned from international travel. Table 15-7 lists the most common illnesses seen in patients presenting with fever after international travel and their associated symptoms. Of these, malaria is the most common and should be considered in all travelers returning from malaria-infested regions with fever. Because the patient spent 6 months in an area with a high prevalence of malaria, she is at significant risk for having contracted the disease. Her presenting symptoms of fever, headache, abdominal pain, vomiting, and diarrhea are all consistent with a diagnosis of malaria. Furthermore, malaria is associated with red blood cell destruction, resulting in hepatosplenomegaly and jaundice, as seen in the patient (Table 15-7).

DIAGNOSIS

The patient had PCR testing for serum EBV, CMV, and adenovirus that were negative. She had titers for hepatitis A and B that were consistent with prior immunization and for hepatitis C that were negative. She had a G6PD assay that was normal.

TABLE 15-7.	Common causes of fever in the returned traveler.		
Diagnosis	*Area of Acquisition*	*Timing of Onset*	*Presenting Symptoms*
Malaria	Africa, Caribbean, Central America, South America, South Asia, SE Asia, Oceania	1 week to several months	Fever, headache, fatigue, chills, myalgias, vomiting, diarrhea
Dengue	Africa, Caribbean, Central America, South America, South Asia, SE Asia, Australia	<1 week	Fever, rash, headache, myalgias, retro-orbital pain, vomiting
Mononucleosis (CMV or EBV)	Worldwide		Fever, pharyngitis, lymphadenopathy, fatigue
Rickettsial Disease (species vary)	Worldwide	2 days to several weeks	Fever, headache, myalgias, rash respiratory symptoms, lymphadenopathy
Typhoid Fever (Salmonella typhi or paratyphi)	Africa, Caribbean, Central America, South America, South Asia, SE Asia	1 week to 2 months	Fever, abdominal pain, rose spots, hepatosplenomegaly, mental status changes, diarrhea, or constipation
Hepatitis A	Worldwide	2 weeks to 2 months	Fever, vomiting, diarrhea, abdominal pain, jaundice
Leptospirosis	Tropical areas	2 days to 1 month	Fever, conjunctiva suffusion, headache, myalgias, rash
Schistosomiasis	Africa, Asia, Latin America	4-8 weeks	Dermatitis ("swimmer's itch") then fever, myalgias, abdominal pain, headache, diarrhea, lymphadenopathy, hepatosplenomegaly, hematuria
Amebic Liver Disease (*Entamoeba histolytica*)	Developing nations	Weeks to months	Fever, abdominal pain, diarrhea

Thick and thin blood smears were sent to pathology for review. They revealed **malaria** with a parasitemia of 2.8 %. The blood smear below demonstrates a red blood cell with a central ring form that was later identified as *Plasmodium vivax* (Figure 15-5, arrow).

INCIDENCE AND EPIDEMIOLOGY

Malaria is caused by the parasite *Plasmodium*, a protozoan transmitted to humans through the bite of the *Anopheles* mosquito. Four species of *Plasmodium* cause human disease: *P. falciparum, P. vivax, P. ovale,* and *P. malariae,* but most infections are due to *P. falciparum* or *P. vivax.* Only *P. falciparum* causes cerebral malaria and it is the species responsible for most malaria-related deaths.

Worldwide, it is estimated that there are 200-500 million cases of malaria per year and approximately 1 million deaths, most of which occur in young children. The vast majority of cases are in developing nations with the highest prevalence found in tropical and subtropical regions, such as sub-Saharan Africa and South Asia. Though malaria is not endemic in the United States, there are roughly 1100-1500 reported annual cases. Most US cases are imported either by immigrants or travelers returning from malaria-endemic regions (Figure 15-6).

Disease occurs after the female *Anopheles* mosquito injects sporozoites into the human bloodstream during a blood meal. These travel to the liver where they mature into schizonts which rupture and release merozoites. Merozoites enter the bloodstream, invade red blood cells (RBCs), and mature into ring-forms known as trophozoites and later into schizonts. During the next 48-72 hours the schizonts rupture, releasing merozoites into the bloodstream and destroying the RBC. Anemia results as more merozoites are released and more RBCs are destroyed. Additionally, the release of

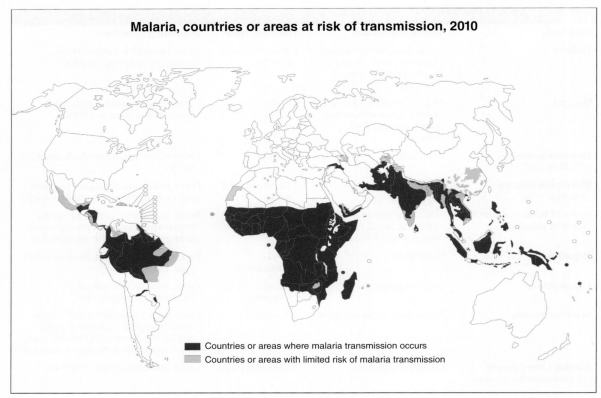

FIGURE 15-6. Global distribution of malaria. *(Reproduced, with permission, from World: Malaria risk areas, 2010. World Health Organization. Published 2011. http://gamapserver.who.int/ mapLibrary/Files/Maps/Global_Malaria_2010.png Accessed April 15, 2013.)* This map is intended as a visual aid only and not as a definitive source of information about malaria endemicity. Source: © WHO 2011. All rights reserved.

merozoites triggers a proinflammatory response with cytokines, such as TNF-alpha, causing fever and systemic symptoms. The diagram below illustrates the various phases of the Plasmodium life cycle (Figure 15-7).

CLINICAL PRESENTATION

Symptoms only occur during the erythrocyte phase of the life cycle, when merozoites are released and RBCs are destroyed. Until then, there is an asymptomatic incubation period which may last from several days to months. On average, the incubation period for *P. falciparum* infections is 9-14 days and 12-17 days for *P. vivax*. Symptoms often begin as a

flu-like prodrome consisting of headache, myalgias, fatigue, diarrhea, and abdominal pain, similar to those seen in the patient. Patients then develop high fevers which classically occur every 48 hours (*P. falciparum, P. vivax,* and *P. ovale*) or every 72 hours (*P. malariae*) in conjunction with the release of the merozoites from the RBCs. However, in practice, these paroxysms of fever may be irregular. Other symptoms include nausea, vomiting, chills, sweats, and cough. As hemolysis progresses, patients develop jaundice and anemia. Hepatosplenomegaly and thrombocytopenia (due to splenic sequestration) may also occur and splenic rupture is possible.

Most cases of malaria are uncomplicated. However some patients develop severe disease, defined

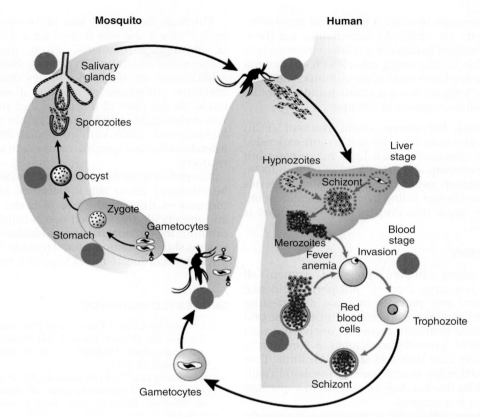

FIGURE 15-7. Plasmodium life cycle. *(Reproduced, with permission, from Shah SS,* Pediatric Practice: Infectious Disease, *New York: McGraw-Hill, 2009.)*

as parasitemia greater than 5%, severe anemia, cerebral involvement, or end-organ dysfunction. Almost all cases of severe disease are due to infection with *P. falciparum* which has several unique characteristics. Unlike the other species of malaria which only invade red blood cells at a particular stage (immature for *P. vivax* and *P. ovale* and mature for *P. malariae*), *P. falciparum* infects RBCs at every stage, resulting in higher levels of parasitemia and more severe anemia. *P. falciparum* is also the only species associated with cerebral malaria which may lead to seizures, coma, or death. Additionally, *P. falciparum* can cause microvascular changes that may lead to acute renal failure and other end organ damage. Other severe complications of malaria include respiratory distress,

hypoglycemia, acidosis, splenic rupture, congenital malaria infection, and death.

DIAGNOSTIC APPROACH

Thick and thin blood smears. Diagnosis of malaria is made through light microscopy of Giemsa-stained thick and thin blood smears. Thick smears are useful in establishing the presence and degree of parasitemia and the thin smears aid in species identification. A negative smear does not exclude a diagnosis of malaria. Due to the cyclic nature of disease, smears should be repeated at 6-, 12-, or 24-hour intervals for the first 48 hours to establish the diagnosis and to follow the density of parasitemia.

Rapid diagnostic testing. A number of rapid diagnostic tests are available. Sensitivities for these tests are highest in detecting *P. falciparum* and are less reliable in diagnosing other species of malaria and detecting lower rates of parasitemia. Additionally, these tests are not quantitative and cannot be used to follow response to therapy.

PCR testing. Polymerase chain reaction (PCR) testing is also available. This test is more expensive and time-consuming than light microscopy but have a sensitivity and specificity of almost 100%. It is particularly useful in detecting very low levels of parasitemia and aiding in species identification, especially when infection by multiple species is suspected.

TREATMENT

Infants, young children, pregnant women, all patients returning from *P. falciparum*-endemic regions and any patients that are ill-appearing should be hospitalized and started on either an oral or parenteral treatment regimen. Any patient with symptoms of severe disease should be admitted to an intensive care unit and started on immediate parenteral therapy. In most cases, consultation with an infectious disease expert or referral to a specialty care center is warranted.

Recommendations for treatment are constantly evolving and vary by species and resistance patterns in the area of disease acquisition. The CDC offers a 24-hour Malaria Hotline (770-488-7788 or 770-488-7100) to assist providers with malaria management. In general, cases of uncomplicated nonfalciparum malaria may be treated with chloroquine. However, there is increasing chloroquine-resistant *P. vivax*, particularly in Indonesia and Papua New Guinea, requiring alternate treatment regimens. Primaquine is often used to prevent relapses in patients with *P. vivax* or *P. ovale*. Chloroquine resistance among *P. falciparum* is so widespread, that almost all cases should be considered resistant. Patients returning from *P. falciparum*-endemic regions should start on an alternate regimen. Several options exist, each with similar efficacy. These include atovaquone-proguanil, quinidine plus doxycycline or clindamycin, artemether-lumefantrine, or mefloquine.

Although the patient was ultimately found to have *P. vivax*, she was started on a 3-day course of atovaquone-proguanil, given the growing chloroquine-resistance in Papua New Guinea. Additionally, she received a 14-day course of primaquine phosphate to prevent disease recurrence. At the time of discharge, her parasitemia was undetectable and her hemoglobin was stable. She followed closely with her pediatrician and an infectious disease specialist and made a complete recovery.

Prevention is the best treatment. Travelers should be educated about the importance of avoiding mosquitoes through the use of insect repellents and insecticide-treated bed nets. Furthermore, all nonimmune patients traveling to malaria-endemic regions should be administered malaria chemoprophylaxis according to the CDC guidelines.

SUGGESTED READINGS

1. Centers for Disease Control and Prevention: Malaria. Centers for Disease Control and Prevention. www.cdc.gov/malaria. Updated August 19, 2011. Accessed September 29, 2011.
2. Freedman DO, Weld LH, Kozarsky PE, et al. Spectrum of disease and relation to place of exposure among ill returned travelers. *New Engl J Med.* 2006;354: 119-130.
3. Laurens MB, Hutter J, Laufer MK. Fever in the returned traveler. In: Shah SS, ed. *Pediatric Practice Infectious Diseases.* New York, NY: McGraw-Hill; 2009:675-686.
4. Miller LH, Baruch DI, March K, Doumbo OK. The pathogenic basis of malaria. *Nature.* 2002;415 (6872):673-679.
5. Murray CK, Gasser RA, Magill AJ, Miller RS. Update on rapid diagnostic testing for malaria. *Clin Microbiol Rev.* 2008;21:97-110.
6. Pickering LK, Baker CJ, Long SS, McMillan JA, eds. *Red Book: 2009 Report of the Committee on Infectious Diseases.* 28th ed. Elk Grove Village, IL: American Academy of Pediatrics; 2009:438-444, 797-802.
7. Ryan ET, Wilson ME, Kain KC. Illness after international travel. *New Eng J Med.* 2002;347:505-516.
8. Sam-Agudu NA, John CD. Malaria. In: Shah SS, ed. *Pediatric Practice Infectious Diseases.* New York, NY: McGraw-Hill; 2009:687-700.
9. World Health Organization. Malaria. World Health Organization. www.who.int/malaria.en. Accessed September 29, 2011.

Nine-Day-Old Boy

STACEY R. ROSE

HISTORY OF PRESENT ILLNESS

A 9-day-old term boy was transferred from a local community hospital for further evaluation and management of sepsis and hyperbilirubinemia.

The infant had been discharged home from the well-baby nursery on the fourth day of life with a bilirubin of 16.7 mg/dL. A bilirubin level 2 days later was 19.4 mg/dL and he was admitted for phototherapy. Within 24 hours of admission he developed emesis and temperature instability. A blood culture and lumbar puncture were performed and ampicillin and gentamicin were started. Additional bilirubin measurements revealed the direct fraction to be 5.2 mg/dL. An ultrasound, performed to assess hepatomegaly, revealed a nondilated biliary system, small gallbladder, and diffuse hepatic enlargement. A nuclear medicine liver scan showed normal bile excretion.

The baby continued to receive breastmilk feedings (with nasogastric tube supplementation required because of poor oral intake) until he experienced blood-tinged emesis. Coagulation studies around this time revealed the PT and PTT to be more than 50 seconds and more than 200 seconds, respectively, for which vitamin K and a dose of fresh frozen plasma were administered. By report, the baby's abdomen was soft and his stool quantity and quality were unremarkable. Transfer to a tertiary care center was arranged.

MEDICAL HISTORY

The infant was born to a 27-year-old G1P0 mother with unremarkable prenatal labs. Delivery was via cesarean section at 37 weeks because of breech presentation. The baby's birth weight was 3.04 kg. He was discharged with his mother on the fourth day of life and was breastfeeding every 3 hours.

PHYSICAL EXAMINATION

T 36.4°C; HR 140 bpm; RR 60/min; BP 83/50 mmHg; Weight 2.7 kg (5th-10th percentile)

Physical examination revealed a 9-day-old term boy who was listless but arousable. His skin demonstrated a yellow-green jaundice but no petechiae, rash, or bruising. He was nondysmorphic and normocephalic with an open, flat fontanelle; his pupils were equal, round, and reactive with red reflexes present bilaterally; mucous membranes were yellow-pink and slightly dry. He was mildly tachypneic but respirations were otherwise unlabored with clear breath sounds bilaterally. Heart examination was normal. The abdomen was soft and nondistended with a smooth, firm liver edge palpable 3 cm below the right costal margin. Examinations of the genitalia and extremities were normal. His tone, power, and primitive reflexes all appeared within normal limits.

DIAGNOSTIC STUDIES

Complete blood count: WBC count, 9400/mm^3 (neutrophils 41%, band forms 1%, lymphocytes 45%); hemoglobin, 16.0 g/dL; platelets, 66000/mm^3. PT and PTT were markedly prolonged at 50 seconds and 112 seconds, respectively. Fibrinogen, 200 mg/dL, fibrin split products were negative. Serum electrolytes: serum bicarbonate, 17 mEq/L; serum glucose, 52 mg/dL; otherwise normal. Hepatic function panel: unconjugated bilirubin, 13.1 mg/dL; conjugated bilirubin, 5.9 mg/dL; alanine aminotransferase, 115 U/L; aspartate aminotransferase, 126 U/L; alkaline phosphatase, 730 U/L; gamma-glutamyl transferase, 255 U/L; albumin, 2.0 mg/dL.

COURSE OF ILLNESS

On admission, the infant received intravenous fluids and antibiotics. In addition he required a second dose of fresh frozen plasma for treatment of his coagulopathy. A repeat liver ultrasound was consistent with the earlier study. An ophthalmology examination was unremarkable. The blood culture from the referring hospital was positive for

Escherichia coli and the baby received a full course of IV antibiotics.

Further testing revealed a specific underlying diagnosis that guided subsequent inpatient management.

DISCUSSION CASE 15-4

DIFFERENTIAL DIAGNOSIS

The differential diagnosis for the systemically ill neonate is quite broad. Given the positive blood culture in the infant, sepsis must be considered first. Sepsis can cause many of the symptoms seen in the infant, including an acidosis, conjugated hyperbilirubinemia, and liver dysfunction. It can also lead to disseminated intravascular coagulation, which should be considered as a cause of this patient's coagulopathy. However, fibrinogen and fibrin split products were normal, suggesting that the elevations in PT and PTT were more likely the result of synthetic liver dysfunction. Infectious etiologies seen in this period include bacterial (e.g., group B *Streptococcus*, staphylococci, *E. coli*, *Listeria monocytogenes*) and viral (e.g., herpes simplex virus, enterovirus) pathogens. Less often, fungi (e.g., *Candida* species) and other classes of organisms (e.g., parasites) are implicated.

Treatment of acute infection is crucial, but there are several other processes to consider when evaluating a critically ill neonate. Cardiac diseases, such as tachydysrhythmias and ductal-dependent anatomic lesions (e.g., coarctation of the aorta, hypoplastic left heart syndrome), may present early in life with profound cardiovascular compromise. Shock can also be seen in severely anemic infants following a placental catastrophe, major intracranial hemorrhage, or significant hemolysis. Multiorgan dysfunction can also result from perinatal asphyxia, neonatal surgical emergencies, and a multitude of endocrine and metabolic abnormalities, including congenital adrenal hyperplasia, glucose and electrolyte derangements, and inborn errors of metabolism.

While sepsis may account for this patient's clinical picture, given the severity of the cholestasis and liver synthetic dysfunction, other causes of conjugated hyperbilirubinemia in the neonate should be considered. Among the possibilities are idiopathic neonatal hepatitis, alpha-1-antitrypsin deficiency, hypothyroidism, bile acid synthesis deficiency, and disorders of hepatobiliary anatomy. Neonatal hepatomegaly can also be seen with congenitally acquired (e.g., TORCH) infections, hydrops or congestive heart failure, tumors, and metabolic disease (e.g., glycogen storage diseases, galactosemia, tyrosinemia, and others).

DIAGNOSIS

Shortly after interhospital transfer, this baby's state newborn screening results revealed him to have **galactosemia**.

INCIDENCE AND PATHOPHYSIOLOGY

Galactosemia is a rare inborn error of metabolism, occurring in 1 per 60 000 infants, caused by defects in galactose metabolism. Classic galactosemia is an autosomal recessive disease. If not recognized and treated, it can be fatal in the neonatal period. Although galactosemia is widely tested for in state newborn screening programs, the onset of life-threatening clinical illness may precede the completion of testing.

Galactosemia results from deficiencies in the enzymes involved in the metabolism of galactose. The hydrolysis of dietary lactose produces glucose and galactose. Galactose is subsequently phosphorylated to galactose-1-phosphate which is then converted by the galactose-1-phosphate uridyl transferase (GALT) enzyme to UDP-galactose. In "classic" galactosemia, GALT activity is completely absent and galactose-1-phosphate accumulates in the tissues leading to signs and symptoms of the disease. However, if partial GALT activity is present, as in a variant known as Duarte galactosemia, individuals may have no long-term clinical sequelae. The GALT gene has been mapped to 9p13 and more than 150 mutations have been identified. The most common allele is Q188R which causes severe disease. A milder form of galactosemia, found primarily in African-Americans, is caused by the S135L allele (Figure 15-8).

Additionally, there are two other types of "nonclassic" galactosemia. Galactokinase (GALK) deficiency, a deficiency of the enzyme necessary for the phosphorylation of galactose, causes cataracts but does not result in mental deficiency. An

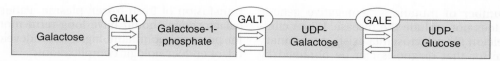

FIGURE 15-8. Simplified pathway of galactose metabolism. GALK, galactokinase; GALT, galactose-1-phosphate uridyltransferase; GALE, uridyl diphosphate galactose 4-epirimase; UDP, uridyl diphosphate.

even rarer type of galactosemia is caused by uridyl diphosphate galactose 4-epimerase (GALE) deficiency. This deficiency causes a spectrum of disease where affected individuals may be completely asymptomatic or may have features similar to those seen in "classic" galactosemia, with the addition of deafness and hypotonia (Table 15-8).

CLINICAL PRESENTATION

Presenting signs in the galactose-exposed, affected neonate can include jaundice, hepatomegaly, seizures, lethargy, vomiting, hypoglycemia, cataracts, and failure to thrive. In addition, babies with galactosemia exhibit a heightened susceptibility to bacterial infection, particularly *E. coli* sepsis. Among the laboratory findings seen with classic galactosemia are conjugated (or combined) hyperbilirubinemia; liver function test and coagulation study abnormalities; elevations of serum and urine amino acids; and a renal tubulopathy with galactosuria, glycosuria, proteinuria, and metabolic acidosis. Plasma galactose and erythrocyte galactose-1-phosphate levels are also elevated.

Unfortunately, even galactosemic children whose diets are restricted very early are at increased risk of developmental delays and learning disabilities. Although the pathophysiology remains unclear, it is thought that continued endogenous production of galactose may contribute to some of these long-term sequelae. Though many children have IQs in the normal range, cognitive, speech, and motor impairments are common. Hypergonadotropic hypogonadism is often observed in girls with galactosemia, and most are infertile as adults. Galactosemic boys demonstrate normal puberty and fertility.

DIAGNOSIS

Newborn screening. Every state in the United States screens for galactosemia. Most states use either a fluorometric assay to detect GALT activity or a bacterial inhibition assay to measure total galactose. Each method is associated with a number of false-positives and false-negatives. Results may be skewed if the infant fed poorly or was given soy formula, received a blood transfusion, or was given antibiotics. The fluorometric assay does not detect GALK or GALE deficiency.

RBC quantitative assay. Definitive diagnosis of classic galactosemia is established by laboratory assay of the GALT enzyme in erythrocytes. If there is clinical suspicion for galactosemia or the infant has had a positive newborn screen (often with a second screen for confirmation), the quantitative assay should be performed. If GALK or GALE deficiency is suspected, RBC assays for GALK and GALE activity should be performed.

Other testing. Prenatal testing for galactosemia is available, as is DNA analysis for some of the more common mutations. However, given the

TABLE 15-8.	Types of galactosemia.
Enzyme Deficiency	**Clinical Features**
GALT (galactose-1-phosphate uridyl transferase)	"Classic" galactosemia Jaundice, vomiting, failure to thrive, lethargy, poor feeding, sepsis, cataracts, liver dysfunction, renal tubular dysfunction Long term: cognitive impairment, speech apraxia, hypergonadotropic hypogonadism
GALK (galactokinase)	Lenticular cataracts Rarely associated with pseudotumor cerebri
GALE (uridyl diphosphogalactose 4-epimerase)	May be asymptomatic or have dysmorphic facial features, sensorineural deafness, developmental delay, poor growth

large number of mutations, a negative genetic screen does not exclude the disease. When clinical suspicion for galactosemia exists, preliminary evidence for that diagnosis can be obtained by testing the infant's urine for nonglucose reducing substances (provided that the infant had recently been exposed to lactose). However, this test is neither sensitive nor specific for galactosemia.

TREATMENT

The removal of galactose from the diet remains the first principle of therapy for galactosemia. Any infant with suspected galactosemia should immediately be changed from breastmilk or a milk-based formula to a soy or hydrolysate formula.

Depending on the degree of illness at the time of presentation, galactosemic neonates often require any number of supportive care measures such as intravenous fluids and antibiotics. Liver synthetic function may be compromised and the sick infant may require supplemental vitamin K or even transfusion of fresh frozen plasma. Patients with galactosemia should have long-term monitoring for potential ophthalmologic, neurodevelopmental, or endocrinologic complications.

SUGGESTED READINGS

1. Bosch AM, Grootenhuis MA, Bakker HD, et al. Living with classical galactosemia: health-related quality of life consequences. *Pediatrics.* 2004;113:e423-e428.
2. Ridel KR, Leslie ND, Gilbert DL. An updated review of the long-term neurological effects of galactosemia. *Pediatr Neurol.* 2005;33:153-161.
3. Shield JPH, Wadworth EJK, MacDonald A, et al. The relationship of genotype to cognitive outcome in galactosemia. *Arch Dis Child.* 2000;83:248-250.
4. Sutton VR. Clinical features and diagnosis of galactosemia. UpToDate. www.uptodate.com/contents/clinical-features-and-diagnosis-of-galactosemia. Updated July 16, 2010. Accessed September 15, 2011.
5. Walter JH, Collins JE, Leonard JV. Recommendations for the management of galactosaemia. *Arch Dis Child.* 1999;80:93-96.

CASE 15-5

Twelve-Year-Old Boy

STACEY R. ROSE

HISTORY OF PRESENT ILLNESS

The patient is a 12-year-old boy with recent onset of scleral icterus. He was in his usual state of good health until 3 weeks ago, at which time his parents noticed yellowing of his eyes. The patient also complained about itching of his arms and legs. He reported having a good appetite but his parents felt that he was eating smaller meals. His stool output had not changed in quantity or quality; there was no history of bloody or dark stool. Urine output was unchanged. There was no history of abdominal pain, vomiting, diarrhea, anorexia, weight loss, fever, fatigue, bleeding, or easy bruisability. There was no joint pain. There was no history of travel, tattooing, or unusual exposures.

The boy was seen in his pediatrician's office where hepatosplenomegaly was detected. He was referred to the hospital for further evaluation.

MEDICAL HISTORY

The boy had no history of hospitalization, surgery, or chronic medical problems. He was a full-term baby. He takes no medications, has no allergies, and is up-to-date with immunizations. The patient has an aunt with ulcerative colitis but family history was otherwise noncontributory. His three siblings were healthy. The boy was a seventh-grader who liked school and did well there.

PHYSICAL EXAMINATION

T 37.2°C; HR 96 bpm; RR 20/min; BP 110/64 mmHg; Weight 37 kg (5th percentile); Height 144 cm (5th percentile)

Physical examination revealed a smiling, pleasant, and cooperative boy. His examination was notable for mildly icteric sclera. The oropharynx was clear. There was no lymphadenopathy. His lungs were clear with unlabored respirations. Heart examination revealed a regular rate and rhythm with a soft I/VI systolic ejection murmur at the left sternal border; peripheral pulses were normal. The abdomen was soft with mild right upper quadrant tenderness. In addition, there was splenomegaly to the level of the umbilicus and the liver edge was palpable 2 cm below the right costal margin. A rectal examination was normal. On genitourinary examination, he was a Tanner I boy without hernia or scrotal swelling. His extremities were warm and well-perfused without edema. Neurologically he was alert and entirely appropriate with a grossly normal examination. His skin examination revealed only multiple chest nevi and some faint scratch marks on his arms.

DIAGNOSTIC STUDIES

Complete blood count: WBCs, 4800/mm³ (segmented neutrophils 41%, lymphocytes 44%); hemoglobin, 12.1 g/dL; platelets, 160000/mm³. Serum electrolytes, normal. Liver function tests: total bilirubin, 3.0 mg/dL, conjugated bilirubin 2.5 mg/dL; ALT, 176 U/L; AST, 228 U/L; alkaline phosphatase, 565 U/L; gamma glutamyl transferase, 345 U/L. Amylase, 67 U/L, lipase, 178 U/dL. Chest radiograph, borderline cardiomegaly but no infiltrates. Abdominal X-ray, no evidence of bowel obstruction.

COURSE OF ILLNESS

Additional laboratory studies were obtained including the following: erythrocyte sedimentation rate, 80 mm/h; prothrombin time, 12.7 seconds; partial thromboplastin time, 31 seconds. Hepatitis B surface antibody was positive. Hepatitis B surface antigen, hepatitis B core antibody, hepatitis A IgM, and hepatitis C polymerase chain reaction were all negative. Abdominal ultrasound showed an enlarged left lobe of the liver, macronodular changes in the liver parenchyma consistent with cirrhosis, a very enlarged spleen, minimal scattered adenopathy, and dilatation of the left bile duct. The child was admitted to the hospital for further evaluation of his hyperbilirubinemia, cirrhosis,

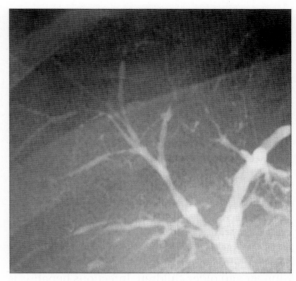

FIGURE 15-9. Cholangiogram. Note the irregular appearance of the biliary tree with multiple strictures and a "pruned-tree" appearance. *(Courtesy of Dr. David Piccoli, The Children's Hospital of Philadelphia. Philadelphia, PA.)*

and bile duct dilatation. Endoscopic retrograde cholangiopancreatography (ERCP) demonstrated irregularity and "beading" of portions of the biliary tract, along with dilatation of the left bile duct (Figure 15-9). These characteristic findings suggested the diagnosis.

DISCUSSION CASE 15-5

DIFFERENTIAL DIAGNOSIS

This boy presented with conjugated hyperbilirubinemia, evidence of liver injury, reflected in the elevation of his transaminases, and left bile duct dilatation. Elevations in conjugated bilirubin, alkaline phosphatase, and GGT levels suggest a cholestatic disorder. The differential diagnosis of cholestatic jaundice in the older child is very different from the list of diseases that present in the first few months of life (Table 15-9). Infants are more likely to have congenital anatomic anomalies (e.g., biliary atresia, cystic malformations) or inborn metabolic disorders (e.g., galactosemia,

TABLE 15-9.	Common causes of cholestasis in the older child or adolescent.	
Infectious	*Anatomic*	*Other*

Viral Hepatitis
Parasitic Infection
• Schistosomiasis
• Leptospirosis
Bacterial Sepsis
	Cholelithiasis
	Choledochal
	  cyst
	Sclerosing
	  cholangitis
	Pancreatitis
	Tumors
		Autoimmune
		  hepatitis
		Toxic hepatitis
		Changes
		  secondary to
		  IBD

Zellweger syndrome, bile acid metabolism deficiencies), whereas older children are more likely to experience acquired or secondary liver diseases, such as autoimmune or toxic hepatitis, or liver impairment related to inflammatory bowel disease. Infection is one area where there is broad overlap between the differential diagnoses of both younger and older children. Infectious hepatitis is among the most common causes of liver disease in older children and adolescents (Table 15-9).

Imaging studies revealed left bile duct dilatation, which implies an obstructive, extrahepatic cause of this patient's conjugated hyperbilirubinemia. Obstructive etiologies to consider in this age group include cholelithiasis, choledochal cysts, sclerosing cholangitis, pancreatitis, and tumors or other anatomic abnormalities along the choledocho-pancreatico-duodenal path.

DIAGNOSIS

Endoscopic retrograde cholangiopancreatography (ERCP) demonstrated irregularity and "beading" of portions of the biliary tract, along with dilatation of the left bile duct (Figure 15-9). An open biopsy of the liver was performed. Tissue pathology revealed cirrhosis, bile duct proliferation, patchy lymphocytic infiltrates, and concentric fibrosis around the bile ducts, confirming the diagnosis of **sclerosing cholangitis** (Figures 15-10 and 15-11). Additional testing to evaluate for an underlying etiology of his condition was negative, and therefore he was presumed to have **primary sclerosing cholangitis (PSC)**.

INCIDENCE AND PATHOPHYSIOLOGY

Sclerosing cholangitis, an inflammatory disease of the hepatobiliary system, is characterized by intra- and

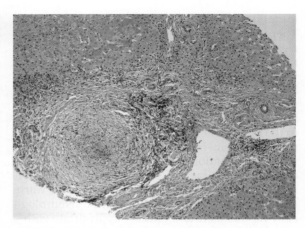

FIGURE 15-10. Liver biopsy specimen showing characteristic "onion-skin" fibrosis.

extrahepatic bile duct inflammation that progresses to areas of obliteration and dilatation. Sclerosing cholangitis is considered *secondary* when it occurs in the setting of cholelithiasis, cystic fibrosis, Langerhans histiocytosis, neoplasia (e.g., Hodgkin disease, ductal carcinoma), anatomic abnormalities (e.g., congenital or postsurgical), immunodeficiencies, and chronic ascending infection. *Primary* sclerosing cholangitis (PSC), however, is diagnosed when no such underlying disease exists.

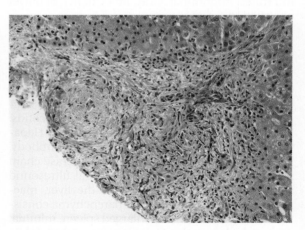

FIGURE 15-11. Liver biopsy specimen showing bile duct proliferation, patchy lymphocytic infiltrates, and concentric fibrosis around the bile ducts.

Primary sclerosing cholangitis is a rare, progressive disease that often results in biliary cirrhosis, portal hypertension, and liver failure. In the year 2000, one study estimated that there were 20.9 cases in 100 000 men and 6.3 out of 100 000 women, though the incidence in children is even lower. PSC is more prevalent in men and has an increased incidence among first-degree relatives. Additionally, there is a strong association between primary sclerosing cholangitis and inflammatory bowel disease (IBD) with ulcerative colitis being prevalent in up to 90% of cases of PSC. However, IBD is not causative. In some cases, the onset of hepatobiliary disease can precede the development of intestinal disease by years, while in others, PSC develops even after proctocolectomy.

The etiology of primary sclerosing cholangitis is not known. Several theories exist, including alterations in immunologic response, bacterial or viral triggers, or ischemia of the biliary tree, although none of these has been proven.

CLINICAL PRESENTATION

Although primary sclerosing cholangitis can develop at any age, adulthood is the most common period of presentation. Patients may be asymptomatic at diagnosis or may present with malaise, anorexia, abdominal pain, diarrhea, and weight loss. Pruritus is another common symptom of extrahepatic cholestasis, though the precise nature of the pruritogen is not well understood. Frank cholangitis may manifest with right upper quadrant pain, jaundice, and fever.

As PSC progresses, biliary obstruction worsens, secondary biliary cirrhosis develops, and ultimately liver failure ensues. Primary sclerosing cholangitis has an unfavorable prognosis and is a common indication for liver transplantation. PSC is associated with numerous complications, as outlined in Table 15-10, and is a risk factor for colon cancer and cholangiocarcinoma in adults.

Children with PSC exhibit many of the same features as their adult counterparts. However, they are more likely to have an overlapping autoimmune hepatitis and tend to have greater elevations in their aminotransferases. Conversely, their risk of developing neoplastic disease is much lower.

TABLE 15-10.	Complications associated with primary sclerosing cholangitis.

Common Complications Associated with Cholestatic Liver Disease and PSC

- Fatigue
- Pruritis
- Fat-soluble vitamin (ADEK) deficiency
- Steatorrhea
- Metabolic bone disease (osteoporosis)
- Recurrent cholangitis
- Dominant biliary stricture
- Cholelithiasis
- Cholangiocarcinoma

DIAGNOSTIC APPROACH

Clinical and biochemical evidence of cholestasis may suggest the possibility of PSC, but these findings alone do not differentiate this disease from other entities. Furthermore, the diagnosis of PSC in patients with established Crohn disease or ulcerative colitis can be confounded by the chronic hepatitis that sometimes accompanies inflammatory bowel disease.

Cholangiography. The definitive diagnosis of sclerosing cholangitis is made by cholangiography. Characteristic hepatobiliary changes include strictures, irregular narrowing of bile ducts, and decreased peripheral branching of intrahepatic ducts. Endoscopic retrograde cholangiography has long been considered the study of choice to establish the diagnosis. However, since it is an invasive procedure associated with potentially severe complications like bacterial cholangitis, magnetic resonance cholangiography is often preferred.

Liver biopsy. Liver biopsy is not definitive but may help support the diagnosis. Histologic changes may include the dilatation and obliteration of bile ducts with concentric, periductal "onion skin" fibrosis. Liver biopsy is carried out in staging of the disease and is helpful in determining prognosis.

TREATMENT

Unfortunately, management options for PSC are limited. The prognosis in children with PSC is unclear but the 10-year survival rate for adult patients is approximately 65%. There is no known effective medical treatment for primary sclerosing cholangitis. Numerous medications, including corticosteroids and other immunosuppressive agents, have been studied but have not demonstrated a definite benefit. Certain treatments, such as ursodeoxycholic acid (UDCA), may improve symptoms and laboratory abnormalities, but have not been proven to slow progression of disease. Furthermore, a recent study looking at the efficacy of high-dose UDCA in adults, suggested an increased risk of death or liver transplant in patients in the treatment group who had advanced disease. More invasive management may be successful, particularly in patients with dominant biliary tract strictures. Although dominant strictures are rare in children, endoscopic or percutaneous dilatation of the biliary tree can effectively alleviate severe focal obstructions. Surgical resection of the extrahepatic biliary tree and a roux-en-Y hepaticojejunostomy are other options that have been successful in certain patients without cirrhosis. However, since there is continued involvement of the intrahepatic bile ducts, this procedure does not halt disease progression and remains controversial. Liver transplantation is the only effective treatment for PSC patients with progressive liver disease. However, recurrence of disease in the graft is possible.

Given the strong association between PSC and ulcerative colitis, all patients should be evaluated for inflammatory bowel disease with colonoscopy and intestinal biopsies. Nutritional support should be optimized. Adult patients should undergo annual colonoscopy and ultrasound of the gallbladder to screen for colon cancer and cholangiocarcinoma. Since rates of malignancy are significantly lower in children with PSC, it is unclear whether such screening is necessary in the pediatric population, but should be strongly considered in the appropriate clinical setting.

SUGGESTED READINGS

1. Bambha K, Kim WR, Talwalker J, et al. Incidence, clinical spectrum, and outcomes of primary sclerosing cholangitis in a United States community. *Gastroenterology.* 2003;125:1364.
2. Chapman R, Fevery J, Kalloo A, et al. Diagnosis and management of primary sclerosing cholangitis. *Hepatology.* 2010;51:660-678.
3. Lee YM, Kaplan MM. Primary sclerosing cholangitis. *New Eng J Med.* 1995;332:924-933.
4. Karlsen TH, Franke A, Melum E, et al. Genome-wide association analysis in primary sclerosing cholangitis. *Gastroenterology.* 2010;138:1102-1111.
5. Kowdley KV. Clinical manifestations and diagnosis of primary sclerosing cholangitis. UpToDate. www.uptodate.com/contents/clinical-manifestations-and-diagnosis-of-primary-sclerosing-cholangitis. Updated January 17, 2011. Accessed September 28, 2011.

CASE 15-6

Two-Month-Old Girl

HISTORY OF PRESENT ILLNESS

A 2-month-old girl was referred to your hospital for evaluation of her jaundice and poor weight gain. Her father felt that she "has been yellow her whole life," starting before she left the newborn nursery. Except for some nasal congestion, the baby seems to be acting and sleeping normally. She has been feeding on cow's milk formula, taking about 2-3 oz every 3 hours, and making 5-6 wet diapers a day. The father describes the baby's stool output as 2-4 "loose" and "pasty" bowel movements a day. There is no history of fever, emesis, diarrhea, travel, or unusual exposures.

MEDICAL HISTORY

The baby was the 3.25 kg product of a term gestation, delivered via cesarean section to a mother with a history of osteoporosis and back pain. The mother took no medications and denied drug and alcohol use during pregnancy. The baby was discharged home with her mother on the second day of life. Her newborn screen was normal.

She lived at home with both parents. There was no family history of cystic fibrosis, cardiac or gastrointestinal disease, or other pediatric illnesses.

PHYSICAL EXAMINATION

T 37.2°C; HR 120 bpm; RR 28/min; BP 80/56 mmHg; Weight 3.9 kg (5th percentile); Length 53 cm (2nd percentile); Head Circumference 37 cm (15th percentile)

The infant appeared small but comfortable in her father's lap. She had an open, flat fontanelle, and a broad forehead; equal and round pupils and scleral icterus. The oropharynx was clear with moist mucous membranes. Respirations were clear and unlabored. Cardiac examination revealed a II/VI systolic murmur loudest at the left sternal border; the rate, rhythm, and distal pulses were all normal. Her abdomen was soft and nondistended with a smooth liver edge palpable 3 cm below the right costal margin; no spleen or other masses were appreciated. The genitourinary, extremity, and neurologic examinations were all normal.

INITIAL DIAGNOSTIC STUDIES

Complete blood count: WBCs, 16700/mm³ (neutrophils: 31%, lymphocytes: 61%); hemoglobin, 9.6 g/dL; platelets, 625000/mm³. Serum electrolytes: blood urea nitrogen, 26 mg/dL; creatinine, 1.1 mg/dL; otherwise normal. Liver function tests: total bilirubin, 11.0 mg/dL; unconjugated bilirubin, 8.0 mg/dL, conjugated bilirubin, 3.1 mg/dL; ALT, 190 U/L; AST, 94 U/L; albumin, 3.0 mg/dL; alkaline phosphatase, 450 U/L. Blood and urine cultures, negative. Evaluations for toxoplasmosis, rubella, cytomegalovirus, and human immunodeficiency virus: negative.

COURSE OF ILLNESS

The baby was admitted to the hospital for further evaluation. A renal ultrasound showed two somewhat small but otherwise unremarkable kidneys, and biochemical measures of her renal function (e.g., BUN, creatinine) trended toward normal during the hospitalization without specific therapy. Echocardiography revealed a structurally normal heart. She had an abdominal ultrasound which showed an enlarged liver but no masses. Hepatobiliary scintigraphy (diisopropyl iminodacetate [DISIDA] scan) was done which showed normal

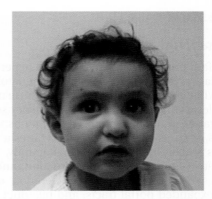

FIGURE 15-12. Photograph of a child with the same condition as the case patient. Note the wide forehead, bulbous nose, and pointed chin. *(Courtesy of Dr. David Piccoli, The Children's Hospital of Philadelphia.)*

tracer uptake but delayed intestinal excretion of the tracer at 4 and 24 h. Given those findings, she underwent immediate cholangiography and liver biopsy. The biopsy showed prominent cholestasis, occasional giant hepatocytes, and a ratio of bile ducts to portal tracts of about 0.5 (normal is around 0.9-1.8). The cholangiogram was normal. The infant had facial features (Figure 15-12) and radiograph findings (Figure 15-13) typical of this condition.

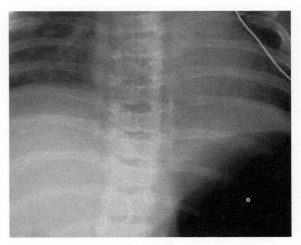

FIGURE 15-13. Butterfly vertebrae that are characteristic of this condition. *(Courtesy of Dr. David Piccoli, The Children's Hospital of Philadelphia.)*

DISCUSSION CASE 15-6

DIFFERENTIAL DIAGNOSIS

This infant presents with a conjugated hyperbilirubinemia and delayed excretion on the hepatobiliary scan. While numerous etiologies may cause neonatal cholestasis, the abnormal hepatobiliary scintigraphy raises immediate concern for an obstructive process, such as extrahepatic biliary atresia. Diagnosis is usually made by cholangiography, which may detect an extrahepatic obstruction, and liver biopsy, which often reveals proliferation of bile ducts, expanded portal tracts, and bile duct plugs. Treatment of extrahepatic biliary atresia (EHBA) by hepatic portoenterostomy (Kasai procedure) is most successful when performed in the first 10-12 weeks of life, so prompt diagnosis and referral to an appropriate surgical center is essential. Even in cases where hepatic portoenterostomy is performed in a timely manner, many patients with EHBA will develop severe liver dysfunction and require liver transplantation.

Normal tracer excretion on a hepatobiliary scan supports bile ducts patency. However, failure to demonstrate hepatic excretion is not diagnostic for biliary atresia. While EHBA must always be considered, the patient had a normal cholangiogram with evidence of bile duct paucity instead of proliferation. Interlobular bile duct paucity is the characteristic, but not unvarying, pathologic finding in Alagille syndrome. In addition, so-called "nonsyndromic" bile duct paucity can be a feature of congenital infections (e.g., CMV, rubella, syphilis), metabolic disorders (e.g., alpha-1-antitrypsin deficiency, defects of bile acid synthesis), sclerosing cholangitis, and idiopathic cholestasis.

DIAGNOSIS

As part of an extensive evaluation, the baby was seen by a geneticist who noted hypertelorism and a pointed mandible (Figure 15-11), in addition to the broad forehead noted on initial examination. The recommended ophthalmologic examination revealed the baby to have posterior embryotoxon, and a review of her admission chest X-ray detected butterfly vertebrae. The baby's constellation of clinical and pathologic findings led to a **diagnosis of Alagille syndrome (AGS)**.

INCIDENCE AND PATHOLOPHYSIOLOGY

Alagille syndrome (also known as syndromic bile duct paucity or arteriohepatic dysplasia) is an uncommon disorder associated with intrahepatic bile duct paucity as well as anomalies of the heart, eyes, kidneys, and skeleton. The disease was first described by Alagille in 1969. Since then more than 600 cases have been reported. The inheritance is autosomal dominant though many cases appear to arise from new mutations. The disease has been mapped to chromosome 20p12, specifically to mutations in *Jagged1* (JAG1), a ligand in the Notch signaling pathway that is important in determining cell fate during embryogenesis. Mutations in *NOTCH2*, the gene for the Notch2 receptor, have also been described. There is wide variability in gene expression in AGS and even patients with identical mutations can have very different features of the syndrome.

CLINICAL PRESENTATION

Alagille syndrome has many manifestations, ranging from subclinical to life-threatening disease that can affect numerous organ systems. The clinical features are summarized in Table 15-11. Although presentation of the disease varies, most patients present with cholestasis in the first months of life. Clinical and laboratory findings of the liver disease include jaundice, hepatomegaly, acholic stools, pruritus, growth failure, conjugated hyperbilirubinemia, and elevations of hepatic enzymes and bile salts. Patients may have mild cholestasis or can progress to portal hypertension, cirrhosis, or liver failure. Bile duct paucity was once considered the hallmark of Alagille syndrome. However, liver biopsies on infants younger than 6 months of age may not yet demonstrate bile duct paucity, and may even show bile duct proliferation. Additionally, an increasing number of patients have been identified with "nonhepatic" AGS, where paucity is never evident and other clinical features predominate (Table 15-11).

Most patients with Alagille syndrome have heart murmurs and the underlying heart conditions range in severity from benign (e.g., mild peripheral pulmonary stenosis) to complex disease requiring surgery (e.g., tetralogy of Fallot). Intracardiac disease is a predictor of poor outcome in AGS and accounts for most early mortality in the syndrome.

TABLE 15-11.	Clinical manifestations of Alagille syndrome.
Body System	**Common Features**
Hepatic	Cholestasis, bile duct paucity, jaundice, pruritis, cirrhosis, liver failure
Cardiac	Peripheral pulmonic stenosis, tetralogy of Fallot, valvular stenosis, truncus arteriosus, VSD, ASD
Facial	Broad forehead, hypertelorism, bulbous nose, large ears
Ocular	Posterior embryotoxon, Rieger anomaly
Skeletal	Butterfly vertebrae, short stature, absent 12th rib, osteopenia, rickets
Renal	Renal insufficiency, renal tubular acidosis, solitary kidney, ectopic kidney, multicystic kidneys
CNS	Intracranial hemorrhage, developmental delay, mental retardation
Other	Failure to thrive, fat-soluble vitamin deficiency, pancreatic insufficiency, xanthomata

Facial and ocular findings are also common characteristics of Alagille syndrome. Patients with AGS often have a distinctive facies that may be detectable as early as infancy. Features can include a triangular face with a broad forehead and pointed chin, deeply set eyes, and a long nose with a bulbous tip (Figure 15-12). The most common ocular finding is posterior embryotoxon, a dysgenesis of the anterior chamber of the eye (best seen on slit-lamp examination) in which there is prominence of Schwalbe ring, a ridge of collagenous fibers surrounding the periphery of Descemet membrane.

Skeletal problems are common, particularly abnormalities such as butterfly vertebrae (Figure 15-13). Other problems associated with Alagille syndrome include renal anomalies (both structural and functional), pancreatic insufficiency, intracranial hemorrhage, and cognitive impairments. Xanthomas are another common physical finding (Figure 15-12).

DIAGNOSTIC APPROACH

Patients known or suspected to have Alagille syndrome require a multidisciplinary initial assessment.

Early evaluation and follow-up by specialists in gastroenterology and nutrition is critical. In addition, cardiology and ophthalmology evaluations should be performed as early as possible.

Liver biopsy. Diagnosis is based on the histopathologic demonstration of bile duct paucity on liver biopsy specimens in the setting of well-recognized clinical associations as described above.

Chest radiograph. X-rays of the chest are necessary to assess for vertebral anomalies ("butterfly" vertebrae and hemivertebrae).

Ophthalmologic evaluation. Ophthalmologic evaluation detects posterior embryotoxon.

Echocardiogram. Recognized cardiac involvement includes peripheral pulmonary artery stenosis and tetralogy of Fallot.

Genetic consultation. As previously noted, most patients afflicted with Alagille syndrome have a characteristic facial appearance. As such, early evaluation by a geneticist can help guide diagnosis and provide appropriate genetic counseling. In addition, genetic testing is now available for *Jagged1* and *NOTCH2* mutations. Recent advances in genetic testing have improved diagnosis of the disease and JAG1 mutations have been found in 94% of patients with AGS.

TREATMENT

Treatment of Alagille syndrome focuses on the medical management of cholestasis, promotion of growth and development, and treatment of any comorbidities (e.g., congenital heart disease). Children with Alagille syndrome suffer from malabsorption and require supplementation of fat-soluble vitamins and provision of sufficient calories for growth, which may require tube feeding. Infants should receive formulas containing medium chain triglycerides, which are absorbable without bile salts. Medications that may benefit Alagille patients (e.g., by promoting bile flow, reducing pruritus, etc.) include phenobarbital, cholestyramine, ursodeoxycholic acid, and anti-histamines.

Long-term follow-up of patients with Alagille syndrome includes monitoring for the development of cirrhosis, portal hypertension, ascites, and liver failure. Twenty-year life expectancy for patients with Alagille syndrome is about 75% overall, though rates are lower for those who require liver transplantation and those with severe associated abnormalities, such as complex congenital heart disease.

SUGGESTED READINGS

1. Emerick KM, Rand EB, Goldmuntz E, Krantz ID, Spinner NB, Piccoli DA. Features of Alagille syndrome in 92 patients: frequency and relation to prognosis. *Hepatology.* 1999;29:822-829.

2. Kamath BM, Thiel BD, Gai X, et al. SNP array mapping of chromosome 20p deletions: genotypes, phenotypes, and copy number variation. *Hum Mutat.* 2008;30: 371-378.

3. Krantz ID, Piccoli DA, Spinner NB. Alagille syndrome. *J Med Genet.* 1997;34:152-157.

4. McDaniell R, Warthen DM, Sanchez-Lara PA, et al. Notch2 mutations cause Alagille syndrome, a heterogeneous disorder of the Notch signaling pathway. *Am J Hum Genet.* 2006;79:169-173.

5. Piccoli DA, Spinner NB. Alagille syndrome and the Jagged1 gene. *Semin Liver Dis.* 2001;21:525-534.

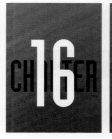

CHAPTER 16

ABNORMAL GAIT, INCLUDING REFUSAL TO WALK

JEANINE RONAN

DEFINITION OF THE COMPLAINT

Children refuse to walk because of pain, neuromuscular weakness, and certain mechanical factors. The list of possible etiologies in this regard is very extensive, consisting of both benign and life-threatening conditions. A systematic approach examining these causes is necessary to ensure a comprehensive evaluation.

A normal gait is a "smooth, mechanical process that advances the center of gravity with a minimum expenditure of energy." The stance phase is the time period when the heel strikes the ground bearing the individual's weight and the ball of the other foot leaves the ground. This requires very strong abductor muscles to stabilize the pelvis. In addition, the swing phase is defined as the time when the foot leaves the ground until the next heel strike.

There are many types of abnormal walking patterns. An *antalgic gait* is the pattern adopted to minimize pain. With this pattern, the patient will shorten the stance or weight-bearing phase on the affected limb, thereby minimizing the amount of time exerted on the painful limb. This will also result in a shortened stride length. A patient with a fracture, soft tissue injury, or infection, will use an antalgic gait. *Circumduction* is the pattern followed to shorten a limb and improve limb clearance. This is commonly seen when there is excessive joint stiffness secondary to spasticity or a leg-length discrepancy. A *Trendelberg gait* is when the muscles on one side of the pelvis are weak causing

pelvic instability; when both sides are involved a *waddling gait* is observed. An *unsteady gait* is suggestive of the presence of ataxia. A *steppage gait* is seen in cases of peripheral neurologic weakness. The foot slaps the ground as the patient walks due to decreased ankle dorsiflexion.

COMPLAINT BY CAUSE AND FREQUENCY

When a child refuses to walk the most common causes may vary based on a child's age (Table 16-1). The primary causes of limp, such as pain, weakness, and mechanical factors, can be further grouped by the following mechanisms: trauma, infectious, inflammatory, congenital, developmental, neurologic, neoplastic, hematologic, metabolic, and non-organic (Table 16-2).

CLARIFYING QUESTIONS

When evaluating a child who refuses to walk or a child with an abnormal gait, a thorough history and physical examination is crucial. Consideration of the patient's age, duration of symptoms, and the presence of systemic complaints allow the examiner to develop the appropriate differential diagnosis for the problem. The following list of questions may be helpful in guiding one to the ultimate diagnosis:

- Is the child's refusal to walk due to pain?
  —Trauma is the most common etiology that will result in a child refusing to walk. This may be due to repetitive or overuse injuries, accidental injury,

TABLE 16-1.	Common causes of refusal to walk in childhood by age.		
Infant/Toddler	*School Age*	*Adolescent*	
Trauma, toddler's fracture	Trauma	Trauma	
Transient synovitis	Transient synovitis	Osteomyelitis/ septic arthritis	
Osteomyelitis/ septic arthritis	Osteomyelitis/ septic arthritis	Slipped capital femoral epiphysis (SCFE)	
Developmental dysplasia of hip	Legg-Calve-Perthes disease	Patellofemoral problems	
Torsional deformities	Juvenile idiopathic arthritis	Overuse injuries	
Foreign bodies	Tumor	Juvenile idiopathic arthritis	
Tumor		Tumor	

TABLE 16-2.	Causes of abnormal gait in childhood by mechanism.
Trauma	Fractures (accidental or child abuse)
	Contusions/soft tissue injuries
	Foreign bodies
	Patellofemoral pain
	Overuse injury
	Spondylolisthesis
Infectious	Septic arthritis
	Osteomyelitis
	Myositis
	Transient synovitis
	Reactive arthritis
	Diskitis
	Lyme arthritis
Inflammatory	Juvenile idiopathic arthritis
	Acute rheumatic fever
	Serum sickness
	Ankylosing spondylitis
	Arthritis due to inflammatory bowel disease
	Kawasaki disease
	Henoch-Schönlein purpura
Congenital	Clubfoot
	Congenital limb abnormalities
Developmental	Developmental dysplasia of hips
	Blount disease
	Limb-length discrepancy
	Avascular necrosis (Legg-Calve-Perthes)
	Slipped capital femoral epiphysis
	Osgood-Schlatter
Neuromuscular	Cerebral palsy
	Peripheral neuropathies
	Muscular dystrophy
	Myelomeningocele
	Charcot-Marie-Tooth
	Guillain-Barré syndrome
	Cerebellar problems
Neoplastic	Benign bone tumors
	Osteoid osteoma
	Malignant bone tumors (osteosarcoma, Ewing sarcoma)
	Neuroblastoma
	Leukemia
Metabolic	Rickets
	Hyperparathyroidism
Hematologic	Sickle cell disease
	Hemophilia
Noninflammatory	Growing pains
	Reflex sympathetic dystrophy
	Conversion disorder

or child abuse. Clues to differentiating between accidental and abuse-related injuries include understanding the mechanism of the injury. Does the explained mechanism for the incident seem appropriate for the developmental age of the child?

Pain may be present because of inflammation and swelling in the bone or joint. Septic arthritis and osteomyelitis are other common causes for limping. A child with juvenile idiopathic arthritis (JIA) or reactive arthritis also complains of pain in his joints and may refuse to walk. Referred pain should also be considered. Commonly, a child with pathology in the hip will complain of knee or medial thigh pain. A child with appendicitis may refuse to walk due to referred pain from the abdomen. Back pain may also present with abnormal gait.

When a child is unable to walk, but denies the presence of pain, one must look hard for neuromuscular, metabolic, congenital, and developmental abnormalities. Developmental dysplasia of the hip may result in a limb-length discrepancy and abnormal walking pattern.

- How did the symptoms evolve? Was there a sudden or gradual onset?
  —In some cases, the parents will notice that the child initially develops an abnormal gait and as symptoms worsen will ultimately refuse to walk. A more gradual onset of symptoms suggests the presence of an inflammatory condition or mechanical cause from overuse. In other cases, a child abruptly is unable to walk which may suggest the presence of an injury or septic joint.

- Are there any associated symptoms?
  —The presence of other symptoms including fever, weight loss, abdominal pain, diarrhea, and rash may be suggestive of other etiologies. Children with leukemia will commonly complain of bone pain as well as weakness, malaise, and fever. A child with undiagnosed inflammatory bowel disease may have diarrhea, weight loss, as well as isolated joint swelling. Systemic JIA presents commonly with fever, weight loss, and rash in a school-aged child.

- Is there the presence of joint swelling and erythema?
  —Associated signs of infection, including toxic appearance, fever, chills, and joint redness, swelling, warmth, and decreased mobility, accompany septic arthritis. Many inflammatory etiologies will also present with joint swelling and increased joint warmth.

- How would you characterize the limp?
  —Does the child refuse to walk due to the presence or absence of pain? Is the child's abnormal walking pattern trying to minimize the amount of time spent on the involved leg? Is the child able to weight bear? Abnormalities in the structure of the lower extremity, for example, torsional deformities or leg-length discrepancies also cause an abnormal walking pattern. In addition, any abnormalities in the muscle such as an increase in tone or the presence of contractures will generate an abnormal walking pattern. A child may also refuse to walk due to neuromuscular weakness. Weakness may be found in the muscle, due to a problem with the peripheral nerves or due to disease within the central nervous system.

- Are there localizing signs on physical examination of the child?

  —If pain is present, try to localize it to the area of maximum tenderness. Point tenderness on a painful extremity is highly suggestive of an infection or acute injury. Point tenderness in a febrile child requires an evaluation for osteomyelitis. Tenderness over the epiphyseal growth plate in addition to a history of trauma increases the possibility of a Salter-Harris type 1 fracture.

- Is the pain referred?
  —The child may have an acute abdomen or torsion of the testes and may refuse to walk to minimize pain. A child with back pain will also have trouble walking due to pain or neurologic weakness. In addition, knee and medial thigh pain is commonly associated with hip pathology.

- Do symptoms vary with the time of day?
  —Rheumatologic disorders are associated with the gelling phenomenon. Symptoms are worse in the morning and improve during the course of the day. When neuromuscular weakness is the etiology, the symptoms tend to progress throughout the day. Pain due to tumors is persistent.

The following cases illustrate the approach to a patient who refuses to walk.

SUGGESTED READINGS

1. Sawyer J, Kapoor M. The limping child: a systematic approach to diagnosis. *Am Fam Physician.* 2009;79(3): 215-224.
2. Hill D, Whiteside J. Limping in children: differentiating benign from dire causes. *J Fam Pract.* 2011;60(4):193-197.
3. Barkin R, Barkin S, Barkin A. The limping child. *J Emerg Med.* 2000;18(3):331-339.
4. Tse S, Laxer R. Acute limb pain. *Pediatr Rev.* 2006;27(5): 170-179.
5. Fleisher GR, Ludwig S. *Textbook of Pediatric Emergency Medicine.* Philadelphia: Lippincott Williams & Wilkins; 2010.

CASE 16-1

Four-Year-Old Boy

AMY T. WALDMAN

HISTORY OF PRESENT ILLNESS

A 4-year-old Caucasian boy presented to the emergency department after a 1-week history of leg pain. Initially, the pain was described as bilateral, primarily surrounding his knees. However, the pain gradually became more diffuse and consistently woke the patient from sleep. In addition, the parents also noted that their son was more clumsy. He had difficulty walking and was dropping objects from both of his hands. Review of systems was significant for constipation, urinary incontinence, and fatigue. Three weeks ago, the patient had an upper respiratory infection, which had resolved.

MEDICAL HISTORY

There was no significant medical history. He had reached all of his developmental milestones on time, and had been walking since 9 months of age.

PHYSICAL EXAMINATION

T 36.3°C; RR 24/min; HR 120 bpm; BP 120/70 mmHg; Height under 5th percentile; Weight 10th percentile

Initial examination revealed an alert and interactive young boy. His cranial nerve examination was normal for cranial nerves II-XII. Notably, extraocular movements were normal and facial weakness was absent. His neurologic examination was remarkable for decreased strength in his lower extremities and hand grip bilaterally. Deep tendon reflexes were not elicited in the upper or lower extremities. His gait was limited by pain and weakness. The remainder of the examination was unremarkable.

DIAGNOSTIC STUDIES

Laboratory analysis included a normal complete blood count and sedimentation rate. Computed tomography of the head demonstrated mild mucosal thickening of the maxillary sinus. Cerebral spinal fluid demonstrated one WBC/mm^3 and 25 RBCs/mm^3. Protein was 106 mg/dL and glucose was 69 mg/dL. He was admitted to the hospital for further evaluation.

COURSE OF ILLNESS

What is the most likely diagnosis?

DISCUSSION CASE 16-1

DIFFERENTIAL DIAGNOSIS

The combination of symptoms including weakness, pain, and areflexia suggests a peripheral neuropathy. There are many causes of peripheral neuropathies. Guillain-Barré syndrome (GBS) is the most common cause of acute generalized weakness. However, at the onset of disease, it is difficult to distinguish GBS from its chronic and relapsing variant, chronic inflammatory demyelinating polyneuropathy. Many drugs have been implicated in inducing neuropathies including isoniazid, vincristine, heavy metals (mercury and lead), and organophosphates. While common in GBS, bilateral facial weakness is not often seen in other neuropathies. In patients with bilateral facial weakness and ataxia but normal or hyperactive reflexes, pathology in the brainstem and cerebellum should also be considered. Asymmetric weakness and sensory symptoms along with urinary retention suggests involvement of the spinal cord as is seen in transverse myelitis. Acute paraparesis or quadriparesis also occurs in the setting of a compressive myelopathy. Myopathies may present with similar symptoms but without sensory involvement and reflexes are preserved. An elevated creatine kinase may also be present in myopathies.

DIAGNOSIS

In this case, the physical finding of absent deep tendon reflexes was very important in establishing the proper diagnosis. The elevated cerebrospinal fluid protein with a normal number of white blood cells (cytoalbuminologic dissociation) was also consistent with the diagnosis of GBS. Electromyography (EMG) showed prolonged distal motor latencies in all motor nerves and a slowed conduction velocity that was consistent with a demyelinating process. **The diagnosis is Guillain-Barré syndrome.** At this point, the patient did not show any signs of respiratory compromise. He was treated with intravenous immunoglobulin (IVIg) and his symptoms gradually improved.

INCIDENCE AND EPIDEMIOLOGY

GBS, the most common cause of acute generalized weakness, occurs in 0.4-1.7/100 000 children. It is an acquired inflammatory disease of the peripheral nervous system. While the exact pathogenesis is unknown, GBS may be mediated by an immune response against myelin antigens of the peripheral nerves, which leads to demyelination and axonal degeneration of motor and sensory nerves. Many cases are postinfectious in which there is a history of gastrointestinal or respiratory illness within 4 weeks of symptom onset. Infections associated with the development of GBS include *Campylobacter jejuni*, varicella, cytomegalovirus, hepatitis, measles, mumps, and *Mycoplasma pneumoniae*.

CLINICAL PRESENTATION

The diagnosis of GBS requires areflexia and the presence of progressive motor weakness of more than one limb. The weakness is usually relatively symmetric and typically ascending, although descending weakness can also occur. Mild sensory loss, including paresthesias, numbness, and diminished position and vibratory sensation, is usually present.

Pain is a surprisingly common finding in children. A review of 29 children hospitalized with GBS demonstrated the presence of pain in 79% of cases. However, in many children the presence of pain obscured the proper diagnosis. The pain hindered accurate neurologic examination and usually caused clinicians to initially suspect a rheumatologic or inflammatory disorder. Adults typically classify the pain as a deep lower limb pain, exacerbated by straight leg raises.

Fever is not a common sign. However, there may be signs of autonomic dysfunction including labile blood pressure, tachycardia or bradycardia, as well as bladder or bowel dysfunction. Respiratory failure may be fairly rapid in onset and is seen in 20% of patients.

The Miller-Fisher variant is characterized by ophthalmoplegia, ataxia, and areflexia and is due to a specific IgG directed at a ganglioside.

DIAGNOSTIC APPROACH

The important step in making the diagnosis is to obtain a detailed history and perform a thorough general and neurologic examination.

Lumbar puncture. Cerebrospinal fluid classically demonstrates cytoalbuminologic dissociation (i.e., an elevated protein with only minimal pleocytosis, typically fewer than 10 WBCs/mm^3); however, an elevated protein may not be present early in the disease course (i.e., during the first week).

Electromyography (EMG). The diagnosis is usually supported by EMG studies, which demonstrate slowed or blocked motor conduction. Within 2 weeks of illness onset, the EMG is abnormal in approximately 50% of patients; more than 85% of patients with GBS ultimately have an abnormal EMG.

Magnetic resonance imaging (MRI) of the spine. Although not usually required for diagnosis, MRI should be performed if spinal compression or central nervous system inflammation (such as transverse myelitis) is suspected. In patients with GBS, MRI frequently reveals spinal nerve root enhancement.

TREATMENT

GBS should be considered a neurologic emergency due to the potential for respiratory and autonomic failure. Patients with suspected or confirmed GBS must be monitored closely for worsening vital capacity and negative inspiratory force as intubation may be required. While spontaneous recovery may occur within 6 months, patients with respiratory compromise or autonomic dysfunction and those unable to walk are typically treated. Plasmapheresis and intravenous immunoglobulin are the current treatment modalities. While plasmapheresis and IVIg are equally effective, IVIg is often easier to initiate. Side effects of IVIg include fever, headache, vomiting, and meningismus. A recent study concluded that 23% of children may continue to have evidence of mild muscle weakness following IVIg therapy. However, in many cases this weakness had no impact on daily function. Children who were young in age and who had a rapid progression of symptoms were more likely to have long-term weakness. Combination therapy (plasmapheresis followed by IVIg) is not superior to either treatment alone and is not recommended. Corticosteroids are not effective and should not be administered in patients with GBS. Recovery from GBS occurs in a descending manner. Physical therapy should be initiated for all patients to assist with timely recovery.

SUGGESTED READINGS

1. Evans OB, Vedanarayanan V. Guillain-Barré syndrome. *Pediatr Rev.* 1997;18:10-16.
2. Gordon PH, Wilbourn AJ. Early electrodiagnostic findings in Guillain-Barré syndrome. *Arch Neurol.* 2001; 58:913-917.
3. Nguyen DK, Agenarioti-Belanger S, Vanasse M. Pain and the Guillain-Barré syndrome in children under 6 years old. *J Pediatr.* 1999;134:773-776.
4. Vajsar J, Fehlings D, Stephens D. Long-term outcome in children with Guillain-Barré syndrome. *J Pediatr.* 2003; 142:305-309.
5. Hughes RAC, Wijdicks EFM, Barohn R, et al. Practice parameter: immunotherapy for Guillain-Barré syndrome: report of the Quality Standards Subcommittee of the American Academy of Neurology. *Neurology.* 2003; 61:736-740.
6. Yuki N, Hartung HP. Guillain-Barré syndrome. *N Engl J Med.* 2012;366:2294-2304.

CASE 16-2

Three-Year-Old Boy

JEANINE RONAN

HISTORY OF PRESENT ILLNESS

A healthy 3-year-old boy presented to the emergency department with significant left ankle swelling and the inability to walk. During the past several months, he has had swelling and tenderness of multiple joints, including his knees, wrists, fingers, and hips. He has also had daily fevers with associated night sweats and an 8-lb weight loss. His mother noted rashes that appeared on his face, back, and chest.

MEDICAL HISTORY

His medical history was unremarkable.

PHYSICAL EXAMINATION

T 38.2°C; RR 24/min; HR 106 bpm; BP 102/64 mmHg; Height 50th percentile; Weight 10th percentile

In general, the boy appeared tired. Musculoskeletal examination revealed multiple painful and swollen joints with limited range of motion, including his right hip, right wrist, and left third digit. His neurologic examination demonstrated intact sensory function and normal deep tendon reflexes. No rash was seen. The remainder of the examination was normal.

DIAGNOSTIC STUDIES

Initial laboratory data revealed a 14 600 WBCs/mm³ with 54% segmented neutrophils, 6% band forms, and 36% lymphocytes. The hemoglobin was 7.9 g/dL and there were 997 000 platelets/mm³. The erythrocyte sedimentation rate was 63 mm/h. Electrolytes, blood urea nitrogen, and creatinine were normal. Liver function tests were normal, except an albumin of 2.9 mg/dL. Blood cultures were subsequently negative. Lyme antibodies and ASO titers were also negative. Radiologic studies were normal including hip and abdominal radiographs.

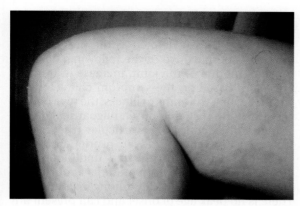

FIGURE 16-1. Photograph of the patient's rash.

TABLE 16-3.	The JONES criteria[a] for acute rheumatic fever.
Major Criteria	**Minor Criteria**
J: Joints (signs of arthritis typically involving knees, ankles, elbows, wrists)	Fever
O: Carditis (involvement can include endocardium, myocardium, epicardium, pericardium)	Arthralgias (if not using arthritis as a major criteria)
N: Subcutaneous Nodules (painless firm nodules over bones)	Prolonged PR interval
E: Erythema Marginatum (well demarcated nonpuritic rash over trunk and extending to extremities)	Acute phase reactants: elevated WBC, CRP, ESR
S: Sydenham Chorea (abrupt purposeless movements, when present is diagnostic)	Previous diagnosis of rheumatic fever

[a]The presence of 2 major criteria or 1 major and 2 minor criteria, and evidence of prior streptococcal infection is used to diagnose acute rheumatic criteria.

COURSE OF ILLNESS

Septic arthritis was considered unlikely given the number of joints involved as well as the chronicity of the problem. Throughout the hospital stay the patient continued to have fevers and joint swelling. A salmon colored rash appeared with each temperature elevation and suggested the diagnosis (Figure 16-1).

DISCUSSION CASE 16-2

DIFFERENTIAL DIAGNOSIS

In a child with fever and refusal to bear weight, infectious causes such as septic arthritis and osteomyelitis must be considered. Children with septic arthritis may have systemic symptoms including irritability and malaise. The affected joint acutely appears erythematous, warm, and tender. Range of motion is typically limited due to pain. In more than 90% of cases, only a single joint is affected. Children with acute hematogenous osteomyelitis manifest symptoms for fewer than 2 weeks. On physical examination there is often erythema, edema, and tenderness over the affected bone. However, the degree of tenderness may be out of proportion to the other findings. The femur, tibia, humerus, and fibula are most commonly involved. Laboratory findings in both septic arthritis and osteomyelitis include leukocytosis and elevation of the erythrocyte sedimentation rate and C-reactive protein. Blood cultures are positive in up to 50% of the children with septic arthritis or osteomyelitis.

Acute rheumatic fever (ARF) may also present with fever. In ARF, the arthritis is classically described as a migratory polyarthritis with pain that is out of proportion to the physical findings and responds quickly to antiinflammatory medication. In addition, there must be evidence of a recent group A *Streptococcus* infection and fulfillment of the Jones criteria (Table 16-3).

Arthritis occurs in late-onset Lyme disease. It should also be considered particularly in areas where Lyme disease is endemic. When occurring, the erythema migrans or bullseye rash develops in early disease and will precede joint swelling. Patients may complain of arthralgias during early-onset disease in addition to fever and generalized malaise. In 80% of cases, Lyme arthritis is monoarticular, typically involving the knee joint, but multiple joints are occasionally involved. The affected joint is erythematous and swollen; pain is relatively mild despite the significant joint effusion.

The constellation of fever, rash, and joint pain also suggests systemic-onset juvenile idiopathic arthritis (JIA). However, in many cases the presentation of systemic-onset JIA can be elusive and is sometimes confused with the presentation of leukemia or lymphoma. The systemic-onset JIA patient may have lymphadenopathy and hepatosplenomegaly. The arthritis and joint symptoms may not be apparent initially.

DIAGNOSIS

In this case, the evanescent salmon colored rash strongly suggested the diagnosis of systemic JIA (Figure 16-1). This rash usually appears while the child is febrile.

INCIDENCE AND EPIDEMIOLOGY

Juvenile idiopathic arthritis is the most common rheumatic disease of childhood. The incidence is 1:10 000, with a prevalence of 1:1000. JIA encompasses a heterogeneous group of disorders. By definition, JIA includes all forms of arthritis that

occur before 16 years of age, persists for greater than 6 weeks, and does not have another known etiology. Arthritis is defined as the presence of a joint effusion plus two of the following: decrease range of motion of the joint, increase in warmth, and pain. Based on the symptom characteristics within the first 6 months of illness, the type of JIA is classified into systemic-onset, oligoarticular (persistent and extended), polyarticular (rheumatoid factor positive and negative), psoriatic arthritis, enthesitis related arthritis, and undifferentiated (Table 16-4). Systemic JIA represents about 10% of all cases and is seen equally among boys and girls. There is no peak age of onset and can present any time throughout childhood. In contrast, oligoarticular JIA is the most common, including about 40% of all JIA cases. Oligoarticular JIA occurs more commonly in girls than boys with a 5:1 ratio. Most children with oligoarticular JIA present between 1 and 6 years of age with a peak at 2-4 years. Polyarticular JIA, which comprises about 25% of JIA

TABLE 16-4.	Subtypes of juvenile idiopathic arthritis.			
Subtype		*Total*	*Age at Onset*	*Characteristics*
Systemic Onset		10%	Childhood	Daily fevers (T > 39°C) Evanesent rash Hepatosplenomegaly Lymphadenopathy Serositis and pericarditis

Oligoarticular
–Persistent (≤4 joints involved
  throughout disease)
–Extended (>4 joint involvement
  after 6 months)
		40%	1-6 years M:F
			ratio 1:6
				Large joint involvement: knees, ankles, elbows
				Hip commonly NOT involved
				High risk for chronic anterior uveitis (30%-50% or
				  patients), especially when ANA positive

Polyarticular
–RF positive
–RF negative
		25%	Late childhood
			and
			adolescence
				Symmetrical arthritis in large and small joints
				Severe degenerative joint disease
				Rh factor positive more common in adolescent
				  females, disease course is similar to adult rheu-
				  matoid arthritis.
				Less risk for uveitis (5%)

Psoriatic Arthritis		2%-11%	Late childhood and adolescence	Patients of first degree relative with psoriasis Nail pitting, onycholysis, dactylitis
Enthesitis-related Arthritis		1%-11%	Peaks: 2-4 years and 6-12 years	Includes IBD related arthritis, reactive arthritis and juvenile ankylosing spondylitis Common involvement of SI joint Associated with HLA-B27 Increase risk for uveitis
Undifferentiated		11%-21%		Does not meet criteria for other categories

cases, is also seen more commonly in girls than boys with a 3:1 ratio. Peak onset of polyarticular JIA occurs between 1-4 years of age and 7-10 years of age until adolescence. The remainder of the cases consists of psoriatic arthritis, enthesitis-related (where tendons and ligaments attach to bone) and undifferentiated.

CLINICAL PRESENTATION

The term juvenile idiopathic arthritis encompasses a group of diseases that involve the infiltration and proliferation of the synovial membrane resulting in joint swelling. JIA is a multifactorial autoimmune disease that develops due to host and environmental susceptibility factors. Immune dysregulation produces cytokines with an increase in inflammatory mediators within the synovium. Tissue inflammation causes remodeling, cartilage degradation, and bony erosions. The pain classically includes morning stiffness and gait disturbance, in contrast to patients with musculoskeletal pain due to mechanical or overuse injuries, which worsen with use and improve with rest. Patients with musculoskeletal pain will have worsening of symptoms during the day or with exercise and have no associated joint effusion.

Systemic-onset JIA. Systemic-onset JIA presents with high spiking fevers, salmon-colored rash that begins in the groin or axilla and extends to the trunk and extremities, hepatosplenomegaly, lymphadenopathy, with or without the arthritis. Supporting laboratory data include an elevated white blood cell count, anemia, thrombocytosis, and elevated ferritin level. Signs of disseminated intravascular coagulation are due to the macrophage activation syndrome. The sedimentation rate is typically greater than 80 mm/h. Chronic uveitis or iriditis does not typically occur.

Oligoarticular JIA. In oligoarticular JIA, the patient presents with less than four joints involved. This category is further divided into patients with persistent disease in which less than four joints are involved throughout the disease course and extended diseases in which more joint involvement develops after the first 6 months. The typical patient is a preschool girl with isolated knee swelling and difficulty walking. The arthritis usually involves the knees, ankles, wrists, or elbows, while sparing the hips. These patients are at high risk for uveitis. In patients with a positive antinuclear antibody (ANA), the risk is about 80%. Chronic anterior uveitis can be asymptomatic initially, but the complications include corneal clouding, cataracts, glaucoma, and vision loss. Serial ophthalmologic examinations are crucial in this population. Treatment may include NSAIDs or intraarticular steroid injections. This is the mildest form of JIA and these patients may go into permanent remission.

Polyarticular JIA. Polyarticular JIA affects five or more joints at the time of presentation. The joint distribution is symmetrical involving small and large joints including joints of the hands, the temporomandibular joint, or cervical spine. Polyarticular JIA is further categorized by the presence of rheumatoid factor. Rheumatoid factor positive polyarticular JIA is seen most commonly in adolescent girls and the disease course is similar to adult rheumatoid arthritis. The risk for uveitis is not as great in this category, but if the ANA is positive, these patients are also at risk for the complications with anterior uveitis.

Psoriatic arthritis. Psoriatic arthritis involves the knees, hands, and feet. It is seen in patients with psoriasis or with first degree relatives with psoriasis. Nail changes including pitting and onycholysis are typically seen along with dactylitis.

Enthesitis-related arthritis. Enthesitis-related arthritis encompasses inflammatory bowel disease associated arthritis, in which arthritis may precede other symptoms, reactive arthritis and juvenile ankylosing spondylitis. Enthesitis describes inflammation at the site of tendon and ligament attachment within the joint capsule. Many of these patients are HLA-B27 positive and develop progressive involvement of the sacroiliac joint.

Undifferentiated arthritis. This includes any arthritis that is not further defined by the above definitions.

DIAGNOSTIC APPROACH

When making the diagnosis of juvenile idiopathic arthritis, by definition the patient must have symptoms for a duration of at least 6 weeks. The history and physical examination should be directed at eliciting clues to changes in gait, the presence of joint effusions, and pain in the joints. It is important to examine all joints including the temporo-mandibular joint and cervical spine for subtle changes. Also, associated symptoms including fever, rash, and adenopathy must be assessed. Looking for signs of psoriasis, nail changes, can also have clues to the diagnosis. Growth parameters should be reviewed. An ophthalmologic examination is also very important. Laboratory data may be a helpful adjunct.

Complete blood count. Patients with systemic JIA often have leukocytosis with neutrophil predominance, thrombocytosis, and anemia.

Antinuclear antibody (ANA). Antinuclear antibody studies are not required for the diagnosis of JIA but are helpful in classifying patients. If JIA patients are ANA-positive, their risk for chronic anterior uveitis is higher. Since chronic anterior uveitis is an asymptomatic condition with devastating complications, including cataracts, glaucoma, and loss of visual acuity, these patients require close ophthalmologic follow-up.

Rheumatoid factor (RF). In general, a positive rheumatoid factor is not helpful in making the diagnosis. In most cases of JIA, the test will be negative with the exception of polyarticular JIA in which approximately 15% of children have a positive result. In this instance, a positive rheumatoid factor is important for prognosis, but not required for the diagnosis, as polyarthritis JIA, RF-positive is most closely related to adult rheumatoid arthritis.

Radiographs. Radiographs are normal early in the course of illness. Radiographs will show joint space narrowing, growth abnormalities of the joint, and bony erosions as persistent arthritis will also lead to bone demineralization and loss of articular cartilage.

Other studies. Erythrocyte sedimentation rate and C-reactive protein will be in most cases of JIA.

TREATMENT

The goals of treatment for JIA are to maintain functional mobility, by controlling inflammation and increasing joint range of motion, as well as limiting the side effects of medications and thereby leading to the normal physical, social, and developmental growth of the patient. Nonsteroidal antiinflammatory drugs (NSAIDs) are the first line of therapy for JIA. NSAIDs are directed at treating the pain and symptoms of JIA but these medications are not disease modulating. NSAIDs can be started at the onset of symptoms prior to classifying the arthritis without resulting clouding the diagnosis. Naproxen is commonly used because it is a twice-a-day medication. The chronic use of NSAIDs requires monitoring of certain data including urinalysis, complete blood count, renal, and liver function tests. A particular skin rash called pseudoporphyria is associated with naproxen. This photosensitive eruption results in small facial vesicles that may lead to permanent scar formation.

Other medications are directed at treating the inflammation and thus are disease modulation. Corticosteroids are used particularly in children with systemic JIA who present with high fevers and severe systemic symptoms. The side effects of systemic corticosteroids make them less appealing for chronic control of inflammation, especially in less severe forms of the disease. In patients with oligoarticular JIA, intraarticular injections with triamcinolone hexacetonide may be very effective treatments.

New data suggest that aggressive therapy at the onset of treatment is more effective in minimizing long-term sequelae. Disease-modifying antirheumatic drugs (DMARDs) including methotrexate are particularly useful in patients with oligoarticular JIA, extended disease, and polyarticular JIA. Methotrexate is usually very safe, but it can be associated with liver toxicity requiring monitoring of hepatic function tests every 4-8 weeks, kidney dysfunction, increase risk of infections, and bone marrow suppression. Folic acid supplementation once a week will decrease the incidence of side effects.

A new area of drug research is focused on targeting inflammatory cytokines to turn off the inflammatory cascade. Biological DMARDs are showing increasing promise in reducing symptoms and altering the disease course. These types of medications include TNF-alpha blocking agents, T-cell co-stimulation modulators, Interleukin 1 blocking agents, Interleukin 6 blocking agents, and B cell depletion agents.

Physical therapy is also crucial for these patients to maintain the most active possible lifestyle. Vitamin D and calcium supplements should be encouraged.

SUGGESTED READINGS

1. Goldmuntz E, White P. Juvenile idiopathic arthritis. *Pediatr Rev.* 2006;27(4):24-32.
2. Prakken B, Albani S, Martini A. Juvenile idiopathic arthritis. *Lancet.* 2011;322(9783):2138-2149.
3. Prince F, Otten M, van Suijlekom-Smit L. Diagnosis and management of juvenile idiopathic arthritis. *BMJ.* 2011;342(c6434):95-102.

CASE 16-3

Two-Year-Old Boy

JEANINE RONAN

HISTORY OF PRESENT ILLNESS

A 2-year-old boy presented with the chief complaint of refusing to walk. The child was in his usual state of health yesterday and was outside playing with his older brother. While looking outside the mother noted that her son had fallen while running on the grass, but he stood up immediately and continued trying to keep up with his older brothers. Over the remainder of the day he seemed to be acting normally. However, when he woke up this morning there was significant swelling over the right lower leg and he was walking with a limp. There has been no history of fever or viral infections.

MEDICAL HISTORY

The medical history was remarkable. He met all his developmental milestones appropriately.

PHYSICAL EXAMINATION

T 36.9°C; RR 28/min; HR 125 bpm; BP 96/70 mmHg; Height 75th percentile; Weight 50th percentile

In general, the child appeared as a happy, well-developed boy. His physical examination was normal with the exception of the right lower extremity. There was an area of focal swelling and discrete tenderness along the lower third of the tibial shaft. His hip, knee, and ankle examination revealed full range of motion. His neurologic examination was normal; however, he refused to bear weight on his right leg. His skin examination did not demonstrate any bruises or unusual marks.

DIAGNOSTIC STUDIES

Complete blood count revealed 8200 WBCs/mm^3 with 54% segmented neutrophils, no band forms 38% lymphocytes, and 8% monocytes. The erythrocyte sedimentation rate and C-reactive protein were normal.

COURSE OF ILLNESS

A radiograph of the right leg revealed the diagnosis (Figure 16-2).

DISCUSSION CASE 16-3

DIFFERENTIAL DIAGNOSIS

When a child presents with the abrupt onset of refusal to walk, acute injury is the most likely etiology. Determining whether the injury is due to an accident or the result of abuse is a challenging diagnostic issue for physicians. In the case of a toddler's fracture, a significant traumatic event may not have occurred. It may result from a minor accident involving a fall while walking or running which may have either been dismissed or not witnessed by the parents. Toddler's fractures typically involve

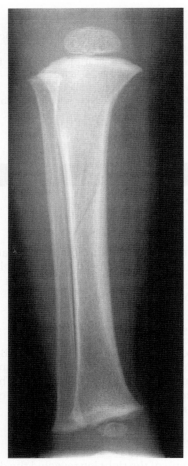

FIGURE 16-2. Radiograph of the tibia.

the distal portion of the tibia, resulting in a spiral or oblique fracture. In contrast, when the fracture results from abuse, usually the midshaft of the tibia is involved because of the large amount of force inflicted while holding the foot and twisting the leg. In the case of child abuse, usually the history will not seem plausible with the injury or the developmental age of the child (Table 16-5). If abuse is considered, a skeletal survey should be carried out to evaluate for any other injuries. Fractures involving the metaphysis and epiphysis (bucket handle fractures), the thoracic cage, scapula and spine, as well as complex skull fractures, should raise the suspicion of child abuse (Table 16-6).

TABLE 16-5.	Common explanations in the history that raise suspicion for child abuse.
No explanation for a significant injury	
Dramatic changes in injury explanation	
An explanation that is not plausible, given the injury	
Different versions of the incident by caregivers	
Mechanism of injury inconsistent with the child's developmental or physical abilities	

In rare cases, unexplained fractures may be a sign of bone disease. The fracture patterns may be similar in child abuse patients and patients with bone disease. Metabolic bone disease is exceedingly rare and should be considered a diagnosis of exclusion. Osteogenesis imperfecta (OI) is the condition most frequently confused with child abuse. OI is a genetic bone disorder due to a mutation in type I collagen. OI should be considered when these features are present: osteopenia, wormian bones on the skull, blue sclera, abnormal dentition, and a family history of "easy" fractures. However, in some milder forms (OI type IV) none of these features may be seen.

DIAGNOSIS

Radiograph of the right leg demonstrated a spiral fracture involving the tibia (Figure 16-2). **The diagnosis is a toddler's fracture.**

INCIDENCE AND EPIDEMIOLOGY

Toddler's fractures are common injuries seen in children between 9 months and 3 years of age. Developmentally, as children start to master walking, they are prone to fall. They can easily twist

TABLE 16-6.	Fractures that raise the suspicion for child abuse.
Multiple fractures and no history of major trauma	
Fractures at different stages of healing	
Rib fractures	
Femur fractures in nonambulatory infants	
Scapula and vertebral fractures without a history of major trauma	
Midshaft humerus fractures	
Epiphyseal fractures	
Metaphyseal fractures and spiral/oblique fractures in nonambulatory infants	
Multiple, complex, or occipital skull fractures	

their lower leg as the foot is fixed on the ground. A toddler's rapid increase in linear growth also contributes to the incidence of this problem. It is very unusual to see a toddler's fracture in the nonambulatory child and this should raise the suspicion of a nonaccidental injury.

CLINICAL PRESENTATION

When a child presents with refusal to walk with isolated swelling of the tibial shaft, one must suspect a toddler's fracture. In many cases, there may be no definitive history of trauma. In some cases, the incident may have seemed so minor that the parents are unable to recall a fall or injury. The physical examination may be completely normal or there may be minimal swelling, increase in warmth and tenderness. Pain may be elicited by gentle twisting of the extremity.

DIAGNOSTIC APPROACH

Radiographs. Initial evaluation of a toddler refusing to walk and concerns for toddler's fractures begins with plain films. The antero-posterior and lateral projections will often show a spiral or oblique fraction extending downward and medially in the distal third of the tibia. These findings are often very subtle. In some cases, initial radiographs will be negative or only show minimal soft tissue swelling. If these projections are negative, an internal oblique view may be useful. If your index of suspicion remains high and plain films are normal, a triple phase bone scan can be performed. In other cases, one may immobilize the leg and repeat the radiograph 2-4 weeks later revealing subperiosteal reaction and new bone formation, confirming the diagnosis.

TREATMENT

Treatment primarily involves immobilization via casting if the fracture is discovered within 2 weeks after symptom onset. These patients should be managed in conjunction with orthopedic surgery colleagues.

SUGGESTED READINGS

1. Shravat B, Harrop S, Kane T. Toddler's fracture. *J Accid Emerg Med.* 1996;13(1):59-61.
2. Kemp AM, Dunstan F, Harrison S, et al. Patterns of skeletal fractures in child abuse: systematic review. *BMJ.* 2008;337:859-862.
3. Cooperman DR, Merten DF. Skeletal manifestations of child abuse. In: Reece RM, Ludwig S, eds. *Child Abuse Medical Diagnosis and Management.* 2nd ed. Philadelphia: Lippincott Williams & Wilkins; 2001:135-139.
4. Pandya N, Baldwin K, Kamath A, Wenger D, Hosalkar H. Unexplained fractures: child abuse or bone disease. *Clini Orthop Relat R.* 2011;469(3):805-812.
5. Kellogg N, the Committee on Child Abuse and Neglect. Evaluation of suspected child physical abuse. *Pediatrics.* 2007;119(6):1232-1241.

CASE 16-4

Two-Year-Old Boy

JEANINE RONAN

HISTORY OF PRESENT ILLNESS

A 2-year-old boy was well until 2 days prior to admission, when he slipped and fell on his right side. After the injury, the parents stated that he began limping. Later that evening he developed fevers to 103°F. He was treated with ibuprofen. During the course of the night he became irritable, particularly when his parents attempted to carry him. He refused to stand. He was taken to a nearby emergency department for evaluation. Radiographs of the right lower extremity were negative and he was sent home with the diagnosis of a knee contusion. The following day, he was able to walk for brief periods but continued to limp. However, during the course of the next few hours, he again stopped walking and became very clingy. He was taken to the hospital for reevaluation.

MEDICAL HISTORY

This child was a healthy boy with no significant medical history. His immunizations were up-to-date. His developmental history was also normal.

PHYSICAL EXAMINATION

T 38.3°C; RR 24/min; HR 110 bpm; BP 98/75 mmHg; Height 25th percentile; Weight 50th percentile

On physical examination, the child was crying and difficult to console. Heart, lungs, and abdomen were normal. There was mild swelling and erythema of the right lower extremity. There was significant tenderness over the length of the tibia. Range of motion was normal at the hip, knee, and ankle. Deep tendon reflexes were present. Perfusion to the right foot was normal. He would only walk with assistance, but he was able to crawl.

DIAGNOSTIC STUDIES

The complete blood count revealed a WBC count of 17 400 cells/mm³ (18% band forms, 77% segmented neutrophils, and 5% lymphocytes), a hemoglobin of 10.7 g/dL, and a platelet count of 578 000/mm³. The erythrocyte sedimentation rate (ESR) was 75 mm/h and his C-reactive protein (CRP) was 9.2 mg/dL. A blood culture was obtained. Repeat radiograph of the right tibia was normal.

COURSE OF ILLNESS

MRI of the right lower extremity confirmed the diagnosis (Figure 16-3).

DISCUSSION CASE 16-4

DIFFERENTIAL DIAGNOSIS

Diagnosing the cause of limp or refusal to walk in a toddler is challenging. A history of overt trauma may be absent or, as in this case, the history of trauma may be misleading. Furthermore, localizing pain in young children may be difficult and the location of the pain may not accurately represent the area of pathology. In these children, the differential

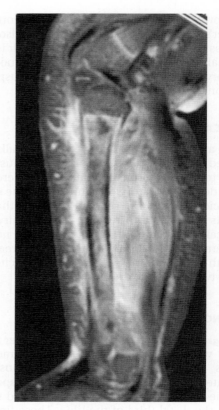

FIGURE 16-3. MRI of the tibia.

diagnosis can be narrowed by assessing associated symptoms. In this child who also has fever, infectious causes must be considered. Septic arthritis is unlikely given the normal examination of the hip, knee, and ankle joints. However, osteomyelitis remains a concern, particularly with associated leg swelling. Cellulitis and myositis are also possible. In addition, one should also consider that this could be the presentation of neoplasms including leukemia, neuroblastoma, or osteoblastoma. Rheumatologic diseases will also present with joint pain and fever. These may include juvenile idiopathic arthritis, reactive arthritis, and acute rheumatic fever.

DIAGNOSIS

MRI of the lower extremity revealed significant soft tissue swelling (Figure 16-3). There was mixed low signal along the entire diaphysis of the tibia consistent with small subperiosteal abscesses surrounded by edema. Edema was also seen circumferentially along the fascia consistent with fasciitis. These findings indicated extensive osteomyelitis of the entire tibia, as well as one large and numerous small subperiosteal collections. Neither the knee nor ankle joint was involved. *Staphylococcus aureus* was isolated from the initial blood culture. The diagnosis was acute hematogenous osteomyelitis of the tibia due to *S. aureus*. In this case, the diagnosis was suspected based on a combination of findings including swelling, erythema, and tenderness over the tibia. The elevated ESR and CRP supported the diagnosis. The MRI confirmed the diagnosis. Initially, the patient was treated with vancomycin based on local resistant patterns for community-acquired methicillin resistant *S. aureus* (CA-MRSA). With clinical improvement, including resolution of fever, being able to weight on his right leg and a substantial decrease in the CRP, the patient was switched to oral clindamycin once antibiotic susceptibilities were available. He was discharged on the sixth day of hospitalization to complete 3-4 weeks of oral antibiotic therapy based on the results of subsequent inflammatory markers. The CRP peaked on the second day after antibiotics were initiated and was normal by the seventh day of treatment. The ESR peaked on the fifth day and normalized 3 weeks after initiation of antibiotics.

INCIDENCE AND EPIDEMIOLOGY

Osteomyelitis in young children is usually due to hematogenous spread of bacteria. Most cases occur within the first 5 years of life, probably due to the rich vascular blood supply at the sites of rapid growth near the growth plates. The valveless sinusoids in the venules at the epiphysis will result in slow nonlaminar blood flow. It is hypothesized that trauma may lead to a hematoma and will be seeded by bacteria during episodes of asymptomatic bacteremia.

In order of decreasing frequency, the affected bones include the femur, tibia, humerus, fibula, and pelvis. The most common organisms causing osteomyelitis vary by age. In neonates, *S. aureus*, group B *Streptococci*, and enteric Gram-negative bacteria predominate. In infants and toddlers, *S. aureus* is by far the most common, but infections may occur due to pneumococcus, group A *Streptococcus*, and *Kingella kingae*. Fungal osteomyelitis due to *Candida* species occurs in premature neonates and intravenous drug abusers. Tuberculous osteomyelitis, due to hematogenous or lymphatic dissemination, occurs in less than 1% of children with active tuberculosis. The spine, femur, and small bones of the hand and feet may be involved with tuberculous osteomyelitis.

Nonhematogenous osteomyelitis usually develops from open fractures, decubitus ulcers, implanted orthopedic equipment, or puncture wounds. Implantable equipment can become infected with *S. aureus* and coagulase-negative staphylococci. In the case of puncture wounds through sneakers, *Pseudomonas aeruginosa* and *S. aureus* are likely pathogens.

CLINICAL PRESENTATION

The presenting signs and symptoms in children with osteomyelitis depend on the site of infection. The typical presentation for patients with osteomyelitis is fever, bone pain, and the inability to bear weight. In many cases, there may be a history of past trauma. Trauma is believed to be a risk factor because of the increase in blood flow to the injured area that occurs after an injury.

Systemic symptoms include fever, malaise, and poor appetite. On physical examination, there may be swelling and erythema of the affected extremity. Often there is point tenderness rather than diffuse bone tenderness. In most cases, the metaphysis of the long bones are the sites of infection. Range of motion should be intact, in comparison to patients with septic arthritis in which micromotion tenderness will be seen. However, the patients may have some limited mobility due to pain or muscle spasm.

A septic hip and shoulder can result in osteomyelitis coinfection, since these joint capsules insert distal to the epiphysis on the femur and humerus. Neonates are unique in that vascular channels extend across the epiphyseal growth plates; thus an osteomyelitis can cause an adjacent joint infection.

DIAGNOSTIC APPROACH

In general, laboratory data may be helpful in supporting the diagnosis of osteomyelitis.

Blood culture. Blood cultures demonstrate the responsible organism in up to 50% of cases. It should be obtained in all cases of suspected osteomyelitis; it should also be obtained prior to the initiation of antibiotics when possible.

Complete blood count. The peripheral white blood cell count can be normal or elevated. It is neither sufficiently sensitive nor specific to aid in diagnosing osteomyelitis. If symptoms have been present for several days, thrombocytosis may also be present.

Inflammatory markers. CRP is elevated at presentation in over 95% of cases. The ESR is elevated in at least 90% of cases at presentation. If the CRP and ESR remain normal for 3 days in a patient with bone pain, the likelihood that the patient has acute osteomyelitis is low. The CRP and ESR can also be used to monitor response to antibiotic therapy. The CRP typically peaks 2 days after initiation of appropriate antibiotic therapy and returns to normal within 7-10 days. The ESR typically peaks by the fifth day after initiation of antibiotics and returns to normal 3-4 weeks later.

Bone biopsy or aspiration of subperiosteal collections. The gold standard for diagnosis is to collect bone aspirate for culture. In 80% of cases, an organism is identified from either the blood, bone, or joint fluids.

Radiologic studies. A plain radiograph will show lytic lesions and periosteal elevation approximately 10-14 days from the onset of symptoms. Radiographs taken before 14 days may be read as normal and should not divert the physician from pursuing the diagnosis.

A technetium-99m-methylene diphosphonate bone scan localizes to areas of hyperemia and early bone resorption. Images are obtained during three time periods: (1) during isotope infusion; (2) 5 minutes after injection ("blood pool" phase) when the isotope has pooled inflamed tissues because of the increased blood flow; and (3) 3 hours later ("bone" phase) after the isotope has left the soft tissues but remains in areas of bone remodeling. Cellulitis causes uptake in the first two phases while osteomyelitis causes update in all three phases. Bone scans may be most helpful in the following situations: (1) vertebral or pelvic

osteomyelitis, (2) neonates, toddlers, and other children who may have difficulty localizing pain, and (3) multifocal involvement. While the sensitivity of the bone scan is high (80%-95%, though lower in neonates), it does not delineate the anatomy and cannot differentiate between trauma, fracture, infection, and infarction. Therefore, the specificity of the technetium bone scan is low.

MRI is the test of choice for diagnosing osteomyelitis with a sensitivity of 92%-100%. It is most useful when symptoms are localized to a specific region. To obtain this study in infants, toddlers, and young children sedation is required.

TREATMENT

Appropriate antibiotic selection depends on many factors including the patient's age, mechanism of acquisition, and local susceptibility patterns for *S. aureus,* because this is the preeminent pathogen in 70%-90% of all cases (Table 16-7). For neonates with osteomyelitis, appropriate therapy includes the combination of an agent for *S. aureus* and a third-generation cephalosporin to treat Gram-negative infections and group B *Streptococcus.* In older children, therapy is directed at CA-MRSA and depending on local resistance patterns may include oxacillin, clindamycin, or vancomycin. Children with underlying hemoglobinopathies should receive cefotaxime or ceftriaxone empirically in addition to clindamycin or vancomycin given the high-risk for *S. aureus* and *Salmonella.* Additional antibiotics can be added to these regimens based on clinical presentation and mechanism of infection. Definitive therapy should be based on clinical response and culture results.

Response to therapy can be monitored by checking serial CRP and ESR levels. The CRP peaks on the second day after initiation of appropriate antibiotic therapy and returns to normal between the seventh and ninth day. Failure of the CRP to substantially decrease by the fourth day of therapy, raises the concern for treatment failure and may require reimaging or changing antibiotic therapy. The ESR generally peaks on the fifth day after initiation of antibiotics and returns to normal by the third or fourth week. Generally, the CRP and ESR are monitored on a weekly basis until therapy is completed.

TABLE 16-7.	The microbiology of osteomyelitis and empiric therapy.	
Patient Characteristics	*Common Organisms*	*Empiric Therapy[a, b]*
Neonate	*Staphylococcus aureus* Group B *Streptococcus* Enterobacteriaceae	Clindamycin or vancomycin + cefotaxime
Infants and Toddlers	*Staphylococcus aureus* Group A *Streptococcus* *Streptococcus pneumoniae* *K. kingae* (less common)	Clindamycin or vancomycin
School-Age Children	*Staphylococcus aureus* Group A *Streptococcus*	Oxacillin or clindamycin or vancomycin
Ill Appearing	*Staphylococcus aureus*	Vancomycin
Patients With Hemoglobinopathies	*Staphylococcus aureus* *Salmonella*	Clindamycin or vancomycin + cefotaxime
Implantable Devices	*Staphylococcus aureus* Coagulase-negative staphylococci	Vancomycin
Foot Puncture Wounds	*Staphylococcus aureus* *Pseudomonas aerginosa*	Oxacillin or clindamycin or vancomycin + cephalosporin with pseudomonas coverage

[a]Initial empiric therapy will ultimately depend on the local CA-MRSA resistance patterns

[b]Once an organism is identified, therapy can be guided by antibiotic susceptibility of the organism

Typically, therapy continues for 3 weeks and up to 6 weeks in more extensive cases. Duration of therapy depends on the causative organism, severity of illness, and clinical and laboratory response. Historically, treatment of *S. aureus* bone infections for less than 4 weeks led to an unacceptably high rate of relapse. Recent data support that this is not necessary. In addition, recent data have supported that early transition to oral therapy is just as effected as prolonged intravenous therapy. In addition, oral therapy is not associated with the risks of central venous catheters including infections and blood clots. When the CRP is decreasing and the signs of acute inflammation have improved including resolution of fever and ability to weight bear, oral therapy may be used. The willingness of the child to take oral medications and the ability of the parents to administer multiple daily doses must also be taken into account.

SUGGESTED READINGS

1. Conrad D. Acute hematogenous osteomyelitis. *Pediatr Rev.* 1995;16:380-384.

2. Roine I, Arguedas A, Faingezicht I, Rodriguez F. Early detection of sequelae–prone osteomyelitis in children with use of simple clinical and laboratory criteria. *Clin Infect Dis.* 1997;24(5):849-853.

3. Peltola H, Unkila-Kallio L, Kallio MJ. Simplified treatment of acute staphylococcal osteomyelitis of childhood. *Pediatrics.* 1997;99:846-850.

4. Jacobs RF, McCarthy RE, Elser JM. *Pseudomonas* osteochondritis complicating puncture wounds of the foot in children: a 10-year evaluation. *J Infect Dis.* 1989; 160(4):657-661.

5. Paakkonen M, Kallio M, Kallio P, Peltola H. Sensitivity of ESR and CRP in childhood bone and joint infections. *Clin Orthop Relat R.* 2010;468(3):861-866.

6. Zaoutis T, Localio A, Leckerman K, Saddlemire S, Bertoch D, Keron R. Prolonged intravenous therapy versus early transition to oral antimicrobial therapy for acute osteomyelitis in children. *Pediatrics.* 2009;123(2): 636-642.

7. Peltola H, Paakkonen M, Kallio P, Kallio MJ. Osteomyelitis-Septic Arthritis Study Group. Short- versus long-term antimicrobial treatment for acute hematogenous osteomyelitis of childhood: prospective, randomized trial on 131 culture-positive cases. *Pediatr Infect Dis J.* 2010;29:1123-1128.

CASE 16-5

One-Year-Old Boy

JEANINE RONAN

HISTORY OF PRESENT ILLNESS

A 1-year-old boy presented to the emergency department 1 day following a fall. His mother was carrying him when she tripped over a foot stool and fell with him in her arms. The child fell forward and landed on a carpet on his stomach and chest. There was no loss of consciousness and the toddler cried immediately. That day, he remained very fussy and refused to use his right leg. He would cry with all diaper changes. Soon she started to notice that there was some increased swelling over the right lower extremity. There was no history of any recent viral infections or skin changes.

MEDICAL HISTORY

The birth history was remarkable for a baby who was small for gestation age, born at 39 weeks via emergent cesarean section. The birth weight was 4 lb and 5 oz. He remained hospitalized for 1 week, in part due to a severe snowstorm that swept through the area in November, shortly after his birth. The child has been treated in the past with iron supplementation for anemia diagnosed at 10 months of age. His developmental history was appropriate. He crawled up steps and cruised while holding onto furniture. He was not walking by himself yet. He was able to take off his own socks. His current diet consisted of breast milk. He did not take many solid foods. He did not receive any medications.

PHYSICAL EXAMINATION

T 37.4°C; RR 24/min; HR 138 bpm; BP 90/50 mmHg; Height 63 cm (<5th percentile); Weight 8.26 kg (<5th percentile)

In general, the child appeared tearful but consolable. His forehead was prominent. His cardiorespiratory examination was normal. The abdominal examination was benign. The musculoskeletal examination revealed some swelling around the distal end of the right femur and some widening of the wrists. His neurologic examination was unremarkable, including normal strength and DTRs.

DIAGNOSTIC STUDIES

The boy's complete blood cell count revealed a WBC of 11400 cells/mm^3 (16% segmented neutrophils, 71% lymphocytes, 3% eosinophils), a hemoglobin of 11.8 g/dL, and a platelet count of 260000 cells/mm^3. His serum electrolytes, blood urea nitrogen, and creatinine were normal. Calcium level was 8.4 mg/L, phosphorus 2.2 mg/dL, and magnesium 2.2 mg/dL. His liver function tests were remarkable for a low serum albumin at 3.3 mg/dL and an elevated serum alkaline phosphatase at 1077 U/L but with a normal AST and ALT.

COURSE OF ILLNESS

Radiograph of the swollen leg revealed both the primary and underlying diagnosis (Figure 16-4).

DISCUSSION CASE 16-5

DIFFERENTIAL DIAGNOSIS

In this case, the differential diagnosis is particularly narrow. The normal white blood cell count and absence of fever make acute osteomyelitis less likely. In this case, fracture following the trauma described was the most likely primary diagnosis.

DIAGNOSIS

Radiologic films of the right lower extremity showed osteopenia, widened metaphyses, irregular metaphyseal, and physeal borders, with an incomplete nondisplaced distal right femur fracture (Figure 16-4). After obtaining further history, it was discovered that the child received very little sunlight exposure and that his diet was very limited consisting only of juice and breast milk. He had not received any multivitamins. The findings on X-ray,

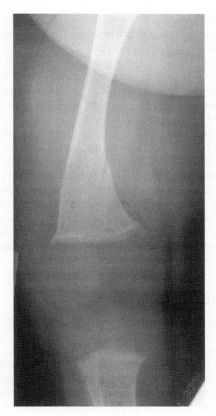

FIGURE 16-4. Radiograph of the femur.

in conjunction with an extremely elevated alkaline phosphatase raised the suspicion of rickets. The diagnosis of rickets was confirmed by a low 25-OH vitamin D level and a normal 1,25-OH vitamin D level. This child had a femur fracture precipitated by trauma in conjunction with nutritional rickets. There was no evidence of an underlying renal or hepatic disease that could have contributed to the development of rickets. An electrocardiogram revealed a normal sinus rhythm and normal intervals. He was placed on vitamin D and calcium supplements orally.

INCIDENCE AND EPIDEMIOLOGY

Rickets is defined as inadequate mineralization of growing bone or osteoid tissue due to a deficiency of vitamin D. Vitamin D receptors are found on the kidney, intestine, bone osteoblasts, and parathyroid gland. Vitamin D_2 (ergocalciferol) is synthesized primarily in plants and with some limited availability in the diet. Vitamin D_3 (cholecalciferol) is made by mammals. It is also found in some foods, but in humans it is naturally synthesized from provitamin form in its skin. Vitamin D_3 is hydroxylated in the liver (25-hydroxylation) forming *calcidiol* (25-hydroxycholecalciferol or $25(OH)D_3$) and again in the renal cortical cells (1-hydroxylation) to produce *calcitriol* (1,25-dihydroxyvitamin D_3 or $1,25(OH)_2D_3$). Rickets develops due to nutritional deficiency of vitamin D or vitamin D transport or metabolism defects ("vitamin D-dependent rickets").

In the past, it was thought that nutritional rickets was seen only in exclusively breastfed infants. Typically, breastmilk has low levels of vitamin D. These infants are not fed other foods rich in vitamin D. In addition, infants have a limited exposure to sunlight which also increases the risk of rickets. However, it has now become known that even formula-fed infants, as well as healthy children, and adolescents can be at risk for vitamin D deficiency. Nutritional rickets may be seen in patients on vegetarian diets. Dietary vitamin D may be found in liver, fish oils, and fatty fish. Many cereals and milk are fortified with vitamin D. In 2003, the American Academy of Pediatrics recommended a daily intake of 400 IU/day of vitamin D for all infants, children, and adolescents. Besides being essential for bone health, vitamin D has also been shown to have an important role in maintaining innate immunity and thereby preventing infection, autoimmune disease, cancer, and diabetes.

For some patients, impaired absorption of vitamin D deficiency may result from malabsorption, including celiac sprue or cystic fibrosis. Also, abnormalities in bile salt metabolism will decrease the absorption of vitamin D.

Nutritional rickets develops because the body tries to maintain a normal serum calcium level. When vitamin D is not present, less calcium is absorbed through the intestine. A lower calcium level causes the secretion of parathyroid hormone and the mobilization of calcium from the bone. Thus, as the body tries to preserve a normal calcium level, the parathyroid hormone becomes elevated, the serum phosphorus level is low, and the alkaline phosphatase enzyme is extremely elevated.

Other causes of rickets occur when there is difficulty with the metabolism of vitamin D. Liver disease may decrease the production of 25-OH cholecalciferol. Certain medications, including phenobarbital, can cause rickets by affecting the liver metabolism of vitamin D. Vitamin D-dependent rickets type I develops from absence of renal hydroxylase. Laboratory data are similar to nutritional rickets with the exception of low calcitriol levels. Symptoms can be overcome with high doses of vitamin D. Vitamin D-dependent rickets type II (vitamin D receptor mutations) occurs when there is a low affinity for vitamin D at the level of receptor. In this case, the calcitriol levels are very high. This too can be overcome by higher doses of vitamin D.

Rickets may also occur in conditions causing chronic acidosis since bone is resorbed to buffer the acid load. Excess phosphate excretion due to defects in renal tubular resorption of phosphate, such as X-linked hyperphosphaturia and Fanconi syndrome, may also lead to rickets.

CLINICAL PRESENTATION

Children with vitamin D deficiency can have a variable presentation. Infants may be asymptomatic, present with signs of hypocalcemia or present with overt signs of rickets and bone demineralization. Clinical signs of hypocalcemia include hypocalcemic seizures, stridor (laryngospasm), tetany, carpopedal spasm, and apnea. The presence of profound hypocalcemia should alert the clinician to vitamin D deficiency, but hypoparathyroidism, 22q11.2 deletion, and pseudohypoparathyroidism should also be considered.

A thorough social and dietary history allows the clinician to identify children who may be at risk of developing rickets. Detailed information regarding the infant feeding method, the timing of solid food introduction, and the use of vitamin D supplements should be collected. It is also necessary to ask about sunlight exposure, medications, family history, and stool consistency to assess for concerns about malabsorption.

The clinical findings will vary based on the child's age, underlying disorder, and duration of the problem. Patients with rickets may present with multiple abnormalities of the musculoskeletal system. Infants and young children may have significant frontal bossing, since the head grows rapidly early in life. Delayed dentition and enamel disruption may be present. The upper extremities and ribs grow quickly during the first year of life, and are therefore the regions to assess for signs of rickets. The child may experience painful and tender bones. The wrists and ankles may be broad and swollen. A rachitic rosary occurs when there is enlargement of the costochondral junctions of the anterior lateral ribs. There will be a prominence of bowing of the lower extremities in an ambulatory child. Some children may have trouble reaching some gross motor milestones, including delayed ambulation. Children with underlying chronic acidosis may present with failure to thrive.

DIAGNOSTIC APPROACH

Radiographs. Rickets may be diagnosed based on radiographic findings. Radiographs of the wrists are usually the most revealing. The metaphysic demonstrates cupping and widening with an increase in the width of radiolucency between the metaphysic and epiphysis. Bone density is decreased and the cortical bone is thin. A Milkman pseudofracture is a ribbon-like radiolucency that extends transversely across the concave side of the long bones. Pathologic fractures may be present. Occasionally, children are diagnosed with rickets by incidental findings on chest radiograph during an evaluation for respiratory distress from bronchiolitis. Chest radiograph findings include demineralization of the skeleton with cupping of the distal end of the ribs and humerus.

Laboratory studies. They can be used to determine the etiology of rickets (Table 16-8). Some important values are discussed below.

Calcium, magnesium, and phosphorus. In vitamin D deficient rickets, the calcium is typically mildly depressed (7-8 mg/dL), but in some cases the calcium may be much lower resulting in symptoms of hypocalcemia; phosphorus levels are normal to low depending on the extent of disease. Other cases of rickets are associated with profoundly low levels of phosphorus. This is usually due to renal

Disorder*	Calcium	iPTH	Phosphate	Creatinine	25(OH)D$_3$	1,25(OH)$_2$D$_3$
TABLE 16-8. Classification of laboratory values in causes of rickets.						
Mild Nutritional Vitamin D Deficiency	Normal/low	Normal/high	Normal/low	Normal	Low	Normal
Severe Nutritional Vitamin D Deficiency	Low	Very high	Low	Normal	Very low	Low
Anticonvulsant-Induced	Low	High	Low	Normal	Low	Normal/low
X-Linked Hypophosphatemic Rickets	Normal	High	Low	Normal	Normal	Low
Liver Disease	Normal/low	Normal	Normal	Normal	Normal	Normal/low
Chronic Renal Failure	Normal/low	Very high	High	High	Normal	Very low
Hereditary Vitamin D Resistant Rickets (mutations in Vitamin D receptor)	Low	High	Low	Normal	Normal	Very high

*Alkaline phosphatase elevated early in all disorders

Abbreviations: iPTH, intact parathyroid hormone; 25(OH)D$_3$, calcidiol; 1,25(OH)$_2$D$_3$, calcitriol

wasting of phosphorus as seen in X-linked hypophosphatemia. Hypomagnesemia is frequently seen when calcium levels are low.

Alkaline phosphatase. Alkaline phosphatase will be elevated even prior to development of hypocalcemia, due to the increase in bone turnover.

Vitamin D metabolites. Both 25(OH)D$_3$ and 1,25(OH)$_2$D$_3$ can be sent. 25(OH)D$_3$ is the most important clinical indicator of nutritional levels. In nutritional rickets, the 25(OH)D$_3$ is low and the 1,25(OH)2D$_3$ may be low or normal depending on the severity of the rickets and the duration of symptoms.

Other studies. Intact parathyroid hormone and serum creatinine are helpful in determining other possible cause of rickets (Table 16-8). Urinary calcium, pH, creatinine, and amino acids can be used to exclude (or diagnose) Fanconi syndrome and proximal renal tubular acidosis.

TREATMENT

Depending on the etiology, the treatment of rickets is aimed at restoring the serum calcium and phosphorus levels and increasing the mineralization of bone. In the case of nutritional rickets, vitamin D and calcium supplementation is the treatment of choice.

Currently, emphasis is placed on prevention of nutritional rickets. All infants, children, and adolescents should take daily vitamin D supplementation. Other natural sources of vitamin D include liver and fish, as well as fortified breakfast cereals and dairy products. Sunlight remains another source to increase the amount of vitamin D; however, the skin cancer risks with sun exposure limit its use.

If the patient has signs of symptomatic hypocalcemia, correction should be carried out immediately in a hospitalized setting. It is important to also monitor the patient's heart rate and rhythm and to evaluate for prolonged QT syndrome. This will improve as the calcium level is restored to normal.

SUGGESTED READINGS

1. Bergstrom WH. Twenty ways to get rickets in the 1990s. *Contemp Pediatr.* 1991;8:88-106.
2. Carpenter TO. Disorders of calcium and bone metabolism in infancy and childhood. In: Becker KL. *Principles and Practice of Endocrinology and Metabolism.* Philadelphia: Lippincott Williams & Wilkins; 1996:631-637.
3. Ryan S: Nutritional aspects of metabolic bone disease in the newborn. *Arch Dis Child.* 1996;74:145-148.
4. Wagner C and Greer F. Prevention of rickets and vitamin D deficiency in infants, children and adolescents. *Pediatrics.* 2008;122(5):1142-1152.
5. Rajah J, Thandrayen K, Pettifor J. Diagnostic approach to the rachititc child. *Eur J Pediatr.* 2011;170:1089-1096.

CASE 16-6

Two-Year-Old Boy

JEANINE RONAN

HISTORY OF PRESENT ILLNESS

A 2-year-old boy with a medical history of asthma initially presented to the emergency department with a fever, cough, and difficulty breathing. The toddler also complained intermittently of back pain. At this time, the physical examination was remarkable only for cervical adenopathy and mild diffuse expiratory wheeze. He was treated with albuterol by metered-dose inhaler and discharged home. One week later, the patient returned to the hospital with an unsteady gait for 2 days. At the time of presentation, he was refusing to walk. He continued to have fevers over the past few days. His activity level was drastically diminished. In addition, he appeared to have focal pain over his lower back. There was no discomfort over any of his extremities. There was no history of trauma. There was no weight loss, night sweats, emesis, or diarrhea.

MEDICAL HISTORY

The boy's birth history was complicated by meconium aspiration syndrome requiring mechanical ventilation for 1 week. He has a history of asthma. He has had several exacerbations treated as an outpatient with albuterol via meter dose inhaler and spacer. He has never received corticosteroids, required hospitalization, or been on daily controller therapy. The family history was unremarkable.

PHYSICAL EXAMINATION

T 38.5°C; RR 24/min; HR 111 bpm; BP 120/70 mmHg; Weight 25th percentile

In general, he appeared comfortable lying with his parents but expressed significant discontent when asked to sit or stand. There was no lymphadenopathy. The heart and lungs were normal. There was no splenomegaly or hepatomegaly. There was mild focal tenderness over the lumbosacral spine with palpation. He was able to flex and extend both lower extremities without difficulty. Deep tendon reflexes were 2+ and symmetric. Cranial nerves appeared intact. His motor strength was symmetrical in all extremities. Sensation appeared intact. There were no cerebellar signs.

DIAGNOSTIC STUDIES

A complete blood cell count of the boy revealed a WBC of 5500 cells/mm^3 (65% segmented neutrophils, 33% lymphocytes), a hemoglobin of 11.2 g/dL, and a platelet count of 225 000 cells/mm^3. The sedimentation rate was elevated at 70 mm/h. The C-reactive protein level was also elevated at 8.5 mg/dL. The lactate dehydrogenase level was high at 2276 U/L (normal range, 470-900 U/L).

COURSE OF ILLNESS

The patient was hospitalized to evaluate for possible vertebral osteomyelitis and diskitis. Given the focal findings on examination, magnetic resonance imaging (MRI) of the lumbar spine was performed (Figure 16-5). The MRI suggested another diagnostic entity and biopsy of the lesion confirmed the final diagnosis.

DISCUSSION CASE 16-6

DIFFERENTIAL DIAGNOSIS

In this case, the initial concern was to evaluate the patient for possible osteomyelitis and diskitis. When this toddler presented with fever, refusal to walk, and elevated markers of inflammation, an infectious etiology must be considered. The most common cause of vertebral osteomyelitis is *Staphylococcus aureus*. Less common causes include group A *Streptococcus*, *Streptococcus pneumoniae*, and enteric Gram-negative rods. Tuberculosis can cause vertebral osteomyelitis. Malignancies should also be considered in this setting. Leukemia and lymphoma often present with nonspecific

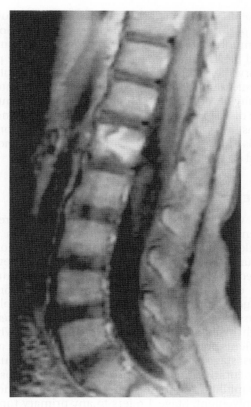

FIGURE 16-5. MRI of the spine.

findings including fever, weight loss, malaise, and refusal to walk. Bone tumors including osteosarcoma or Ewings sarcoma are other possible etiologies. Metastatic neuroblastoma often presents with bone pain and fever. Neuroblastoma can also present with local effects, including an isolated thoracic or abdominal mass.

DIAGNOSIS

The MRI (Figure 16-5) demonstrated a heterogeneous bone marrow signal with marked contrast enhancement of approximately 1 cm in the anterior aspect of the vertebral body. The lesion did not extend into or disrupt the disk space. There was no associated soft tissue edema or abscess. These MRI findings were not consistent with osteomyelitis. When there is an infectious cause, soft tissue edema and disk space involvement should be

seen. Given these concerns, biopsies of the vertebral lesion and bone marrow were performed. **The pathology results showed metastatic neuroblastoma.** Further radiologic studies, including computed tomography of the head, abdomen, and chest, were unable to determine a primary lesion. The patient received chemotherapy for stage 4 neuroblastoma.

Neuroblastoma is an embryonal tumor derived from the neural crest cells that form sympathetic ganglia and adrenal medulla. As in this case, the diagnosis is suspected based on history and radiographic findings, but confirmed by pathology. Histologically, neuroblastoma typically is made up of areas of calcification and hemorrhage surrounding small round cells with cytoplasmic granules. The cells may form together into shapes like rosettes, which are called Homer Wright rosettes.

INCIDENCE AND EPIDEMIOLOGY

Neuroblastoma, the most common extracranial solid tumor of childhood, accounts for about 10% of all childhood cancers. There are about 500 new cases in the United States every year. Most cases are diagnosed before 4 years of age with the median age of 17 months at the time of diagnosis. Most tumors (80%) are located below the diaphragm and approximately 50% of all neuroblastoma tumors arise from the adrenal gland.

CLINICAL PRESENTATION

Neuroblastoma presents in a wide variety of ways depending on the tumor location and extent of disease. It can arise throughout the body from developing tissues of the sympathetic nervous symptoms. Tumors can develop in the adrenal medulla or paraspinal ganglia, and in the neck, chest, abdomen, and pelvis. A thoracic mass may be seen as a hard, painless lump in the neck or chest, or may present with signs of superior vena cava syndrome due to compression from large mediastinal tumors. In some cases, a young child may present with an enlarging abdominal mass. Depending on location, the patient may be asymptomatic, and show signs of bowel obstruction, or liver involvement. If compression occurs on renal vasculature due to an enlarging adrenal tumor, the patient may develop hypertension. If the tumor involves cells from the sympathetic ganglia, a paraspinal mass may be present. These patients may experience back pain and nerve compression resulting in bladder or bowel dysfunction or gait disturbance. If cervical sympathetic ganglia are involved, a unilateral Horner syndrome (ptosis, miosis, anhidrosis) may be seen. Common sites of metastatic disease include regional lymph nodes and bone marrow and liver via the hematopoietic system.

There are some unique presentations with neuroblastoma. A paraneoplastic syndrome, called opsoclonus-myoclonus or "dancing eyes," may develop. This involves jerky and chaotic eye movements and myoclonic jerks. If this is detected, it is important to look for the primary source of the tumor. In most cases, the opsoclonus and myoclonus improve with treatment. However, some patients continue to have issues even after eradication of the tumor. Occasionally, metastases may deposit in the periorbital region causing proptosis and periorbital ecchymosis. This finding resembles "raccoon eyes." Excess catecholamine secretion from the tumor leads to other systemic signs including flushing, tachycardia, hypertension, and diarrhea.

DIAGNOSTIC APPROACH

The first step to the diagnostic approach is to consider the possibility of neuroblastoma. Consider the diagnosis in patients with nonspecific systemic signs and bone pain. Physical examination findings may involve a palpable abdominal mass and lymphadenopathy. It is also important to pay attention to the patient's blood pressure.

Complete blood count. Pancytopenia suggests bone marrow involvement.

Urinary catecholamines. In more than 90% of cases, urine catecholamines, such as homovanillic acid (HVA) and vanillylmandelic acid (VMA), will be elevated. These should be collected via a 24-h urine collection since random "spot" samples may yield false-positive results.

Bone marrow biopsy. Bone marrow aspirates are necessary to determine metastatic involvement of the bone marrow.

Radiologic studies. Skeletal radiographs should be performed to detect metastatic bone lesions. Computed tomography of the chest, abdomen, and pelvis should be performed to detect the primary site and possible metastatic sites of involvement. Meta-iodobenzylguanidine (MIBG) scintography is very helpful in determining the extent of the disease. It is taken up by the sympathetic neurons in 90%-95% of patients with neuroblastoma. This study can be used with the initial diagnosis and as a means to monitor treatment.

TREATMENT

As with many oncologic diseases, the treatment and prognosis is determined based on the patient's stage at presentation. The International Neuroblastoma Staging System (INSS) was developed based on clinical, radiographic, and surgical evaluation of children with neuroblastoma. Stage 1 represents localized tumor with complete gross excision. Stage 2 refers to localized disease with ipsilateral lymph node involvement. When patients present with localized disease (stage 1 and most stage 2), surgical removal of the tumor is usually curative. Stage 3 occurs when disease crosses the midline and there is contralateral lymph node involvement. Stage 4 refers to any primary tumor with dissemination to distant lymph nodes, bone, bone marrow, liver, skin, or other organs (except as defined for stage 4S). Stage 4S refers to localized primary tumor with dissemination limited to skin, liver, or bone marrow in infants younger than 1 year. Patients with stage 4S disease are frequently classified into the low-risk category. However, this classification has had its limitations in its ability to address the appropriate therapy for patients who fall between the extremes. The International Neuroblastoma Risk Group (INRG) has developed a new system based on the prognostic risk factors associated with the tumor, including patient age, tumor stage, tumor differentiation, DNA ploidy, and amplification of the *MYC-N* oncogene. This further classification system will hopefully be able to better define therapy with the best chance for cure. For more favorable prognostic factors, ways to reduce toxicity may be identified. For more aggressive tumors, intensification of the chemotherapy can be evaluated.

Treatment for patients with high-risk neuroblastoma includes an induction phase of remission, consolidation phase, and a maintenance phase. Autologous hematopoietic stem cell transplant after myeloablative chemotherapy has been shown to improve the disease-free survival. Aggressive induction therapy is imperative as 50%-60% of high-risk patients will have a relapse and currently there are no curative salvage treatment plans. Isotretinoin has been shown to differentiate neuroblastoma cell lines and is now part of standard therapy. Future developments are investigating ways to treat children with high-risk neuroblastoma including the possibility of ^{131}I-labeled MIBG. Patients with low-risk neuroblastoma (asymptomatic stages 2a or 2b) have excellent survival rates after surgery alone; overall survival is 97% and event-free survival (absence of progressive disease, relapse, secondary malignancy, or death from any cause) is approximately 90%. Chemotherapy may be restricted to the minority of patients with low-risk neuroblastoma such as older children with stages 2b disease and those with unfavorable tumor histology or diploid tumors.

Survival rates exceed 98% in those children categorized as low risk and approaches 90%-95% in those children categorized as intermediate risk. Unfortunately, those considered high risk have a survival rate of only 40%-50%.

SUGGESTED READINGS

1. Castleberry RP. Biology and treatment of neuroblastoma. *Pediatr Clin N Am*. 1997;44:919-937.
2. Strother DR, London WB, Schmidt ML, et al. Outcome after surgery alone or with restricted use of chemotherapy for patients with low-risk neuroblastoma: results of Children's Oncology Group study P9641. *J Clin Oncol*. 2012;30:1842-1848.
3. Behrman RE, Kliegman RM, Arvin AM. *Nelson Textbook of Pediatrics*. Philadelphia: W.B. Saunders Company; 1996.
4. Maris J. Recent advances in neuroblastoma. *N Engl J Med*. 2010;362:2202-2011.

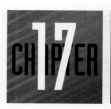

DIARRHEA

CHRISTINA L. MASTER

DEFINITION OF THE COMPLAINT

Diarrhea is one of the most common conditions for which patients seek medical care. It is a condition that continues to be associated with significant morbidity and mortality worldwide, despite medical advances. It is characterized by an increase in the frequency, volume, or liquid content of stool as compared to any given individual's usual pattern.

Diarrhea may also be further characterized by the duration of the symptoms, with acute episodes of diarrhea generally resolving within 2 weeks, while chronic diarrhea generally lasts longer than 2 weeks. Another important distinction in the type of diarrhea is based on whether it is secretory or osmotic in nature. Agents that disrupt the normal absorption of intestinal luminal fluid at the cellular level generally cause a profuse and voluminous secretory diarrhea that continues regardless of the patient's oral intake. Osmotic diarrhea, however, is the result of poorly absorbed substances that draw fluid into the intestinal lumen. This type of diarrhea tends to improve with fasting on the part of the patient.

The most common causes of diarrhea are infectious, with viral etiologies occurring more frequently than bacterial. The differential diagnosis of diarrhea, however, is quite extensive and includes some rare causes. Many cases of diarrhea occur in children who are otherwise well appearing, while some cases of diarrhea present in children who are ill appearing, due to either poor nutrition, hydration, or other systemic reasons.

COMPLAINT BY CAUSE AND FREQUENCY

There are myriad causes of diarrhea that can be stratified by age (Table 17-1) or diagnostic category (Table 17-2).

CLARIFYING QUESTIONS

A thorough history can provide clues to facilitate an accurate diagnosis in the child who presents with diarrhea. Consideration of the age and appearance of the patient, the length and course of the illness, and associated clinical features provides a useful framework for creating a differential diagnosis. The following questions may help provide clues to the diagnosis:

- How long has the diarrhea lasted?
  —Diarrhea that has lasted less than 2 weeks is acute diarrhea, rather than chronic. Acute diarrhea is more likely to be infectious (viral or bacterial) in etiology. Chronic diarrhea raises the concern over other diagnoses such as malabsorptive conditions (cystic fibrosis, celiac disease), although infectious (parasitic) and postinfectious (postinfectious carbohydrate malabsorption) causes are still possible.

- Is there any blood or mucus in the stool?
  —In the acute setting, blood or mucus in the stool increases the possibility of an enteroinvasive agent (enteroinvasive *Escherichia coli*, *Salmonella* spp. or *Shigella* spp.). In the chronic setting, inflammatory bowel disease should be considered. In a systemically ill-appearing child, hemolytic uremic syndrome must be considered.

TABLE 17-1.	Causes of diarrhea by age.	
Prevalence	*Neonate/Infant*	*School Age/ Adolescence*
Common	Systemic infections	Infectious gastroenteritis
	Infectious gastroenteritis	Nonspecific diarrhea of childhood
	Necrotizing enterocolitis	Antibiotic-associated
	Antibiotic-associated	Encopresis
	Overfeeding	Carbohydrate malabsorption
	Carbohydrate malabsorption	Food poisoning
Less Common	Hirschsprung enterocolitis	Inflammatory bowel disease
	Milk protein allergy	Lactose intolerance
	Cystic fibrosis	Cystic fibrosis
	Celiac disease	Laxative abuse
Uncommon	Congenital lactase deficiency	Secretory tumors
	Congenital villous atrophy	Hyperthyroidism
	Secretory tumors	Intestinal lymphangiectasia
	Congenital adrenal hyperplasia	

- Is there abdominal pain or cramping? Tenesmus?
  —Acute infectious gastroenteritis can present with abdominal cramping, while a chronic history of cramping or tenesmus raises the concern for inflammatory bowel disease.

- Is there any vomiting?
  —Vomiting may be associated with acute infectious gastroenteritis. However, if bilious vomiting is noted, especially in a neonate or an infant, an anatomic condition (malrotation, incarcerated hernia) must be considered.

- Is there a fever?
  —Presence of a fever acutely may indicate either an enteroinvasive infectious agent or systemic illness (pneumonia) with an associated nonspecific diarrhea. In a toxic-appearing child, sepsis and toxic shock syndrome must be considered. In a patient with a chronic history of diarrhea with acute exacerbations associated with fever, inflammatory bowel disease is a distinct possibility.

TABLE 17-2.	Causes of diarrhea by diagnostic category.
Diagnostic Category	*Specific Cause*
Infectious	Viral —Rotavirus —Enteric adenovirus —Astrovirus —Norovirus —Calicivirus Bacteria —*Salmonella* species —*Shigella* species —*Escherichia coli* —*Campylobacter jejuni* —*Yersinia enterocolitica* —*Vibrio cholerae* —*Clostridium difficile* Parasitic —*Giardia lamblia* —*Cryptosporidium* species
Dietary	Sorbitol Fructose Food poisoning
Malabsorptive	Celiac disease Cystic fibrosis Carbohydrate malabsorption, postinfectious
Oncologic	Neuroblastoma Ganglioneuroma
Endocrine	Hyperthyroidism Hyperparathyroidism Congenital adrenal hyperplasia Adrenal insufficiency
Toxicologic	Medication side effect Antibiotic-associated Laxatives
Allergic	Milk protein allergy
Immunologic	Immune deficiencies AIDS Inflammatory bowel disease
Anatomic	Short bowel syndrome Malrotation Hirschsprung disease
Congenital	Congenital lactase deficiency Congenital villous atrophy
Vasculitis	Henoch-Schönlein purpura Hemolytic uremic syndrome
Miscellaneous	Irritable bowel syndrome Chronic nonspecific diarrhea of childhood Overfeeding Encopresis

- Does the patient appear systemically ill?
  —In acute diarrhea, a systemically ill-appearing child should raise the concern for sepsis (*Salmonella* spp., *E. coli*, especially in a neonate or infant). If oliguria is also present, hemolytic uremic syndrome must be considered, in addition to simple dehydration associated with diarrheal losses. In patients who have a history of chronic diarrhea and failure to thrive, superimposed episodes of acute diarrhea can make them appear systemically ill, as in cases of inflammatory bowel disease, celiac disease, or cystic fibrosis.

- Is there failure to thrive?
  —A chronic history of diarrhea associated with failure to thrive raises the concern for malabsorptive conditions such as cystic fibrosis and celiac disease. Neuroendocrine tumors that cause a secretory diarrhea may present with significant weight loss. Inflammatory bowel disease also commonly presents with linear growth arrest in addition to poor weight gain.

- Are there ill contacts with diarrhea?
  —Close contacts with similar symptoms may indicate an outbreak with a common source of contamination (e.g., daycare, family reunion, restaurant), whether toxin-associated food poisoning, or fecal-oral contamination.

- Is there any unusual food exposure?
  —In particular, undercooked foods, specifically beef, are of concern as a source for *E. coli* O157:H7 resulting in hemolytic uremic syndrome (HUS). Improperly stored food is another potential source for food poisoning. New foods may not be tolerated well and be the source of transient diarrhea or may cause bloody diarrhea, as in the case of milk-protein allergy in infants.

- Any recent history of travel?
  —Foreign travel increases the concern over travelers' diarrhea, often due to unfamiliar strains of *E. coli*, or unusual organisms, such as *Entamoeba histolytica*, as a cause of chronic diarrhea. Other parasites such as *Giardia lamblia* and agents such as hepatitis A may also be acquired during travel.

- What is the water source?
  —Untreated or contaminated water sources can harbor *Giardia lamblia* or *Cryptosporidium*. Cases of *E. coli* O157:H7 transmission have also been known to occur with exposure in water sources such as swimming pools or lakes.

- Are there any pets? Any exposure to animals?
  —Pets such as lizards, turtles, and iguanas may harbor *Salmonella*, which can then cause diarrhea in children who play with them. Farm animals and petting zoos are also potential sources for *E. coli* O157:H7 and epidemic cases of hemolytic uremic syndrome.

- Is there a history of recent antibiotic use?
  —Antibiotic-associated diarrhea, including *Clostridium difficile* colitis, may occur.

- Is there any significant medical history?
  —Failure to thrive is of particular concern with either superimposed acute or chronic diarrhea. Former premature infants who had surgical necrotizing enterocolitis may have subsequent chronic diarrhea due to short bowel syndrome. Other conditions may also have diarrhea associated (human immunodeficiency virus infection and other immune compromising conditions) as well as endocrinologic disorders (e.g., hyperthyroidism).

- Is there a significant family history?
  —Patients with inflammatory bowel disease may present with family members with similar symptoms. Cystic fibrosis and celiac disease have traditionally been associated with Northern European ancestry, although patients of other ethnicities can also carry these diagnoses.

- Is the diarrhea worse with oral intake? Is it improved with fasting?
  —This question will help to differentiate osmotic diarrhea, which characterizes most cases of diarrhea, from secretory diarrhea, which is much less common and often is associated with otherwise occult oncologic conditions.

- Is there a rash?
  —A petechial, purpuric rash would be indicative of Henoch-Schönlein purpura, although, in an ill-appearing child, sepsis would also have to be considered. Other rashes, such as dermatitis herpetiformis, can be seen in chronic conditions, such as celiac disease. Rashes may also develop due to nutritional deficiencies.

- Is the weight loss intentional?
  —Teenagers who are overly concerned with body image may be using laxatives to lose weight.

CASE 17-1

Two-Month-Old Boy

CHRISTINA L. MASTER

HISTORY OF PRESENT ILLNESS

The patient is a 2-month-old boy who presents with vomiting and diarrhea. The patient had been recently discharged from the hospital 3 days ago. During that previous hospitalization, he had been diagnosed with gastroesophageal reflux by pH probe and upper gastrointestinal series. He had been discharged to home on ranitidine and had been doing well until the evening prior to presentation when he developed vomiting and diarrhea. He had 12 episodes of nonbloody, nonbilious vomiting with eight episodes of loose stools. There was no fever or associated upper respiratory symptoms. He had normal urine output. His mother reports that he was more fussy than usual and she noted a lump in his groin on the day of presentation to the hospital.

MEDICAL HISTORY

The patient was a full-term baby with an uncomplicated pregnancy, labor, and delivery history. He was hospitalized only once, diagnosed with gastroesophageal reflux, and placed on ranitidine.

PHYSICAL EXAMINATION

T 36.9°C; RR 32/min; HR 136 bpm; BP 100/54 mmHg

Weight 5th percentile

On examination, the infant was alert and in no acute distress. His head, neck, cardiac, and respiratory examination were unremarkable. He was well hydrated with a nontender and non-distended, soft abdomen. There was no hepatosplenomegaly or abdominal masses. He had normal male genitalia, with bilaterally descended testicles. A tender, firm, and erythematous mass measuring 5 cm × 3 cm was palpable in the right inguinal region.

DIAGNOSTIC STUDIES

The complete blood count revealed a WBC count of 10 100 cells/mm^3 (11% segmented neutrophils, 76% lymphocytes), a hemoglobin of 10.8 g/dL with a mean corpuscular volume of 87 fL and a platelet count of 387 000 mm^3. Serum electrolytes, blood urea nitrogen, and creatinine were normal.

COURSE OF ILLNESS

An abdominal radiograph obtained on his previous admission suggested a cause for the current complaint (Figure 17-1). A surgical consultation was requested.

DISCUSSION CASE 17-1

DIFFERENTIAL DIAGNOSIS

In this case, diarrhea was associated with vomiting and a critical physical finding, that of an inguinal mass. This essential finding directs the differential diagnosis toward causes of inguinal or scrotal swelling. An important distinction to make is between a painful or painless mass. A hydrocele is a common entity that causes painless inguinal or

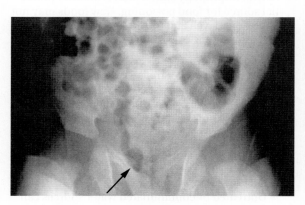

FIGURE 17-1. Abdominal radiograph.

scrotal swelling. It is primarily differentiated from an inguinal hernia by the ability to palpate above the mass, revealing discontinuity between the mass and the inguinal canal. The mass, as a result, does not change in size with straining or crying. In addition, a hydrocele is not reducible and usually transilluminates, although the ability to transilluminate the mass does not exclude the possibility of an incarcerated hernia.

Another cause of a painful scrotal mass is testicular torsion. There often is no history of a prior scrotal mass, and in fact may be associated with a history of undescended testis. This mass is very tender and does not extend into the inguinal canal.

Torsion of the appendix testis results in a painful scrotal mass that may present as a tender blue nodule on the upper pole of the testis which, itself, is not tender. Inguinal lymphadenopathy may be tender or painless but the key to diagnosis is the lateral and inferior location of these nodes in relation to the inguinal canal. Signs of infection in the area of lymphatic drainage are also important in making this diagnosis. An inguinal hernia is usually characterized by a painless swelling in the inguinal area often increasing in size with crying or straining. Incarceration of the hernia results in extreme pain and signs of bowel obstruction. If strangulation occurs, bloody diarrhea may occur.

DIAGNOSIS

A thorough history and physical examination are the keys to this diagnosis. In this case, the painful nature and inguinal location of this mass are the essential findings. Abdominal radiograph from the previous admission revealed a right inguinal hernia (Figure 17-1, arrow) that is now incarcerated. **The diagnosis is incarcerated inguinal hernia.** The hernia was reduced in the emergency department by pediatric surgical staff. No hernia was noted on the left side on physical examination. The patient was admitted for intravenous fluids and observation to allow the bowel edema from the incarceration to resolve. The patient manifested no signs or symptoms of bowel necrosis during 2 days in the hospital after which he was taken to the operating room. Intraoperatively, bilateral inguinal hernias were found and repaired without any complications.

INCIDENCE AND EPIDEMIOLOGY OF INGUINAL HERNIA

The incidence of inguinal hernia is estimated to be anywhere from 1% to 5%, which is approximately 10-20 per 1000 live births. The incidence in premature infants is significantly higher, approaching 30%. The ratio of boys to girls is 6:1. In boys, the right side is more frequently involved than the left, presumably due to the embryologic origin of inguinal hernias through a patent processus vaginalis and the fact that the right testis descends later during gestation than the left. In both boys and girls, 60% of inguinal hernias occur on the right, 30% on the left, and 10% bilaterally. Inguinal hernias are usually diagnosed during the first year of life, most frequently in the first month of life. There is often a family history of inguinal hernia. Undescended testes may also be associated with inguinal hernias. Other conditions associated with inguinal hernias include Ehlers-Danlos syndrome, cystic fibrosis, congenital cytomegalovirus infection, and testicular feminization. There is no apparent ethnic or racial predisposition to inguinal hernia. Incarcerated inguinal hernias occur most frequently in those younger than 6 months of age, are less common after 2 years of age, and are rare after 5 years of age.

CLINICAL PRESENTATION OF INGUINAL HERNIA

An inguinal hernia usually presents as an asymptomatic swelling in the scrotal or labial area that increases in size with any increase in intra-abdominal pressure, as occurs with crying or straining. Reducible hernias disappear spontaneously or with minimal pressure. An incarcerated hernia develops when a loop of bowel becomes trapped and is accompanied by severe pain and signs of bowel obstruction, such as bilious emesis. Strangulation of the herniated loop of bowel occurs when the blood supply to the bowel is compromised and may develop within 2 hours of incarceration. Urgent medical attention is necessary in cases of incarceration and emergency surgical intervention may be necessary in cases of strangulation.

DIAGNOSTIC APPROACH

The key to diagnosis of inguinal hernia lies in the index of suspicion in the appropriate historical context, which is then confirmed by physical examination. In distinguishing an incarcerated hernia, an awareness of the other important entities in the differential diagnosis is important. The diagnosis itself is primarily founded on the history and physical examination as well as a thorough knowledge of the disease process.

Abdominal radiograph. An abdominal radiograph may show signs of bowel obstruction and may serve as an adjunctive supportive piece of evidence in making the diagnosis.

TREATMENT

In cases of incarcerated hernia, time is of the essence. Compromised blood flow to the affected loop of bowel may result in strangulation and bowel necrosis within 2 hours, hence medical intervention is necessary. Attempt at reduction of the incarcerated hernia by experienced pediatric surgical staff is optimal. A gentle attempt at reduction using pressure on the scrotum with simultaneous counterpressure above the external inguinal ring is indicated, but should never be forcefully done. Intravenous hydration and nasogastric tube decompression, in anticipation of definitive surgical management, is also indicated. Immediate surgical correction is necessary if the incarcerated

hernia is not reducible. If the incarcerated loop of bowel is reduced, surgery may be postponed for 12-36 h to allow the bowel edema to resolve.

Elective repair of an asymptomatic inguinal hernia should be performed as soon as possible after diagnosis to avoid complications, such as incarceration. All inguinal hernias require surgical correction as they do not resolve spontaneously. In boys, undescended testes may be associated with inguinal hernia and require orchiopexy. There is still ongoing debate as to the importance of surgical exploration of the contralateral side in search of an occult inguinal hernia not detected by physical examination, as did occur with the patient in this case. This decision is left to the individual surgeon, but contralateral exploration is performed in the majority of cases.

SUGGESTED READINGS

1. Clarke S. Pediatric inguinal hernia and hydrocele: an evidence based review in the era of minimal access surgery. *J Laparoendosc Adv Surg Tech A.* 2010;20(3):30-39.
2. Brandt ML. Pediatric hernias. *Surg Clin North Am.* 2008;88(1):27-43, vii-viii.
3. Katz D. Evaluation and management of inguinal and umbilical hernias. *Pediatr Ann.* 2001;30:729-735.
4. Kapur P, Caty M, Glick P. Pediatric hernias and hydroceles. *Pediatr Clin North Am.* 1998;45:773-789.
5. Irish M, Pearl R, Caty M, Glick P. The approach to common abdominal diagnoses in infants and children. *Pediatr Clin North Am.* 1998;45:729-772.

CASE 17-2

Two-Year-Old Boy

CHRISTINA L. MASTER

HISTORY OF PRESENT ILLNESS

The patient is a 2-year-old boy, who had been previously well until 3 days prior to presentation to the hospital with watery diarrhea and decreased appetite. The next day, he also developed vomiting at which point he was seen by his primary physician who treated him with trimethobenzamide hydrochloride (Tigan) suppositories which

provided no relief. The symptoms progressed to 20 episodes of diarrhea, now with blood and mucus and abdominal cramping on the day of presentation. The patient was admitted to an outside hospital for presumed bacterial gastroenteritis. There were no known ill contacts, no known ingestion of undercooked foods, no recent travel, and no recent exposure to antibiotics.

MEDICAL HISTORY

The boy's history was significant only for one hospital admission for an asthma exacerbation. There was no surgical history, no medications. His mother has a history of irritable bowel syndrome.

PHYSICAL EXAMINATION

T 37.5°C; RR 30/min; HR 150 bpm; BP 105/50 mmHg

Weight 50th percentile

The patient was alert, but quiet and ill appearing. His eyes were mildly sunken. He had dry mucous membranes. There was no lymphadenopathy. The remainder of his head and neck examination was unremarkable. His cardiac examination revealed tachycardia, but no murmur or gallop. There was tachypnea, but no rales or wheezing. His neurologic examination was nonfocal. His skin turgor was diminished.

DIAGNOSTIC STUDIES

Complete blood count revealed a WBC count of 16 600 cells/mm³ with a differential of 62% segmented neutrophils, 24% band forms, 10% lymphocytes, 3% monocytes, and 1% atypical lymphocytes. Hemoglobin was 14.2 g/dL and platelet count was 381 000 cells/mm³. White blood cells were present on Gram stain of the stool. Routine bacterial and viral stool cultures were sent which eventually returned negative. Serum electrolytes were significant for a chloride of 100 mmol/L and a bicarbonate of 19 mmol/L. Blood urea nitrogen was 73 mg/dL and creatinine was 1.2 mg/dL.

COURSE OF ILLNESS

The patient was admitted to the hospital for intravenous fluid rehydration and given nothing by mouth after failing of repeated oral clear liquid challenges while continuing to have diarrhea. A Foley catheter was placed to monitor urine output (Figure 17-2). On the second day of hospitalization the patient developed a fever to 39°C with increased abdominal pain, particularly in the

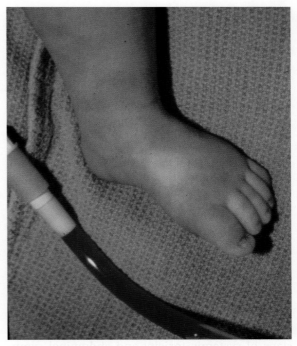

FIGURE 17-2. Photo of the patient's leg (note the poor perfusion) that also includes a portion of the urinary catheter drainage.

periumbilical region and right lower quadrant. His abdominal examination now revealed hypoactive bowel sounds and an abdominal radiograph demonstrated ileus. An abdominal ultrasound showed a small amount of ascites. Ampicillin, gentamicin, and clindamycin were started intravenously. A sigmoidoscopy was performed to 50 cm, demonstrating a normal appearing colon. A biopsy was obtained which showed signs of chronic inflammation. Later that day, the patient was taken for an exploratory laparotomy due to worsening abdominal pain and signs of an acute abdomen. Surgery revealed a leathery thickening of the descending colon, possibly consistent with chronic inflammation, without involvement of the transverse colon or distal sigmoid. A large amount (500 mL) of clear yellow ascitic fluid was also removed. A central venous catheter was placed, given the anticipated need for prolonged intravenous fluids and medications.

DISCUSSION CASE 17-2

DIFFERENTIAL DIAGNOSIS

The key to this diagnosis is having the appropriate level of suspicion in the right clinical context. During the initial prodrome of bloody diarrhea, any of the other bacterial causes of enteroinvasive diarrhea would be on the list of differential diagnoses. *Salmonella*, *Shigella*, and *Campylobacter* species would be among some of the etiologies. In fact, HUS has been associated with *Shigella* infection, as a result of elaboration of Shiga toxin. All of these bacterial causes would be routinely screened for in most stool cultures. It is important to remember that *E. coli* O157:H7 may not be routinely screened for, although it may now be the most common cause of bloody diarrhea in the United States. *Clostridium difficile* colitis could also present in this manner and testing for toxins A and B would be important in distinguishing this entity, as would a prior history of recent antibiotic use.

Inflammatory bowel disease could also present in this fashion, especially as an acute flare with signs of systemic toxicity and abdominal symptoms severe enough sometimes to warrant surgical exploration.

DIAGNOSIS

The Foley catheter revealed bloody urine (Figure 17-2). The patient's lower extremity, also included in the photograph, revealed evidence of poor perfusion. Postoperatively the patient was noted to be edematous while on maintenance intravenous fluids. Repeat laboratory studies revealed a serum sodium of 133 mmol/L, chloride 114 mmol/L, bicarbonate 11 mmol/L, blood urea nitrogen 24 mg/dL, and creatinine 3.0 mg/dL. The hemoglobin decreased to 11.3 g/dL and the platelet count was 118 000 cells/mm^3. The peripheral smear showed the presence of schistocytes, suggesting a hemolytic process. Liver function tests were significant for an aspartate aminotransferase of 532 U/L, alanine aminotransferase 287 U/L, lactate dehydrogenase 4290 U/L, and albumin 1.7 g/dL. The partial thromboplastin time was slightly elevated at 37.4 seconds. During the next 3 hours, the patient's urine output stopped completely. He was given 25% albumin intravenously with intravenous

fluids followed by furosemide which resulted in only 10 cc of urine output. At this point, the patient was transferred to our institution for continuous arteriovenous hemoperfusion. A stool culture sent specifically for detection of *E. coli* O157:H7 returned positive. **This culture confirmed the diagnosis of hemolytic uremic syndrome (HUS) secondary to infection with *E. coli* O157:H7, otherwise known as D(+) HUS, in that it is associated with diarrhea.** During his 4-week hospitalization, his blood urea nitrogen level peaked at 101 mg/dL and creatinine at 9.9 mg/dL. His hemoglobin nadir was 4.7 g/dL and platelet count nadir was 103 000/mm^3. He required continuous arteriovenous hemoperfusion for most of the remainder of his hospitalization. Upon discharge, his blood urea nitrogen was 74 mg/dL and his creatinine was 5.5 mg/dL.

INCIDENCE AND EPIDEMIOLOGY OF HEMOLYTIC UREMIC SYNDROME

HUS is one of the most common causes of acute renal failure in children, and in turn, *E. coli* O157:H7 infection is the most common cause of HUS. As a member of the enterohemorrhagic group of *E. coli*, it causes a hemorrhagic colitis and elaborates a verotoxin that is similar to Shiga toxin, produced by *Shigella dysenteriae* type 1. In the United States, it appears to be one of the most common causes of bloody diarrhea. Cases can occur on a sporadic as well as epidemic basis, which has appeared to be increasing in the last decade. There is a seasonal pattern to infection, in that cases are more common in the summer months, although cases do sometimes occur in the winter. This may also be associated with the fact that cattle and their undercooked meat products or unpasteurized dairy products are the most significant factors in transmission and are more likely to be consumed during the summertime.

The highest attack rates occur at the extremes of the age spectrum—the very old and the very young appear to be at greatest risk. In particular, children younger than 4 years of age are at great risk of contracting *E. coli* O157:H7 infection and are also at greater risk for developing HUS as a result. HUS occurs in approximately 10% of patients who acquire sporadic infection with *E. coli* O157:H7 and appears to occur at a higher attack rate of up to 40% of patients infected in an outbreak. The mortality rate is approximately 5% and another 5% of patients suffer from severe neurologic sequelae or end-stage renal failure. Extremely poor prognostic factors include a high leukocyte count, a severe gastrointestinal prodrome, age younger than 2 years, and early onset of anuria.

CLINICAL PRESENTATION OF HEMOLYTIC UREMIC SYNDROME

Infection with *E. coli* O157:H7 begins as a non-bloody diarrhea that progresses to bloody diarrhea, often a few days after the onset of illness. Vomiting occurs in half of the patients and a fever in approximately one-third. Fecal leukocytes are often present. The hemorrhagic colitis is otherwise nonspecific and may appear indistinguishable clinically from many other colitides. Abdominal symptoms may become severe enough to mimic an acute abdomen, prompting surgical intervention. Complications include intussusception, perforation, or stricture. The classic triad of microangiopathic hemolytic anemia, thrombocytopenia, and acute renal failure follows the gastrointestinal prodrome. Leukocytosis develops, as can cerebral edema with seizure activity. Irritability progressing to stupor and coma may also develop. Cortical blindness and stroke may occur as well.

HUS may present in a D(–) form which is not associated with diarrhea. Cases of D(–) HUS, otherwise known as atypical HUS, have been associated with medications, familial patterns of inheritance, recurrent episodes of HUS, and bacterial infections, such as *Streptococcus pneumoniae*. In general, patients with D(–) HUS have a higher incidence of neurologic sequelae in addition to the renal sequelae and overall have worse outcomes than patients with D(+)HUS.

HUS is occasionally associated with *S. pneumoniae*. Children with pneumococcal HUS typically present with pneumonia complicated by empyema. Blood cultures are typically positive. In one multicenter case series of children with pneumococcal HUS, 4 of 37 patients have concomitant pneumococcal meningitis. Up to one-third of children with pneumococcal HUS have residual renal dysfunction, including elevated creatinine, proteinuria, and hypertension.

DIAGNOSTIC APPROACH

Clinical and laboratory findings. The key to diagnosis is recognition of the clinical syndrome in the appropriate context. An abnormal complete blood count with thrombocytopenia and anemia with schistocytes and red blood cell fragments on the peripheral smear in the context of fluid overload and oliguria or anuria with a rising serum creatinine confirm the diagnosis of this syndrome.

Microbiology. Stool culture is important to rule out other infectious causes of colitis, but specific biochemical tests are necessary to identify the specific serotype, O157:H7, and in some laboratories, may not be routinely performed and must be specifically requested.

Enzyme immunoassays. New, rapid methods to detect *E. coli* O157:H7 lipopolysaccharide and shiga toxin are very useful in diagnosing infection in a timely manner.

TREATMENT

Current therapy remains supportive in nature; however, prevention is essential by ensuring complete cooking of all beef products, particularly ground beef, thorough hand-washing when interacting with animals which may be carriers, and avoidance of unpasteurized dairy or other products. Patients who develop HUS require significant volume-support with careful fluid and electrolyte management. Transfusion may be necessary due to significant gastrointestinal blood loss and microangiopathic hemolytic anemia. Hypertension and renal failure must be anticipated in the clinical management and patients often require dialysis. Neurologic complications, such as seizures, may require antiepileptic therapy. There is no evidence that antibiotics are helpful and they may be potentially harmful, by causing increased release of toxin. Antimotility agents are also contraindicated because of the increased absorption of toxin.

SUGGESTED READINGS

1. Loirat C, Fremeaux-Bacchi V. Atypical hemolytic uremic syndrome. *Orphanet J Rare Dis.* 2011;6:60.
2. Zoja C, Buelli S, Morigi M. Shiga toxin-associated hemolytic uremic syndrome: pathophysiology of endothelial dysfunction. *Pediatr Nephrol.* 2010;2(11):2231-2240.

3. Bitzan M, Schaefer F, Reymond D. Treatment of typical (enteropathic) hemolytic uremic syndrome. *Semin Thromb Hemost.* 2010;36(6):594-610.

4. Malina M, Orumenina LT, Seeman T, et al. Genetics of hemolytic uremic syndromes. *Presse Med.* 2012;41(3Pt2): e10-e14.

5. Scheiring J, Rosales A, Zimmerhackl LB. Clinical practice: today's understanding of haemolytic uremic syndrome. *Eur J Pediatr.* 2010;169(1):7-13.

6. Palerma MS, Exeni RA, Fernandez GC. Hemolytic uremic syndrome: pathogenesis and update of interventions. *Expert Rev Anti Infect Ther.* 2009;7(6): 697-707.

7. Copelovitch L, Kaplan BS. *Streptococcus pneumoniae-*associated hemolytic uremic syndrome. *Pediatr Nephrol.* 2008;23(11):191-196.

8. Iijima K, Kamioka I, Nosu K. Management of diarrhea-associated hemolytic uremic syndrome. *Clin Exp Nephrol.* 2008;12(1):16-19.

9. Banerjee R, Hersh AL, Newland J, et al. *Streptococcus pneumoniae*-associated hemolytic uremic syndrome among children in North America. *Pediatr Infect Dis J.* 2011;30:736-739.

10. Waters AM, Kerecuk L, Luk D, et al. Hemolytic uremic syndrome associated with invasive pneumococcal disease: the United Kingdom experience. *J Pediatr.* 2007;151:140-144.

CASE 17-3

Seventeen-Year-Old Boy

AMY FELDMAN

HISTORY OF PRESENT ILLNESS

The patient is a 17-year-old boy who presents with 7 months of loose nonbloody stool and 1 week of fever to 39.5°C, severe abdominal pain, and bloody diarrhea. The patient was well until 7 months ago when he began having 3-4 loose stools per day whenever he ingested food. During those 7 months, he had no fevers, abdominal pain, nausea, emesis, bloody stool, rash, or arthritis. One week prior to admission, he developed intermittent fevers to a maximum of 39.5°C, periumbilical abdominal pain with ingestion of food, and multiple episodes per day of grossly bloody stool. On admission, the patient had just completed a 10-day course of oral clarithromycin for sinusitis. He denied recent travel outside the country, ingestion of undercooked food, or sick contacts. He did admit to a 7-lb weight loss during the past 7 months that had been unintentional.

MEDICAL HISTORY

Medical history is significant for seasonal allergic rhinitis for which the patient takes loratadine (Claritin) as needed. There is no known family history of any gastrointestinal or bleeding disorders.

PHYSICAL EXAMINATION

T 37°C; RR 18/min; HR 60 bpm; BP 120/65 mmHg

Weight 55 kg, 10th percentile; Height 170 cm, 25th percentile

Physical examination revealed a lean but non-emaciated boy in no acute distress. He was anicteric with moist mucous membranes. Cardiac and respiratory examinations were normal. His abdomen was soft, nontender, and nondistended without hepatosplenomegaly or palpable masses. He had normoactive bowel sounds. On external anal examination he had no visible fissures, tags, or masses. Rectal examination revealed grossly heme-positive soft stool in the rectal vault. There were no palpable rectal masses. His skin examination revealed no rashes, petechiae, or purpura. Neurologic examination was normal.

DIAGNOSTIC STUDIES

Serum electrolytes, glucose, blood urea nitrogen, and creatinine were all normal. A complete blood count (CBC) revealed a WBC count of 23 700 cells/mm^3, hemoglobin of 11.7 g/dL, and a platelet count of 302 000/mm^3. Coagulation factors including PT, PTT, and INR were all normal. The erythrocyte sedimentation rate (ESR) was 5 mm/h and the C-reactive protein (CRP) was 1.5 mg/dL. A hepatic function panel was normal except for a serum albumin that was low at 2.4 g/dL and a serum alkaline phosphatase that was low at 58 U/L. Stool samples were negative for *Clostridium difficile*, bacterial pathogens, viral pathogens, and ova and parasites.

COURSE OF ILLNESS

The patient was initially admitted to an outside hospital where he underwent flexible sigmoidoscopy, which reportedly showed inflammation that the physicians believed to be consistent with inflammatory bowel disease. The patient was placed on mesalamine enemas as well as oral mesalamine, omeprazole, and prednisone. He had some improvement in stool frequency, consistency, and amount of fecal blood and was discharged home.

Five days after discharge, the patient presented to our hospital with recurrence of bloody diarrhea and abdominal pain. After rehydration he underwent a complete endoscopy and colonoscopy that revealed multiple polyps in the small bowel and throughout the colon (Figure 17-3). Several polyps were removed and were sent to pathology for review. Due to findings seen on pathology, a retinal examination was performed which suggested a diagnosis.

DISCUSSION CASE 17-3

DIFFERENTIAL DIAGNOSIS

Chronic or persistent diarrhea (lasting more than 2 weeks) can occur in several conditions. In neonates and young infants, the most common etiologies of chronic diarrhea are infection, cow's milk protein or soy protein intolerance, cystic fibrosis, disaccharidase deficiency, or immunodeficiency. In older children and adolescents, the most likely etiologies of chronic diarrhea are infection, celiac disease, lactose deficiency (primary or secondary), or inflammatory bowel disease. Other less common causes of chronic diarrhea to consider in children are disorders of the pancreas (cystic fibrosis, Shwachman-Diamond syndrome,

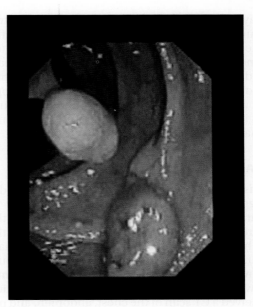

FIGURE 17-3. Colonic polyps. *(Reproduced, with permission, from McQuaid KR. Gastrointestinal disorders. In: Papadakis MA, McPhee SJ, Rabow MW, eds. CURRENT Medical Diagnosis & Treatment 2013. New York: McGraw-Hill; 2013. http://www.accessmedicine.com/content.aspx?aID=6395. Accessed April 25, 2013.)*

Johanson-Blizzard syndrome, Pearson syndrome, pancreatic enzyme deficiency, or pancreatitis), bile acid disorders (secondary to cholestasis, terminal ileum resection, or bacterial overgrowth), altered gastrointestinal anatomy (Hirschsprung disease, small bowel obstruction, malrotation), hyperthyroidism, or malignancy (VIPoma).

DIAGNOSTIC TESTS

To investigate chronic diarrhea, one should begin with an examination of the stool for red blood cells, white blood cells, fat, and reducing substances. The stool should be examined for bacterial, viral, and parasitic pathogens. The stool should also be tested for *C. difficile*, particularly if the patient has a history of recent antibiotic use. Hematologic and biochemical studies can also be useful in determining etiology. A CBC may show anemia suggesting chronic blood loss through the GI tract. An elevated white blood cell count and elevated CRP may suggest acute infection. An elevated platelet count and elevated erythrocyte sedimentation rate (ESR) may suggest a chronic inflammatory condition such as inflammatory bowel disease. Endoscopy and colonoscopy should be performed to obtain histologic clues as to etiology. An upper GI with small bowel follow through can be useful in identifying anatomic abnormalities seen in small bowel Crohn disease.

DIAGNOSIS

This patient had negative stool infectious studies suggesting against an infectious etiology for his diarrhea. Examination of the colonic polyps that were removed during colonoscopy revealed that he had adenomatous polyposis with carcinoma in situ. An upper GI with small bowel follow through showed multiple polyps throughout the small bowel. Due to the carcinoma in situ, the patient received a CT scan of the chest, abdomen, and pelvis which showed no signs of metastasis. **Formal**

ophthalmologic examination revealed congenital hypertrophy of the retinal pigment epithelium. The patient was diagnosed with Gardner syndrome. The patient underwent total proctocolectomy, given the high risk of malignancy.

INCIDENCE AND EPIDEMIOLOGY OF GARDNER SYNDROME

Gardner syndrome is a phenotypic variant of familial adenomatous polyposis, an autosomal dominant disease characterized by numerous adenomatous polyps in the GI tract which have a high potential for malignant transformation. The prevalence has been estimated to be 1:5000 to 1:17000. Patients may have anywhere from only a few adenomatous polyps to thousands of polyps throughout the colon. The average age of onset of adenomatous polyposis is 16 years, and progression to carcinoma is likely to occur by the fifth decade of life. The presence of upper gastrointestinal polyps is associated with an increased risk of malignancy (Table 17-3).

TABLE 17-3. Polyposis syndromes in children.

	Genetic Mutation	Clinical Findings
Adenomas		
Familial adenomatous polyposis (FAP)	APC gene	1. 100s-1000s of colonic polyps that inevitably become malignant
Gardner syndrome	APC gene	1. Adenomatous gastrointestinal polyps 2. Dental and ocular abnormalities 3. Soft tissue tumors, osseous abnormalities 4. Extraintestinal malignancies
Turcot syndrome	APC or mismatch-repair genes (hMLH1 or hPMS2)	1. Colonic adenomatous polyps 2. Brain tumors
Hamartomas		
Peutz Jeghers syndrome	STK11 or LKB1	1. Intestinal hamartomatous polyps 2. Mucocutaneous melanotic pigmentation 3. Pancreatic, breast, ovarian, testicular, thyroid malignancy
Juvenile polyposis syndrome	SMAD 4 or BMPR 1A	1. Multiple juvenile polyps within the gastrointestinal tract 2. Increased risk of colon, stomach, and duodenal cancer
Cowden syndrome and Bannayan-Riley-Ruvalcaba syndrome	PTEN	1. Gastrointestinal hamartomas 2. Mucocutaneous lesions 3. Macrocephay and neurologic abnormalities 4. Breast, thyroid, and genitourinary cancers

In addition to adenomatous colonic polyps, patients with Gardner syndrome can have a number of extraintestinal manifestations. Commonly, patients may have osteomas of the mandible, skull, and long bones. They may have cutaneous manifestations including epidermal inclusion cysts, sebaceous cysts, or skin tumors. Dental abnormalities including impacted teeth, supernumerary teeth, or mandibular cysts can be seen. One characteristic finding on ophthalmologic examination is multiple, bilateral, pigmented ocular fundus lesions, also known as congenital hypertrophy of the retinal pigment epithelium. This finding can be seen in up to 90% of Gardner patients. Desmoid tumors of the abdomen, chest, and extremities are found in approximately 8%-18% of patients with Gardner syndrome. These tumors can result in bowel obstruction, bowel perforation, and intra-abdominal abscesses. Patients with Gardner syndrome are at risk for several malignancies including colorectal adenocarcinomas, duodenal carcinomas, adrenal adenomas, hepatoblastoma, pancreatic cancer, and thyroid cancer. The association of malignant brain tumors in patients with Gardner syndrome or familial adenomatous polyposis is known as Turcot syndrome.

Gardner syndrome is inherited in an autosomal dominant fashion, although spontaneous mutations can be seen in about one-third of cases. The molecular defect causing the occurrence of the multiple adenomatous colonic polyps is a mutation in the adenomatous polyposis coli (APC) tumor suppressor gene located on chromosome 5q21.

TYPICAL PRESENTATION OF GARDNER SYNDROME

The clinical presentation of Gardner syndrome can vary greatly, from painless rectal bleeding to chronic abdominal pain with diarrhea. Asymptomatic iron-deficiency anemia from occult gastrointestinal blood loss may be seen. Colocolic intussusception is possible, with an adenomatous polyp serving as the lead point. Alternatively, patients may present primarily with extraintestinal manifestations. Exostoses of the mandible or long bones, or dental abnormalities such as

supernumerary teeth, should raise the index of suspicion for Gardner syndrome.

DIAGNOSTIC RATIONALE

Endoscopy and colonoscopy. Endoscopy and colonoscopy should be performed on every patient to visualize and remove polyps.

Upper gastrointestinal series with small bowel follow through. This radiologic study may help identify upper gastrointestinal polyps not detected by endoscopy or colonoscopy.

Roentgenograms of long bones and mandible. These radiographs can help identify the exostoses often associated with Gardner syndrome.

Computed tomography (CT). CT of the abdomen, chest, and pelvis may be helpful in identifying desmoid tumors or metastases.

Complete ophthalmologic examination. A thorough retinal examination is important in detecting the presence of congenital hypertrophy of the pigment epithelium which can help confirm a diagnosis of Gardner syndrome.

Genetic testing. Genetic testing can be performed using peripheral blood lymphocytes in an in vitro protein truncation assay; 80%-90% of affected patients are detected by this assay.

TREATMENT

For patients with Gardner syndrome, prophylactic total proctocolectomy is the treatment of choice due to the unavoidable progression to neoplasia. Colectomy is recommended shortly after the diagnosis is confirmed. Oral calcium may help to inhibit future proliferation of the rectal epithelium. Sulindac and tamoxifen can be used if rectal polyps develop after colectomy.

Patients with Gardner syndrome need to be screened on a frequent basis for extracolonic malignancies. Patients should undergo screening for thyroid cancer (serum thyroid tests and thyroid ultrasound), brain cancer (brain MRI), liver cancer (LFTs, abdominal ultrasound, and alpha fetoprotein levels), skin cancer (frequent skin examinations by a dermatologist), and adrenal and small bowel cancer (abdominal CT).

Once an individual has been diagnosed with Gardner syndrome, screening of other family members should take place. Genetic testing is the method of choice under these circumstances. The general consensus is that children should undergo genetic testing around 8-10 years of life.

SUGGESTED READINGS

1. Corredor J, Wambach J, Barnard J. Gastrointestinal polyps in children: advances in molecular genetics, diagnosis, and management. *J Pediatr.* 2001;138(5):621-628.

2. Giardiello FM, Yang VW, Hylind LM, et al. Primary chemoprevention of familial adenomatous polyposis with sulindac. *N Engl J Med.* 2002;346(14):1054-1059.

3. Juhn E, Khachemoune A. Gardner syndrome: skin manifestations, differential diagnosis, and management. *Am J Clin Dermatol.* 2010;11(2):117-122.

4. Rustgi A. Hereditary gastrointestinal polyposis and nonpolyposis syndromes. *New Engl J Med.* 1994;331 (25):1694-1702.

5. Traboulsi E, Krush AJ, Gardner EJ, et al. Prevalence and importance of pigmented ocular fundus lesions in Gardner's syndrome. *N Engl J Med.* 1987;316: 661-667.

CASE 17-4

Fifteen-Month-Old Boy

CHRISTINA L. MASTER

HISTORY OF PRESENT ILLNESS

The patient is a 15-month-old boy who presents with watery diarrhea for the last 3 months associated with weight loss. At 12 months of age he developed diarrhea characterized by six to eight watery brown stools per day accompanied by significant flatulence. There was no associated emesis or blood in the stool. He continued to have a good appetite despite frequent stooling. Dietary changes including bananas, rice, apples, toast diet (BRAT diet) as well as a lactose-free diet were introduced, without any improvement in the diarrhea. Occasional low-grade fevers were noted. There was no history of foreign travel or ill contacts. There are two cats and one dog in the home. He has lost three pounds in the last 3 months.

MEDICAL HISTORY

The boy was a full-term infant with a birth weight of 3900 g who was fed cow's milk-based commercial formula without any problems. He had normal weight gain and developmental milestones. He was introduced to rice cereal, baby foods, and adult table foods without any problems. He was taking no medications.

PHYSICAL EXAMINATION

T 36.8°C; RR 26/min; HR 100 bpm; BP 102/53 mmHg

Weight below 5th percentile; 50th percentile for a 6-month old; Height 10th percentile

The initial examination revealed a quiet, gaunt-appearing child. His eyes were sunken but the rest of the head, eyes, ears, nose, mouth, and throat examination was unremarkable. His cardiac and respiratory examinations were normal. His abdominal examination revealed no masses; his liver edge was palpable at the right costal margin. There was no clubbing of his fingers. He had dry skin around his nose and lips. He had very little subcutaneous fat. His neurologic examination was nonfocal.

DIAGNOSTIC STUDIES

Laboratory analysis revealed 11 100 WBCs/mm^3 with 29% segmented neutrophils, 66% lymphocytes, 5% monocytes. The hemoglobin was 12.2 g/dL and there were 492 000 platelets/mm^3. Electrolytes were significant for serum potassium of 2.8 mmol/L, serum bicarbonate 16 mmol/L. His erythrocyte sedimentation rate was 4 mm/h. Urinalysis was negative with a urine specific gravity of 1.005. Serum alkaline phosphatase was low at 115 U/L, while alanine aminotransferase was elevated at 59 U/L, aspartate aminotransferase at 64 U/L, and lactate dehydrogenase at 845 U/L.

COURSE OF ILLNESS

The patient was admitted and started on hyperalimentation for his nutritional status and to correct his hypokalemia. Blood culture and stool culture were both negative. A sweat test was normal. Stool sample tested negative for *Clostridium difficile* toxins. Stool for ova and parasites revealed Indian meal moth larvae. Colonoscopy was performed on the sixth day of hospitalization that revealed nonspecific lymphoid hyperplasia. Despite taking nothing by mouth, he continued to have mucousy diarrhea which became heme positive. Stool osmolality was normal at 298 mOsm/kg H_2O. Chest radiograph (Figure 17-4) suggested a diagnosis that was confirmed by biopsy.

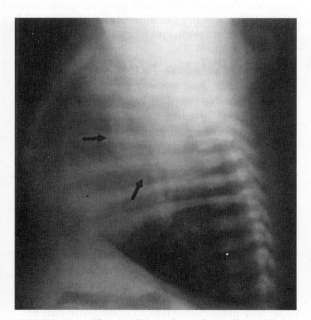

FIGURE 17-4. Chest radiograph similar to that of the patient's. *(Reproduced, with permission, from Swischuk LE. Imaging of the Newborn, Infant, and Young Child. 4th ed. Baltimore: Williams & Wilkins; 1997, p. 144.)*

DISCUSSION CASE 17-4

DIFFERENTIAL DIAGNOSIS

The chronic nature of his diarrhea for the last 3 months, associated with weight loss, moves the differential diagnosis away from the diagnosis of acute infectious diarrhea, due to either bacterial or viral causes. A prolonged bout of postinfectious diarrhea due to disaccharidase deficiency is possible, but unlikely. Chronic diarrhea due to infection with *C. difficile* or ova and parasites is a possibility even without history of antibiotic use, bloody diarrhea, foreign travel, or use of untreated water sources. The key observation in making this diagnosis occurred while in the hospital: the patient took nothing by mouth but continued to produce profuse voluminous watery diarrhea. This finding indicates the presence of secretory, rather than osmotic, diarrhea. In this differential diagnosis, the list is rather brief, including rare congenital and paraneoplastic conditions. Congenital defects in chloride or sodium transport are more likely to present in infancy. Infectious causes of secretory diarrhea include small bowel overgrowth or infection with immunoadherent *Escherichia coli* stimulating gastrointestinal secretions. Any cause of villous atrophy, whether congenital, autoimmune, or secondary to immune deficiency, such as severe combined immunodeficiency (SCID) or HIV may also present with this picture. Neuroblastoma, or other tumors of neural crest origin, such as ganglioneuroma, may secrete vasoactive intestinal peptide, resulting in secretory diarrhea.

DIAGNOSIS

Chest radiograph revealed a large posterior mediastinal mass (Figure 17-4). Computed tomography of the chest performed on the seventh day of hospitalization confirmed a 4 cm × 4 cm right posterior mediastinal mass. The urine vanillylmandelic acid level was 498 mg/g of creatinine and the homovanillic acid level was 245 mg/g of creatinine, which were both extremely elevated. Surgical excision revealed neuroblastoma with a favorable histology. **These findings were consistent with the diagnosis of neuroblastoma causing secretory diarrhea.**

INCIDENCE AND EPIDEMIOLOGY OF NEUROBLASTOMA

The incidence of neuroblastoma is approximately eight per million per year in children younger than 15 years of age. The median age at diagnosis is 22 months and 95% of cases are usually diagnosed by the age of 10 years. Neuroblastoma accounts for approximately 6% of all pediatric tumors. There is a slight male preponderance with a boy:girl ratio of 1.2:1. There also appear to be familial cases, which present at a younger age (median age, 9 months). These tumors derive from postganglionic sympathetic cells found in the paraspinal sympathetic ganglia and the adrenal chromaffin cells. Neuroblastoma and ganglioneuroblastoma represent the malignant forms of these neural crest tumors, while ganglioneuroma represents the most benign form, with no metastatic potential. The primary tumor is located in the abdomen in most (approximately two-thirds) children with neuroblastoma.

CLINICAL PRESENTATION

Most pediatric patients with neuroblastoma are diagnosed by 5 years of age and most are intra-abdominal in location. Signs and symptoms as well as outcomes vary with the site of presentation. Patients diagnosed in the first year of life have a higher incidence of intrathoracic and cervical tumors compared with those diagnosed after 1 year of age. Seventy-five percent of cases in children older than 1 year of age present with a disseminated advanced stage of disease; children presenting at this late stage account for a significant proportion of neuroblastoma-associated mortality. Infants younger than 1 year tend to present with lower stage disease, resulting in high cure rates. Some tumors in this latter group even undergo spontaneous regression. One percent of patients will have no detectable primary tumor. Neuroblastoma metastases occur in 35% of children to the regional lymph nodes which then qualifies as disseminated disease. Hematogenous spread to bone, bone marrow, liver, and skin also occurs. Late metastases are seen in the brain and lung. Patients may present with a large abdominal mass or respiratory distress secondary to the intra-abdominal mass. Intrathoracic tumors are often incidentally found. Opsoclonus-myoclonus

is a well-defined but uncommon presenting syndrome for neuroblastoma; fewer than 2% of cases present with opsoclonus-myoclonus syndrome. Presentation as severe secretory diarrhea, as in the case of our patient, is known as Verner-Morrison syndrome.

DIAGNOSTIC APPROACH

Clinical observation. The observation of continued, intractable watery diarrhea while the patient takes nothing by mouth is key to the ultimate diagnosis. Whether this is accomplished by obtaining a very thorough history or by observation while in the hospital, this piece of information is vital to making the ultimate diagnosis.

Radiographs. Radiographs may localize calcifications and often provide the first indication of the presence of such a tumor as an incidental finding. Skeletal surveys may show bone involvement and are used in tumor staging.

Computed tomography or magnetic resonance imaging. Three-dimensional imaging more accurately delineates the location of the tumor, which is usually retroperitoneal or adrenal and also assists in staging. Occasionally, tumors may be found along the sympathetic chain in the thoracic or cervical region.

Vasoactive intestinal peptide level. Elevated plasma vasoactive intestinal peptide levels may be elaborated by tumors of neural crest origin and may cause secretory diarrhea.

Urinary (or serum) catecholamine levels. Elevation of urinary homovanillic or vanillylmandelic acid in conjunction with diagnostic pathologic features is diagnostic of neuroblastoma. These levels may also be used to follow disease activity.

Surgical removal. Complete surgical excision provides a pathologic specimen for further identification and characterization of the tumor and is also therapeutic, especially with regard to the secretory diarrhea. It is also important in the staging process, especially in assessing lymph node involvement.

Bone scintigraphy. A bone scan is important in detecting possible metastases and is used in the staging process.

Radionuclide scan. Radiolabeled metaiodobenzylguanidine is taken up by catecholamine-secreting cells and is useful for staging in detecting bone and soft tissue involvement.

TREATMENT

Surgical resection is usually performed in all patients. Low-risk patients may not need any additional therapy. Radiotherapy and chemotherapy are used depending on the stage of the disease. Patients with high-risk disease may have some improvement in short-term survival with autologous bone marrow transplantation, but longer term outcome is still poor. Surgical removal of the tumor usually cures the secretory diarrhea. The use of somatostatin analogs also has a therapeutic effect on the secretory diarrhea, but the definitive therapy for the diarrhea remains surgical removal of the primary tumor.

SUGGESTED READINGS

1. Gera PK, Kikrios CS, Charles A. Chronic diarrhoea: a presentation of immature neuroblastoma. *ANZ J Surg.* 2008;78(3):218-219.
2. Gesundheit B, Smith CR, Gerstle JT, Weitzman SS, Chan HS. Ataxia and secretory diarrhea: two unusual paraneoplastic syndromes occurring concurrently in the same patient with ganglioneuroblastoma. *J Pediatr Hematol Oncol.* 2004;26(9):549-552.
3. Posner JB. Paraneoplastic syndromes in neuroblastoma. *J Pediatr Hematol Oncol.* 2004;26(9):33-34.
4. Bown N. Neuroblastoma tumour genetics: clinical and biological aspects. *J Clin Pathol.* 2001;54:897-910.
5. Alexander F. Neuroblastoma. *Urol Clin N Amer.* 2000; 27:383-392.

CASE 17-5

Five-Year-Old Girl

CHRISTINA L. MASTER

HISTORY OF PRESENT ILLNESS

The patient is a 5-year-old girl with a recent diagnosis of cystic fibrosis who presents with several weeks of watery stools. She has been treated with pancreatic enzyme supplements for pancreatic insufficiency associated with cystic fibrosis. Increasing the pancreatic enzyme supplementation did not alter her stooling pattern. There was also no improvement of her diarrhea while on a clear liquid diet. She was started on metronidazole 2 days prior to admission for possible parasitic infection. Stool tests for ova and parasites, Giardia antigen by enzyme-linked immunosorbent assay, and *Clostridium difficile* toxins A and B were negative. Her symptoms worsened with increased abdominal distension and lethargy. She has had a 2-kg weight loss during the last 3 weeks. She has no fever or vomiting. She has normal urine output.

MEDICAL HISTORY

The girl was the product of a full-term uncomplicated pregnancy. She did not have meconium ileus at birth. She was diagnosed with cystic fibrosis 9 weeks prior to this admission. She presented at that time with failure to thrive with foamy, foul-smelling stools. Her diagnosis was delayed due to the finding of *Dientamoeba fragilis*, which was treated with iodoquinol, and *Blastocystis hominis*, which was treated with metronidazole, 5 months prior to the diagnosis of cystic fibrosis. Despite treatment and follow-up stool tests, which were negative, she did not gain weight, although her diarrhea had transiently resolved until the past several weeks. Her current medications include metronidazole, albuterol, nebulized cromolyn sodium, pancrelipase capsules, and vitamins A, D, E, and K. Her family history is significant for an older sibling who has a history of constipation and poor growth.

PHYSICAL EXAMINATION

T 37°C; RR 32/min; HR 147 bpm; BP 109/68 mmHg

Weight and height are far below the 5th percentile

Physical examination revealed a lean girl with no rhinorrhea, slightly dry mucous membranes. The remainder of her head and neck examination was normal. Her cardiac and respiratory examinations were normal except for mild tachycardia. Her abdomen was protuberant but otherwise unremarkable. Her rectal examination revealed a minimal amount of stool, which was heme negative. Her extremities were wasted with very little subcutaneous fat. There were no skin rashes. Her neurologic examination was nonfocal.

DIAGNOSTIC STUDIES

Chest radiograph revealed mildly increased interstitial markings but no focal infiltrates. A complete blood count revealed a WBC count of 13 100 cells/mm³ (40% segmented neutrophils, 46% lymphocytes, 14% monocytes), and a hemoglobin of 12.7 g/dL, and a platelet count of 472 000 cells/mm³. Her erythrocyte sedimentation rate was 5 mm/h. Serum electrolytes, blood urea nitrogen, serum creatinine, and serum glucose were normal. Her serum alanine aminotransferase was mildly elevated at 56 U/L as was her aspartate aminotransferase at 68 U/L. Her serum alkaline phosphatase was low at 72 U/L, as was her serum albumin at 1.9 g/dL, and total protein at 3.8 g/dL.

The girl's stool pH was 6.0 and her routine stool cultures were negative. Stool examination was negative for ova and parasites and assays for *C. difficile* toxins A and B were negative. Tests for *Giardia lamblia* antigen and *Cryptosporidium* were negative.

COURSE OF ILLNESS

All feeding attempts resulted in abdominal distension and pain. Abdominal radiograph showed the presence of stool, dilated loops of small bowel with air fluid levels. Upper gastrointestinal barium study with small bowel follow through suggested the diagnosis (Figure 17-5).

DISCUSSION CASE 17-5

DIFFERENTIAL DIAGNOSIS

In the context of her recent diagnosis of cystic fibrosis, this patient has many symptoms of chronic

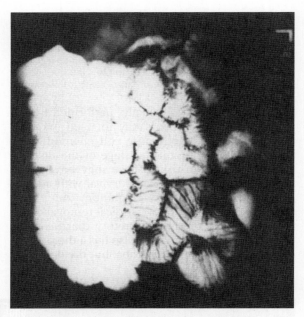

FIGURE 17-5. Upper gastrointestinal study with small bowel follow-through similar to that of the patient's. *(Reproduced, with permission, from Avery ME, First LR, eds.* Pediatric Medicine. *Baltimore: Williams & Wilkins; 1989, p. 435.)*

malabsorption, including poor weight gain, chronic diarrhea, and abdominal distension. Inadequate management of her cystic fibrosis could account for her symptoms, as could infectious causes of chronic diarrhea superimposed on the diagnosis of cystic fibrosis. *Clostridium difficile, G. lamblia,* and *Cryptosporidium* are potential culprits. Celiac sprue should be considered in the differential due to reports of an association with cystic fibrosis.

DIAGNOSIS

The upper gastrointestinal barium study revealed thickened, dilated small bowel loops with prominent valvulae conniventes resulting from the dilatation (Figure 17-5). This finding suggested the diagnosis of celiac sprue. Duodenal bulb biopsies showed intense lamina propria inflammatory cells with villous blunting and ulceration with almost complete villous flattening and inspissated secretions in some crypts. Antigliadin IgG >140 mg/dL (normal <15 mg/dL), IgA >136 mg/dL (normal

<4 mg/dL). Antiendomysial IgA titer was 1:320. **The diagnosis is celiac sprue in the setting of cystic fibrosis.**

INCIDENCE AND EPIDEMIOLOGY OF CELIAC SPRUE

Celiac disease, also known as celiac sprue or gluten-sensitive enteropathy, is a multifactorial autoimmune disorder occurring in genetically susceptible persons. The disease results from abnormal immune responses to the enzyme tissue transglutaminase. In the United States, the prevalence has been estimated at 1 per 3000 in the population. However, recent seroprevalence studies suggest that the prevalence may be as high as 1 in 120 to 1 in 300 persons in Europe and North America. There is an ethnic predisposition in Western Europeans and their descendants. It rarely occurs among people from an African-Caribbean, Chinese, or Japanese background. Girls are slightly more frequently affected than boys. There is a familial predisposition, with approximately 10% of patients with affected first-degree relatives and greater than 95% of patients with celiac sprue express a specific HLA-DQ heterodimer. In a cohort of children with cystic fibrosis from Norway and Sweden, the prevalence of celiac disease of 1.2% (1:83) was found to be approximately threefold higher than the general population of those countries.

CLINICAL PRESENTATION

Celiac sprue is a malabsorptive condition caused by an autoimmune T-cell-mediated response against gluten that results in severe inflammation in small bowel mucosa. The classic presentation is in infants who develop diarrhea, abdominal distension, and failure to thrive as cereals are introduced into their diet, typically between 6 months and 2 years of age. Vomiting, anorexia, and abdominal pain may be associated. Affected infants may develop iron-deficiency anemia and rickets secondary to the malabsorption. Older children and adolescents may not present with malabsorptive symptoms, but rather with hyper-transaminasemia, short stature, pubertal delay, or recurrent aphthous ulcers. Adults may present with a history of symptoms that date back to childhood, or may present with no previous symptoms

whatsoever. Diarrhea with lactose-intolerance and steatorrhea are common, as is steatorrhea. Weight loss with flatulence and abdominal distension also occur. Adults may be otherwise asymptomatic and present only with anemia due to iron-deficiency or recurrent aphthous ulcers.

Extraintestinal manifestations may be present without significant gastrointestinal symptoms. Dermatitis herpetiformis, a pruritic papulovesicular rash on the extensor surfaces of the extremities and trunk, is associated with dermal IgA deposits; the lesions resolve with withdrawal of gluten from the diet. Other extraintestinal manifestations include dental enamel hypoplasia, hepatitis, arthritis or arthralgias, seizures (from intracranial calcifications), and other autoimmune conditions, including thyroiditis and type I diabetes mellitus.

Patients with refractory celiac disease are at increased risk for developing enteropathy-associated T cell lymphoma. These patients have severe symptoms despite adherence to a gluten-free diet for at least 6 months. This condition often requires treatment with corticosteroids or immunosuppressants. Strict adherence to a diet free from gluten can decrease the risk of cancers associated with celiac disease.

DIAGNOSTIC APPROACH

Endoscopy. Endoscopy with biopsy of the small intestine remains the reference standard for diagnosis. Pathologic specimens reveal the presence of absent or flattened villi with hyperplastic crypts and a significant presence of inflammatory lymphocytes and plasma cells. These findings generally resolve after withdrawal of gluten from the diet, but the resolution of pathologic findings generally lags behind signs of clinical improvement. Currently, repeat biopsies are not necessary due to the highly accurate nature of the available serologic tests.

Serologic tests. Serologic tests have high sensitivity and specificity for the diagnosis of celiac disease. IgA antiendomysial antibodies are reported to be 85%-98% sensitive and 97%-100% specific compared with intestinal biopsy. Antigliadin IgA and IgG are much less specific and have moderate sensitivity and can be seen in adults with nonspecific gastrointestinal inflammation and are not as useful. In children younger than 2 years of age, however, IgA antigliadin is the most useful serologic marker. All of these markers respond to withdrawal of gluten and often become undetectable within 3-6 months after initiation of the appropriate dietary regimen. Serologic tests are currently used to identify children who warrant intestinal biopsy for confirmation of celiac disease.

Radiographic studies. Abdominal radiographs and upper gastrointestinal series using barium are no longer necessary in making the initial diagnosis, given the high sensitivity and specificity of serologic testing combined with endoscopy findings. Radiographic imaging, including computed tomography may be helpful, however, in evaluating patients with refractory celiac disease, especially for signs of intestinal lymphoma.

Tests of malabsorption. Measurement of fecal fat or oral D-xylose absorption are not specific and therefore, not necessary, and merely serve to confirm the malabsorptive nature of the condition.

Gluten withdrawal. Empiric elimination of gluten from the diet is not indicated because the results of intestinal biopsy following this intervention may be equivocal and serologic tests are less reliable when gluten has been eliminated from the diet.

TREATMENT

The definitive therapy for celiac disease is lifetime avoidance of gluten in the diet. Complete avoidance is probably impossible due to the widespread presence in processed foods, but elimination of products that contain wheat gluten, barley, or rye

is important. Oats should also be avoided initially but may be slowly reintroduced in some patients without serious consequences. Studies have documented the safety of oats for patients with celiac disease. However, cross-contamination is a concern because oats are often harvested and processed in facilities used for preparing wheat-based flours. Dairy products are also initially avoided due to a secondary lactase deficiency and may be reintroduced in the diet a few months later. A multivitamin is also important, in addition to correcting any severe vitamin deficiencies that may be present. Patients with hyposplenism should receive antibiotic prophylaxis for invasive procedures.

SUGGESTED READINGS

1. Ludvigsson JF, Green PH. Clinical management of coeliac disease. *J Intern Med.* 2011;269(6):560-571. doi:10.1111/j.1365-2796.2011.02379.x.
2. Mansoor DK, Sharma HP. Clinical presentations of food allergy. *Pediatr Clin North Am.* 2011;58(2):315-326, ix.
3. Tack GJ, Verbeek WH, Schreurs MW, Mulder CJ. The spectrum of celiac disease: epidemiology, clinical aspects and treatment. *Nat Rev Gastroenterol Hepatol.* 2010;7(4):204-213. [Epub 2010 Mar 9.]
4. Smlimoglu MA, Karbiber H. Celiac disease: prevention and treatment. *J Clin Gastroenterol.* 2010;44(1):4-8.
5. Zawahir S, Safta A, Fasano A. Pediatric celiac disease. *Curr Opin Pediatr.* 2009;21(5):655-660.
6. Barker JM, Liu E. Celiac disease: pathophysiology, clinical manifestations, and associated autoimmune conditions. *Adv Pediatr.* 2008;5:349-365.
7. Fluge G, Olesen HV, Gilljam M, et al. Co-morbidity of cystic fibrosis and celiac disease in Scandinavian cystic fibrosis patients. *J Cyst Fibros.* 2009;8:198-202.

CASE 17-6

Two-Year-Old Boy

CHRISTINA L. MASTER

HISTORY OF PRESENT ILLNESS

The patient is a 2-year-old boy who was well until 5 months prior to admission when he developed intermittent watery diarrhea. He has had more than three large watery stools per day, sometimes

up to 10 such stools per day. As an outpatient, he was seen and examined. A stool culture was negative as were tests for *Clostridium difficile* and ova and parasites. Other blood tests sent at that time were also normal according to his mother. Since then, he has been seen once in an emergency department where he was treated for an intestinal parasite without any improvement in his symptoms. He had been otherwise well appearing during these last 5 months until the day prior to presentation to the hospital when he had significantly decreased oral intake, has had decreased activity, and has been acting cranky. On the day of admission to the hospital he had three episodes on nonbloody and nonbilious emesis. He also has developed a tactile temperature and is refusing to walk. He has not had any rash or weight loss according to his mother. She is unsure about his urine output.

MEDICAL HISTORY

The boy is a former premature infant born at 33 weeks gestation and did not require endotracheal intubation. Surgical procedures included patent ductus arteriosus ligation, inguinal hernia repair, and removal of a vocal cord cyst. He was hospitalized 6 months ago for pneumonia and has had recurrent episodes of otitis media (6 episodes). His only medication is a multivitamin. His family history is significant only for type 2 diabetes mellitus and asthma.

PHYSICAL EXAMINATION

T 38.5°C; RR 24/min; HR 117 bpm; BP 108/54 mmHg

Weight 25th percentile

The boy's examination revealed an ill-appearing but responsive toddler. His head and neck examinations were significant only for tacky mucous membranes. His cardiac and respiratory examinations were normal. His abdomen was soft and nontender without any organomegaly. His rectal examination was normal and the stool was heme negative. His extremity examination was unremarkable and his neurologic examination was nonfocal, but he continued to refuse to walk.

DIAGNOSTIC STUDIES

A complete blood count revealed a WBC count of 9600 cells/mm³ (66% segmented neutrophils; 24% lymphocytes; 9% monocytes; 1% eosinophils), a

hemoglobin of 15.1 g/dL, and a platelet count of 291 000 cells/mm³. Serum electrolytes were significant for potassium 2.1 mmol/L, bicarbonate 11 mmol/L, and alkaline phosphatase was 214 U/L. Cerebrospinal fluid (CSF) analysis revealed no WBCs/mm³ and 4 RBCs/mm³. CSF protein and glucose were normal. His urinalysis was significant for moderate blood with 5-10 RBCs/hpf and 0-2 WBCs/hpf.

COURSE OF ILLNESS

The patient took nothing by mouth while in the hospital, but continued to make more than 2 L per day of diarrhea for the next 3 days. Despite intravenous fluid repletion, his serum bicarbonate never rose above 18 mmol/L. Repeat stool cultures for bacteria and viruses, stool examination for ova and parasites, and assays for *C. difficile* toxins A and B were all negative. Stool antigen testing for *Giardia* and *Cryptosporidium* were also negative. An abdominal radiograph (Figure 17-6) and CT (Figure 17-7) directed further testing.

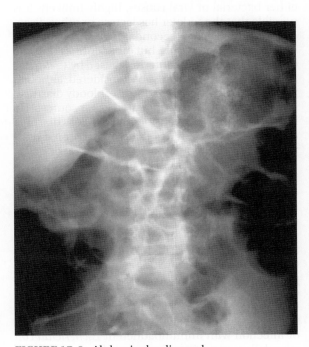

FIGURE 17-6. Abdominal radiograph.

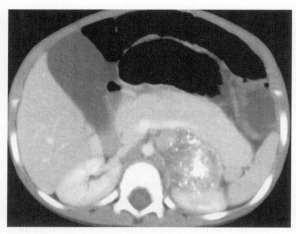

FIGURE 17-7. Abdominal CT.

DISCUSSION CASE 17-6

DIFFERENTIAL DIAGNOSIS

The chronic nature of his diarrhea for the last 5 months makes acute infectious diarrhea, due to either bacterial or viral causes, highly unlikely. It is possible that the toddler has lactase or other disaccharidase deficiency secondary to an episode of infectious gastroenteritis, but other entities must be considered. Infectious enteritis caused by *C. difficile* and ova and parasites must be considered, although there is no history of antibiotic use, bloody diarrhea, foreign travel, or use of untreated water sources. He is too ill appearing to consider the toddler's diarrhea as a cause. Other entities that cause chronic diarrhea such as inflammatory bowel disease or celiac disease are considerations, but there is a key finding during the patient's hospital stay that quickly directs us down another path. While in the hospital, the patient took nothing by mouth but continued to produce profuse voluminous watery diarrhea which indicated the presence of secretory, rather than osmotic, diarrhea. In this differential diagnosis, the list is rather brief, including rare congenital and paraneoplastic conditions. Congenital defects in chloride or sodium transport are unlikely to present in a 2-year old in this fashion. Infectious causes of secretory diarrhea include small bowel overgrowth or infection with immunoadherent *Escherichia coli* stimulating gastrointestinal secretions. Any cause

of villous atrophy, whether congenital, autoimmune, or secondary to immune deficiency, such as severe combined immune deficiency or human immunodeficiency virus (HIV) infection may also present with chronic diarrhea. Neuroblastoma, or other tumors of neural crest origin, such as ganglioneuroma, may secrete vasoactive intestinal peptide, resulting in secretory diarrhea.

DIAGNOSTIC TESTS

An abdominal radiograph showed calcifications above the left kidney (Figure 17-6) and subsequent computed tomography revealed a large left adrenal mass (Figure 17-7). Surgery was performed and the mass was completely resected and was identified as a ganglioneuroblastoma on pathology. The vasoactive intestinal peptide (VIP) level returned at 195 (normal <70).

DIAGNOSIS

These findings were consistent with the diagnosis of VIP-secreting ganglioneuroblastoma causing secretory diarrhea. Immediately following surgery, his diarrhea resolved and a repeat VIP level was normal.

INCIDENCE AND ETIOLOGY

Most VIP-secreting tumors in childhood are neurogenic in origin, as opposed to those in adults, most of which are of pancreatic islet cell origin. Pediatric patients usually present during the first 10 years of life. Most pediatric tumors are adrenal or retroperitoneal in location and ganglioneuromas or ganglioneuroblastomas are common.

TYPICAL PRESENTATION

Generally speaking, pediatric patients will present as this child did, with profuse, watery, secretory diarrhea, and not with a palpable mass. The biochemical profile is that of hypokalemia and achlorhydria due to the effect of VIP on the gastrointestinal tract to promote secretion of water and electrolytes and inhibiting gastric acid secretion. Calcifications may also be noted incidentally on X-ray and thus prompt further investigation.

DIAGNOSTIC RATIONALE

Clinical observation. The observation of continued, intractable watery diarrhea while the patient takes nothing by mouth is key to the ultimate diagnosis. Whether this is accomplished by obtaining a very thorough history or by observation while in the hospital, this piece of information is vital to making the ultimate diagnosis.

Radiographs. Radiographs may localize calcifications and often provide the first indication of the presence of such a tumor as an incidental finding.

Computed tomography. Computed tomography will more accurately delineate the location of the tumor, which is usually retroperitoneal or adrenal. Occasionally, tumors may be found along the sympathetic chain in the thoracic region.

Peptide panel. Elevated plasma VIP levels are diagnostic. Other peptides that are tested include gastrin, somatostatin, calcitonin, and serotonin. These peptides are elaborated by tumors not commonly found in the pediatric population (gastrinoma, carcinoid syndrome, medullary thyroid carcinoma, mastocytosis, and villous adenoma of the rectosigmoid colon).

Surgical removal. Complete surgical excision provides a pathologic specimen for further identification and characterization of the tumor and is also therapeutic, especially with regard to the secretory diarrhea.

TREATMENT

Complete surgical excision is necessary and sufficient to cure the secretory diarrhea. Somatostatin analogs have been shown to decrease diarrhea due to the inhibitory effect on gastrointestinal secretions, but surgery remains the definitive treatment. Subsequent chemotherapy is then determined based on the type of tumor and the tissue pathology as well as other information, such as the presence of molecular amplification of oncogenes.

SUGGESTED READINGS

1. Zella GC, Israel EJ. Chronic diarrhea in children. *Pediatr Rev.* 2012;33(5):207-218.
2. Husain K, Thomas E, Demerdash Z, Alexander S. Mediastinal ganglioneuroblastoma-secreting vasoactive intestinal peptide causing secretory diarrhoea. *Arab J Gastroenterol.* 2011;12(2):106-108.
3. Bourdeaut F, de Carli E, Timsit S, et al; Neuroblastoma Committee of the Société Française des Cancers et Leucémies de l'Enfant et de l'Adolescent. VIP hypersecretion as primary or secondary syndrome in neuroblastoma: a retrospective study by the Societe Francaise des Cacers de l'Enfant (SCFE). *Pediatr Blood Cancer.* 2009;52(5):585-590.
4. Keating JP. Chronic diarrhea. *Pediatr Rev.* 2005;26(1):5-14.
5. Nikou GC, Toubanakis C, Nikolaou P, et al. VIPomas: an update in diagnosis and management in a series of 11 patients. *Hepatogastroenterology.* 2005;52(64):1259-1265.
6. Rodriguez M, Regalado J, Zaleski C, Thomas C, Tamer A. Chronic watery diarrhea in a 22-month-old girl. *J Pediatr.* 2000;136:262-265.
7. Murphy M, Sibal A, Mann JR. Persistent diarrhoea and occult vipomas in children. *BMJ.* 2000;320:1524-1526.

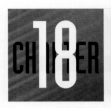

SYNCOPE

SAMIR S. SHAH

DEFINITION OF THE COMPLAINT

Syncope is generally thought of as a temporary, but sudden, loss of consciousness and postural tone. It is due to a reversible interruption of cerebral perfusion, typically caused by a deficit of cerebral oxygen or glucose delivery. The deficit in oxygen delivery may be caused by decreased cardiac output, peripheral vasodilatation, or obstruction of cerebral blood flow. It is important to differentiate the episode of syncope from other etiologies that appear like syncope, such as seizure and near syncopal episodes. Painful events, episodes of micturition or defecation, and stress frequently precede syncope. Sweating and nausea prior to the episode are common as well. Seizures frequently have no prodromal period; however, they may be associated with an aura prior to the event. Seizures are frequently associated with tonic-clonic movements during the event; however, syncopal events that last 20 seconds or longer can also be associated with very brief tonic-clonic movements. Confusion after the event, prolonged return to normal state of consciousness, and unconsciousness lasting longer than 5 minutes suggests seizure activity. During near syncopal episodes the patient feels as though they are about to lose consciousness, but do not actually become unconscious.

Syncope is a common complaint in pediatrics. Approximately 15% of children will have a syncopal episode by the time they reach adulthood.

COMPLAINT BY CAUSE AND FREQUENCY

Pediatric causes of syncope are generally benign, but syncope may signal serious life-threatening causes, particularly if it is recurrent or if there is a family history of sudden cardiac arrest. In children, common causes of syncope include vasovagal episodes, orthostatic hypotension, and breath-holding spells (Table 18-1). In contrast, most adult syncope is due to a cardiac cause. The goal in evaluating syncope is to differentiate benign causes from a more worrisome etiology (Table 18-2).

CLARIFYING QUESTIONS

- Were there any palpitations or "funny heart beats"?
  —If the child reports palpitations, then a cardiac dysrhythmia should be considered.

- Did it occur with activity?
  —Syncope that occurs with activity is particularly concerning for idiopathic hypertrophic cardiomyopathy.

- Did it occur without warning?
  —Syncope that occurs suddenly and without warning should raise concern for a cardiac arrhythmia.

- Were there prodromal symptoms?
  —Acute orthostatic intolerance (e.g., simple faint) typically occurs in the context of known precipitants (e.g., standing, heat, emotion) and prodromal symptoms (e.g., nausea, blurred vision, headache).

- Did it happen on standing?
  —Orthostatic hypotension is associated with syncope on standing.

- Was there pain, fear, or some disturbing visual sight prior to the syncope?

TABLE 18-1.	Differential diagnosis by age.		
Disease Prevalence	**Infant/Toddler**	**School Age**	**Adolescent**
Common	Breath-holding spell Arrhythmia Mimickers of syncope	Vasovagal syncope Breath-holding spell Anemia Arrhythmia Mimickers of syncope	Vasovagal syncope Mimickers of syncope Anemia Arrhythmia Pregnancy Dysautonomia disorders*
Uncommon	Structural heart disease Hypoglycemia Hypoxemia	Structural heart disease Hypoglycemia Hypoxemia	Structural heart disease Hypoglycemia Hypoxemia Adrenal insufficiency

*Includes familial dysautonomia and postural orthostatic tachycardia syndrome.

TABLE 18-2.	Differential diagnosis of syncope by etiology.
Autonomic	Vasovagal syncope Increased vagal tone Orthostatic hypotension (volume depletion) Breath-holding spell Situational syncope (cough, micturition, defecation) Pregnancy
Structural Heart Disease	Outflow obstruction (IHSS, valvular aortic stenosis, primary pulmonary hypertension, Eisenmenger syndrome, atrial myxoma) Dilated cardiomyopathy Pericarditis with tamponade
Arrhythmias	Long QTc syndrome (congenital or acquired) Supraventricular tachycardia Ventricular tachycardia Atrioventricular block Sinus node disease
Vascular	Vertebrobasilar insufficiency
Metabolic	Hypoglycemia Hypoxia Hyperammonemia Carbon monoxide poisoning
Mimickers of Syncope	Seizures Migraines Hysteric faints Malingering Hyperventilation Panic disorder Depression

—Strong emotional impulses may stimulate a vasovagal response and ultimately syncope.

- Was there any seizure-like activity?
—Brief seizure-like motor activity can occur with vasovagal syncope. Prolonged seizure activity should prompt a more thorough seizure workup. There is no significant postictal period with the seizure-like activity associated with syncope.

- How long did it take to return to baseline?
—Vasovagal syncope is associated with a relatively quick (minutes) return to baseline mental status as soon as cerebral blood flow is restored. If there is a delay in assuming a recumbent position, there may be a longer delay in return to baseline mental status. Increased duration of unconsciousness or confusion suggests seizures rather than syncope.

- Was there a history of trauma?
—A recent history of head trauma raises concern for intracranial hemorrhage.

- Is there a family history of sudden death, including common causes such as drowning or auto accidents?
—A family history of sudden death should raise suspicion for cardiac arrhythmias.

- Is there a history of anemia?
—Anemic patients may be more likely to have a syncopal episode because of decreased cerebral oxygen delivery.

Seventeen-Year-Old Girl

SAMIR S. SHAH

HISTORY OF PRESENT ILLNESS

A 17-year-old girl presented to the emergency department after her second episode of passing out in a week. The first episode happened 7 days ago while she was walking home from school. She experienced a prodromal period of everything around her blackening and then awoke on the sidewalk with her friends around her. Her friends took her home that day. The next episode occurred shortly prior to presentation. She had just finished dinner and was walking into another room when a similar episode of darkening occurred and then she awoke on the floor. On review of systems, she was found to have had occasional episodes of shaking chills, tactile temperatures, and a 5-lb weight loss during a 2-week period. She was a senior in high school and planning on going to college. She was sexually active, but used protection every time. Her last menstrual period, which occurred 1 week ago, was normal.

MEDICAL HISTORY

The girl has been a healthy child and had never been hospitalized. She has three brothers who are also healthy. Her immunizations were up-to-date, including the human papilloma virus vaccine.

PHYSICAL EXAMINATION

T 38.2°C; HR 90 bpm; RR 20/min; BP 95/58 mmHg

Weight 75th percentile and Height 20th percentile

On examination she was alert and cooperative in no distress. She did not appear pale. Her head and neck examination was normal. Her lungs were clear to auscultation. Her cardiac examination was normal. Her abdomen was soft and there was no organomegaly or masses detected. Her neurologic examination was normal. Her skin examination revealed rashes all over her body (Figure 18-1).

DIAGNOSTIC STUDIES

A complete blood count revealed a WBC count of 12 000 cells/mm^3 (6% bands, 30% segmented neutrophils, 42% lymphocytes, 19% atypical lymphocytes, 3% monocytes), hemoglobin of 12.2 g/dL, and a platelet count of 14 000/mm^3.

COURSE OF ILLNESS

She was admitted to the hospital for further evaluation. Due to the thrombocytopenia, fever, and weight loss, a bone marrow aspirate was performed.

DISCUSSION CASE 18-1

DIFFERENTIAL DIAGNOSIS

The presence of intermittent fever, petechial rash, thrombocytopenia, and 5-lb weight loss raise concern for neoplastic disorders, such as leukemia or lymphoma. Blast forms on peripheral smear are occasionally mistaken for atypical lymphocytes. However, they are also a marker for a potential Epstein-Barr virus (EBV) infection. More broadly,

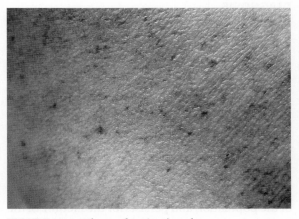

FIGURE 18-1. Photo of patient's rash.

thrombocytopenia may be caused by increased platelet destruction or consumption or by impaired or ineffective platelet production. Infectious causes of platelet destruction include EBV, cytomegalovirus, human immunodeficiency virus, hepatitis B or C, toxoplasmosis, leptospirosis, syphilis, rickettsioses (e.g., Rocky Mountain spotted fever, ehrlichiosis, human granulocytic anaplasmosis), and bacterial sepsis. Idiopathic thrombocytopenic purpura is a frequent cause of thrombocytopenia in children that can have both an acute and chronic course. However, the incidence of ITP peaks at 3-5 years of age. Other immunologic causes of platelet destruction include systemic lupus erythematosus, autoimmune hemolytic anemia (Evan syndrome), and hyperthyroidism. Nonimmunologic causes include hemolytic-uremic syndrome and Kasabach-Merritt syndrome. Drug-induced thrombocytopenia should be considered if the patient is taking any medication, particularly sulfonamides, digoxin, quinine, quinidine, or chemotherapeutic agents. Disorders of impaired platelet production include marrow infiltrative processes such as leukemias, nutritional deficiencies (e.g., iron, folate, vitamin B_{12}), and infection-associated suppression (e.g., EBV, HIV, parvovirus B9). Thrombocytopenia can occur after vaccination with MMR vaccine. Rare genetic disorders such as Fanconi anemia, Hermansky-Pudlak syndrome, thrombocytopenia with absent radii syndrome (TAR), Wiskott-Aldrich syndrome, May-Hegglin anomaly, and Bernard-Soulier disease are possibilities as well.

DIAGNOSIS

The petechial rash was consistent with her thrombocytopenia (Figure 18-1). The bone marrow aspirate revealed a normal marrow with increased megakaryocytes. The interpretation is that this is a clinical picture consistent with viral consumption of platelets. The EBV titers were positive for IgM and IgG antibody to viral capsid antigen. No Epstein-Barr nuclear antigen (EBNA) was detected. **The diagnosis is EBV infection.**

INCIDENCE AND EPIDEMIOLOGY

EBV is close to ubiquitous. It infects more than 90% of the population and persists for the lifetime of the host. Infection occurs at a later age in developed countries than in developing countries. This differential may be due to improved sanitary conditions and reduced population density in developed countries. The incidence of EBV infection is 50 per 100 000 individuals overall; however, it is 1 per 1000 individuals aged 15-25 years. The incubation period may last up to 30 days.

EBV is linked to infectious mononucleosis, Burkitt lymphoma, nasopharyngeal carcinoma, as well as other cancers. The virus is a member of the herpesvirus family. EBV binds to the CD21 molecule on the B-cell and gains entry into the cell. After infection of an epithelial cell in the oropharynx, the virus replicates and the cell ultimately dies. When EBV infects the B-cell, the virus becomes latent. However, unlike other herpesvirus infections, EBV does not recur. Infection is spread from person to person with contact of oral secretions. Transmission by aerosol or fomites is uncommon. The incubation period during which the virus may be communicated but the patient is asymptomatic is approximately 4 weeks; however, transmission rates are relatively low as evidenced by the absence of widespread EBV epidemics.

CLINICAL PRESENTATION

Young children with EBV exhibit no or few symptoms. Symptoms, when present, typically mimic viral respiratory infections with fever, cough, and rhinitis. While acute EBV infection is not synonymous with infectious mononucleosis ("mono"), infectious mononucleosis is the most commonly recognized clinical manifestation of EBV infection. Infectious mononucleosis typically presents with the triad of fever, tonsillopharyngitis, and lymphadenopathy. The pharyngitis is typically exudative. Lymphadenopathy is nontender and symmetrically involves the posterior cervical chains. Nausea, vomiting, and anorexia frequently occur which likely reflects the high prevalence of hepatitis (90% of patients may have a mild hepatitis). More than half of all patients with EBV infection will have splenomegaly; however, hepatomegaly is much less frequent. The acute symptoms resolve within 2 weeks, though fatigue may persist longer.

A minority of patients will have rashes which may be petechial, maculopapular, scarlatiniform, or urticarial. Other less common systemic presentations of EBV infection include Guillain-Barré syndrome, facial nerve palsy, aseptic meningitis, meningoencephalitis, metamorphopsia ("Alice in Wonderland" syndrome in which there are bizarre perceptual distortions in shape or spatial relationships), transverse myelitis, peripheral neuropathy, optic neuritis, hemophagocytic lymphohistiocytosis, and, in boys, orchitis.

Complications from EBV infection include the possibility of a diffuse morbilliform rash if the patient is administered a penicillin drug, splenic rupture, upper airway obstruction, and lymphoproliferative disorders. Splenic rupture, which is more common in boys, has been reported to occur in 1 in 1000 cases typically on day 4-21 after the onset of symptoms. It may occur spontaneously and should be considered in any patient with left upper abdominal pain that radiates to the left shoulder. Airway obstruction is very rare, but carries significant morbidity and mortality. The airway compromise can be treated with steroids if necessary. Lymphoproliferative disorders can occur if there is decreased cellular immunity. It is the T-cell and natural killer cells that keep the latent EBV infection in check.

DIAGNOSTIC APPROACH

The diagnosis of an EBV infection is based on the correct clinical picture with supporting laboratory evidence.

Complete blood count. The complete blood count typically reveals a leukocytosis, though neutropenia is relatively common; the differential count usually reveals lymphocyte predominance with greater than 10% atypical lymphocytes. Other viruses that cause atypical lymphocytes include cytomegalovirus, human immunodeficiency virus, hepatitis, and measles; however, only EBV and cytomegalovirus have greater than 10% atypical lymphocytes. Mild thrombocytopenia is common; the platelet count rarely decreased below 100 000 platelets/mm^3. Anemia is typically not associated with EBV, but if present consider autoimmune hemolysis (which occurs in less than 1% of patients) or splenic rupture.

Hepatic transaminases. Hepatic transaminases may be mildly elevated (two- to threefold).

Heterophile antibodies. Heterophile antibodies (e.g., Monospot), which agglutinate sheep or horse red blood cells, may be positive. These antibodies typically appear within 2 weeks of infection and may persist for as long as 6 months. Younger children are less likely than older children to have heterophile antibodies. False-positive monospot results may occur with leukemia, lymphoma, and Gaucher disease.

EBV-specific antibodies. EBV antibody titers may be sent for confirmation of disease. IgM and IgG antibodies directed against viral capsid antigen (anti-VCA IgM and IgG) appear first and are always present during the symptomatic phase (Table 18-3). The IgM is transient, disappearing within 2-3 months, while the IgG antibodies persist. Antibodies against EBV early antigen (anti-EA) typically increase several weeks after infection and disappear by 12 months. Anti-Epstein-Barr virus nuclear antigen antibody (anti-EBNA) appears last (usually >6 weeks after infection) and persists indefinitely. The presence of anti-EBNA antibodies excludes the possibility of acute infection.

TABLE 18-3.	Interpretation of Epstein-Barr virus antibodies.		
	Acute Infection	*Recent Infection*	*Past Infection*
Anti-Viral Capsid Antigen IgM	Present	Present/absent	Absent
Anti-Viral Capsid Antigen IgG	Present[a]	Present	Present
Anti-Early Antigen	Absent/present[b]	Present	Present/absent
Anti-Epstein-Barr Nuclear Antigen	Absent	Absent/present[c]	Present

[a]Increases early in illness, always elevated when symptoms are present and persists for life.
[b]Increases weeks to months after symptom onset.
[c]Increases later in illness, typically more than 4 weeks after symptom onset.

EBV polymerase chain reaction. EBV polymerase chain reaction (PCR) has limited utility in the acute infectious stage. It may be transiently positive in acute infections, but it is also usually positive in those who have had a past EBV infection in whom the current symptoms may be unrelated to EBV. It is most useful in immune compromised hosts at risk for lymphoproliferative disorder.

TREATMENT

The mainstay of treatment is supportive care including adequate rest, fluids, and antipyretics. Although antivirals such as acyclovir demonstrate in vitro activity against EBV, there is no clinical benefit in uncomplicated mononucleosis in an otherwise healthy child. In the absence of concurrent bacterial infection, antibiotics should not be used. If antibiotic therapy is necessary, aminopenicillins (e.g., amoxicillin, ampicillin) should be avoided as these agents cause a rash, typically manifesting after the first few days of therapy. The rash is maculopapular, pruritic, and prolonged. Its appearance is not a contraindication to future aminopenicillin

use. Systemic corticosteroids are not routinely recommended, but can be considered when there are complications such as tonsillar hypertrophy causing airway obstruction, massive splenomegaly, myocarditis, pericarditis, or significant hemolysis. Because of the possibility of splenic rupture, patients should avoid contact sports for at least 1 month or until the resolution of the splenomegaly.

SUGGESTED READINGS

1. Marshall BC, Koch WC. Mononucleosis syndromes. In: Shah SS, ed. *Pediatric Practice: Infectious Diseases.* New York: McGraw-Hill Medical; 2009:658-664.
2. Cohen JI. Epstein-Barr virus infection. *New Engl J Med.* 2000;343:481-492.
3. Durbin WA, Sullivan JL. Epstein-Barr virus infection. *Pediatr Rev.* 1994;15:63-68.
4. Straus SE, Cohen JI, Tosato G, Meier J. Epstein-Barr virus infections: biology, pathogenesis, and management. *Ann Intern Med.* 1993;118:45-58.
5. Schneider H, Adams O, Weiss C, Merz U, Schroten H, Tenenbaum T. Clinical characteristics of children with viral single- and co-infections and a petechial rash. *Pediatr Infect Dis J.* 2012 [PMID 23249918].

CASE 18-2

Fifteen-Year-Old Boy

SAMIR S. SHAH

HISTORY OF PRESENT ILLNESS

A 15-year-old boy felt the acute onset of his heart beating fast while he was on the phone with a friend. He became dizzy and lightheaded and fell backward onto his bed. He was not sure whether he lost consciousness, but remembered calling for his mother to help him. He was taken to the community emergency department for assistance. On arrival, he had some mild mid-sternal chest pain. He denied fever, nausea, vomiting, diarrhea, and cough. The remainder of his review of systems was negative.

MEDICAL HISTORY

He has been a healthy child with no significant illnesses. He was a good student at school and

active in sports. His family history did not reveal any episodes of sudden unexplained death. Of note, his sister had coarctation of the aorta that required repair in infancy. He did not take any medications. He has received all of his childhood immunizations.

PHYSICAL EXAMINATION

T 37.2°C; HR 230 bpm; RR 20/min; BP 105/68 mmHg

Weight 50th percentile and Height 90th percentile

On examination he was awake, but anxious appearing. His head and neck examination was normal. His lungs were clear to auscultation. His cardiac examination was significant for profound tachycardia with a rate that could not be counted manually. There was no jugular venous distention. His perfusion was adequate with a capillary refill of 1 second at the fingertip. His pulses were palpable throughout. His abdomen was soft without any enlargement of his spleen or liver. His extremities were well perfused. His neurologic examination was normal.

DIAGNOSTIC STUDIES

WBC count revealed 12 400 cells/mm³ (54% segmented neutrophils, 1% bands, 38% lymphocytes); hemoglobin, 13.2 g/dL; and platelets, 278 000/mm³. Measurement of serum chemistries revealed the following: sodium, 138 mEq/L; potassium, 4.3 mEq/L; chloride, 106 mEq/L; bicarbonate, 22 mEq/L; calcium, 9.2 mg/dL; and magnesium, 2.9 mg/dL.

COURSE OF ILLNESS

Chest roentogram (CXR) revealed a normal heart size and no pulmonary edema. The initial

(Figure 18-2A) and subsequent (Figure 18-2B) electrocardiograms (ECG) revealed the acute and underlying diagnoses.

DISCUSSION CASE 18-2

DIFFERENTIAL DIAGNOSIS

The initial ECG (Figure 18-2A) revealed a narrow complex tachycardia with a rate of almost 300 bpm. The patient had paroxysmal supraventricular tachycardia (SVT). Features consistent with the diagnosis of SVT included a compatible history, lack of heart rate variability, heart rate greater than 180 bpm, and absence of P waves on the ECG. Supraventricular tachycardia may be due to structural heart disease (e.g., Wolff-Parkinson-White syndrome), acute heart disease (e.g., myocarditis, pericarditis), hyperthyroidism, excessive caffeine consumption, pregnancy, illicit drug use (e.g., cocaine), and prescription medications (e.g., digitalis, beta-agonists).

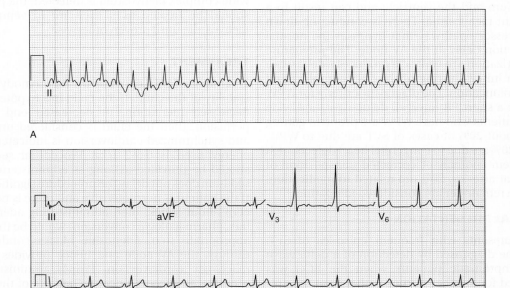

FIGURE 18-2. **A.** Initial ECG. **B.** Subsequent ECG.

DIAGNOSIS

Vagal maneuvers were unsuccessful so the patient received two doses of adenosine. When these failed to convert his rhythm, synchronized cardioversion using a dose of 0.5 J/kg and then 2 J/kg was performed and normal rhythm was restored. **On subsequent ECGs he was found to have a short PR interval (<0.12 seconds) and a delta wave (slurring of the QRS complex) consistent with Wolff-Parkinson-White syndrome (WPW) (Figure 18-2B). The diagnosis is SVT due to WPW.**

INCIDENCE AND EPIDEMIOLOGY

SVT encompasses three diagnostic etiologies, atrial tachycardia, nodal tachycardia, and AV reentrant tachycardia. Most episodes of SVT are caused by AV reentrant tachycardias. Ectopic tachycardias are rare in pediatrics. Nodal tachycardias originate from the AV node and tend to have slower rates (150-200 bpm) than the tachycardias that arise from above the node.

WPW is a form of preexcitation that results from an anomalous conduction pathway between the atrium and the ventricle and can result in a reentrant tachycardia. There is conduction down the accessory pathway that bypasses the normal conduction delay at the AV node. The premature depolarization of a ventricle produces a delta wave (i.e., an initial slurring of the QRS complex) and QRS prolongation. The diagnostic criteria for WPW include a short PR interval, delta wave, and wide QRS. Patients who have WPW are prone to getting SVT. About 20% of cases of SVT are due to WPW, about 20% are due to congenital heart defects such as Ebstein anomaly or corrected transposition of the great arteries, 20% are related to medication, and the remainder are considered idiopathic.

CLINICAL PRESENTATION

WPW presents with frequent episodes of SVT. It can be diagnosed by detection of a delta wave in asymptomatic patients when the ECG was obtained for another purpose other than the episode of SVT. SVT is the most common arrhythmia in childhood, with 40% presenting in the first 6 months of life and 30% presenting in the school age years. An infant who presents with SVT will typically be more fussy than usual, may have difficulty feeding, and may have episodes of grunting. Frequently, the infant will be in SVT for a longer period of time until there are behavioral changes that alert the caretaker that something is wrong with the infant. As the time spent in SVT continues, there is an increased chance the child will begin to show symptoms of heart failure. When the heart rate is actually measured, it will be in the range of 220-320 bpm. An older child who is verbal will be able to report the acute onset of a rapid heartbeat. Many children describe the feeling as having butterflies in their chest.

DIAGNOSTIC APPROACH

Electrocardiogram. An ECG obtained during an episode of SVT will reveal a tachycardia, narrow QRS complex, and P waves that are either partially obscured by the ST segment or not even visible at all. In infants, the typical rates are in the range of 220-320 bpm. In older children and adolescents, the rates are in the 150-250 bpm range. If the SVT is aberrantly conducted, the QRS complex will be wide and resemble ventricular tachycardia. If a wide complex tachycardia is detected, the patient should be treated as if they are in ventricular tachycardia until proven otherwise.

TREATMENT

Treatment of SVT depends on the hemodynamic stability of the child. If the child has hypotension, decreased mentation, or decreased end organ perfusion, then the child is considered unstable and synchronized cardioversion is indicated. The energy used is 0.5-2 J/kg. Procedural sedation should be provided as long as administering the sedation does not delay the procedure significantly. If the patient is normotensive and there is no concern about shock, then administering adenosine (i.e., pharmacologic conversion) would be the next appropriate step. Adenosine blocks conduction through the AV node and hence provides pharmacologic cardioversion. Proper administration is critical to success since the half-life of the drug is short, less than a minute. Two syringes should be connected to a T-connector or stopcock; give adenosine rapidly with one syringe and immediately flush with 5 mL or more of normal saline with the other. Verapamil is used frequently in older children and adults with SVT, but should be avoided in young children because it can cause profound vasodilatation and cardiovascular collapse. If the patient has recalcitrant SVT, slow infusion of procainamide or amiodorone should be considered.

Treatment of WPW typically involves radiofrequency catheter ablation. Patients at high risk for ablation-related complications may receive pharmacotherapy with class I (e.g., flecainide) or class III (e.g., amiodarone) antiarrhythmic medications to slow accessory pathway conduction.

SUGGESTED READINGS

1. Ganz LI, Friedman PL. Supraventricular tachycardia. *New Engl J Med*. 1995;332:162-173.
2. Kleinman ME, Chameides L, Achexnayder SM, et al. Part 14: pediatric advanced life support: 2010 American Heart Association Guidelines for Cardiopulmonary Resuscitation and Emergency Cardiovascular Care. *Circulation*. 2010;122:s876-s908.
3. Trohman RG. Supraventricular tachycardia: implications for the intensivist. *Crit Care Med*. 2000;28:N129-N135.

CASE 18-3

Fourteen-Year-Old Boy

SAMIR S. SHAH

HISTORY OF PRESENT ILLNESS

A 14-year-old boy was brought to the emergency department after collapsing at school. He was at basketball practice when he collapsed to the ground. The paramedics were called and brought him to the emergency department. He awoke within a few minutes of the fall. There was no seizure activity reported. He did not complain of shortness of breath, palpitations, or chest pain. He denied fever, cough, and rhinorrhea. He has no complaints at present. He denied having taken any illicit drugs.

MEDICAL HISTORY

The boy has been healthy with no significant medical history. There was no family history of early cardiac deaths in children or young adults. He takes no medications and all his immunizations are up-to-date.

PHYSICAL EXAMINATION

T 37.0°C; HR 112 bpm; RR 20/min; BP 124/78 mmHg

Weight 90th percentile and Height 75th percentile

On examination he was awake and in no acute distress. His mucous membranes were moist. His lungs were clear to auscultation. His cardiac examination revealed a regular rate and rhythm with a normal S1 and S2 and an S3 gallop rhythm. No murmur could be detected. His abdomen was soft without any hepatosplenomegaly. His extremities were warm and well perfused with strong peripheral pulses. His neurologic examination was normal.

DIAGNOSTIC STUDIES

Because of the syncopal episode, he had a bedside glucose level checked which returned at 108 mg/dL. Electrolytes and a complete blood count were normal. The chest radiograph revealed a top-normal sized cardiothymic silhouette.

COURSE OF ILLNESS

An ECG (Figure 18-3) suggested the diagnosis.

DISCUSSION CASE 18-3

DIFFERENTIAL DIAGNOSIS

This case of syncope is probably caused by a cardiac etiology due to the abnormal physical examination findings as well as the ECG and chest

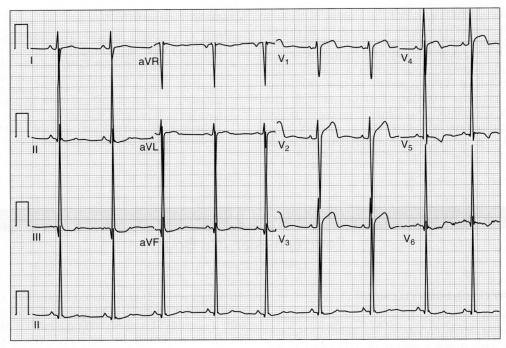

FIGURE 18-3. ECG.

radiography abnormalities. Of all the abnormalities present, **the left ventricular hypertrophy seen on the ECG is the most concerning** (Figure 18-3). Etiologies to consider include systemic hypertension, aortic valvular stenosis, and hypertrophic cardiomyopathy. Metabolic disorders such as glycogen storage disease, type II may also cause left ventricular hypertrophy.

DIAGNOSIS

Echocardiography revealed a large intraventricular septum and a top-normal sized left ventricular end-diastolic dimension. There was no left ventricular outflow obstruction detected. Exercise stress testing did not reveal any arrhythmias; however, there was a 3-mm ST segment depression during maximal exercise. **The diagnosis is hypertrophic cardiomyopathy.** He was started on a beta-blocker to reduce the pressure gradient across the left ventricular outflow tract. He was also counseled to avoid strenuous competitive athletic activity and strenuous physical exertion. An implantable cardioverter defibrillator (ICD) was considered to prevent sudden arrhythmic death.

INCIDENCE AND EPIDEMIOLOGY

Hypertrophic cardiomyopathy (HCM), a relatively common genetic disease, is the leading cause of sudden cardiac death in preadolescent and adolescent children. There is autosomal dominant inheritance with variable penetrance; approximately 50% of cases are familial. There is a considerable heterogeneity of clinical expression and prognosis even in familial cases. The prevalence of HCM is not well defined. It is detected in 0.5% of outpatients referred for echocardiography. However, population-based studies report a much lower incidence of 1 in 500 or 0.2% of the general adult population. Furthermore, a substantial proportion of patients in the general population probably have a mutant gene for HCM, yet are undetected due to lack of clinical due to lack of clinical symptoms.

CLINICAL PRESENTATION

HCM is frequently suspected because of a heart murmur, positive family history, new clinical symptoms (e.g., syncope), or an abnormal ECG. The physical examination of patients with HCM is often normal because most (>75%) affected patients do not have outflow tract obstruction; abnormal findings on physical examination are usually related to left ventricular outflow tract obstruction. If an outflow tract obstruction is present, a murmur can be heard. The murmur is louder with increasing outflow obstruction such as valsalva maneuvers and softer with relief of the obstruction such as can be seen with squatting.

Complications of HCM include congestive heart failure, ventricular and supraventricular arrhythmias, atrial fibrillation with mural thrombus, and sudden death. The overall rate of sudden cardiac death is approximately 1% per year. ICDs prolong life by effectively terminating life-threatening ventricular arrhythmias. In contrast, pharmacologic therapy does not appear to protect against sudden cardiac death.

DIAGNOSTIC APPROACH

The American College of Cardiology Foundation and the American Heart Association have published practice guidelines to assist healthcare providers in clinical decision-making.

Echocardiogram. HCM is defined as left ventricular hypertrophy (maximal wall thickness ≥15 mm) without left ventricular dilatation and without cardiac or systemic conditions that can explain the extent of hypertrophy. Transthoracic echocardiography should be performed in the initial evaluation of all patients with suspected HCM. Transthoracic echocardiography should also be repeated if any change in clinical status occurs, including new cardiovascular events.

Electrocardiogram. An ECG can be of benefit in the diagnosis of HCM. It is abnormal in 75% or more of patients and has a wide range of patterns. Twenty-four-hour ambulatory (Holter) ECG monitoring should be repeated every 1-2 years in patients with HCM who have no previous evidence of ventricular tachycardia to identify patients who may be candidates for implantable cardioverter defibrillator therapy.

Clinical screening. Clinical screening, including ECG and echocardiography, is recommended for all first-degree relatives of patients with HCM.

Genetic screening. Evaluation of familiar inheritance and genetic counseling is recommended as part of the assessment of patients with HCM. Genetic testing is reasonable in the index patient to facilitate identification of first-degree family members at risk for developing HCM. For those with pathogenic mutations who do not express the HCM phenotype, serial ECGs, transthoracic echocardiograms and clinical assessment is required every 12-18 months for children and every 5 years for adults. However, ongoing screening is not indicated in genotype-negative relatives in families with HCM.

Myocardial biopsy. Biopsy specimens of HCM hearts reveal cellular disarray patterns in sections of the heart that are affected by the disease.

TREATMENT

The treatment for patients with HCM is as variable as their presentation. Patients with HCM should not participate in intense competitive sports (e.g., basketball, soccer, football), whether or not they have left ventricular outflow tract obstruction. The main goal of pharmacologic therapy is to alleviate symptoms of exertional dyspnea, palpitations, and chest discomfort. Beta-blockers are the main pharmacologic therapy because of their negative inotropic effects and their ability to attenuate adrenergic-induced tachycardia. Patients unresponsive to or unable to tolerate beta-blockers may receive calcium channel blockers for symptomatic relief. ICDs prevent sudden cardiac death. Patients with HCM and at sufficient risk of sudden cardiac death should be offered ICD placement. Septal reduction therapy should be considered in patients with severe, drug-refractory symptoms and a resting or provoked left ventricular outflow tract gradient of 50 mmHg or greater. Surgical septal myectomy is preferred over alcohol septal ablation.

SUGGESTED READINGS

1. Gersh BJ, Maron BJ, Bonow RO, et al. 2011. ACCF/AHA guideline for the diagnosis and treatment of hypertrophic cardiomyopathy. A report of the American College

of Cardiology Foundation/American Heart Association Task Force on Practice Guidelines. *J Thorac Cardiovasc Surg.* 2011;142:e153-e203.

2. Berger S, Dhala A, Friedberg DZ. Sudden cardiac death in infants, children, and adolescents. *Pediatr Clin N Am.* 1999;46:221-234.
3. Maron BJ. Hypertrophic cardiomyopathy: a systematic review. *JAMA.* 2002;287:1308-1320.
4. Maron BJ, Gardin JM, Flack JM, et al. Prevalence of hypertrophic cardiomyopathy in a general population

of young adults. Echocardiographic analysis of 4111 subjects in the CARDIA study: coronary artery risk development in (young) adults. *Circulation.* 1995;92:785-789.

5. McKenna WJ, Behr ER. Hypertrophic cardiomyopathy: management, risk stratification, and prevention of sudden death. *Heart.* 2002;87:169-176.
6. Spirito P, Seidman CE, McKenna WJ, Maron BJ. The management of hypertrophic cardiomyopathy. *N Engl J Med.* 1997;336:775-785.

CASE 18-4

Fourteen-Year-Old Boy

SAMIR S. SHAH

HISTORY OF PRESENT ILLNESS

A 14-year-old boy is taken to the emergency department by paramedics after "passing out" at school. The history provided by the paramedics is that he had a nosebleed and stood up. Shortly after standing, he became lightheaded and passed out, falling to the ground. The paramedics found him to be unresponsive. They placed him in a cervical collar, inserted an intravenous line, and administered naloxone and dextrose en route to the emergency department. There was no response from either of the medications.

MEDICAL HISTORY

The boy has been a healthy teenager who only suffers from seasonal allergies. One year prior to this presentation he had testicular torsion and underwent an orchiopexy. Otherwise, he is currently not taking any medications and is also not allergic to any medications. His immunization status is up-to-date. He lives at home with his parents and sister. He is in the eighth grade and is a B/C student. He denies the use of any illicit drugs.

PHYSICAL EXAMINATION

T 37.9°C; HR 110 bpm; RR 16/min; BP 129/72 mmHg

Weight more than 95th percentile and Height 50th percentile

On examination he was somnolent, but arousable to verbal stimuli. Shortly after stimulation, he fell asleep. His head and neck examination revealed 5 mm pupils that were briskly reactive to 2 mm bilaterally. His extraocular muscles were intact. He has dried blood in his right nares and an eschar on the anterior nasal septum. The cervical collar was in place; there was no spinal tenderness elicited. His lungs were clear to auscultation. His cardiac examination had no murmurs or abnormal heart sounds. His pulse was regular and strong. His abdominal, rectal, extremity, and skin examinations were entirely normal. On neurologic examination he was found to be arousable to verbal stimuli. He was oriented to person, time, place, and situation. He followed simple commands and was able to count backwards from 100 by 7. His deep tendon reflexes were 2+ and symmetric. His sensation was intact. However, his motor strength was rated 2/5 in both arms and legs. He was able to move his extremities in the plane of the bed, but could not lift them against gravity.

DIAGNOSTIC STUDIES

A complete blood count and basic metabolic panel returned with normal values. His urine and serum drug screens were negative. A head CT did not reveal intracranial pathology. A chest radiograph was normal. An electrocardiogram revealed a normal sinus rhythm with normal intervals. A lumbar puncture was performed with an opening pressure of 17 cm H_2O, 1 WBC/mm^3 and 0 RBC/mm^3, protein and glucose normal, and Gram stain with no bacteria and no WBCs present.

COURSE OF ILLNESS

The patient underwent the above studies while in the emergency department. He did not regain his strength or return to baseline mental status after several hours and was admitted to the inpatient service.

DISCUSSION CASE 18-4

DIFFERENTIAL DIAGNOSIS

This patient presents with a change in mental status with a history of syncope. The differential diagnosis for the change in mental status can be discussed using the mnemonic AEIOU TIPS: **A**lcohol; **E**lectrolytes and endocrine; **I**nsulin, intussusception and intoxication; **O**xygen; **U**remia (and other metabolic causes); **T**rauma, tumors, and temperature; **I**nfection; **P**sychiatric; and **S**troke (Table 18-4). The clinician should consider vascular events such as cerebral thromboembolism or intracranial bleeding. Intussusception may cause depressed mental status or somnolence infants and toddlers. Trauma, including nonaccidental trauma, should always be considered a possibility with resultant cerebral contusion and concussions. Toxic ingestions may include medications (e.g., sulfonylurea), illicit drugs, and heavy metals. Metabolic disorders such

TABLE 18-4.	Causes of altered mental status.
Initial	*Cause*
A	Alcohol
E	Electrolytes and endocrine
I	Insulin, intussusceptions, and intoxication
O	Oxygen
U	Uremia (and other metabolic causes)
T	Trauma, tumors, and temperature
I	Infection
P	Psychiatric
S	Stroke

as hypoglycemia and other electrolyte abnormalities can present with decreased mental status. Infectious etiologies such as meningitis and encephalitis should always be considered. Neoplasms in the brain can produce depressed mental status as well as a cancer that produces profound anemia. And finally, seizures are a frequent cause of depressed mental status whether the patient is postictal or in subclinical status epilepticus.

DIAGNOSIS

This patient was admitted to the inpatient service. The sudden and prolonged weakness that began after a syncopal episode was difficult to explain. His neurologic examination was normal. On further questioning, it became evident that he was under a significant amount of stress at school. His grades were poor, he had been in several fights recently, and felt that there is a group of kids at school who were "out to get him." **The diagnosis is malingering.**

INCIDENCE AND EPIDEMIOLOGY

Malingering is described as the intentional production of or gross exaggeration of physical or psychological symptoms. It is frequently motivated by external incentives such as avoidance of school, work, and military obligations. Malingering differs from factitious disorder in that there is no external incentive in factitious disorders. There is a clearly definable goal for the malingering patient. The actual incidence of malingering is unknown; however, it is a rare phenomenon in children. It is more common in patients who are in a restrictive environment such as incarceration or the armed forces. Malingering represents a conscious attempt to avoid an unpleasant situation. Somatoform disorders, such as conversion disorders, are much more common in children and represent an unconscious attempt to handle unpleasant emotions without an obvious external incentive. Malingering is not considered a mental disorder.

CLINICAL PRESENTATION

Many malingering patients appear aloof and hostile toward the physician in an attempt to delay the discovery of their deception. They will readily submit to painful diagnostic procedures. By contrast, patients who have conversion disorders tend to be very friendly and appropriately concerned about diagnostic procedures.

DIAGNOSTIC APPROACH

Psychologic evaluation. According to the DSM-IV, malingering should be suspected when any of the following are noted, particularly in combination: (1) medicolegal context, that is, the patient was referred to the physician by an attorney; (2) there is an obvious discrepancy between the patient's claimed stress and disability and the objective findings; (3) there is a lack of cooperation during the examination and with the recommended treatment; and (4) the presence of an antisocial personality disorder.

Other studies. Most patients who present with malingering have vague and subjective complaints such as headache, pain in a body part, dizziness, amnesia, anxiety, or depression. These symptoms are difficult to disprove. Objective tests such as audiometry, EMG, nerve conduction studies, or evoked potential studies may be of benefit for particular symptoms.

TREATMENT

The patient suspected of malingering should be thoroughly evaluated in an objective manner. Merely linking the symptoms to psychosocial stressors may be therapeutic. Unfortunately, in the adult patients, confrontation frequently occurs which results in either the end of the doctor-patient relationship or the patient becomes more on guard and proof of the deception becomes impossible. Careful evaluation of the patient and environment often reveals the cause of the symptoms without the need for a confrontation. Preservation of the doctor-patient relationship is important to arrive at the correct diagnosis and long-term care of the patient. Of note, in malingering, symptom relief is not obtained by suggestion or hypnosis as it is in the somatoform disorders. Psychiatric referral may be warranted.

SUGGESTED READINGS

1. American Psychiatric Association. *Diagnostic and Statistical Manual of Mental Disorders.* 4th ed. Washington, DC, American Psychiatric Association; 1994:683.
2. Prazar G. Conversion reactions in adolescents. *Pediatr Rev.* 1987;8:279-286.
3. DeMaso DR, Beasley PJ. The somatoform disorders. In: Klykylo WM, Kay J, Rube D, eds. *Clinical Child Psychiatry.* Philadelphia, PA: W.B. Saunders Company; 1998;429-437.
4. Nemzer ED. Somatoform disorders. In: Lewis M, ed. *Child and Adolescent Psychiatry: A Comprehensive Textbook.* 2nd ed. Philadelphia, PA: Williams & Wilkins; 1996:693-702.

CASE 18-5

Eleven-Year-Old Boy

GIL BINENBAUM

SAMIR S. SHAH

HISTORY OF PRESENT ILLNESS

An 11-year-old boy was brought to the emergency department after having a syncopal episode at school. He was feeling "short of breath" and was being escorted to the school nurse when he "blacked out." The event occurred suddenly and without a prodromal phase. A teacher who witnessed the event reported a transient loss of consciousness. Further discussion with his parents revealed a 1-month history of fatigue, malaise, and progressive dyspnea with exertion. He had also complained of blurry vision and mild photophobia.

MEDICAL HISTORY

The child was born at term. He had not had any prior episodes of syncope.

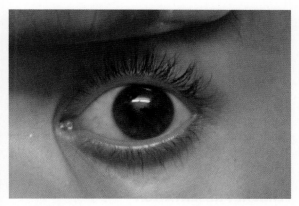

FIGURE 18-4. Photograph of the patient's eye. Note the conjunctival injection and irregularly shaped pupil.

PHYSICAL EXAMINATION

T 37.6°C; HR 40 bpm; RR 26/min; BP 110/48 mmHg

Weight 25th percentile and Height 50th percentile

On examination he was tired-appearing. Pen light examination of the left eye revealed conjunctival injection and an irregularly shaped pupil (Figure 18-4). There was a I/VI systolic ejection murmur. The lungs were clear to auscultation. There was palpable, nontender axillary lymphadenopathy.

DIAGNOSTIC STUDIES

The electrocardiogram (ECG) revealed second degree AV block (2:1) with a prolonged PR interval and right ventricular hypertrophy. The complete blood count revealed a WBC count of 4200/mm³ with 65% neutrophils, 30% lymphocytes, and 5% monocytes. The hemoglobin was 12.6 g/dL and the platelet count was 256 000/mm³. Hepatic transaminases were mildly elevated with an alanine aminotransaminase (ALT) of 250 U/L and an aspartate aminotransferase (AST) of 200 U/L. Serum electrolytes, including calcium, and uric acid levels were normal. Chest radiograph revealed mild cardiomegaly and bilateral hilar lymphadenopathy.

COURSE OF ILLNESS

Tuberculin skin test, histoplasma urinary antigen, and human immunodeficiency virus tests were all negative. The findings on eye examination, combined with the clinical presentation and abnormalities on ECG and chest radiograph, suggested a narrow range of possible diagnoses. The diagnosis was confirmed on lymph node biopsy.

DISCUSSION CASE 18-5

DIFFERENTIAL DIAGNOSIS

In Figure 18-4, the iris at the pupillary margin appeared scarred to the anterior capsule of the lens, which sits directly posterior to the iris. These adhesions are known as posterior synechiae and are a sign of uveitis or intraocular inflammation. The inflamed iris scars down to the surface of the lens. The pupil then appears misshapen with dilation in dim light because the scarred areas of the pupil do not dilate, while the unscarred areas do. If the synechiae are extensive, the result could be poor dilation altogether. Synechiae are an important sign for the pediatrician because the irregular pupil is visible to the naked eye. Therefore, whenever a red eye is being examined, the shape of the pupil should be assessed. Synechiae persist even after resolution of the acute episode of uveitis.

The finding of uveitis helps to narrow the differential diagnosis of the nonocular findings. Potential causes of uveitis include infection, systemic inflammation, neoplasia, trauma, and idiopathic disease (Table 18-5). A systemic laboratory and radiologic workup is indicated for bilateral, recurrent unilateral, or severe unilateral cases; posterior ocular involvement; or suspicion of systemic disease based on a detailed review of systems, medical history, and physical examination.

While many lung infections can cause hilar adenopathy, some infections and other conditions can cause hilar lymphadenopathy with minimal parenchymal disease (Table 18-6).

DIAGNOSIS

The serum angiotensin-converting enzyme (ACE) level was elevated with a value of 75 U/mL. **Biopsy of the axillary lymph node revealed noncaseating granulomas which confirmed the diagnosis of sarcoidosis.**

TABLE 18-5.	Differential diagnosis of uveitis.
Disease Category	**Condition**
Infection	Herpes simplex virus
	Varicella zoster virus
	Cytomegalovirus
	Toxoplasmosis
	Human immunodeficiency virus
	Syphilis
	Tuberculosis
	Lyme disease
Systemic Inflammation	Sarcoid
	Bechet disease
	Juvenile idiopathic arthritis
	Inflammatory bowel disease
	HLA-B27-associated diseases
Malignancy	Retinoblastoma
	Leukemia
	Lymphoma
Trauma	Accidental or non-accidental trauma
Idiopathic	—

TABLE 18-6.	Causes of hilar lymphadenopathy often with minimal lung parenchymal disease.
Disease Category	**Condition**
Infection	*Mycobacterium tuberculosis*
	Nontuberculous mycobacteria
	Mycoplasma pneumoniae
	Bartonella henselae
	Bordetella pertussis
	Yersinia enterocolitica
	Brucella spp.
	Francisella tularensis
	Histoplasma capsulatum
	Coccidioides immitis
	Paracoccidioides brasiliensis
	Blastomyces dermatitidis
	Cryptococcus neoformans
	Toxoplasma gondii
Chronic Inflammation	Bronchiectasis
	Cystic fibrosis
Other Conditions	Hodgkin lymphoma
	Non-Hodgkin lymphoma
	Leukemia
	Chronic granulomatous disease
	Langerhans cell histiocytosis
	Sarcoidosis
	Castleman disease

INCIDENCE AND EPIDEMIOLOGY

Sarcoidosis, a systemic disease of unknown cause, is characterized by noncaseating granulomas; the term noncaseating refers to the absence of necrosis within the granuloma. The disease occurs more commonly in blacks (approximately 35 per 100 000 per year) compared with whites (approximately 10 per 100 000 per year). Sarcoid is less common in children than in adults. Most pediatric cases occur in adolescents, though toddlers are occasionally diagnosed with the disease.

CLINICAL PRESENTATION

The clinical presentation of sarcoid varies considerably because extrapulmonary symptoms often cause the most prominent symptoms of the disease. Common sites of involvement in children include the lungs, eyes, skin, and lymph nodes. The heart, liver, and spleen are occasionally involved. Initial symptoms are usually nonspecific with children complaining of fever, malaise, fatigue, and weight loss. Older children will typically present with multisystem disease, while younger children present with the early-onset form with a triad of uveitis, rash, and arthritis.

Pulmonary. Symptoms of pulmonary sarcoidosis may include cough, dyspnea, wheezing, and, occasionally, chest pain. However, up to one-half of patients with pulmonary sarcoidosis are asymptomatic; in these instances, the disease is detected incidentally on chest radiograph. Lung auscultation is usually normal; crackles are infrequently present.

Ocular. Uveitis refers to inflammation of the uveal tract, which consists of iris, ciliary body, and choroid. Anterior uveitis, or iritis, is one subtype and remains the most common ocular manifestation of sarcoidosis. Clinical symptoms of uveitis include eye redness, pain, photophobia, and sometimes decrease in vision, all of which may be absent in some children. Most patients with anterior uveitis have concomitant systemic symptoms. Up to one-third of patients with posterior uveitis may have no signs of anterior segment inflammation. Sarcoid may also manifest as conjunctival nodules which are visible in the inferior fornix by pulling down the lower eyelid.

Lymph nodes. One-half to two-thirds of affected children have peripheral or hilar lymphadenopathy. The peripheral lymph nodes are usually firm, nontender, and moveable.

Cutaneous. Skin lesions on the face are papular and red or brown in color. Skin lesions on the trunk and extremities are usually violaceous and plaque-like. Erythema nodosum may also occur; these nodules are erythematous and tender and appear on the anterior legs. Sarcoid granulomas, though more common in adults, occasionally manifest in children; these granulomas typically infiltrate sites of scarring (i.e., "scar sarcoidosis").

Other sites. As occurred in the current case, cardiac sarcoidosis can cause left ventricular dysfunction and arrhythmias. Cardiac involvement is far more common in adults than in children with sarcoidosis. Hepatomegaly and splenomegaly may be present, but severe liver or spleen dysfunction is uncommon. Renal involvement is relatively uncommon in children with sarcoidosis. Joint involvement may lead to joint pain or effusions. Bone lesions are relatively uncommon but when present tend to involve the hands and feet. Neurosarcoid in children manifests with seizures in one-third of affected children; in contrast to adults with neurosarcoid, cranial nerve palsies are uncommon.

DIAGNOSTIC APPROACH

Slit lamp examination of the eye. Uveitis is diagnosed by examination of the eye with a slit lamp biomicroscope, which permits direct visualization of inflammatory cells floating in the anterior chamber, and a fundus examination. Synechiae with a resultant irregular pupil are not common, but when present are visible without a slit lamp. Severe inflammation may also cause a grossly visible, white crescent of aggregated cells in front of the inferior iris, termed a "hypopyon." The red reflex may be dull or absent with anterior or posterior uveitis. All patients with suspected uveitis require a dilated fundus examination to check for findings such as optic disc swelling, chorioretinitis, or vasculitis, as well as to rule out a life-threatening malignancy, such as retinoblastoma. The finding of uveitis should prompt consideration of underlying systemic causes, including sarcoid.

Angiotensin-converting enzyme (ACE) level. ACE is produced in the epithelioid cells of granulomas; ACE levels are elevated in more than 75% of children with sarcoidosis. Epithelioid cells within the granulomas are thought to be the source of ACE. While ACE levels may decrease with corticosteroid therapy, ACE levels do not necessarily correlate with symptoms. Other conditions that may produce elevated ACE levels include leprosy, Gaucher disease, hyperthyroidism, and disseminated granulomatous infections such as miliary tuberculosis.

Biopsy. Biopsy is performed to confirm the diagnosis of sarcoidosis. While enlarged peripheral lymph nodes are the preferred source given their accessibility, biopsy of skin lesions, central lymph nodes (e.g., mediastinal), lung, liver, or bone marrow may be required if peripheral lymph nodes are not enlarged. Microscopic examination classically reveals non-caseating granulomas; noncaseating refers to the absence of necrosis within the granuloma. Biopsy should be performed on the most readily accessible site. In children, the yield from palpable peripheral lymph nodes is typically high. Microscopic examination should also be performed to exclude infectious causes (e.g., tuberculosis, histoplasmosis, blastomycosis). Conjunctiva may offer a less invasive biopsy option than other body sites if the child is old enough to undergo the procedure without the need for general anesthesia; the biopsy site heals quickly and there is minimal discomfort to the child. Some experts recommend a "blind" biopsy (i.e., no conjunctival nodules or follicles) which has a sensitivity of approximately 50% before pursuing more invasive procedures (e.g., biopsy of mediastinal lymph nodes).

Chest radiograph. Chest radiographs should be obtained in all children in whom sarcoidosis is a diagnostic consideration. The chest radiograph often reveals bilateral hilar lymphadenopathy and interstitial pulmonary infiltrates; nodular infiltrates have also been described. Serial chest radiographs are sometimes used to follow the course of lung involvement.

Pulmonary function testing. Approximately half of all affected children have evidence of restrictive lung disease.

Complete blood count. Anemia and leukopenia with eosinophilia may occur.

Other studies. Serum chemistries may reveal elevated blood urea nitrogen (BUN) and creatinine values as well as hypercalcemia. Urinalysis may reveal proteinuria and hematuria. Hypercalciuria may also be present. C-reactive protein and other inflammatory markers are usually elevated, though this is a nonspecific finding.

TREATMENT

Uveitis is a sight-threatening condition, which requires prompt management by an ophthalmologist. Management of uveitis includes treating the underlying cause as well as the use of topical steroids, topical cycloplegic (dilating) drops, and systemic steroids; immunosuppressive, steroid-sparing agents may be required for recalcitrant cases. Collaborative management by pediatric ophthalmologists and rheumatologists is common and beneficial. Pediatricians should refer any child with a red eye and a history of uveitis for ophthalmologic evaluation to rule out recurrent disease. Vision-threatening complications include cataract, glaucoma, and macular edema.

Treatment of sarcoid with multisystem involvement typically includes systemic corticosteroids.

Corticosteroid therapy (typically prednisone) continues until clinical manifestations improve; the corticosteroids are then tampered over a period of several months to the lowest dose that controls disease activity. Immunosuppressive agents such as methotrexate are used for steroid nonresponsive cases and when side effects of corticosteroids are not tolerated. Other immunosuppressive agents such as azathioprine, cyclophosphamide, cyclosporine, and antitumor necrosis factor alpha are less well studied in the treatment of pediatric sarcoidosis.

SUGGESTED READINGS

1. Shetty AK, Gedalia A. Sarcoidosis in children. *Curr Probl Pediatr.* 2000;30:149-176.
2. Shetty AK, Gedalia A. Childhood sarcoidosis: a rare but fascinating disorder. *Pediatr Rheumatol.* 2008;6:16.
3. Baumann RJ, Robertson WC Jr. Neurosarcoid presents differently in children than in adults. *Pediatrics.* 2003;112:e480-e486.
4. Dempsey OJ, Paterson EW, Kerr KM, Denison AR. Sarcoidosis. *BMJ.* 2009;339:b3206.
5. Haimovic A, Sanchez M, Judson MA, Prystowsky S. Sarcoidosis: a comprehensive review and update for the dermatologist: part II. Extracutaneous disease. *J Am Acad Dermatol.* 2012;66:719e1-719e10.

SEIZURES

AMY T. WALDMAN

DEFINITION OF THE COMPLAINT

Seizures, a common neurologic disorder that occurs in childhood, affect 4%-6% of all children. A seizure is defined as a transient, involuntary alteration of consciousness, behavior, motor activity, sensation, and/or autonomic function caused by an excessive rate and hypersynchrony of discharges from a group of cerebral neurons. Epilepsy is diagnosed after two or more unprovoked seizures. In other words, recurrent seizures only occurring with precipitating events such as illness, fever, or acute head trauma are typically not considered epilepsy, even though antiepileptic drugs may be used to treat the seizures acutely. The first step in formulating a differential diagnosis in a child who presents with "seizures" is to characterize the type of event. Seizures are classified into generalized seizures (such as a tonic-clonic seizure affecting the entire body simultaneously) or focal seizures (arising from a specific area or areas of the cortex, with or without spread to the entire brain). The underlying cause is divided into three categories: genetic, structural/metabolic, and unknown cause. Genetic epilepsy is defined by seizures caused by a known or presumed genetic defect (e.g., *SCN1A* mutation). Structural/metabolic seizures are due to a lesion, such as stroke or tumor, but may also include infection. Tuberous sclerosis complex, while caused by a genetic mutation, is classified in this category because it is the structural changes in the brain, rather than being directly caused by

the mutation itself, that result in epilepsy. The etiology of epilepsy that does not have a recognized genetic or structural/metabolic cause is classified as unknown.

This chapter will discuss possible causes of seizures. However, seizures should be differentiated from other childhood paroxysmal events that can mimic seizure activity. For example, prolonged syncope and clonic jerks occurring in the setting of a syncopal event may resemble a generalized tonic-clonic seizure. Syncope is the most common alternative diagnosis assigned to otherwise healthy patients who fall to the ground without warning. Atonic seizures or "drop attacks" in which a child loses muscle tone are rare and typically occur in children with other seizure types as well (e.g., myoclonic and tonic seizures). Gastroesophageal reflux with opisthotonic posturing (Sandifer syndrome) frequently mimics seizures in infancy. Breath-holding spells, which occur in approximately 4% of infants, can resemble seizures and are also associated with cyanosis. A variety of movement disorders, such as benign myoclonus of infancy and Tourette syndrome, may also be mistaken for seizures. Additionally, seizure activity is often subtle, making seizures difficult to diagnose. For example, in the neonatal period seizures may present with horizontal eye movements, repetitive sucking, or pedaling and stepping motions that are difficult to distinguish from normal newborn infant activity. In older children, childhood absence epilepsy is characterized by a brief impairment of consciousness manifesting as a stare or behavioral arrest and is often mistaken for attention deficit disorder.

COMPLAINT BY CAUSE AND FREQUENCY

It is important to remember that a seizure does not constitute a diagnosis but is a symptom of an underlying pathologic process that requires a thorough evaluation. The causes of seizures and development of epileptic syndromes in childhood vary by age (Table 19-1). Many of the diagnoses in this table, such as infections and drug toxicities, are not specific to one age group. However, they were included with certain age categories due to increased susceptibility within that age group. While the etiology of seizures should be classified as genetic, structural/metabolic, or unknown, it is often helpful to develop a differential diagnosis by classifying the cause of seizures by category (Table 19-2).

TABLE 19-1.	Selected causes of seizures or epilepsy in childhood by age.			
	Neonatal	**Infancy/Toddler**	**School Age**	**Adolescent**
Common	Hypoxic-ischemic encephalopathy	Febrile seizures	Childhood absence epilepsy	Juvenile myoclonic epilepsy
	Intracranial hemorrhage	Drug toxicity (accidental ingestion)	Benign epilepsy with centrotemporal spikes (BECTS, formerly benign rolandic epilepsy)	Juvenile absence epilepsy
	Ischemic stroke	Infantile spasms (West syndrome)		
	CNS infections	Tuberous Sclerosis Complex		
	Metabolic abnormalities			
Less Common	Inborn errors of metabolism	Lennox-Gastaut syndrome		
	Maternal drug withdrawal	Landau Kleffner (acquired epileptic aphasia)	Panayiotopoulos syndrome (benign childhood occipital epilepsy)	
Uncommon	Neonatal epileptic syndromes –Ohtahara syndrome –Early myoclonic encephalopathy –Benign familial neonatal convulsions –Benign nonfamilial neonatal convulsions –Benign idiopathic neonatal convulsions (fifth day fits)	Myoclonic-astatic epilepsy (Doose syndrome)	Rasmussen encephalopathy	
	Metabolic deficiencies –Pyridoxine dependency –Pyridoxal phosphate dependency –Folinic acid responsive seizures	Mitochondrial disorders –Myoclonic epilepsy with ragged red fibers (MERRF)	Childhood Occipital Epilepsy of Gastaut	
		Neuronal ceroid lipofuscinosis (NCL)		
		Severe myoclonic epilepsy of infancy (Dravet syndrome)	Autosomal dominant nocturnal frontal lobe epilepsy	
		Sturge-Weber syndrome		

TABLE 19-2.	Causes of seizures in childhood by etiology.	
	Primary Neurologic Etiologies	**Secondary or Systemic Etiologies**
Vascular	Ischemic stroke	Disruption of blood flow or oxygen to the brain (hypoxic/ischemic causes)
	Sinovenous thrombosis	
	Intracerebral hemorrhage	
	Vascular malformations (arteriovenous malformations)	
	Hyperperfusion syndrome	
	Hypertensive encephalopathy	
Infectious	Encephalitis	Systemic infection (i.e., TORCH infections)
	Meningitis	
	Abscess	
	Parasites	
Inflammatory	Acute disseminated encephalomyelitis	Systemic lupus erythematosus
	Primary angiitis of the CNS	
	Rasmussen syndrome (Rasmussen encephalitis)	
Neoplastic	Primary brain tumors	Metastatic disease
Congenital	Cortical dysplasia or brain malformations	
	–Hemimegalencephaly	
	–Polymicrogyria	
	–Cortical dysplasia	
	Neurocutaneous syndromes	
	–Neurofibromatosis 1	
	–Tuberous Sclerosis Complex	
	–Hypomelanosis of Ito	
	–Incontinentia pigmenti	
	–Klippel-Trenaunay Weber	
	–Sturge-Weber syndrome	
Chromosomal Disorders		1p36 deletion
		4p deletion syndromes
		–Wolf-Hirschhorn syndrome
		–Pitt-Roger-Danks syndrome
		Chromosome 15 disorders
		–Angelman syndrome
		Inv dup 15
		Chromosome 20 (Ring chromosome syndrome)
		Trisomy 21
		Fragile-X
Traumatic	Contusion	
	Depressed skull fracture	
	Epidural hematoma	
	Subdural hematoma	
Toxic/Metabolic		Drug withdrawal
		–Includes antiepileptic withdrawal
		Drug toxicity
		–Prescription medications (includes accidental ingestions)
		–Drugs of abuse
		Pesticides

(Continued)

TABLE 19-2.	Causes of seizures in childhood by etiology. (Continued)
Primary Neurologic Etiologies	**Secondary or Systemic Etiologies**
Toxic/Metabolic (Cont.)	Electrolyte abnormalities –Hypo/hyperglycemia –Hyponatremia –Hypophosphatemia Hepatic failure Uremia Metabolic disorders –Amino acidopathies –Organic acidurias –Mitochondrial encephalopathies –Storage diseases –Urea cycle disorders –Pyridoxine (Vitamin B_6) deficiency –Folic acid responsive seizures

CLARIFYING QUESTIONS

Thorough history taking is essential to arrive at an accurate diagnosis in a child who presents with seizures. Consideration of seizure type, precipitating factors, and associated clinical features provides a useful framework for creating a differential diagnosis. The following questions may help to provide clues to the diagnosis:

- Did the seizure involve the entire body or only a portion?
—Focal (or partial) seizures reflect initial involvement from a localized lesion or lesions in the cerebral hemisphere(s). Focal seizures were previously classified on the basis of whether consciousness was impaired (complex partial seizure) or unaffected (simple partial seizure); however, these terms have been removed from the most recent classification recommendations for epilepsy. Although focal seizures are likely due to localized lesions, such structural causes are only found on magnetic resonance imaging (MRI) in 30%-50% of cases.

- Was there a preceding illness or fever?
—Febrile seizures occur most commonly in children 6 months to 5 years old. Febrile seizures occur in the setting of a systemic illness, such as a respiratory infection. Central nervous system infections, such as meningitis or encephalitis, are not considered febrile seizures but rather a separate category of primary central nervous system infection.

- Is there an ingestion or toxin exposure?
—Many medications and environmental toxins can lead to seizures including anticonvulsant medications, hypoglycemic agents, isoniazid, lithium, methylxanthines, heavy metals (e.g., lead), and tricyclic antidepressants.

- Is there recent headache, vomiting, lethargy, weakness, or alteration in gait?
—These symptoms suggest underlying central nervous system pathology and the need for neuroimaging. In neonates, the early onset of lethargy, vomiting, and seizures should prompt an evaluation for an underlying metabolic disorder, such as an aminoacidopathy, organic aciduria, and urea cycle defect; examples include phenylketonuria and maple syrup urine disease.

- Is there a history of previous seizures, febrile or afebrile, or neurologic abnormality?
—One-third of children with a simple febrile seizure will have a second episode. A previous afebrile seizure or existing neurologic abnormality increases the likelihood of a seizure disorder or epileptic syndrome.

- Is there a history of head trauma?
—Head trauma can result in epilepsy at any age. Seizures can occur within 1-2 weeks after the injury (early posttraumatic seizures), as an acute reaction to head trauma, or after intervals of several months or even years (late posttraumatic seizures). The risk of developing seizures

is related to the severity of the head injury. The child with a mild head injury (transient loss of consciousness without evidence of skull fracture or neurologic abnormality) is not at a significantly higher risk than the general population. Moderate head injuries are associated with an increased risk of epilepsy ranging from 2% to 10%. Children with severe head injuries, such as intracerebral hematoma or a history of unconsciousness more than 24 hours, have a 30% risk of developing epilepsy.

- Is there a history of a remote neurologic insult?
  —A history of anoxic birth injury, cerebral palsy, stroke, intracranial hemorrhage, or meningitis places the child at increased risk for a seizure disorder. Intrauterine infection with cytomegalovirus, toxoplasma, or rubella is known to cause abnormal brain development and predispose the child to seizures.

- Are there skin abnormalities on physical examination, such as café-au-lait or ash leaf spots, or cutaneous vascular malformations?
  —These findings suggest an underlying neurocutaneous disorder including neurofibromatosis, tuberous sclerosis complex, and Sturge-Weber syndrome.

- What is the child's head morphology?
  —Microcephaly suggests an underlying neurologic abnormality. A full or bulging fontanelle can signify elevated intracranial pressure due to meningitis, trauma, malignancy, or hydrocephalus.

- Is there a family history of seizures?
  —Both febrile and afebrile seizures can be hereditary.

The following cases represent less common causes of seizures in childhood.

CASE 19-1

Eight-Day-Old Girl

MATTHEW TEST

SAMIR S. SHAH

HISTORY OF PRESENT ILLNESS

An 8-day-old girl presented to the emergency room after an episode of irregular, rapid breathing followed by stiffening of her body and shaking of her extremities that lasted several seconds. On arrival, the infant was lethargic, cyanotic, and bradycardic with minimal spontaneous respirations. She underwent emergent endotracheal intubation and received multiple boluses of normal saline, with improvement in her perfusion and heart rate. She then had a generalized seizure and received intravenous lorazepam. Ampicillin and cefotaxime were administered after a blood culture was obtained. According to the family, she had fed poorly that day and had been sleeping more than usual. The infant had been afebrile and had normal stooling and urine output. There was no vomiting, diarrhea, or rashes. There were no ill contacts.

MEDICAL HISTORY

The infant weighed 3400 g at birth and was the product of a full-term gestation. She was born by spontaneous vaginal delivery after an uncomplicated pregnancy. Maternal serology was negative. The infant's postnatal course was remarkable only for mild jaundice that did not require phototherapy. The mother denied a history of genital herpes simplex virus (HSV) infection. There was no family history of seizures.

PHYSICAL EXAMINATION

T 39.0°C; RR 20/min; HR 180 bpm; BP 86/45 mmHg; SpO$_2$ 100% in room air

Weight 25th percentile; Head Circumference 50th percentile

Examination revealed a mechanically ventilated infant. She was sedated but withdrew to painful stimuli. The fontanelle was bulging. There were no head lacterations or skull depressions. The sclera were anicteric, and the pupils were 1.5 mm and symmetrically reactive. There were no cardiac murmurs, and the femoral pulses were weakly palpable. The lungs were clear to auscultation. The abdomen was soft, and the umbilical stump was well healed without erythema or discharge. There were two pustules in the perineal area.

DIAGNOSTIC STUDIES

Laboratory results were as follows: sodium, 132 mEq/L; potassium, 3.3 mEq/L; chloride, 99 mEq/L; bicarbonate, 23 mEq/L; glucose, 73 mg/dL; calcium, 8.9 mg/dL; and magnesium, 2.1 mg/dL. The complete blood count revealed 8000 WBCs/mm^3, including 33% band forms, 18% segmented neutrophils, 35% lymphocytes, and 10% monocytes. The hemoglobin and platelet count were normal. On cerebrospinal fluid (CSF) examination, there were 879 WBCs/mm^3 (48% segmented neutrophils, 19% lymphocytes, and 33% monocytes) and 1739 RBCs/mm^3; no organisms were seen on Gram staining. The CSF glucose was 36 mg/dL, and the protein concentration was 400 mg/dL. CSF was sent for bacterial culture and detection of HSV by polymerase chain reaction (PCR). There were no abnormalities on chest radiograph.

COURSE OF ILLNESS

In the intensive care unit, the patient received ampicillin, gentamicin, and acyclovir. A head computed tomogram (CT) was normal, and the patient's neurologic examination improved quickly during the next day. She was extubated on the second day of hospitalization but required replacement of the endotracheal tube due to multiple episodes of apnea. Electroencephalogram (EEG) revealed status epilepticus. Sustained seizure control was observed only after the addition of phenobarbital and phenytoin. Because HSV was not detected in the CSF by PCR, acyclovir was discontinued. Growth of an organism from the CSF on the third day of hospitalization guided additional therapy.

DISCUSSION CASE 19-1

DIFFERENTIAL DIAGNOSIS

Seizures are a feature of almost all brain disorders in the newborn. The time of onset of the first seizure is helpful in determining the cause. The cause of neonatal seizures occurring after the first 72 hours of life includes intracranial infection, intracranial hemorrhage, metabolic abnormalities, developmental defects, and drug withdrawal. Intracranial infections occur in 5%-10% of neonatal seizures. Common bacterial causes in the age group include group B *Streptococcus* (GBS) and *Escherichia coli*; *Listeria monocytogenes* is less common. *E. coli* may cause ventriculitis or brain abscesses (Figure 19-1). Early-onset GBS infection typically includes bacteremia, pneumonia, and meningitis. Late-onset GBS infection (infection beyond the first week of life) may include meningitis with other foci of infection, such as osteomyelitis (Figure 19-2), arthritis, and cellulitis-adenitis

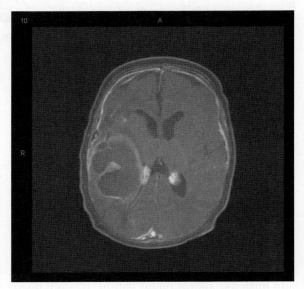

FIGURE 19-1. Brain MRI of an infant with meningitis caused by *Escherichia coli*. The MRI shows a large multiseptated cystic lesion within the right cerebral hemisphere with irregular peripheral enhancement. There is inflammation of the adjacent lateral ventricle and choroid with mass effect.

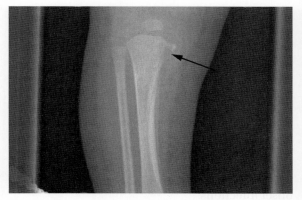

FIGURE 19-2. Lower leg radiograph of an infant with late onset group B *Streptococcal* osteomyelitis. The radiograph demonstrates an area of focal bony erosion (arrow) at the medial metaphyseal region of the proximal right tibia associated with faint periosteal reaction.

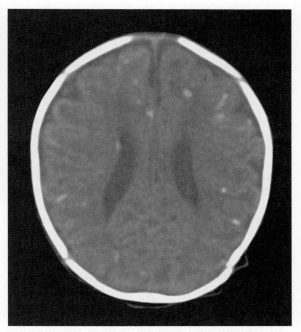

FIGURE 19-3. Computed tomography of the head in an infant with congenital toxoplasmosis. There are scattered intracranial calcifications, predominantly involving the cortex and subcortical white matter.

syndrome. Seizures with HSV typically occur during the second week of life and 30% of infected infants present with a vesicular rash. Congenital infections, particularly cytomegalovirus and *Toxoplasma gondii*, may present with seizures in the context of intracranial calcifications. The calcifications tend to be periventricular for cytomegalovirus and diffuse for toxoplasmosis (Figure 19-3). Intracranial hemorrhages are frequently associated with hypoxic-ischemic or traumatic birth injury. Intraventricular hemorrhages principally occur in the premature infant, and subarachnoid and subdural hemorrhages usually occur in the term infant. Metabolic abnormalities include disturbances of glucose, calcium, magnesium, and sodium. Hypocalcemia is associated with low birth weight, asphyxia, maternal diabetes, transient neonatal hypoparathyroidism, and microdeletions of chromosome 22q11. Other metabolic abnormalities include inborn errors of metabolism, especially aminoacidurias, because protein and glucose feedings have been initiated. Aberrations of brain development are usually related to a disturbance of neuronal migration such as lissencephaly, pachygyria, and polymicrogyria. Passive addiction of the newborn and drug withdrawal may involve narcotic-analgesics (methadone), sedative-hypnotics (shorter-acting barbiturates), cocaine, alcohol, and tricyclic antidepressants. In the case described, the results of CSF analysis suggested an intracranial infection, but interpretation of the Gram stain was misleading.

DIAGNOSIS

The diagnosis is meningitis due to *L. monocytogenes*, a Gram-positive rod. On the fourth day of hospitalization, the organism was noted to have only intermediate susceptibility to ampicillin. The patient was switched to intravenous vancomycin, and gentamicin was continued. CSF from the lumbar puncture, repeated on the sixth day of hospitalization, was sterile. Head CT was repeated on the eighth day of hospitalization and revealed bilateral frontal, parietal, and temporal lobe infarcts but no ventriculomegaly. Mechanical ventilation was required until the ninth day of hospitalization. The infant was discharged after 21 days of antibiotic therapy.

INCIDENCE AND EPIDEMIOLOGY

Listeria monocytogenes, a motile Gram-positive rod, was first isolated in 1926 during an investigation of epidemic perinatal infection among a colony of rabbits. It is a common veterinary pathogen that causes meningoencephalitis in sheep and cattle. It is widespread in the environment and is found commonly in soil and decaying vegetation. Many foods are contaminated with this organism; it has been recovered from raw vegetables, fish, poultry, beef, prepared meats, unpasteurized milk, and certain types of cheese. The organism has been isolated from the stools of 5% of healthy adults, and higher rates of recovery have been reported for household contacts of patients with clinical infection. Infection in humans is uncommon but occurs most frequently in neonates, pregnant women, and elderly or immunosuppressed patients. Human infection occurs most commonly following ingestion of contaminated food, but it can also occur through direct animal contact, as has been documented in veterinaries and farmers, and through vertical transmission from mother to neonate, either transplacentally or through an infected birth canal. Approximately 30% of all *L. monocytogenes* infections occur in neonates.

CLINICAL PRESENTATION

Neonatal *L. monocytogenes* infection, like group B streptococcal infection, manifests in both an early- and late-onset form. Clinical manifestations of *L. monocytogenes* infection are similar to those of other neonatal bacterial infections. Signs of infections include temperature instability, respiratory distress, irritability, lethargy, and poor feeding.

In early-onset disease, transplacental transmission after maternal bacteremia or ascending spread from vaginal colonization leads to intrauterine infection with *L. monocytogenes.* The neonate can also acquire the infection during passage through an infected birth canal. Pregnancy complications, including preterm labor, spontaneous abortion, and stillbirth, are common among infants with early-onset *L. monocytogenes* infections; length of gestation is less than 35 weeks in approximately 70% of cases. There is often

evidence of an acute febrile maternal illness, with symptoms of fatigue, arthralgias, and myalgias preceding delivery by 2-14 days. Blood cultures are positive for *L. monocytogenes* in 35% of mothers of infants with early-onset listeriosis.

Early-onset infection classically develops within the first or second day of life. Bacteremia (75%) and pneumonia (50%) are usually seen with early-onset infection. Meningitis is seen in 25% of early-onset cases. In severe infection, a granulomatous rash is associated with disseminated disease (granulomatosis infantiseptica). The mortality rate, including stillbirths, is 20%-40% in early-onset infections.

In late-onset infection, the mode of transmission is poorly understood but mechanisms unrelated to maternal carriage may be involved. Late-onset infection develops during the second to eighth week of life, often in full-term infants following uncomplicated delivery. The most common form of *L. monocytogenes* infection during this period is meningitis, which is present in approximately 95% of cases. Bacteremia (20%) and pneumonia (10%) are less common. Mortality of late-onset infection is generally low (15%) if the infection is diagnosed early and treated appropriately. The presentation of late-onset infection can be subtle, and may be characterized by temperature instability, irritability, poor feeding, and lethargy.

A nosocomial outbreak occurred when nine newborn infants were bathed in mineral oil contaminated with *L. monocytogenes.* The affected infants developed bacteremia (two cases), meningitis (two cases), or both (five cases); one infant died. Signs of infection developed within 1 week after exposure to the mineral oil.

DIAGNOSTIC APPROACH

Lumbar puncture. Isolation of the organism from culture of CSF is the only reliable means of diagnosing meningitis due to *L. monocytogenes.* The finding of short, sometimes coccoid, Gram-positive rods on microscopic examination of the CSF strongly supports the diagnosis of *L. monocytogenes* meningitis. However, because of the low concentrations of organisms, most (60%) Gram-stained smears of CSF from infants with *L. monocytogenes* meningitis do not reveal bacteria, as occurred with the infant in this case.

Furthermore, *L. monocytogenes* sometimes does not stain clearly as Gram positive. In such cases, variable decoloration on Gram staining may cause the organism to appear as a Gram-negative rod and be confused with *H. influenzae,* especially with long-standing disease or when the patient has received prior antibiotics. In other instances, *Listeria* has been mistaken for *Streptococcus pneumoniae* or *Corynebacterium* spp. CSF glucose is normal in more than 60% of cases of *L. monocytogenes* meningitis. CSF is often purulent with mononuclear cells predominance in one-third of cases. CSF protein is often elevated, with increasing levels correlated with a poor prognosis.

Additional studies. PCR probes and antibodies to listeriolysin O, the major virulence factor of the organism, have not proved useful for acute diagnosis of invasive disease.

TREATMENT

Ampicillin is the preferred agent in the treatment of *L. monocytogenes* infections. Based on synergy studies in vitro and in animal models, most authorities suggest adding gentamicin to ampicillin for the treatment of meningitis due to *L. monocytogenes.* There appears to be partial synergy with combinations of ampicillin or vancomycin with rifampin. Vancomycin alone has been used successfully in

a few penicillin-allergic adult patients, but others have developed listerial meningitis while receiving the drug. Trimethoprim-sulfamethoxazole is effective in penicillin-allergic patients, but should not be used in neonates because of the concern for bilirubin toxicity. Cephalosporins are not active against *L. monocytogenes.* Once susceptibility studies become available, changes in therapy may be necessary. The recommended duration of therapy for *L. monocytogenes* meningitis is 14-21 days.

Corticosteroids should be avoided, if possible, because impairment of cellular immunity due to corticosteroid therapy is a major risk factor for the development of listeriosis. A maternal history of a previous infant with perinatal listeriosis is not an indication for intrapartum antibiotics.

SUGGESTED READINGS

1. Lorber B. *Listeria monocytogenes.* In: Long SS, ed. *Principles and Practice of Pediatric Infectious Diseases.* 4th ed. Philadelphia, PA: W.B. Saunders Company; 2012;762-767.
2. Lorber B. Listeriosis. *Clin Infect Dis.* 1997;24:1-11.
3. Posfay-Barbe KM, Wald ER. Listeriosis. *Semin Fetal Neonatal Med.* 2009;14:228-223.
4. Schuchat A, Lizano C, Broome CV, et al. Outbreak of neonatal listeriosis associated with mineral oil. *Pediatr Infect Dis J.* 1991;10:183-189.
5. Southwick FS, Purich DL. Mechanisms of disease: intracellular pathogenesis of listeriosis. *New Engl J Med.* 1996; 334:770-776.

CASE 19-2

Ten-Day-Old Boy

REBECCA TENNEY-SOEIRO

HISTORY OF PRESENT ILLNESS

The patient is a 10-day-old boy who was well until the day of admission when he had a sudden onset of left arm and leg shaking while sleeping. The episode lasted about 1 minute and was accompanied by eyelid fluttering. After spontaneous cessation of the episode, the infant continued sleeping but was aroused

easily. He was brought to the emergency department for evaluation. He did not have fevers or cyanosis. There was no recent vomiting or diarrhea. His oral intake had been unchanged during the past several days, consisting exclusively of cow-milk-based formula every 2.5-3 h. The parents were uncertain about urine output since the maternal grandmother had cared for the infant the day prior to admission.

MEDICAL HISTORY

The infant weighed 3600 g, born by spontaneous vaginal delivery after an uncomplicated pregnancy. The infant required phototherapy briefly on the second day of life for hyperbilirubinemia with a peak total bilirubin level of 15.5 mg/dL. The mother had vaginal colonization with group B *Streptococcus* and received two doses of penicillin during labor. She also had a history of genital herpes simplex virus infection. Although no lesions were noted at delivery, she did develop lesions on the seventh postpartum day.

PHYSICAL EXAMINATION

T 37.5°C; HR 124 bpm; RR 40/min; BP 75/45; SpO$_2$ 100% in room air

Weight 50th percentile; Length 25th percentile; Head Circumference 25th percentile

The infant appeared alert. There were no vesicles on the scalp or skin. His anterior fontanelle was open and flat. His conjunctivae were pink and anicteric. Red reflex was present bilaterally. There was no murmur on cardiac examination and femoral pulses were strong. The spleen tip was just palpable and there was no hepatomegaly. The Moro reflex was symmetric. The remainder of the examination was normal.

DIAGNOSTIC STUDIES

Complete blood count revealed 8800 WBCs/mm^3 (16% segmented neutrophils, 70% lymphocytes; 11% monocytes; and 3% atypical lymphocytes);

hemoglobin, 13.4 g/dL; and platelets, 511000/mm^3. Serum chemistries included sodium, 139 mmol/L; potassium, 5.5 mmol/L; chloride, 104 mmol/L; and bicarbonate, 28 mmol/L. The blood urea nitrogen and creatinine were normal. Serum alanine and aspartate aminotransferases were normal. Serum albumin was 3.3 g/dL. Examination of the cerebrospinal fluid revealed the following: WBCs, 12/mm^3; RBCs, 1834/mm^3; glucose, 45 g/dL; and protein, 124 g/dL. There were no bacteria on Gram stain.

COURSE OF ILLNESS

They infant was treated empirically with ampicillin, cefotaxime, and acyclovir while awaiting the results of CSF bacterial culture and CSF HSV PCR. An ECG (Figure 19-4) suggested a cause of the seizures, which was confirmed by additional blood tests in both the infant and his mother.

DISCUSSION CASE 19-2

DIFFERENTIAL DIAGNOSIS

Many neonatal seizures are idiopathic. The most common definable etiologic agents include asphyxia, intracranial infection, trauma, nontraumatic hemorrhage, strokes, metabolic disorders, central nervous system malformations, and maternal drug abuse. Seizures due to perinatal asphyxia typically occur within the first 24 hours of life. Common infectious causes in the first week of life include bacterial meningitis due to group B *Streptococcus* and *Escherichia coli*. Neonates with herpes simplex meningitis typically present during the second week of life

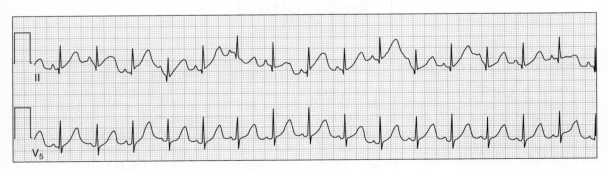

FIGURE 19-4. Electrocardiogram.

but up to 40% develop symptoms within the first 5 days of life. Intracranial hemorrhage of any cause can provoke seizures. Neonatal seizures related to birth trauma with subsequent subarachnoid hemorrhage or subdural and epidural hematomas usually occur within the first 72 hours of life. Non-traumatic causes of intracranial hemorrhage including ruptured arteriovenous malformations and underlying disorders of coagulation can occur at any time. Metabolic disorders include hypocalcemia, hypoglycemia, and pyridoxine dependency. Neonatal hypocalcemia occurring after the third day of life is usually due to transient relative hypoparathyroidism. The immature neonatal parathyroid may be unable to handle an excessive phosphate load, particularly when the infant is fed a formula with a relatively low ratio of calcium to phosphorus. Rarely, prolonged phototherapy induces hypocalcemia. Phototherapy decreases melatonin secretion, which in turn decreases glucocorticoid secretion, which leads to an increase in bone calcium uptake with subsequent hypocalcemia. Multiple defects in urea cycle and organic acid metabolism may cause seizures during the neonatal period. Infants with these disorders usually have unexplained stupor, coma, and vomiting in addition to seizures. Infants born to mothers who have used heroin or methadone may have seizures, although other symptoms such as poor feeding, diarrhea, sweating, jitteriness, and irritability are more common.

DIAGNOSIS

Bacterial cultures and HSV PCR of the CSF were negative. The ECG demonstrated QTc prolongation (QTc = 0.47 seconds) characteristic of hypocalcemia (Figure 19-4). The infant's serum calcium was 6.6 mg/dL (normal range 8.8-10.1 mg/dL); ionized calcium, 0.83 mmol/L (normal range 1.00-1.17 mmol/L); phosphate, 10.6 mg/dL (normal range 4.8-8.2 mg/dL); and magnesium, 1.1 mg/dL (1.5-2.5 mg/dL). Additional testing included intact parathyroid hormone, 9.7 pg/mL (normal range 10-55 pg/mL); 25-hydroxy vitamin D, 7 ng/mL (normal range 5-42 ng/mL); and active vitamin D (1-alpha-25-dihydroxy-cholecalciferol) $(1,25(OH)_2D)$, 114 pg/mL (normal range 8-72 pg/mL). See Table 19-3 for the differential diagnosis of hypocalcemia in an infant. Although the mother

TABLE 19-3	Differential diagnosis of neonatal hypocalcemia.
Early (within 2-3 days of birth)	*Late (often occurs at end of first week)*
Prematurity	Hypoparathyroidism
Infants of diabetic mothers	–Excess phosphorus intake is most common
Perinatal asphyxia	–May occur as part of a
Intrauterine growth restriction	syndrome-DiGeorge, Kearns-Sayre or Kenny-Caffey
Severe maternal vitamin D deficiency	Maternal hyperparathyroidism
	Hypomagnesemia
	Phototherapy for hyperbilirubinemia
	Acute renal failure
	Rotavirus infection

was asymptomatic, her calcium level was elevated to 12.8 mg/dL. The mother was subsequently diagnosed with hyperparathyroidism related to a parathyroid adenoma. The infant was diagnosed with transient neonatal hypoparathyroidism secondary to maternal hyperparathyroidism. The infant was initially treated with intravenous calcium gluconate followed by oral calcium and vitamin D supplementation, which were weaned over the subsequent 3 weeks.

INCIDENCE AND EPIDEMIOLOGY OF TRANSIENT NEONATAL HYPOPARATHYROIDISM

Hyperparathyroidism has a prevalence rate of 0.15% with a peak incidence between 30 and 50 years of age. Approximately 80% are due to a solitary adenoma that requires resection and 15% are due to chief cell hyperplasia. Maternal symptoms are not apparent until the serum calcium level exceeds 12-13 mg/dL. However, even mild maternal hypercalcemia leads to chronic fetal hypercalcemia, which in turn suppresses fetal PTH production. After birth, calcium levels decrease but PTH production cannot be rapidly increased. In this condition, neonatal hypoparathyroidism is transient, lasting only several days to several weeks. Eventually, as the parathyroids become more active, increasing PTH levels stimulate vitamin D production and extra calcium absorption from the plentiful supply in the gut. Clinically detectable hypocalcemia develops in 15%-25% of infants born to mothers with hyperparathyroidism. As in this case, neonatal seizures or tetany often lead to a search that identifies a maternal parathyroid adenoma.

CLINICAL PRESENTATION OF TRANSIENT NEONATAL HYPOPARATHYROIDISM

Signs of hypocalcemia usually develop within the first 3 weeks of life. Signs of neonatal hypocalcemia are often nonspecific and may be seen in a variety of other conditions. Tremors and jitteriness are most commonly seen. Other signs include irritability, hyperreflexia, facial twitching, carpalpedal spasm, seizures, cyanosis, and, rarely, laryngospasm. More importantly, other disorders that can present with hypocalcemia should be considered. Features of 22q11 deletion syndromes include cleft palate, micrognathia, ear anomalies, bulbous nasal tip, and conotruncal heart defects. Findings associated with Albright hereditary osteodystrophy (pseudohypoparathyroidism type Ia) include round face, short distal phalanges of the thumbs, subcutaneous calcifications, and a family history of developmental delay and dental hypoplasia. Sensorineural deafness, renal dysplasia, and mental retardation are also associated with syndromes that include hypoparathyroidism.

DIAGNOSTIC APPROACH

Serum calcium and ionized calcium. Both calcium and ionized calcium levels are low with symptomatic hypocalcemia.

Serum albumin. Since approximately 45% of serum calcium is protein bound, low serum albumin levels lead to low serum calcium levels but normal ionized levels. Symptoms of hypocalcemia develop only when ionized calcium is low. The following correction factor approximates whether a low measured serum calcium level is due solely to hypoalbuminemia: Corrected serum calcium = measured serum calcium + [(Normal serum albumin − measured serum albumin) × 0.8].

When the corrected serum calcium is less than normal (<8.8 mg/dL), the ionized calcium may also be low, increasing the likelihood of symptomatic

hypocalcemia. In this patient, the corrected serum calcium was calculated as follows: [6.6 mg/dL + (4.0 mg/dL − 3.3 mg/dL) × 0.8] = 7.1 mg/dL = Corrected calcium.

Serum magnesium. Magnesium deficiency can lead to neonatal hypocalcemia through functional hypoparathyroidism and pseudohypoparathyroidism. In most cases, it is seen in neonates born to magnesium-deficient mothers, such as those with poorly controlled diabetes mellitus. In magnesium deficiency, magnesium replenishment leads to increases in both calcium and PTH levels. In hypoparathyroidism of any other cause, magnesium administration does not lead to changes in the calcium and PTH levels.

Serum phosphorus. Phosphorus levels are elevated with both phosphate-induced neonatal hypocalcemia and with hypoparathyroidism.

Serum PTH. PTH levels are low with hypoparathyroidism. However, in phosphate-induced neonatal hypocalcemia, serum PTH is appropriately elevated.

Active vitamin D. Levels of $1,25(OH)_2D$ are low with hypocalcemia due to vitamin D deficiency but normal or high with underlying hypoparathyroidism.

Other tests. Infants who were treated with bicarbonate or other alkali to correct acidosis can develop very significant hypocalcemia, therefore, an arterial blood gas should be considered. A chest radiograph can document a normal thymic shadow in neonates when 22q11 deletion syndromes are a concern. When neonatal risk factors for hypocalcemia are absent, consider measuring maternal serum calcium, phosphorus, and PTH levels.

TREATMENT

Emergency treatment for neonatal hypocalcemia consists of intravenous 10% calcium gluconate infusion with continuous electrocardiographic monitoring. Additionally, 1,25-dihydroxycholecalciferol (vitamin D_3; calcitriol) should be given. Once the QTc interval on ECG is normal, therapy can be continued with oral calcium and vitamin D_2 (ergocalciferol), which is less costly than calcitriol.

Serum calcium levels should be measured frequently in the early stages of treatment to determine the appropriate dosing. If hypercalcemia occurs, therapy should be discontinued and resumed at a lower dose after the serum calcium level has returned to normal. When maternal hyperparathyroidism is the cause of neonatal hypoparathyroidism and hypocalcemia, supplementation with calcium and vitamin D analogs is only required for 3-4 weeks.

SUGGESTED READINGS

1. Hsieh YY, Chang CC, Tsai HD, et al. Primary hyperparathyroidism in pregnancy: report of three cases. *Arch Gynecol Obstetrics.* 1998;261:209-214.

2. Kaplan EL, Burrington JD, Klementschitsch P, Taylor J, Deftos L. Primary hyperparathyroidism, pregnancy, and neonatal hypocalcemia. *Surgery.* 1984;96:717-722.

3. Rubin, LP. Disorders of calcium and phosphorus metabolism. In: Taeusch HW, Ballard RA, eds. *Avery's Diseases of the Newborn.* 7th ed. Philadelphia, PA: WB Saunders Company; 1998:1189-1191.

4. Mimouni FB, Root AW. Disorders of calcium metabolism in the newborn. In: Sperling MA, ed. *Pediatric Endocrinology.* Philadelphia, PA: W.B. Saunders Company; 1996:95-115.

5. Morrison A. Neonatal seizures. In: Pomerance JJ, Richardson CJ, eds. *Neonatology for the Clinician.* Norwalk, CT: Appleton & Lange; 1993:411-423.

6. Romagnoli C, Polidori G, Cataldi L, Tortorolo G, Segni G. Phototherapy induced hypocalcemia. *J Pediatr.* 1979;94: 815-816.

CASE 19-3

Eight-Month-Old Boy

AMY T. WALDMAN

HISTORY OF PRESENT ILLNESS

The patient is an 8-month-old boy who was well until 1 week prior to admission when he was found by his mother having a "seizure." He had shaking and jerking of all extremities that did not stop when his extremities were held. He did not respond to touch or stimulation. There was no cyanosis. The episode lasted approximately 15 minutes. On arrival of Emergency Medical Services, the patient was alert and feeding from a bottle. He was not taken to the hospital. His last feeding was approximately 3 hours prior to the event. Two days later the patient was evaluated by his primary physician who performed the following laboratory evaluation: Glucose (during feeding), 121 mg/dL; alanine aminotransferase (ALT), 73 U/L; aspartate aminotransferase (AST), 93 U/L; gamma glutamyl transferase (GGT), 28 U/L; and cholesterol, 423 mg/dL. These labs were repeated 2 days later with similar results except that the glucose was 16 mg/dL. Head CT and EEG were normal. He was hospitalized for additional evaluation.

MEDICAL HISTORY

The patient was born at 38 weeks gestation with a birth weight of 3400 g. His delivery was complicated by meconium aspiration. He was treated with supplemental oxygen and empiric antibiotics for 3 days. He also had hypoglycemia requiring intravenous dextrose and bottle feedings every 1.5 hours. This resolved and he was discharged home on the fourth day of life. He received oral antibiotics for otitis media diagnosed at 3 months of life. There is no family history of seizures or mental retardation.

PHYSICAL EXAMINATION

T 36.2°C; RR 20/min; HR 90-110 bpm; BP 120/55 mmHg; SpO_2 100% in room air

Height 25th percentile; Weight 10th percentile; Head Circumference 25th percentile

On examination, he was thin but playful. The anterior fontanelle was open and flat. The heart sounds were normal and the lungs were clear to auscultation. His abdomen was slightly protuberant with a liver edge that was firm and palpable 6 cm below the right costal margin. The spleen tip was just palpable below the left costal margin. There was no ascites or palpable abdominal mass. The infant was circumcised and had normal male genitalia. The neurological examination was normal. The child was awake and alert and interactive with the parents and examiner. He made excellent eye contact and babbled during the examination. Pupils were equal, round, and reactive to light. Funduscopic examination was normal. He tracked in all directions without nystagmus. Facial movements were symmetric. The gag reflex was intact. He had antigravity movements and normal axial and appendicular tone with passive range of motion and vertical and horizontal suspension. The infant was able to sit without support. He withdrew to pain in all extremities. Deep tendon reflexes were 2+ throughout and symmetric. The plantar responses were flexor (upgoing Babinski, normal for age). There were no hyper- or hypopigmented skin lesions.

DIAGNOSTIC STUDIES

Serum chemistries included sodium, 137 mmol/L; potassium, 5.5 mmol/L; chloride, 100 mmol/L; bicarbonate, 13 mmol/L; calcium, 10.5 mg/dL; phosphorous, 6.5 mg/dL; and serum glucose 20 mg/dL. The cholesterol and triglycerides were 465 mg/dL and 4070 mg/dL, respectively. Hepatic function tests included AST, 125 U/L; ALT, 155 U/L; GGT, 564 U/L; total bilirubin 0.6 mg/dL; and albumin 4.0 g/dL. Serum and urinary ketones were present. White blood cell count, hemoglobin, and platelet count, as well as prothrombin and partial thromboplastin times were normal. Blood, urine, and stool cultures were obtained.

COURSE OF ILLNESS

The patient underwent a fasting study which revealed the diagnosis within approximately 4 hours.

DISCUSSION CASE 19-3

DIFFERENTIAL DIAGNOSIS

This infant had seizures related to hypoglycemia. Hypoglycemia in an infant, defined as a blood glucose concentration ≤40 mg/dL, warrants immediate treatment followed by appropriate investigation. Many inborn errors of metabolism are responsible for hypoglycemia present in the first year of life, while milder defects of glycogen degradation and gluconeogenesis manifest only in childhood after prolonged periods of fasting. Causes of hypoglycemia in an infant include hyperinsulinism, hormone deficiency, and defects in branched-chain amino acid metabolism, fatty acid oxidation, and hepatic enzymes.

Urinary ketones are absent or low in children with hyperinsulinism and fatty acid oxidation defects who present with hypoglycemia. Hypoglycemia secondary to hyperinsulinism most commonly appears during the first year of life. It is usually associated with islet-cell dysplasia and rarely with islet-cell adenomas. Insulin level are elevated (>5 μU/mL) and injection of glucagon elicits a rapid rise in blood glucose levels. Children with disorders of fatty acid metabolism can present with hypoglycemia and profound disturbance of consciousness that may not improve when the plasma glucose is normalized. In addition to hyperketonemia, they have high plasma free fatty acid concentrations, elevated ALT and AST, rhabdomyolysis, cardiomyopathy, and cerebral edema.

The presence of urinary ketones usually suggests hormone deficiency, glycogen storage disease, or defects in gluconeogenesis. Hypoglycemia is a common presentation for an infant with panhypopituitarism, isolated growth hormone deficiency, and absolute (adrenal hypoplasia, Addison disease, adrenoleukodystrophy) or relative (congenital adrenal hyperplasia) glucocorticoid deficiency. Midline defects such as cleft lip or palate, optic dysplasia, and microphallus suggest anterior pituitary hormone deficiency. Hyperpigmentation associated with Addison disease rarely occurs in young children. Addison disease is occasionally associated with hypoparathyroidism (hypocalcemia). Severely compromised adrenal function, as in congenital adrenal hyperplasia, may lead to serum electrolyte disturbances or ambiguous genitalia.

Children with branched-chain ketonuria (maple syrup urine disease) excrete urinary ketoacids that impart the characteristic odor of maple syrup. Clinically, these infants have frequent hypoglycemic episodes, lethargy, vomiting, and muscular hypertonia. Glycogen storage diseases are inherited autosomal recessive defects characterized by either deficient or abnormally functioning enzymes involved in the formation or degradation of glycogen. Hepatomegaly, growth failure, hyperlipidemia, and hyperuricemia are common clinical features. Other disorders to consider include galactosemia, especially in children with hepatosplenomegaly, jaundice, and mental retardation, and fructose-1,6-diphosphatase deficiency, in children with hepatomegaly due to lipid storage but only mildly abnormal liver function studies.

DIAGNOSIS

After 4 hours, the glucose was 16 mg/dL; lactate, 32 mg/dL (normal range 5-18 mg/dL); and uric acid 14.2 mg/dL (normal range 2-7 mg/dL). He received intravenous glucagon (30 mcg/kg) after which the blood glucose concentration was 22 mg/dL and the lactate level increased to 44 mg/dL. He then received oral glucose and his blood glucose increased to 65 mg/dL and the lactate decreased to 24 mg/dL. These findings suggested type IA glycogen storage disease (von Gierke disease). Liver biopsy demonstrated increased glycogen content and deficient G6P enzyme activity (2 nmol/min/mg protein; normal range, 20-70 nmol/min/mg protein).

INCIDENCE AND EPIDEMIOLOGY OF GLYCOGEN STORAGE DISEASE

The glycogen storage diseases (GSDs) or glycogenoses comprise several inherited diseases caused by deficiency in one of the enzymes that regulate the synthesis or degradation of glycogen. The end result is abnormal accumulation of glycogen in various tissues. GSD type I has an estimated incidence of 1 in 200 000 births. GSD type IA is due to deficiency of the enzyme glucose-6-phosphatase (G6P), which catalyzes the breakdown of stored glycogen into glucose for use by the body. At least 56 different mutations in the gene for G6P enzyme (chromosome 17q21) have been found in patients with GSD type Ia. GSD types IB and IC are caused by failure of the G6P transporter (type IB) and microsomal phosphate transporter (type IC), which ultimately impair G6P activity. The three types of GSD result in similar clinical and biochemical disturbances. G6P is expressed in the liver, kidneys, and intestines.

CLINICAL PRESENTATION OF GLYCOGEN STORAGE DISEASE

GSD type I is characterized by severe hypoglycemia within 3-4 hours after a meal. Although symptomatic hypoglycemia may appear soon after birth, most patients are asymptomatic as long as they receive frequent feeds that contain sufficient glucose to prevent hypoglycemia. Symptoms of hypoglycemia appear only when the interval between feedings increases, such as when the child begins to sleep through the night or when an intercurrent illness disrupts normal feeding patterns.

Patients may have hyperpnea from lactic acidosis. Untreated patients have poor weight gain and growth retardation. Most patients have a protuberant abdomen and hepatomegaly due to glycogen deposition and fatty infiltration. Social and cognitive development are normal unless the infant suffers neurologic impairment after frequent hypoglycemic seizures. Xanthomas may appear on the extensor surfaces of the extremities and buttocks. Older children develop gout.

DIAGNOSTIC APPROACH

Fasting study. In GSD, the liver fails to release sufficient glucose from hepatic stores to meet peripheral tissue demands. The consequence of this "fasting state" is hypoglycemia, which causes lipolysis and protein breakdown. Therefore, in GSD, hypoglycemia is accompanied by elevated lactic acid, uric acid, and metabolic acidosis. Serum insulin level is low but serum and urinary ketones are markedly elevated. Glucagon does not significantly alter glucose level and actually increases lactic acid levels. An oral glucose load increases serum glucose and decreased lactic acid levels. At the time of hypoglycemia, serum should be collected for insulin, C-peptide, growth hormone, beta-hydroxybutyrate, lactate, and free fatty acids. Urine may be analyzed for organic acids, ketones, and reducing substances. This combination of studies allows for the diagnosis of GSD as well as the exclusion of other disorders that present with hypoglycemia.

Liver function tests. Mild elevations of AST and ALT occur.

Lipid profile. Markedly elevated serum triglycerides, free fatty acids, and apolipoprotein C-III. Infants with triglyceride levels greater than 1000 mg/dL are at high risk for developing acute pancreatitis. Despite the hypertriglyceridemia, the risk for cardiovascular disease is not increased.

Complete blood count. Neutropenia develops with GSD type IB but not with type IA.

Bleeding time. Although this test is not routinely performed, most children with GSD type I have impaired platelet function due to systemic metabolic abnormalities. This bleeding tendency, manifested by recurrent epistaxis and prolonged bleeding after surgery, resolves with correction of the metabolic abnormalities.

Urinalysis. Glycosuria and proteinuria indicate proximal renal tubular dysfunction that improves with correction of metabolic abnormalities.

Abdominal ultrasound. Hepatic adenomas occur in the majority of patients by the second decade of life but may be noted before puberty. Women also usually have polycystic ovaries, a finding whose clinical significance remains unclear.

Other studies. Measurement of G6P enzyme activity in a fresh liver biopsy specimen can be used to diagnose GSD IA. Molecular analysis to identify mutations on the G6P gene is a reliable alternative to liver biopsy.

TREATMENT

Treatment consists of providing a continuous dietary source of glucose to prevent hypoglycemia. When hypoglycemia is prevented, the biochemical abnormalities and growth improve and liver size decreases. Infants require frequent feeding, approximately 2-3 hours during the day and every 3 hours at night. A variety of methods can be followed to provide a continuous source of glucose at night in older children, including intravenous dextrose infusion, continuous intragastric feeding via a nasogastric or gastrostomy tube, and the use of low glycemic index foods such as cornstarch. Orally administered uncooked cornstarch seems to act as an intestinal reservoir of glucose that is slowly absorbed into circulation. It has been used successfully in infants as young as 8 months of age and may obviate the need for continuous intragastric infusion of formula overnight. It can be mixed with water, formula, or artificially sweetened fluids in 4-6-hour intervals overnight. The optimal schedule requires validation by serial glucose monitoring. Allopurinol and lipid-lowering agents are used for severe uric acid and lipid abnormalities. Hepatocyte infusion and liver transplantation may be curative, but the long-term complications in children with GSD are not yet known.

SUGGESTED READINGS

1. Lee PJ, Patel A, Hindmarsh PC, Mowat AP, Leonard JV. The prevalence of polycystic ovaries in the hepatic glycogen storage diseases: its association with hyperinsulinism. *Clin Endocrinol.* 1995;42:601-606.
2. Rake JP, ten Berge AM, Visser G, et al. Glycogen storage disease type Ia: recent experience with mutation analysis, a summary of mutations reported in the literature and a newly developed diagnostic flow chart. *Eur J Pediatr.* 2000;159:322-330.
3. Sperling MA, Finegold DN. Hypoglycemia in the child. In: Sperling MA, ed. *Pediatric Endocrinology.* Philadelphia, PA: W.B. Saunders Company; 1996;265-279.
4. Willi SM. Glycogen storage diseases. In: Altschuler SM, Liacouras CA, eds. *Clinical Pediatric Gastroenterology.* Philadelphia, PA: Churchill Livingstone; 1998;377-383.
5. Wolfsdorf JI, Holm IA, Weinstein DA. Glycogen storage diseases. *Endocrinol Metabol Clinics.* 1999;28:801-823.
6. Taub KS, Abend NS. Seizure disorders. In: Stockwell JA, Preissig CM, eds. *Comprehensive Critical Care: Pediatric.* Mount Prospect, IL: Society of Critical Care Medicine; 2012:447-468.
7. Berg AT, Berkovic SF, Brodie MJ, et al. Revised terminology and concepts for organization of seizures and epilepsies: report of the ILAE Commission on Classification and Terminology, 2005-2009. *Epilepsia.* 2010; 51(4):676-685.

Three-Year-Old Boy

PRATICHI K. GOENKA

HISTORY OF PRESENT ILLNESS

The patient was a 3-year-old boy with a history of developmental delay who was in his usual state of health until 1 day prior to admission when he developed a tactile fever and had one episode of nonbloody, nonbilious emesis. On the day of admission, he was noted to have poor oral intake and decreased activity. The evening of admission he was found lying on the kitchen floor. He had abnormal eye movements and twitching of his mouth. According to his mother, this episode lasted for 20 minutes and was followed by a period of somnolence. He was taken to a nearby hospital where he was lethargic, responding only to noxious stimuli. There he had several generalized seizures that were treated with lorazepam. He was noted to have very poor respiratory effort. An arterial blood gas obtained at that time revealed pH 6.9, $PaCO_2$ 146 mmHg, PaO_2 311 mmHg, and base deficit of 6.4 mmol/L. The patient was transferred to our institution after endotracheal intubation. There was no history of trauma or ingestion. Additional history revealed that he required evaluation by his primary physician for irritability and poor appetite approximately 2 weeks prior to admission but was otherwise well.

MEDICAL HISTORY

The patient was a full term 3100 g product of an uncomplicated pregnancy. He had speech delay and a history of pica. He received mineral oil periodically during the past 2 months due to constipation but he did not require any other medication. His immunization status was not known. There was no family history of mental retardation or seizures.

PHYSICAL EXAMINATION

T 37.5°C; RR 10/min; HR 110 bpm; BP 130/80 mmHg

Height 25th percentile (estimated); Weight 50th percentile

On examination, the patient was sedated, endotracheally intubated, and minimally responsive to stimulation. His pupils were sluggishly reactive. The optic discs were sharp and there was no papilledema. The left tympanic membrane was mildly erythematous without bulging or retraction. The oropharynx was moist. The neck was supple. Heart sounds and femoral pulses were normal. Auscultation of the lungs revealed symmetric air entry without wheezing or rales. The Glasgow coma score was 7. His gag reflex was intact. Deep tendon reflexes were 3+ but symmetric. There was sustained left ankle clonus and toes were upgoing on Babinski.

DIAGNOSTIC STUDIES

The complete blood count revealed a WBC count of 11300 cells/mm³ (74% segmented neutrophils, 20% lymphocytes, 5% monocytes, and 1% eosinophils), a hemoglobin of 6.6 g/dL, and 473000 platelets/mm³. The reticulocyte count was 5.1%. Serum electrolytes and calcium were normal. The blood urea nitrogen was 15 mg/dL and creatinine 0.3 mg/dL. Serum glucose was 170 mg/dL. Serum alanine and aspartate aminotransferases were 83 U/L and 118 U/L, respectively. Ammonia was mildly elevated at 64 mcg/dL. Urinalysis revealed moderate amounts (2+) of glucose and protein, 5-10 WBCs/hpf, 0 RBCs/hpf, and no ketones. Head CT showed diffuse cerebral edema and decreased gray/white differentiation but no masses or intracranial hemorrhage. Opening pressure measured during lumbar puncture was 46 mm H_2O. Cerebrospinal fluid analysis revealed 15 WBCs/mm³ and 15 RBCs/mm³. CSF glucose was 85 mg/dL and protein was 42 mg/dL. No bacteria were seen on Gram stain. Urine and serum toxicology screens were negative.

COURSE OF ILLNESS

Electroencephalogram showed paroxysmal epileptiform activity with generalized slowing of the

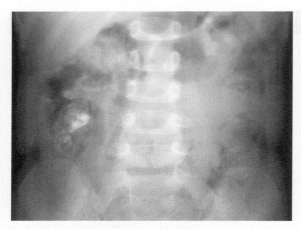

FIGURE 19-5. Abdominal radiograph

background electrical activity. The seizures were controlled with phenytoin infusion. Examination of the abdominal radiograph suggested a diagnosis (Figure 19-5).

DISCUSSION CASE 19-4

DIFFERENTIAL DIAGNOSIS

Encephalopathy refers to a diffuse neurologic disturbance in the absence of CNS inflammation. Acute encephalopathy may present with seizures, delirium, or coma. The diagnosis of encephalopathy is usually inferred from clinical examination. The ultimate distinction between encephalopathy and encephalitis requires neuropathologic examination but CSF pleocytosis is generally absent in children with encephalopathy. The differential diagnosis of encephalopathy and seizures in this patient includes CNS infection. Viral causes to consider include herpes simplex virus, influenza virus, and enteroviruses, the most common cause of central nervous system infection in children. Bacterial causes in this age group may be suggested by appropriate exposures and include *Bartonella henselae* (cat scratch disease), *Rickettsia rickettsii* (Rocky Mountain spotted fever), and *Borellia burgdorferi* (Lyme disease). Children with *Mycoplasma pneumoniae* encephalitis may have a concurrent respiratory infection. *Salmonella* species, *Shigella* species, and *Campylobacter jejuni* have all been

reported to cause toxic encephalopathy accompanied by diarrhea. Postinfectious encephalitis may be seen with measles, mumps, rubella, and varicella but knowledge of the patient's immunization history is important. Substrate deficiencies such as hypoglycemia, while possible, were not suggested by the laboratory findings in this case. Ingestion of medications or toxins (e.g., phenothiazines, anticonvulsants, lead, organophosphates) may cause an acute encephalopathy. Organ failure causing hepatic coma or hypertensive encephalopathy should be considered. Diabetes mellitus should be considered but is unlikely in this case due to the absence of urinary ketones. Trauma with accompanying intracranial hemorrhage must always be excluded as a cause of seizures and encephalopathy in an infant. Anemia with reticulocytosis makes sickle cell disease with stroke, coagulopathy with intracranial hemorrhage, and lead intoxication possible. The absence of rash, ketonuria, diarrhea, and exposure to pets makes several of the above diagnostic considerations unlikely.

DIAGNOSIS

In this case, abdominal radiograph revealed a radiodensity in the right lower quadrant in the area of the cecum, consistent with lead or other foreign substance ingestion (Figure 19-5). **This finding raised the possibility of lead ingestion and subsequent lead encephalopathy.** Additional findings on complete blood count included the following: mean corpuscular volume, 50 fL; and red cell distribution width, 12.4. The serum lead level was 375 mcg/dL and the free erythrocyte protoporphyrin was 260 mcg/dL. Other findings of lead poisoning were present and included glucosuria, aminoaciduria, reticulocytosis, mild CSF pleocytosis, elevated CSF protein, and elevated opening pressure on lumbar puncture.

INCIDENCE AND EPIDEMIOLOGY OF LEAD POISONING

Although the hazards of lead exposure have been recognized for some time, lead intoxication remains the most common metal poisoning encountered today. Sources of lead that contribute to poisoning include interior paint removal in older homes and soil contamination from lead pipes and leaded fuel—lead was a gasoline additive until 1996. Folk medicines (azarcon in Mexican cultures) and cosmetics (kohl in Asian-Indian cultures) may also contain substantial quantities of lead. Children are particularly vulnerable to lead poisoning for a variety of reasons. First, the frequent hand-to-mouth activity of young children increases the likelihood of lead ingestion. Once ingested, children absorb a greater proportion of lead from the gastrointestinal tract than do adults; approximately 70% for children compared with approximately 20% for adults. Iron deficiency, calcium deficiency, and a fasting state can increase the GI absorption of lead. Lead in the body can either be excreted by the kidney or into the biliary system, or retained in blood, soft tissues, or bone. Children younger than 2 years of age retain up to one-third of absorbed lead, whereas adults retain about 1%.

Before 1991, lead levels more than 25 mcg/dL were considered elevated. Meta-analyses of epidemiologic studies found that even blood lead levels of 10-20 mcg/dL were associated with attentional impairment, aggressive behavior, and cognitive deficits, suggesting that the public health significance of low-level lead exposure may be substantial. In 1991, these findings prompted the CDC to consider a childhood blood lead concentration of more than or equal to 10 mcg/dL as a level of concern. The percentage of children younger than 6 years of age with lead levels more than or equal to 10 mcg/dL varies by state and ranges from 2.7% to 14.9%.

CLINICAL PRESENTATION OF LEAD POISONING AND ENCEPHALOPATHY

The signs and symptoms of lead poisoning depend on the blood lead level and the age of the patient. Most children with mildly elevated lead levels are asymptomatic. Some may have mild neurocognitive deficits or behavioral problems. As the lead level increases above 50 mcg/dL, young children gradually develop anorexia, apathy, lethargy, anemia, irritability, poor coordination, constipation, abdominal pain, and sporadic emesis. Regression of newly acquired skills, especially speech, may be reported. These complaints increase in severity over 3-6 weeks. Children with lead levels more than 80 mcg/dL are most susceptible to encephalopathy. The onset of encephalopathy is heralded by the development of ataxia, persistent emesis, periods of lethargy, and, finally, intractable seizures.

Physical examination findings include ataxia, tremor, and peripheral motor weakness, particularly the extensors of the fingers and wrists. Pallor of the skin and mucosa develop with severe anemia. Children with chronic lead exposure may develop dark deposits of lead sulfide at the interface of the teeth and gums, resulting in the gingival "lead line." This finding can be an important clue to the presence of high lead exposure but must be differentiated from normal pigmentation in dark-skinned children.

DIAGNOSTIC APPROACH

Blood lead. Because blood samples obtained by fingerstick may be contaminated by exogenous lead on the finger, elevated capillary blood lead levels should be confirmed in blood obtained by venipuncture.

Free erythrocyte protoporphyrin (FEP) and Zinc protoporphyrin (ZPP). Elevated FEP and ZPP reflect lead-induced inhibition of heme synthesis. FEP and ZPP levels are increased 2-6 weeks after elevation of lead levels above approximately 15 mcg/dL.

Complete blood count and reticulocyte count. Hemolysis occurs after acute, high-dose lead exposure. Chronic lead exposure causes a slowly developing hypochromic, microcytic, or normocytic anemia. Anemia usually develops when the lead level is greater than 40-50 mcg/dL. Microscopic inspection of the peripheral blood smear may reveal basophilic stippling (aggregation of ribosomal fragments) as a consequence of lead-induced inhibition of cellular ribonucleases. Reticulocytosis is usually present.

Renal function tests. Urinalysis may be unremarkable or reveal mild to moderate proteinuria. A Fanconi-like syndrome with aminoaciduria, glucosuria, and hypophosphatemia with relative hyperphosphaturia occurs after acute, high-dose lead exposure. Interstitial nephritis is occasionally detected on renal biopsy in patients with lead-induced renal dysfunction.

Lumbar puncture. Elevated opening pressure and CSF protein are characteristic of lead encephalopathy. CSF white blood cell count may be normal or mildly elevated (up to 15 WBCs/mm³).

Head CT or MRI. CNS imaging reveals symmetrically narrowed ventricles and effacement of the cerebral gyri consistent with diffuse cerebral edema.

Other tests. Abdominal radiographs may reveal radiopaque lead fragments within the gastrointestinal tract. Radiographs of long bones reveal transverse linear opacities at the metaphyseal ends, which represent hyperdense calcium deposits that accumulate due to lead-induced inhibition of calcified cartilage reabsorption. These "radiographic lead lines" are seen in children 2-6 years of age with lead levels greater than approximately 70 mcg/dL. They will not persist, nor first develop, during late childhood.

TREATMENT

Lead encephalopathy constitutes a medical emergency requiring intensive care unit management. Optimal treatment of lead poisoning combines decontamination, supportive care, and chelation. Consider whole bowel irrigation for inorganic lead compounds and activated charcoal after recent ingestion. Surgical or endoscopic removal of solitary lead objects in the gastrointestinal tract is important, especially when there is evidence of ongoing lead absorption. Goals of supportive care include: (1) normalization of intracranial pressure; (2) transfusion of packed red blood cells, when clinically indicated, for severe anemia; (3) treatment of seizures; and (4) maintenance of adequate urine output to permit renal lead excretion.

Chelating agents are used to decrease blood lead concentration and increase urinary lead excretion. Children with lead encephalopathy require combination therapy with dimercaprol (British anti-Lewisite; BAL) (75 mg/m²) and calcium disodium edetate (EDTA) (1500 mg/m²/24 h). Lead levels in children with lead encephalopathy seem to decrease more rapidly in children given the combination, rather than calcium EDTA alone. The duration of dimercaprol plus calcium EDTA therapy

is limited to 5 days to diminish the risk of nephrotoxicity. In one series of 130 children with lead poisoning who were treated with the combination of dimercaprol and calcium EDTA, 13% developed nephrotoxicity and 3% developed reversible acute renal failure. After completion of combination parenteral therapy, children should receive succimer (dimercaptosuccinic acid; DMSA), an orally administered water-soluble analog of dimercaprol, for 14 days.

Blood levels are repeated after 24-48 hours to ensure that the levels are declining. Failure of levels to decline by at least 20% over 48 hours suggests either ongoing external lead exposure, significant lead retention in the gastrointestinal tract, renal insufficiency, or noncompliance with chelation therapy. Blood lead levels should be repeated at weekly intervals during and after succimer therapy. Children with lead encephalopathy have a high body lead burden and redistribution of lead from bone to soft tissues following cessation of chelation often results in a rebound of blood lead concentration to within 20% of pretreatment values. Repeat courses of chelation are frequently necessary.

SUGGESTED READINGS

1. American Academy of Pediatrics, Committee on Drugs. Treatment guidelines for lead exposure in children. *Pediatrics.* 1995;96:155-160.
2. Bellinger DC, Stiles KM, Needleman HL. Low-level lead exposure, intelligence and academic achievement: a long-term follow-up study. *Pediatrics.* 1992;90:855-861.
3. Centers for Disease Control and Prevention. Blood lead levels in young children-United States and selected states, 1996-1999. *MMWR.* 2000;49:1133-1137.
4. Chisolm JJ Jr. The use of chelating agents in the treatment of acute and chronic lead intoxication in childhood. *J Pediatr.* 1968;73:1-38.
5. Kosnett MJ. Lead. In: Ford MD, Delaney KA, Ling LJ, Erickson T, eds. *Clinical Toxicology.* Philadelphia, PA: W.B. Saunders Company; 2001:723-736.
6. Moel DI, Kumar K. Reversible nephrotoxic reactions to a combined 2,3-dimercapto-1-propanol and calcium disodium ethylenediaminetetraacetic acid regimen in asymptomatic children with elevated blood lead levels. *Pediatrics.* 1982;70:259-262.
7. Ziegler EE, Edwards BB, Jensen RL, Mahaffey KR, Fomon SJ. Absorption and retention of lead by infants. *Pediatr Res.* 1978;12:29-34.

CASE 19-5

Eleven-Year-Old Boy

MATTHEW TEST

SAMIR S. SHAH

HISTORY OF PRESENT ILLNESS

An 11-year-old boy was well until the day of admission, when he stood up and fell, striking his head on a desk at school. Approximately 1 hour later, he developed head twitching, eye blinking, and tonic-clonic movements of his right arm that lasted approximately 20 minutes. During this episode, he had bowel and bladder incontinence. The school nurse found him confused, combative, and unable to follow simple commands. He was taken to the emergency department for evaluation. His family reported that the patient had been intermittently febrile during the past 2 weeks but denied any history of headache, vomiting, rash, visual problems, alteration in gait, travel, ill contacts, and use of alcohol or illicit drugs.

MEDICAL HISTORY

The boy did not have any underlying medical conditions. His growth and development had been normal. His older brother had died from complications related to acquired immunodeficiency syndrome several years earlier, after becoming infected with human immunodeficiency virus (HIV) through intravenous drug use. There was no family history of seizures, metabolic disorders, or sickle cell disease. His maternal grandmother and father both died of complications related to hypertension. He lived at home with his mother and stepfather. They had two healthy kittens at home but no reptiles or birds. He had received all required immunizations, including the meningococcal conjugate vaccine. He did not require any medications.

PHYSICAL EXAMINATION

T 38.6°C; HR 110 bpm; RR 18/min; BP 136/80 mmHg; SpO$_2$, 96% in room air

Weight 50th percentile; Height 75th percentile

On examination, he was agitated and combative. There was a small contusion over his left eyebrow but no other signs of trauma. There were no scleral hemorrhages. There was no hemotympanum. Pupils were symmetrically reactive (6 mm-4 mm). His neck was supple. There was a 2-cm right cervical lymph node without surrounding erythema or drainage (Figure 19-6). There were no murmurs or rubs on cardiac examination. Lungs were clear to auscultation. No other lymphadenopathy was appreciated. His abdomen was soft without hepatosplenomegaly. He was incontinent of urine and

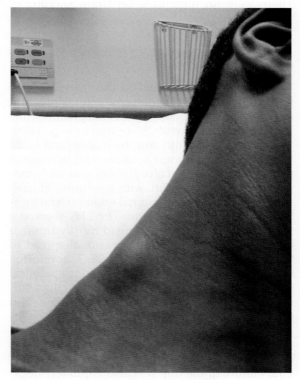

FIGURE 19-6. Photo of the patient's neck.

stool. There were no petechiae. Neurologic assessment was difficult to obtain. The child cried and shouted but his speech was unintelligible. He did not follow simple commands. He thrashed his arms and legs spontaneously and purposefully.

DIAGNOSTIC STUDIES

Complete blood count revealed 5300 WBCs/mm³ (51% segmented neutrophils, 32% lymphocytes, 13% monocytes, and 5% eosinophils); hemoglobin, 11.6 g/dL; and 333 000 platelets/mm³. Serum ALT and AST were 152 U/L and 114 U/L, respectively. Serum electrolytes, blood urea nitrogen, calcium, magnesium, phosphorus, creatinine, and albumin were normal. Serum glucose was 106 mg/dL. Serum and urine toxicology screens were negative. CT of the head did not reveal any hemorrhage, mass lesions, or ventriculomegaly. Examination of the CSF revealed 24 WBCs/mm³; 1 RBC/mm³; glucose, 77 mg/dL; and protein, 19 mg/dL. There were no organisms on Gram staining of the CSF.

COURSE OF ILLNESS

The patient was admitted to the intensive care unit and received vancomycin, cefotaxime, and acyclovir as empiric therapy for encephalitis while the results of additional CSF testing were pending. Two hours after admission, he had several additional right-sided motor seizures with occasional generalization. He received phenytoin and multiple doses of lorazepam, with resolution of each seizure. He ultimately required endotracheal intubation for respiratory failure. The EEG showed a right temporal focus that spread mostly through the right hemisphere, with occasional spread to the left hemisphere. Continuous EEG monitoring demonstrated a total of 75 clinical and subclinical seizures over the next 24 hours, despite the addition of Tegretol (carbamazepine), valproate, and phenobarbital. CSF PCR for *Borrelia burgdorferi* (Lyme disease), HSV (repeated twice), and enterovirus were negative, as were cultures for bacteria and stains for fungi and acid-fast bacilli. Viral culture of the CSF was also ultimately negative. Serum acute and convalescent IgM and IgG

titers were undetectable for Lyme disease, Rocky Mountain spotted fever, and human granulocytic ehrlichiosis. Metabolic studies including serum and urine organic acids, serum amino acids, and serum and CSF lactate and pyruvate were within normal limits. Findings on physical examination combined with results of the abdominal CT suggested a diagnosis (Figure 19-7).

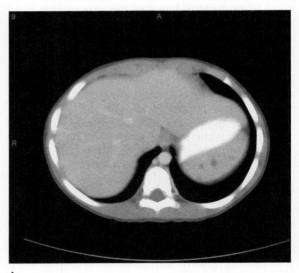

A

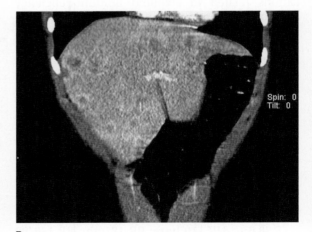

B

FIGURE 19-7. CT of the patient's abdomen demonstrates lesions in the **A.** Spleen. **B.** Liver.

DISCUSSION CASE 19-5

DIFFERENTIAL DIAGNOSIS

Encephalitis occurs in 0.5 per 100 000 individuals in the United States. In late childhood, a variety of agents cause encephalitis, although viruses are most commonly implicated. HSV is a serious but potentially treatable cause of viral encephalitis. Viral culture is frequently negative in cases of HSV encephalitis; therefore, HSV PCR is considered the gold standard diagnostic test. Enteroviruses are the most common cause of CNS infection in children, but predominant encephalitis without meningitis is an unusual manifestation. Encephalitis occurs in approximately 1 of every 1000 cases of Epstein-Barr virus-associated mononucleosis; children frequently have a history of antecedent fatigue and pharyngitis. Other viral causes of encephalitis in the United States include human herpesvirus 6, arboviruses (Eastern and Western equine encephalitis), hepatitis viruses A and B, HIV, and rabies virus. Postinfectious encephalitis often occurs after respiratory infections, especially those caused by influenza virus or *M. pneumoniae*. The incidence of encephalitis related to measles, mumps, and varicella has declined due to widespread immunization. Encephalitis in the summer months should raise suspicion for Rocky Mountain spotted fever, Lyme neuroborreliosis, and enterovirus infection. Exposure to kittens raises the possibility of *B. henselae* encephalitis. Few pyogenic bacteria cause encephalitis without overt meningitis. Syphilis, leptospirosis, brucellosis, tuberculosis, and listeriosis are rare causes of encephalitis but should be considered when an appropriate exposure has been documented.

DIAGNOSIS

The abdominal CT revealed multiple hypodense hepatic and splenic lesions (Figure 19-7). These findings, in conjunction with cervical lymphadenopathy (Figure 19-6) and history of contact with a kitten, suggested infection with *B. henselae*, the causative agent of cat-scratch disease (CSD). *Bartonella henselae* antibody titers were 1:2,048. **These findings supported the diagnosis of hepatosplenic CSD with encephalitis.** The patient's

seizures continued for more than 1 week despite aggressive anticonvulsant therapy. He received rifampin and macrolide antibiotics for his CSD. Unfortunately, his hospital course was complicated by disseminated fungal infection, including *Candida albicans* retinitis and meningitis, and chronic respiratory failure requiring a tracheostomy. He was discharged after 8 months of hospitalization with impaired vision, developmental delay, and recurrent seizures. His poor neurologic outcome was most likely related to prolonged seizures and disseminated candidiasis.

INCIDENCE AND EPIDEMIOLOGY

CSD, a well-recognized and self-limited cause of regional lymphadenitis in children, is often associated with systemic symptoms such as fever and malaise. Approximately 24 000 cases are reported in the United States each year; the highest age-specific incidence occurs in children younger than 10 years of age. CSD predominantly occurs in the fall and winter, possibly related to temporal changes in animal behavior and reproduction. History of contact with a cat can be established in more than 90% of cases of CSD, and clustering of cases has occurred within families upon acquisition of new pet cats. The infection may be transmitted through licks, scratches, or bites. Cats which transmit CSD are not ill and have no distinctive features, although most are kittens (younger than 1 year of age). In a study of 1200 patients with CSD, 64% reported contact with only a kitten, and 25% reported contact with both kittens and adult cats. Up to 50% of domestic cats demonstrate antibodies to *B. henselae*.

Approximately 10% of children with CSD develop atypical features, including Parinaud's oculoglandular syndrome, neuroretinitis, erythema nodosum, pulmonary nodules, osteomyelitis, and encephalitis or encephalopathy. Encephalitis or encephalopathy complicates approximately 2% of cases of CSD.

CLINICAL PRESENTATION OF CAT-SCRATCH DISEASE AND CAT-SCRATCH ENCEPHALITIS

The clinical manifestations of CSD depend on the site of inoculation and infection. Fever and localized, tender lymphadenopathy is the most common presentation of CSD. The most frequently involved sites include the axillary and epitrochlear nodes (46%), the neck and jaw (28%), and the groin (18%).

Children with hepatosplenic CSD often complain of fever, malaise, and abdominal pain. Physical examination findings include hepatomegaly (30%), hepatosplenomegaly (16%), and lymphadenopathy (25%)—usually a single enlarged lymph node. A scratch or papule identifies the probable site of inoculation in 60%-90% of cases. Recently, *B. henselae* has been identified as an important cause of fever of unknown origin (FUO), accounting for up to 5% of patients with FUO.

Children with CSD-associated encephalitis often present with complaints of fever, malaise, and lymphadenopathy. Two to three weeks later, they develop headache, alterations in mental status, and seizures. Patients may also present with weakness, nuchal rigidity, and alterations in tone and reflexes. Less common manifestations of this rare event include hallucinations, hemiplegia, aphasia, cerebellar ataxia, and sixth cranial nerve palsy. In Florida, a cluster of five children with acute CSD encephalopathy occurred within a 6-week period in 1994. All presented with status epilepticus and required endotracheal intubation but subsequently recovered without sequelae. In one series of 76 patients with neurologic symptoms attributable to CSD, encephalopathy occurred 1-6 weeks after onset of lymphadenopathy; seizures occurred in 46% of these patients. More than 90% of children with CSD encephalitis or encephalopathy experience complete and spontaneous resolution of symptoms, although recovery has often taken up to 8 weeks and can take as long as 1 year.

DIAGNOSTIC APPROACH

Bartonella henselae IgG antibodies. Serologic testing is the standard method of diagnosis and should be considered for patients who present with status epilepticus, adenopathy, and history of feline contact. A single elevated indirect immunofluorescence assay titer or enzyme immunoassay value for IgG antibodies is usually sufficient to confirm CSD, because initiation of a humoral immune response usually precedes or is concurrent with symptom onset. IgG levels rise during the first 2 months after onset of illness, followed by a gradual decline. The sensitivity is reported to be greater than 98%; however, IgG titers remain elevated for up to 1 year following acute infection, often complicating the identification of acute infection. An IgG titer greater than 1:64 is consistent with recent infection. An increase in antibody titers between acute and convalescent (2 weeks later) may be confirmatory. Paired sera are particularly useful in cat owners who may have a background rate of *B. henselae* antibody seropositivity greater than the general population. IgM levels are less useful in the diagnosis of CSD, since IgM antibodies have a short duration of detection and have frequently cleared by the time of presentation.

Bartonella henselae DNA polymerase chain reaction. PCR may be performed on tissue samples (lymph node aspirates, liver or spleen tissue, bone biopsies). It is available on a limited basis at some commercial laboratories as well as from the Centers for Disease Control and Prevention. PCR has specificity as high as 100% in the identification of *B. henselae*; however, sensitivity ranges from 43% to 76%, making it less useful in uncomplicated cases.

Lumbar puncture. CSF analysis may be normal, but some patients have a mild pleocytosis (fewer than 30 WBCs/mm^3). CSF protein may be slightly elevated, but CSF glucose is normal. PCR assays to exclude other potential causes of encephalitis, including HSV, enteroviruses, and arboviruses, should be considered.

Abdominal CT. Abdominal CT is usually not warranted but may demonstrate granulomata in the liver and spleen which, as in this case, may help establish the diagnosis.

Central nervous system imaging. Head CT is normal but should be performed to exclude CNS lesions that can cause seizures. Head MRI may reveal focal or diffuse white matter changes that are not specific for CSD.

Other studies. *Bartonella henselae* can be cultured from blood, lymph nodes, and other tissues, but it grows slowly and requires a 6-week incubation period. Additionally, isolation of *B. henselae* from tissues can be difficult, particularly in patients with limited disease. A presumptive diagnosis can be made based on microscopic examination of tissues by demonstrating the bacilli with the use of

Warthin-Starry silver impregnation staining. Other histologic findings depend on duration of illness. Early findings in affected lymph nodes include lymphocytic infiltration and epithelioid granuloma formation. Later changes include neutrophil infiltration and necrotizing granulomas. The cat-scratch skin test is no longer used. Studies to exclude other causes of encephalopathy should be performed.

TREATMENT

In the immunocompetent child with hepatosplenic CSD, the benefit of antimicrobial therapy is unclear, because the illness is self-limited in most cases. Patients who receive rifampin appear to have more rapid resolution of fever, but no controlled trial had been conducted, so the efficacy of any antibiotic regimen in the treatment of hepatosplenic CSD is not known. In a study by Bass et al., a 5-day course of azithromycin hastened resolution of lymphadenopathy, causing an 80% reduction in lymph node volume in 50% of azithromycin-treated patients compared with 7% of patients receiving placebo. However, there was no difference in time to complete resolution between the azithromycin- and placebo-treated groups. Although antimicrobial therapy is not recommended for mild-to-moderate infection, azithromycin can be considered in patients with extensive lymphadenopathy. Trimethoprim-sulfamethoxazole, erythromycin, clarithromycin, doxycycline, ciprofloxacin, and gentamicin may also be effective in treating patients with severe illness. Beta-lactam agents appear ineffective despite favorable in vitro susceptibility. Immunocompromised patients with CSD show a much more significant response to antimicrobial therapy, and these patients should receive antibiotics for a minimum of 3 months. Erythromycin ethylsuccinate is the preferred agent in children, but doxycycline, isoniazid, azithromycin, gentamicin, and rifampin have shown benefit.

Experience with antimicrobial therapy in CSD encephalitis is limited to anecdotal reports. Most children appear to recover without CSD-specific therapy, and conservative, symptomatic management, including anticonvulsants for seizure activity, is recommended. The poor outcome for the patient in this case was probably related to disseminated fungal infection rather than CSD.

SUGGESTED READINGS

1. Arisoy ES, Correa AG, Wagner ML, Kaplan SL. Hepatosplenic cat-scratch disease in children: selected clinical features and treatment. *Clin Infect Dis.* 1999;28: 778-784.
2. Armengol CE, Hendley JO. Cat-scratch disease encephalopathy: a cause of status epilepticus in school-aged children. *J Pediatr.* 1999;134:635-638.
3. Bass JW, Freitas BC, Freitas AD, et al. Prospective randomized double blind placebo-controlled evaluation of azithromycin for treatment of cat-scratch disease. *Pediatr Infect Dis J.* 1998;17:447-452.
4. Bass JW, Vincent JM, Person DA. The expanding spectrum of *Bartonella* infections: II. Cat-scratch disease. *Pediatr Infect Dis J.* 1997;16:163-179.
5. Carithers HA, Margileth AM. Cat-scratch disease: acute encephalopathy and other neurologic manifestations. *Am J Dis Child.* 1991;145:98-101.
6. Florin TA, Zaoutis TE, Zaoutis LB. Beyond cat scratch disease: widening spectrum of *Bartonella henselae* infection. *Pediatrics.* 2008;121(5):e1413-e1425.
7. Klotz SA, Ianas V, Elliott SP. Cat-scratch disease. *Am Fam Physicians.* 2011;83(2):152-155.
8. Margileth AM. Antibiotic therapy for cat-scratch disease: clinical study of therapeutic outcome in 268 patients and review of the literature. *Pediatr Infect Dis J.* 1992;11:474-478.
9. Noah DL, Bresee JS, Gorensek MJ, et al. Cluster of five children with acute encephalopathy associated with cat-scratch disease in South Florida. *Pediatr Infect Dis J.* 1995;14:866-869.

CASE 19-6

Twelve-Year-Old Boy

MATTHEW TEST

SAMIR S. SHAH

HISTORY OF PRESENT ILLNESS

A 12-year-old boy had difficulty rising from a sitting position when asked to do so at a basketball game 2 days before admission. He was able to stand only after several minutes, and he attributed this episode to fatigue. Later that evening, while lying on the couch at home, he again had difficulty standing and required assistance from his mother. He was eventually able to walk upstairs unassisted. His mother found him several minutes later, lying on the floor, staring, open-mouthed, and drooling. He had spontaneous respirations but was unresponsive to verbal stimuli. He was taken to a nearby hospital by ambulance.

On arrival, the patient was somnolent but arousable, with a Glasgow coma score of 10. He then experienced an episode of staring, unresponsiveness to verbal stimuli, and right hand shaking that lasted 10 minutes, stopping only after administration of rectal diazepam followed by intravenous lorazepam (0.05 mg/kg) and phenytoin. Unenhanced CT imaging of the head revealed normal-sized ventricles without evidence of midline shift. Opening pressure on the lumbar puncture was 18 mmH$_2$O. After a CSF sample was sent for laboratory analysis, the patient received ceftriaxone intravenously.

He was transferred to another institution for additional management. Discussion with family members did not reveal a history of fevers, night sweats, vomiting, behavior or personality changes, or ataxia. There was no history of witnessed ingestion or trauma.

MEDICAL HISTORY

The patient was born in Mexico and emigrated to the United States when he was 9 years old. His perinatal history was unremarkable. Specifically, there were no maternal infections during pregnancy. The patient was born at term gestation after an uncomplicated delivery. He had never been hospitalized and did not take any prescription medications. There was no family history of seizures.

PHYSICAL EXAMINATION

T 36.7°C; RR 18/min; HR 60 bpm; BP 111/67 mmHg

Height 50th percentile; Weight 5th percentile

On examination, the patient was somnolent but easily arousable and was able to answer questions appropriately. His appearance was thin but not cachectic. There was no papilledema or scleral icterus. His pupils were symmetrically reactive to light. His neck was supple. There was no hepatomegaly, splenomegaly, or lymphadenopathy. There were no hypopigmented or hyperpigmented skin lesions. The remainder of the physical examination, including the neurologic examination, was normal.

DIAGNOSTIC STUDIES

The complete blood count revealed 11 400 WBCs/mm^3 (86% segmented neutrophils, 9% lymphocytes, and 5% monocytes); hemoglobin, 12.2 g/dL; and platelets, 257 000/mm^3. Serum electrolytes, calcium, blood urea nitrogen, and creatinine were normal. The serum glucose was 166 mg/dL, and the phenytoin level was 18.1 mg/L (normal therapeutic range, 10-20 mg/L).

Examination of the CSF revealed no WBCs and only 1 RBC/mm^3. The protein concentration was 11 mg/dL, and glucose was 93 mg/dL. There were no organisms on Gram stain of the CSF. An acid-fast stained smear of CSF was negative. An ECG demonstrated sinus bradycardia but was otherwise normal. Echocardiogram and EEG were also normal.

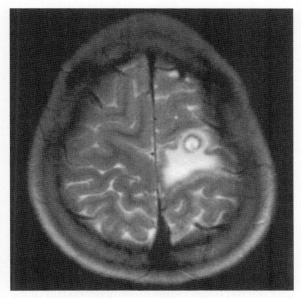

FIGURE 19-8. Intravenous gadolinium-enhanced magnetic resonance image of the head.

COURSE OF ILLNESS

The patient continued taking phenytoin and did not have any further complex partial seizures. MRI of the head performed, with intravenous gadolinium (Figure 19-8), was considered diagnostic.

DISCUSSION CASE 19-6

DIFFERENTIAL DIAGNOSIS

Partial seizures are less common in children than in adults, accounting for about 45% of all childhood seizure disorders. In contrast to adults, most complex partial seizures in children are idiopathic. These typically occur as manifestations of one of the so-called benign focal epilepsy syndromes of childhood. The differential diagnosis in this patient also includes early-onset posttraumatic epilepsy, which is associated with partial seizures in the older child. Onset is within 24 hours of the injury in 50% of cases. The incidence of traumatic epilepsy is relatively small in closed-head injuries. Infectious causes of partial seizures should always be considered in this age group. Viral encephalitis due to HSV or Epstein-Barr virus is possible. Subacute

sclerosing panencephalitis, associated with measles infection, is less likely, but knowledge of the patient's immunization history is important. Parasitic infection of the CNS may result in partial seizures. Neurocysticercosis has a high prevalence in developing areas of Central and South America, and echinococcosis is hyperendemic in areas of South America, central Asia, and the western United States. Tuberculosis with tuberculoma formation in the brain continues to be a problem in some parts of the world. Less common causes of partial seizures in this age group include brain tumors, which are present in fewer than 10% of children with partial seizures. Nevertheless, focal seizures accompanied by a history of headaches may be caused by a CNS tumor. Cerebrovascular disease causing a partial seizure is unlikely unless predisposing factors such as sickle cell disease or an inherited thrombotic disorder (e.g., factor V Leiden mutation, protein C or S deficiency) are present. Bacterial endocarditis with cerebral emboli can cause partial seizures but is usually associated with persistent fever and an abnormal echocardiogram. An important clue to the diagnosis in this case was the patient's history of emigration from Mexico, an area of high prevalence for certain parasitic diseases.

DIAGNOSIS

Intravenous gadolinium-enhanced head MRI revealed a 10-mm ring-enhancing lesion in the left parietal white matter with surrounding vasogenic edema and localized mass effect (Figure 19-8). There was no evidence of elevated intracranial pressure. **These findings were consistent with the diagnosis of neurocysticercosis.** Intravenous dexamethasone, which was started before his arrival at the current institution, was discontinued. Cultures of blood and CSF were negative, and antimicrobial therapy was discontinued. Cysticidal therapy was not recommended. The patient was discharged on phenytoin after a period of observation. On follow-up 1-year later, he had remained seizure free.

INCIDENCE AND EPIDEMIOLOGY OF NEUROCYSTICERCOSIS

Neurocysticercosis is the most common parasitic infection of the CNS. It is caused by the pork tapeworm *Taenia solium*. The disease is highly endemic in Latin America, Mexico, Eastern Europe, Asia, Africa, and Spain. In the United States, the infection is most common among immigrants from endemic areas and children in contact with these immigrants, and it is estimated that there are more than 1000 new cases of neurocysticercosis in the United States each year. Cysticercosis can affect humans at any age including infection by the transplacental route. It is most common during the third and fourth decades of life; only 10% of individuals with neurocysticercosis are children. The estimated serologic prevalence of cysticercosis in Mexican adults is 3.6%, with positive confirmation at autopsy in 1.9%.

Taenia solium is a gastrointestinal tapeworm (cestode) that causes two types of disease syndromes. Intestinal infection with the adult tapeworm occurs when infective larvae are ingested in undercooked pork. Cysticercosis occurs when humans ingest food contaminated with feces containing *T. solium* eggs. The eggs hatch in the intestine, liberating embryos. The embryos penetrate through the intestinal mucosa and are disseminated by the blood to brain (neurocysticercosis), subcutaneous tissues, muscle, and eye, where they develop into cysticerci. Cysterci are often 5 mm in diameter, but may enlarge to 50 mm. Within the brain, cysts are most commonly located in the parietal lobes.

CLINICAL PRESENTATION OF NEUROCYSTICERCOSIS

The clinical manifestations in children are different from those in adults. The initial sign of neurocysticercosis in children is usually (>80% of cases) the new onset of focal or generalized seizures. Rare presentations in children include hemiparesis, increased intracranial pressure with headache and vomiting, encephalitis, meningitis, and simulation of a psychotic illness with delirium or hallucinations. Although some children have several parenchymal cysts, most children (75%) have a solitary lesion.

Adolescents and young adults who develop seizures due to neurocysticercosis often have a calcified brain granuloma. The cysticerci remain clinically silent during the natural course of infection, immune reaction, parasite destruction, and

granuloma formation. After several years, as evidenced by calcification of the granuloma, the patient develops epilepsy. Adult disease with acute presentation is characterized by multiple brain cysts and an intense immune response. Approximately 30% of adults present with signs of increased intracranial pressure.

DIAGNOSTIC APPROACH

Head CT or MRI. Contrast-enhanced CT and MRI of the head are diagnostic. CT most commonly reveals single, small cysticerci (ring-enhancing) with surrounding edema, granuloma, or calcification. Disseminated infection with multiple parenchymal cysts is identified by a "starry sky" appearance. MRI is the best imaging test overall for the diagnosis and should be performed on all patients for whom the clinical history and CT scan suggest the diagnosis of neurocysticercosis. The cysticerci may not be clearly visible on noncontrast CT of the head.

Enzyme-linked immunotransfer blot (EITB). EITB of serum or CSF can assist in confirming a presumptive clinical and radiographic diagnosis. The specificity is approximately 100%. In patients with more than two lesions, the sensitivity is greater than 90%. However, the test is often negative in patients with solitary or calcified lesions (75% of children). Excretory secretory (ES) antigens are a mixture of protein products of live tapeworm larvae, and an immune response to these antigens is thought to indicate the presence of live parasite. Recent use of ES antigen in EITB showed a sensitivity of 85.6% in the identification of solitary lesions (n = 111) and 100% in the identification of calcified lesions (n = 5). However, the specificity was 64%.

Stool testing for ova and parasites. All children with neurocysticercosis and their contacts should have their stool examined for *T. solium* ova on three consecutive daily specimens. The source of infection in children is frequently infected stools of family members or other close contacts. Such testing may prevent further exposure and transmission of the disease.

EEG. An EEG should be performed to assist in localizing seizures in all children with partial seizures.

Lumbar puncture. Examination of the CSF often reveals elevated protein and a mild lymphocytic pleocytosis (mean, 59 WBCs/mm^3).

TREATMENT

In children, an isolated cystic lesion in the brain parenchyma usually does not require treatment. In these patients, ring enhancement demonstrated on contrast-enhanced CT is associated with inflammation around a dead or dying parasite. Because a solitary lesion usually disappears spontaneously within 2-3 months, the use of antihelminthic therapy in this setting is controversial (Table 19-4). A 2010 Cochrane Review identified studies comparing albendazole therapy to no treatment. The authors found that, in children with nonviable (enhancing on neuroimaging) lesions, administration of albendazole was associated with significant reduction in seizure recurrence but no change in cyst persistence. In those adults with viable (nonenhancing on neuroimaging) lesions, there was no change in seizure recurrence, but albendazole

administration was associated with decreased cyst persistence. There were no trials involving viable lesions in children. A recent study demonstrated no benefit of albendazole and praziquantel combination therapy over albendazole monotherapy in lesion eradication or seizure prevention. Children with the highest risk of chronic seizures are those with a calcified granuloma (indicating a dead parasite) that remains as a permanent sequelae of the cysticercus.

Those with multiple lesions or viable cysticerci without radiographic evidence of inflammation need therapy. Albendazole for 28 days is the recommended cysticidal therapy and in most cases results in complete disappearance or significant regression in cyst volume. If albendazole results in only a partial response, praziquantel may be given for 14 days. Individuals whose stool examination reveals adult *T. solium* should be treated with a single dose of praziquantel to prevent transmission.

Initiation of cysticidal therapy may result in cerebral edema. Therefore, dexamethasone should

TABLE 19-4.	Randomized controlled trials in children with neurocysticercosis presenting with nonviable lesions.		
Study	*Participants*	*Intervention*	*Conclusions*
Baranwal (1998)	n = 63	Albendazole vs placebo	Albendazole was associated with decreased seizure recurrence at 4 weeks and reduced lesion size on CT at 1 and 3 months
Gogia (2003)	n = 72	Albendazole vs placebo	No difference between treatment groups in seizure recurrence or lesion reduction at 6 month follow-up
Kalra (2003)	n = 123	Albendazole plus dexamethasone vs no treatment	Albendazole and dexamethasone were associated with decreased seizure recurrence at 3 and 6 months and reduced lesion size at 3 months
Kaur (2009)	n = 103	Albendazole plus praziquantel vs albendazole plus placebo	No difference between treatment groups in seizure recurrence at 6 months or lesion reduction on CT at 1, 3, and 6 months
Singhi (2003)	n = 122	Albendazole, 7-day duration vs 28-day duration	No difference between treatment groups in seizure recurrence or lesion reduction on CT at 2 year follow-up
Kaur (2010)	n = 120	Albendazole, 7-day duration vs 28-day duration	No difference between treatment groups in seizure recurrence at 6 months or lesion reduction on CT at 3 and 6 months
Singhi (2004)	n = 110	Albendazole alone vs. corticosteroids alone vs albendazole plus corticosteroids	Children in the corticosteroids alone group had a significantly increased risk of seizure recurrence at 18 months; there was no difference between treatment groups in lesion reduction at 3 and 6 months

be given 2 days before cysticidal therapy and continued during therapy and shortly after its completion. Dexamethasone therapy should not be given in the absence of antihelminthic drugs, as dexamethasone alone has been associated with increased seizure recurrence. Of note, dexamethasone lowers plasma levels of praziquantel by as much as 50% but raises the level of albendazole by 50%. Anticonvulsant therapy is also often required. In children with degenerating cysts, anticonvulsant therapy may be withdrawn when the lesion disappears and the EEG is normal. In those patients with calcified or viable parasites, anticonvulsant therapy should be continued for a 1-year seizure-free interval.

Neurosurgical resection is used as a last resort for lesions causing significant neurologic impairment. Resolution of lesions with medical management alone is superior, and the reliance on surgical intervention has decreased over time. Less invasive, neuroendoscopic resection has been used for removal of protracted lesions. Brain biopsy should be considered in cases in which the diagnosis remains questionable and the lesion has not resolved.

CNS-imaging studies should be repeated at 2-month intervals (with continued therapy) until the parenchymal brain cysticerci are successfully eliminated. The outcome for neurocysticercosis is generally good. The majority of patients weaned from anticonvulsants remain seizure free. However, there is a 10% mortality with neurocysticercosis, and others may have recurrent seizures or deterioration of higher cerebral functions.

SUGGESTED READINGS

1. Abba K, Ramaratnam S, Ranganathan LN. Anthelmintics for people with neurocysticercosis. *Cochrane Database Syst Rev.* 2010;3:CD000215.
2. Baranwal AK, Singhi PD, Khandelwal N, Singhi SC. Albendazole therapy in children with focal seizures and single small enhancing computerized tomographic lesions: a randomized, placebo-controlled, double blind trial. *Pediatr Infect Dis J.* 1998;17:696-700.
3. Del Brutto OR, Rajshenkhar V, White AC, et al. Proposed diagnostic criteria for neurocysticercosis. *Neurology.* 2001;57(2):177-183.
4. Garcia HH, Evans CA, Nash TE, et al. Current consensus guidelines for treatment of neurocysticercosis. *Clin Microbiol Rev.* 2002;15:747-756.
5. Gogia S, Talukdar B, Choudhury V, Arora BS. Neurocysticercosis in children: clinical findings and response to albendazole therapy in a randomized, double-blind, placebo-controlled trial in newly diagnosed cases. Trans R Soc Trop Med Hyg 2003;97:416-421.
6. Hotez PJ. Cestode infections. In: Jenson HB, Baltimore RS, eds. *Pediatric Infectious Diseases: Principles and Practice.* Norwalk, CT: Appleton and Lange, 1995;509-516.
7. Kalra V, Dua T, Kumar V. Efficacy of albendazole and short-course dexamethasone treatment in children with 1 or 2 ring-enhancing lesions of neurocysticercosis: a randomized controlled trial. J Pediatr 2003;143:111-114.
8. Kaur P, Dhiman P, Dhawan N, Nijhawan R, Pandit S. Comparison of 1 week versus 4 weeks of albendazole therapy in single small enhancing computed tomography lesion. Neurol India. 2010;58:560-564.
9. Kaur S, Singhi P, Singhi S, Khandelwal N. Combination therapy with albendazole and praziquantel versus albendazole alone in children with seizures and single lesion neurocysticercosis: a randomized, placebo-controlled double blind trial. *Pediatr Infect Dis J.* 2009; 28(5):403-406.
10. Singhi P, Dayal D, Khandelwal N. One week versus 4 weeks of albendazole therapy for neurocysticercosis: a randomized, placebo-controlled, double blind trial. Pediatr Infect Dis J 2003;22:268-272.
11. Singhi P, Singhi S. Topical review: neurocysticercosis in children. *J Child Neurol.* 2004;19:482-492.
12. St. Geme JW III, Maldonado YA, Enzmann D. Consensus: diagnosis and management of neurocysticercosis in children. *Pediatr Infect Dis J.* 1993;12:455-461.
13. Sotelo J, del Brutto OH, Penagos P, et al. Comparison of therapeutic regimen of anticysticercal drugs for parenchymal brain cysticercosis. *J Neurol.* 1990;237:69-72.
14. Vazquez V, Sotelo J. The course of seizures after treatment for cerebral cysticercosis. *New Engl J Med.* 1992;327:696-701.
15. White AC Jr. Neurocysticercosis: a major cause of neurological disease worldwide. *Clin Infect Dis.* 1997;24:101-113.

INDEX

Page numbers followed by *f* and *t* indicate figures and tables, respectively.

Encephalitis
  bacterial, 290–291
  in cat-scratch disease, 494. *See also* Cat-scratch disease
  cryptococcal. *See* Cryptococcal infections
  differential diagnosis of, 210, 290–291, 493
  M. pneumonia. See Mycoplasma pneumoniae encephalitis
  viral, 291
Encephalopathy. *See also* Altered mental status
  differential diagnosis of, 488
  HIV-related, 291
  lead. *See* Lead encephalopathy
Endocarditis, prophylaxis guidelines, 101
Entamoeba histolytica, 387*t*
Enterocolitis
  Hirschsprung-associated, 80–81, 309
  infectious causes of, 132
Enterovirus infections, 255, 299
Ependymoma, spinal cord
  case history, 322–323
  clinical presentation of, 323–324
  diagnosis of, 324
  differential diagnosis of, 323
  pathophysiology of, 323
  treatment of, 324
Epidural abscess, spinal. *See* Spinal epidural abscess
Epilepsy. *See* Seizures
Epilepsy, posttraumatic, 497
Epstein-Barr virus (EBV) infections
  case history, 455
  clinical presentation of, 361, 456–457
  diagnosis of, 456, 457–458, 457*t*
  differential diagnosis of, 455–456
  encephalitis with, 493
  epidemiology of, 461
  incidence of, 456
  mononucleosis, 360–361, 387
  myocarditis, 358–361, 360*f,* 362
  pathophysiology of, 456
  treatment of, 458
Erosion, 224, 227*t*
Erythema, 224
Erythema chronicum migrans, 225*f,* 299*f,* 300. *See also* Lyme disease
Erythema marginatum, 144, 409*t*
Erythema multiforme, 230*f*
Erythema nodosum, 226*f*
Erythrocyte adenosine deaminase (eADA), 262

Erythroderma, 228*t*
Erythromycin, side effects of, 116
Escherichia coli
  in epidural abscess, 121*t*
  in meningitis, 476, 476*f*
Escherichia coli O157:H7, 431, 436. *See also* Hemolytic uremic syndrome
Esophageal atresia
  diagnosis of, 20
  etiology of, 19
  incidence of, 18
  treatment of, 20
  types of, 18, 19*f*
Ethambutol, side effects of, 108
Excoriation, 224, 228*t*
Extrahepatic biliary atresia, 400
Extremity pain. *See* Joint or extremity pain

F
Failure to thrive
  causes of, 147, 149*t*
  definition of, 147
  with diarrhea, 431
  with diarrhea and fever, 148–150
  differential diagnosis of, 150, 155, 161, 164–165, 167
  with heart failure and liver mass, 160–161, 160*f*
  indications for hospitalization in, 148*t*
  with malabsorption symptoms, 154–155
  with normal calorie intake, 157–158
  psychosocial causes of, 168–170, 169*f,* 170*f*
  questions about history of, 147–148
  with vomiting, 164–165
  with weight loss, 166–167
Familial adenomatous polyposis, 440, 440*t*
Familial Mediterranean fever, 198*t*
Fanconi anemia
  case history, 232–233, 233*f*
  clinical presentation of, 233–234, 233*t,* 261
  diagnosis of, 234, 261
  genetic factors in, 233
  incidence of, 233
  treatment of, 234
Fanconi syndrome. *See also* Cystinosis
  case history, 68–69, 69*f*
  clinical presentation of, 283*t*
  diagnosis of, 70, 70*t*
  differential diagnosis of, 69–70